AF881030

The Buffalo (*Bubalus bubalis*) – Production and Research

Edited by

Giorgio A. Presicce

ARSIAL – Regione Lazio, Rome, Italy

advertisements or ideas contained in the Work.

Limitation of Liability:

In no event will Bentham Science Publishers, its staff, editors and/or authors, be liable for any damages, including, without limitation, special, incidental and/or consequential damages and/or damages for lost data and/or profits arising out of (whether directly or indirectly) the use or inability to use the Work. The entire liability of Bentham Science Publishers shall be limited to the amount actually paid by you for the Work.

General:

1. Any dispute or claim arising out of or in connection with this License Agreement or the Work (including non-contractual disputes or claims) will be governed by and construed in accordance with the laws of the U.A.E. as applied in the Emirate of Dubai. Each party agrees that the courts of the Emirate of Dubai shall have exclusive jurisdiction to settle any dispute or claim arising out of or in connection with this License Agreement or the Work (including non-contractual disputes or claims).
2. Your rights under this License Agreement will automatically terminate without notice and without the need for a court order if at any point you breach any terms of this License Agreement. In no event will any delay or failure by Bentham Science Publishers in enforcing your compliance with this License Agreement constitute a waiver of any of its rights.
3. You acknowledge that you have read this License Agreement, and agree to be bound by its terms and conditions. To the extent that any other terms and conditions presented on any website of Bentham Science Publishers conflict with, or are inconsistent with, the terms and conditions set out in this License Agreement, you acknowledge that the terms and conditions set out in this License Agreement shall prevail.

Bentham Science Publishers Ltd.
Executive Suite Y - 2
PO Box 7917, Saif Zone
Sharjah, U.A.E.
Email: subscriptions@benthamscience.org

BENTHAM
SCIENCE

CONTENTS

FOREWORD

Buffaloes are members of the kingdom Animalia, phylum Chordata, class mammalian, order Artiodactyla and family Bovidae. They are further classified into two main species, the African wild buffalo (*Syncerus*) and the Asian buffalo (*Bubalus*). The Asian buffalo is further classified into the river (*Bubalus bubalis*) and swamp type (*Bubalus carabensis*) species. The study related to their origins indicate that swamp buffaloes may have originated in China and were domesticated about 4,000 years ago, while the river type may have originated from India some 5,000 years ago. Thus, the buffalo has been domesticated more recently as compared to *Bos taurus* and *Bos indicus* cattle, both domesticated ~10,000 years ago.

According to the FAO, the total population of buffaloes in the world during 2013 was 193.8 million. Asia alone accounts for the majority of heads, 187.9 million buffaloes that constitute 96.96 % of the total population. Because of its usefulness, the buffalo has been moved to Africa (4.2 million; 2.17%), America (1.34 million; 0.71%), Europe (0.43 million; 0.22%) and Oceania (210 numbers), and it is becoming popular in many non-buffalo rearing countries of these subcontinents. India possesses the largest number (109.4 million: 56.4%) and most of the best breeds of buffaloes (such as Murrah, Nili-Ravi, Banni, Mehsana, Bhadavari, Jafarabadi, Surti *etc.*).

Buffaloes are very important animals in Asian farming with milk, meat and hides as their major contribution to the zoo-economy, together with other forms of contribution within field-work such as pumping water, ploughing, planting and cultivation of crops, puddling of rice fields, hauling carts to carry various materials and people, thrash grains and crush sugar canes, *etc.* Buffaloes are also used for social and cultural events, sports and religious purposes. It contributes to about 55% of the milk produced in India and about 10% of the total global milk production. Buffalo milk has a high level of nutrients, and many consumers prefer it because of its white color, high fat content and flavor. Similarly, buffalo meat is amazingly tender, juicy with a slightly sweet flavor and it is lower in fat, calories and cholesterol than cattle beef, and higher in protein. The buffalo has an intrinsic ability to efficiently convert poor quality forages and crop residues of marginal areas into high quality milk and meat and it has exceptionally long productive life; in fact a healthy female may have as many as nine to ten lactations. Because of its colour and immense economic value, the buffalo is often called "Black Gold", and today more human beings depend on them than on any other domestic animal.

Depending on the geographical situations and the purpose for which they are used, buffaloes are managed differently all over the world. Slowly buffalo rearing is changing from the backyard to commercial enterprises and is following the path of cattle industry. Buffalo has an excellent potential for milk and meat production, and therefore development and application of simple technologies to overcome deficiencies in breeding, nutrition, healthcare, management and welfare and simultaneously judicious application of current technologies such as genomics, proteomics, reproductive biotechnologies, nanotechnology, bioinformatics *etc.*, may lead to its faster development.

Scientific literature on buffaloes has mushroomed in the last two decades, covering various aspects of buffalo production. In order to maximize productive and reproductive performances, newly developed technologies have been implemented in buffalo farming and management, and in some instances with excellent results. This book has 15 chapters, from the contribution of selected renowned educators / scientists from different buffalo rearing countries, dealing with the most recent advances ranging from reproductive physiology to nutrition, welfare, milk production and genetics. The book is aimed at magnifying the importance of this species in the world, and highlights areas of research that need to be explored urgently.

I am sure this book will be a valuable reference for researchers, policy experts, professionals, and above all, educators as well as under-graduate and post-graduate students interested in the bubaline species.

Prof. AK Misra
Vice-Chancellor
Maharashtra Animal and Fishery Sciences University
Seminary Hills
Nagpur-440 001
Maharashtra, India

PREFACE

Scientific literature on buffaloes (*Bubalus bubalis*) has skyrocketed in the last two decades, ranging from production to reproduction issues. Buffaloes have played an instrumental role in so-called emerging countries of the Asian continent, especially thanks to their intrinsic ability to convert poor quality forages and crop residues of marginal areas, into high quality milk and meat. A special focus of interest has been addressed from researchers to the river subspecies, being the most productive across countries of the European as well as the Asian continents. In fact, in some countries, the river buffalo has shown over the years, an increasing trend in the number of available heads, whereas in others, swamp buffaloes have decreased dramatically. In order to maximize productive and reproductive performances, newly developed technologies have been implemented in buffalo farming and management, and in some instances with excellent results. This book, presenting the most recent advances in buffalo production and research, aims at magnifying the importance of this species in the world and at highlighting areas of research still in need to be more deeply explored.

Giorgio A. Presicce
ARSIAL – Regione Lazio,
Rome,
Italy

List of Contributors

Pietro Sampaio BARUSELLI	Departamento de Reprodução Animal, FMVZ-USP, São Paulo, SP, Brazil
Giovanna BIFULCO	Department of Veterinary Medicine and Animal Production, Federico II University, V. Delpino 1, 80137, Naples, Italy
Antonio BOSCO	Department of Veterinary Medicine and Animal Productions, University of Naples Federico II, CREMOPAR Regione Campania, Italy
Ada BRAGHIERI	Scuola di Scienze Agrarie, Forestali, Alimentari ed Ambientali, Università della Basilicata, *Via* dell'Ateneo Lucano 10, 85100, Potenza, Italy
Narongsak CHAIYABUTR	Dairy Cattle Physiology Division, National Dairy Research, Institute, Karnal-13200, Haryana, India
Vongpasith CHANTHAKHOUN	Department of Animal Science, Faculty of Agriculture and Forest Resources, Souphanouvong University, Laos
Giuseppe CRINGOLI	Department of Veterinary Medicine and Animal Productions, University of Naples Federico II, CREMOPAR Regione Campania, Italy
Libertado C. CRUZ	Philippine Carabao Center (PCC), Science City of Muñoz 3120, Nueva Ecija, Philippines
Gautam Kumar DEB	Division of Applied Life Science (BK21 Program), Graduate School of Gyeongsang National University and Animal Production Research Division, Bangladesh Livestock Research Institute, Savar, Dhaka–1341, Bangladesh
Giuseppe DE ROSA	Dipartimento di Agraria, Università di Napoli Federico II, *Via* Università 133, 80055 Portici (NA), Italy
Bianca GASPARRINI	Department of Veterinary Medicine and Animal Production, Federico II University, *Via* F. Delpino 1, 80137 Naples, Italy
Fernando GRASSO	Dipartimento di Agraria, Università di Napoli Federico II, *Via* Università 133, 80055 Portici (NA), Italy
Alessandra IANNUZZI	National Research Council (CNR), Institute of Animal Production Systems in Mediterranean Environment (ISPAAM), Laboratory of Animal Cytogenetics and Gene Mapping, Naples, Italy
Leopoldo IANNUZZI	National Research Council (CNR), Institute of Animal Production Systems in Mediterranean Environment (ISPAAM), Laboratory of Animal Cytogenetics and Gene Mapping, Naples, Italy

Pichad KHEJORNSART
Tropical Feed Resources Research and Development Center (TROFREC), Department of Animal Science, Faculty of Agriculture, Khon Kaen University, Khon Kaen, 20004, Thailand

Il Keun KONG
Division of Applied Life Science (BK21 Program), Graduate School of Gyeongsang National University and Institute of Agriculture and Life Sciences, Jinju 660-701, Gyeongnam, Republic of Korea

Maria Paola MAURELLI
Department of Veterinary Medicine and Animal Productions, University of Naples Federico II, CREMOPAR Regione Campania, Italy

Claro N. MINGALA
Philippine Carabao Center (PCC), Science City of Muñoz 3120, Nueva Ecija, Philippines

Fabio NAPOLITANO
Scuola di Scienze Agrarie, Forestali, Alimentari ed Ambientali, Università della Basilicata, *Via* dell'Ateneo Lucano 10, 85100, Potenza, Italy

Gianluca NEGLIA
Department of Veterinary Medicine and Animal Production, Federico II University, V. Delpino 1, 80137, Naples, Italy

Egil Robert ORSKOV
International Feed Resource Unit, Macaulay Land Use Research Institute, UK

Corrado PACELLI
Scuola di Scienze Agrarie, Forestali, Alimentari ed Ambientali, Università della Basilicata, Via dell'Ateneo Lucano 10, 85100, Potenza, Italy

Rangsun PARNPAI
Embryo Technology and Stem Cell Research Center, School of Biotechnology, Suranaree University of Technology, Nakhon Ratchasima 30000, Thailand

Alfredo PAUCIULLO
National Research Council (CNR), Institute of Animal Production Systems in Mediterranean Environment (ISPAAM), Laboratory of Animal Cytogenetics and Gene Mapping, Naples, Italy

Ruangyot PILAJUN
Tropical Feed Resources Research and Development Center (TROFREC), Department of Animal Science, Faculty of Agriculture, Khon Kaen University, Khon Kaen, 20004, Thailand

Giorgio Antonio PRESICCE
ARSIAL, Regione Lazio, *Via* R. Lanciani, 38 - 00161, Rome, Italy

Laura RINALDI
Department of Veterinary Medicine and Animal Productions, University of Naples Federico II, CREMOPAR Regione Campania, Italy

Marina SANSINENA
Technical Department of Argentine Buffalo Breeders Association, International Consultant, Arcos 1325, 1426, Buenos Aires, Argentina

Vo Thi Kim THANH
Department of Animal Physiology, Hue University of Agriculture and Forestry, Vietnam

Ramesh C. UPADHYAY Dairy Cattle Physiology Division, National Dairy Research Institute, Karnal-13200, Haryana, India

Marvin A. VILLANUEVA Philippine Carabao Center (PCC), Science City of Muñoz 3120, Nueva Ecija, Philippines

M. WANAPAT Tropical Feed Resources Research and Development Center (TROFREC), Department of Animal Science, Faculty of Agriculture, Khon Kaen University, Khon Kaen, 20004, Thailand

Marco ZAVA Technical Department of Argentine Buffalo Breeders Association, International Consultant, Arcos 1325, 1426, Buenos Aires, Argentina

Luigi ZICARELLI Dipartimento di Medicina Veterinaria e Produzioni Animali - Università "Federico II" - Napoli, *Via* Delpino, 1 - 80137 Napoli, Italy

DEDICATION

To my mother, to my father always with me, to my children. To my sources of inspiration.

Reproduction and Production of Water Buffaloes (*Bubalus bubalis*) Around the World

Editor: Giorgio A. Presicce

eISBN (Online): 978-1-68108-417-6

ISBN (Print): 978-1-68108-418-3

First published in 2017.

CHAPTER 1

River and Swamp Buffaloes: History, Distribution and their Characteristics

Claro N. Mingala[*], **Marvin A. Villanueva** and **Libertado C. Cruz**

Philippine Carabao Center, Science City of Muñoz 3120, Nueva Ecija, Philippines

Abstract: Water buffalo, whether it belongs to the swamp or river type, is an important animal resource aside from cattle, whose great potential as source of products of animal origin and as a tool for research has been widely recognized. With a population of about 168 million, buffaloes are widely distributed in many countries around the world, mainly in the Asian continent as an important source of milk, meat, hide and draft power. This paper presents the history, world distribution, breeds, the characteristics of the two types of buffaloes, and the genetic improvement achieved in this species.

Keywords: Breed, Crossbreeding, Draft, Milk, River and swamp buffalo.

1. INTRODUCTION

The water buffalo and the men, who have been raising it with love for centuries, have been closely related and dependent on each other, so the buffalo has acquired a great social and cultural importance to human beings. The buffalo appears in the legends and folk arts of many people, especially the Asian, becoming an inseparable part of human life.

2. HISTORY

The Asian buffalo or the water buffalo (*Bubalus bubalis*) belongs to class Mammalia, sub-class Ungulata, order Artiodactyla, sub-order Ruminantia, family

[*] **Corresponding author Claro N. Mingala:** Philippine Carabao Center, Science City of Muñoz 3120, Nueva Ecija, Philippines; Tel: +63 44 4560731; Fax: +63 44 4560730; E-mail: cnmingala@hotmail.com

Giorgio A. Presicce (Ed.)

Bovidae, sub-family Bovinae, and tribe Bovini. Under the tribe Bovini three groups are included, the Bovina (cattle), Bubalina (the Asian buffalo), and Syncerina (the African buffalo). The Asian and the African buffaloes are classified under the genus names *Bubalus* and Syncerus, respectively, which are generally similar despite some anatomic differences between them.

The African buffalo (Syncerina group) includes only one species (*Syncerus caffer*) and some subspecies. The Asian buffalo (*Bubalus*) includes three different buffalo species: Anoa (*Bubalus depressicornis*) from the Island of Celebes, Tamaraw (*Bubalus mindorensis*) from the Island of Mindoro in the Philippines and Arni (*Bubalus arnee*) or the Indian wild buffalo. Of these four species of African and Asian buffaloes only the Indian wild buffalo, Arni has been domesticated and received the species name *bubalis*. The other three types have not been domesticated. The domestic buffalo is presently raised in the world under the name water buffalo and is classified as *Bubalus bubalis* [1].

Information about the origin and domestication period of the Indian wild buffalo is lost back in ancient times, although archeological evidence shows that both Asia and Europe have relied on water buffaloes for a very long time. According to Shalash [2], there is archeological evidence of buffalo domestication dating back to 2,000 BC in Mesopotamia and the valley of Indus. In 1980, Prof. Sieh Chen-Hsia of Nanking Agricultural College, China, however, reported on more recent archeological investigations in China (Chekiang Province) which give grounds to the assumption that the domestication of the buffalo has started 7,000 years ago. On the contrary, Bhat [3] believes that this has happened about 5,000 years ago on the Indian sub-continent, more precisely in the valley of Indus. Their horns, coarse skin, wide muzzles, and low-carried heads have been represented on seals struck since 5,000 years ago in the Indus Valley, suggesting that in India and Pakistan such animals had been already domesticated since that time. Accordingly, the domestication of swamp buffaloes also took place in China independently about 1,000 years later [4].

Water buffalo did spread widely all over Asia and was introduced in parts of Europe, the Near East and Egypt, the Caucasian region of the former USSR and later in South America. Buffaloes were probably unknown to ancient Egyptians,

Romans and Greeks and this is possibly the reason why such animals have not been mentioned in their literature or seen in their arts; nevertheless buffaloes were used in China 4,000 years ago. Arabs began moving the buffaloes from Mesopotamia around 600 A.D. to the Near East (today Syria, Israel and Turkey), whereas the same animals were introduced by pilgrims and crusaders from their return from the Holy Land into Europe in the Middle Ages. Buffaloes adapted well to the malaric Pontine marshes characterizing the southeast area of Rome and south of Naples, and established themselves also in other territories today known as Hungary, Romania, Yugoslavia, Greece and Bulgaria, and stayed there ever since. In Egypt, medieval villagers began adopting and using the buffaloes, and have remained since then even in modern Egypt the most important domestic animals, in fact doubling the population up to a million heads in the course of the last 50 years [1, 4].

Since 84 years ago, Brazil invested into buffalo production by importing groups of animals mostly from Italy and India. A similar attitude has been witnessed also in nearby countries like Trinidad by importing buffaloes from India in the early 90s, whereas other countries like Venezuela, Colombia and Guyana have become familiar with buffalo import much more recently. Similarly, some remaining countries of the American continent like Costa Rica, Ecuador, Cayenne, Panama and Suriname began importing small herds of buffaloes in the 70s.

Even in Papua New Guinea, the buffaloes have been imported and the new environment has been fitting the new species very well. Comforted by such good results, in the 60s scientists evaluated buffalo performances in Papua New Guinea and more animals were imported from Australia. As a result, the whole lot of buffaloes introduced have been performing so well that they have out-performed the cattle counterpart both in terms of born calves and meat produced. In fact, buffaloes differently from cattle, as it also happens elsewhere, are able to maintain their physiological functions and appetite, despite the heat and humidity typical of the region. For these reasons the government of Papua New Guinea has since decided to import additional water buffaloes along the years, reaching today a total of almost 3,500 heads.

Buffaloes have not been recognized for their potential for a long time in the

United States, until the first herd of 50 heads was imported for commercial farming at the end of the 70s. Such animals with time showed their potential along the farm fields of Florida and Louisiana, and have now become the center of interest in many U.S. Universities and farm circles.

The domestication of the Indian wild buffalo went on with different intensity through the ages and is not over yet. Most of these buffaloes have been fully domesticated and their existence is closely related to human life since ancient times while others have been only tamed and used to satisfy basic human needs in some parts of the world. Together, these two groups of the Indian wild buffalo represent the total water buffalo world population. Currently, however, there are still some carefully maintained Indian wild buffalo herds in India and in some other countries and its non-domesticated type is widely spread in Australia [1, 4].

3. DISTRIBUTION

In the world, the buffalo (*Bubalus bubalis*) population is around 168 million heads, of which the majority can be found in Asia with 161 million (95.8%), in Africa, almost entirely in Egypt, with 3.7 million (2.2%), in South America with 3.3 million (1.9%), in Australia with 40,000 (0.02%) and in Europe with 500,000 (0.3%).

A comprehensive study on the distribution of water buffaloes across the world was done by Borghese [5], which can be briefly summarized below:

Asia

- India is the first country in the world with regard to the number of buffalo heads (95 million – 56.5% of the total world buffalo population) and milk production with 134 million tons produced. In this country some of the best and more productive River milk breeds are originated, such as Murrah, Nili-Ravi, Surti and Jaffarabadi. In addition, this country in Asia can be considered the first and most important one in terms of scientific and technological development in several areas of enquiry such as nutrition, production, reproductive technologies and genetic improvement.
- **China** developed a huge variety of buffalo genetic resources belonging all to the

swamp type. They are distributed in different regions (*i.e.*, those that live in lowlands and in mountains). Breeds of the lowlands are the Binhu breed (461,000 heads) in the Hunan province, the Xinyang breed (290,000 heads) in the Henan province, the Enshi breed (77,000 heads) in Hubei, the Fuan breed (70,000 heads) in the Fujian province, the Yanjin breed (45,000 heads) in Yunnan, the Xinglong breed (24,000 heads) in Hainan and the Wenzhou breed (10,000 heads) in Zhejiang [6].

Two further breeds inhabit the lowlands and can also be found along the saline seaside shores of the east sea: these are the Haizi breed (65,000 heads) in Jiangshu and the Shanghai breed (36,000 heads) around the city of Shanghai.

The most numerous breed in China is the Guizhou (1.46 million), a mountain breed of the Guizhou province: raised on natural pasture and of varying body size according to environmental conditions. With regard to the other mountain breeds, there are the Fuling (415,000 heads) in Sichuan, the Dehong (390,000 heads), the Diandong (220,000 heads) in Yunnan, the Dechang (190,000 heads) in Sichuan, the Xilin (59,000 heads), the Fuzhong (57,000 heads) in Guanxi and the Dongliu (27,000 heads) in the Anhui province.

- **Pakistan** has 22 million head of buffaloes wherein 76 percent of which are found in the Punjab and the remaining 24 percent are located in Sind, North West Frontier Provinces and Baluchistan. The buffalo is considered as the main dairy animal in the country.
- The **Philippines** has 3.2 million Carabao buffaloes, where 99 percent belong to small farmers.
- **Bangladesh** had a total buffalo population of 772,764 heads in 2003. These buffaloes are found in the Bramhaputra-Jamuna flood plain of central Bangladesh, the Ganges-Meghna flood plain of southern Bangladesh and in institutional herds.
- The buffalo population in **Thailand** at present is about 1.7 million and is tending to decrease gradually. In the past Thailand had the second largest number of swamp buffaloes in the world. However this buffalo population drastically declined from 4.7 million in 1990 to 1.9 million in 1998.
- In 1985, the total buffalo population in **Indonesia** was 3,245,000, whereas in 1993, the total population was 3,238,000, with Jawa Barat 487,000, DI Aceh 454,000, Sulawesi Selatan 342,000, Sumatra Utara 265,000, Jawah Tengah

232,000, Sumatra Barat 228,000, Nusa Tenggara Barat 227,000, Nusa Tenggara Timur 167,000, and Sumatra Selatan 152,000, while the remaining population in each province was less than 100,000.

- The total buffalo population in **Malaysia** is about 170,000, of which 60 percent is mostly concentrated in the rice growing states of Kelantan, Terengganu, Kedah and Pahang in West Malaysia. Buffaloes in Malaysia belongs also to the river and swamp types. The population of river buffaloes is less than 2,000 heads of Murrah from India.

Mediterranean Area

In the Mediterranean region comprising European countries and countries of the Near East, the buffalo population is around 5.5 million heads, which is 3.4% of the total buffalo world population.

- According to FAO statistics available in 1974, there were around one million heads in Turkey. A decrease in the buffalo population of 65% has been noted from 1984 to 1997, as a consequence of a preference in breeding practices in cattle as compared to buffalo in the Egean and Marmara regions, where many buffaloes were originally raised. As of today, only 110,000 buffalo heads remain in Turkey belonging to the Anatolian breed.
- **Azerbaijan** has approximately 300,000 buffaloes, which is the most valuable buffalo gene pool to be found in the USSR.
- There are about 1,000 buffaloes in **Armenia**.
- In Iran in the 1930s there were around 1,500,000 buffaloes, with a steadily reduction to 500,000 by 1995. Buffaloes are mostly found (80%) in the north and north-west (Azerbaijan province), and a remaining 18% in the south of the country. Nowadays, the buffalo population increases at about a rate of 1.3 percent annually.
- In **Iraq** there were 98,000 total River Khuzestani or Iraqi buffaloes.
- The total number of buffaloes in **Egypt** reached about 3,717,000 in 2003, of which 42 percent were cows, 6 percent buffalo bulls, 32 percent heifers less than two years old and 20 percent male calves less than two years old.
- The buffalo population in **Romania** was more than 200,000 heads in 1996 [7]. At present there are about 100,000 animals of the Mediterranean breed,

sometimes crossbred with Bulgarian Murrah.

- The Bulgarian Murrah, which is the new buffalo population in **Bulgaria,** was created through crossing of Indian Murrah and indigenous Mediterranean, with a total population of 9,200 heads.
- In Italy there are approximately 400,000 heads of the Mediterranean breed.

America

According to recent data, the buffalo population in Venezuela is 200,000 and 70,000 in Argentina. The present population all over America is about 3,415,000.

Australia

Buffaloes, which are not native in Australia are estimated to be less than 40,000 – 50,000 heads, with 20,000 in managed herds confined by fences and the remainder ranging over uncontrolled areas (monitored negative for TB) in southern and south eastern Arnhemland (an Aboriginal reserve), east of Katherine and along the south coast of Darwin.

Africa

The total population of buffalo in Africa is about 2-3 million.

4. BREEDS AND THEIR CHARACTERISTICS

There are two main types of water buffalo: the swamp and river buffalo. River type buffaloes are raised as dairy animals, but they express also good meat qualities. They are raised mainly for milk, although they can be also used for dual and triple productive purposes. These animals love to bathe in rivers, irrigation canals, artificial lakes and swamps.

These types of buffalo include different breeds, usually have curled horns, and are widely spread in many countries of the world, either as pure breed or used for crossing. River buffaloes have a diploid complement of 50 chromosomes, whereas swamp type have a diploid complement of 48 chromosomes.

In terms of reproduction, river buffaloes have higher calf mortality, later maturity in both sexes, delayed resumption of the ovarian cycle after calving, seasonal influence on reproduction, reduced sperm quality of buffalo bulls, and lower conception rate when deep frozen semen is used, compared to swamp buffaloes. A river buffalo also matures sooner and reaches breeding age faster than swamp buffalo.

Based on Egyptian and Bulgarian studies, the full spermatogenic cycle of young buffalo bulls takes place at about 12 months of age but their first ejaculates can be obtained at a later age. The active breeding life of the buffalo bulls is from 3-4 to 10 years. Usually, the normal sexual activity goes up to 12 and more years of age but after about the seventh year the sexual potential starts declining and after the 15th year senile traits are observed. The age of first estrus in buffalo cows varies within extremely wide limits depending on the breed, management conditions, nutrition level, season and other factors.

The age at first calving of river buffalo breeds among different countries is quite high, from 34 to 54 months with extremely large individual variability. In terms of service period, buffalo cows have a considerably longer service period which is usually over 100-120 days. Buffaloes also have a longer pregnancy within limits of 281 to 334 days, being 300 to 320 days for most of them and some ranging from 299 to 346 days.

Compared to swamp buffaloes, river type buffaloes have 2 to 4 times higher average milk yield per lactation but lower fat content in milk. They also have longer lactation period than the swamp buffalo, which is nevertheless shorter compared to cattle. It has been found out that the first lactation period is the longest and it decreases with each consecutive lactations.

On the other hand, swamp type buffalo is used mainly for draught and meat production. It has a very low milk yield which is hardly enough to feed the buffalo calves. It is described as a breed with a great number of varieties, created in accordance with the environmental conditions of the countries and areas where they are raised. This buffalo type forms the basic buffalo populations of the East Asian countries. Interestingly, crosses between river and swamp buffaloes have 49 chromosome complement [8].

Most of the swamp buffaloes are dark gray. A comparatively small part of them though is albinoid. There are also black-and-white buffaloes in some regions of Indonesia. It is characteristic of the gray water buffaloes that most of them have two white chevrons: one is under the lower jaw and the other around the chest. Some of the animals, however, have only one chevron under the neck.

Usually, swamp buffaloes have bigger and longer horns than cattle. However, there are also polled buffaloes. The horn size and setting vary to a great extent. In most of these animals, horns extend outwards and then curl backwards into a semi-circle but remain in the forehead plane. Some individuals may also have drooping horns. Buffalo horns are usually long, flat and thick. In some cases they can be short and thick.

The average birth weight of buffalo calves is 26-30 kg, at 8 months of age is around 125-150 kg and at 1 year is between 135 and 205 kg. The average daily gain for the period prior to weaning varies within 340-410 g and after weaning 340-750 g. The growth rate of male buffalo calves is insignificantly higher than females. The average live weight of mature swamp buffalo cows is 350-450 kg and that of mature buffalo bulls is 450-650 kg. This trait can vary extremely within the population of each country but there are no significant differences in the average values among different countries.

Limited exterior measurements of mature swamp buffaloes show that the average height at withers of buffalo cows from different countries is within 120-126 cm, and within 121-136 cm for buffalo bulls, with an average body length of 121-151 cm and 123-157 cm, respectively, while the average chest girth is within 179-202 cm and 183-209 cm, respectively.

The swamp buffalo has an excellent draught capacity but the intensity of its utilization varies to a great extent in different countries. Usually the use for draught starts at about 4 years of age and comes to a close at 12 years and in some cases even 20 years of age. The average daily working time is 5 hours and the average annual record is between 20 and 146 days. The draught effort equals to 10-14% of their weight. Usually, Asian farmers select the buffaloes for draught at an age of about 3-3.5 years, the criteria being the body size and height at withers. In some cases the bulls are castrated before their draught training.

Swamp buffaloes usually reach sexual maturity at 4 years of age. In many cases, however, it starts much earlier. The first estrus of buffalo heifers takes place on the average at about 1.6-3.0 years of age with a very big variation and the first calving is usually reported at an average age of 3.5-4.7, up to 5-6 years. On average, the estrus cycle is 20-34 days and the estrus duration is 24-42 hours, the latter ranging from 12 hours to 3-5 days. Compared to the river buffaloes, the swamp type has a longer pregnancy period which varies between 308 and 341 days on average, according to different studies. Most authors, however, accept an average duration of 330 days. The range for calving interval is 370-670 days. The conception rate of buffalo cows is lower compared to the river type. The percentage of calves born varies within extremely large limits from 23 to 82%. Twins are rare, 0.001-0.015 per 100 buffalo cows.

Along with its main use for draught, the swamp buffalo is also used for meat production in all countries. Usually, old buffaloes are slaughtered after they have lost or decreased their work ability; therefore, the meat is characterized by very low quality. In recent years, however, certain steps have been taken to improve meat quality. Many buffaloes that were previously slaughtered at an age of 15-20 years at 380 kg live weight after losing their work ability, are now being fattened for 7-8 months before slaughter. Fattening of young bulls has started in order to obtain higher meat quality. Studies of carcass traits of slaughtered swamp buffaloes at a pre-slaughter weight of 300-600 kg show that the average dressing percent is lower than cattle with a variation between 43 and 53%. The proportion of net meat is on average 73-75%, carcass length of 111-118 cm and the area of *musculus longissimus dorsi* varies within an average of 33,059 cm^2. Swamp buffaloes have a very low milk yield which satisfies mainly the needs of buffalo calves. Most of the studies show that the daily milk yield of recorded buffalo cows is only 1-2 kg plus the milk additionally sucked by buffalo calves. In most Asian countries the average milk yield of swamp buffalo for the lactation period is 250-500 kg.

Many Asian and Latin American countries crossbreed swamp to river buffaloes, producing a progeny with 49 chromosomes [1]. This practice shows that crossing the two buffalo types can produce fertile progeny, although some studies have shown that male crossbred progeny sometimes display fertility problems while female progeny may manifest longer calving intervals only in the case of further backcross [6].

A list of different river and swamp breeds are detailed below:

SWAMP TYPE

Breed: PHILIPPINE CARABAO
Origin: Philippines
Color/Description: Light gray with two stripes or chevron distinct on the ventral side of the neck, one near the brisket and the other near the jaw. Color is lighter on the legs and underside of the body and the ears. Horns are generally curved outward and inward to form the base of the head. The upper surface of the hornes are characterized by grooves. The body is sufficiently well built to be considered a type of animal for draft and meat
Average mature weight: 500 kg (male); 420 kg (female)
Milk production: 1.45-2.64 kg/day
Sources [1, 9]

Breed: INDONESIAN BUFFALO Tedong Bonga
Origin: Sulawesi Island, Indonesia
Description: Black and white in color, especially large, with strong muscles
Height at withers of adult male: 127-130 cm
Height at withers of adult female: 124-125 cm
Average body weight: 450-600 kg, can reach up to 800 kg
Sources [1, 5]

Breed: CHINESE BUFFALO (Binhu breed, Xinyang breed, Enshi breed, Fuan breed, Yanjin breed, Xinglong breed, Wenzhou breed, Haizi breed, Shanghai breed, Guizhou breed, Fuling breed, Dehong breed, Diandong breed, Dechang breed, Xilin breed, Fuzhong breed, Dongliu breed)
Origin: China
Population size: 22,759 million
Description: Most buffalo breeds tolerate all ranges of temperature, from 0°C in the winter to 30°C and over in the summer. All buffaloes have long horns. Coat color is grey, with varying intensities: from deep grey and blackish grey to brown,

hoar and light grey. The majority of the breeds also have white spots either in the form of stripes on the breast or in the form of rings on the neck. Chinese buffaloes are used for draught, often as their only task.

Height at withers of adult female: 120.1-123.8 cm (hill and mountain type)

Average body weight: 607.8 kg (Haizi), 616.5 kg (Shanghai), 400.5-496.1 kg (hill and mountain type)

All lactation total yield: 441-1,031 kg

All lactation length: 210-300 days

Sources [1, 5]

Breed: VIETNAMESE BUFFALO (Nghe-an, Thanh-hoa, Thuan-hai)

Origin: Vietnam

Description: They are divided ecologically into the mountainous and plain buffalo. They are mainly raised for work and meat. Vietnamese buffaloes are characterized by an extremely high work ability, disease resistance and good growth rate. Puberty takes place after 3 years of age.

Average body weight: 400-420 kg (heifer), 370-420 kg, others may reach up to 500-600 kg (buffalo cow)

All lactation total yield: 500 kg per lactation

Sources [1, 5]

Breed: THAILAND BUFFALO

Origin: Thailand

Description: Swamp buffaloes are indigenous in Thailand, and most of them are completely black in color, with only few exceptions of white coat. Such animals are not albino, because their white color is due to some peculiar genetic effects.

Average mature weight: 450 – 600 kg (mature male)

Source [10]

RIVER TYPE

Breed: AMERICAN MURRAH

Origin: USA

Description: This breed has well expressed body forms, characteristic of a meat-type animal; the growth rate and fattening ability are good, with broad, massive

body conformation. This breed has no record yet as an individual breed of buffalo.
Milk yield: 3-4 kg/day
Sources [1, 9]

Breed: ANATOLIAN
The Anatolian buffalo originated from Indian migration (7th century) in correspondence with the expansion of Islam, and was raised in Turkey for centuries.
Description: Black in color, long hair, with variation in tail length and frequent white switch.
Height at withers of adult male: 138 cm, body weight is 200-500 kg
Height at withers of adult female: 138 cm, body weight is 200-500 kg
Average slaughter weight: 300-350 kg, at the age of 18-20 months
Lactation duration: 220-270 days
Milk yield: 700-1,000 kg
Milk fat: 6.6-8.1 percent
Milk protein: 4.2-4.6 percent
Source [5]

Breed: AZERI or CAUCASIAN
This breed originates from the Indo valley (Indian buffalo). There is some evidence that buffaloes were raised in Lorestan (Iran) in the 9th Century B.C. since six engraved buffalo heads have been found on a bronze stick from this period.
Origin: Azerbaijan
Description: Overall impression is strong and coarse, but dragged rump, small udder, inadequate leg setting and poor muscles are some exterior disadvantages. Buffaloes are medium size and have different appearance; color ranges within dark brown, dark gray and black with black and red hues, often with lighter legs; similar to Surti by appearance; horns are thick, medium sized, pointed backwards with the top pointed forwards and inwards; chest is deep but medium wide; legs are stout and coarse; udder is bell-shaped but not very well developed, being small in most cases.
Height at withers of adult male: 137 cm, body weight is 400-600 kg
Height at withers of adult female: 133 cm, body weight is 400-600 kg

Average mature weight: 550-600 kg (female)
Lactation duration: 200-220 days
Milk yield: 1,200-1,300 kg
Milk fat: 6.6 percent
Sources [1, 5]

Breed: BANGLADESHI
Population size: 5,000
Description: Black in color, white spot on the forehead and tail-switch in some cases. Curled and short horns. Indigenous Bangladeshi buffaloes of the river type are found in the South-West. In the remaining parts of the country they are either swamp or crosses with exotic breeds: Nili-Ravi and Murrah type.
Source [5]

Breed: BHADAWARI
This is an improved local breed. It is the result of selection of Indian breeds of buffalo. It is considered the best breed of buffalo in Uttar Pradesh.
Description: Copper coloured coat, scanty hair which is black at the roots and reddish brown at the tip. Sometimes it is completely brown. The neck presents the typical white color ring. Tail switch is white or black and white. Horns are short and grow backwards.
Height at withers of adult male: 128 cm, body weight is 475 kg
Height at withers of adult female: 124 cm, body weight is 425 kg
Average body weight: 385.5 kg
Age at first calving: 48.6±0.58 months
First lactation 305 days or less yield: 711±25 kg
All lactation 305 days or less yield: 812±23 kg
All lactation total yield: 781±29 kg
All lactation length: 272±4 days
Average fat: 7.2±0.4 to 13 percent
Average dry period: 297±24 days
Sources [1, 5]

Breed: BUFALYPSO
Description: The only meat breed of the river type water buffalo that was created

by crossing 6-7 different famous breeds of the river water buffalo from the Indian subcontinent Nili, Ravi, Jafarabadi, Surti, Nagpuri, Bhadawari, and Murrah. It has a well expressed body forms, characteristic of a meat type animals. Growth rate and fattening ability are very good; at the same time, it also has very good meat qualities, fat is white, the meat is marbled, very tasty and there is almost no difference from beef. Hair coat is usually brown to copper-brown with an occasionally gray hair color of the legs. Some have white spots on the forehead and a small white strip on the tailhead; horns are small and curled wider, they are flat, compact, pointed backwards, upwards, and inwards with slightly sharp ends; neck is thick, the withers is high, back line is straight and rump is slightly dragged.

Overall growth rate: 726 g

Source [1]

Breed: BULGARIAN MURRAH

From 1962 to 1990, Murrah buffaloes from India were imported into Bulgaria and a new population of buffalo was created by upgrading the local buffalo.

Origin: Bulgaria

Description: Developed by upgrading Bulgarian Mediterranean buffalo with Indian Murrah (75%). It is very similar to the Indian Murrah by type and conformation and sometimes cannot be differentiated from it. The neck is long, thin, and with very thin folds; the chest is wide and deep; the rump is straight, medium, long and wide; the body is long, bones are prominent and strong; the milk veins are well shaped; the udder is well shaped and developed. Gray to rusty brown hair; horns coil downward and upward to form a hook; wedge shaped conformation. In bulls, the front is more developed while the hind portion is narrow; two streaks of white markings are evident around the jaw from ear to ear and the other lower down the brisket.

Body weight of adult male: 700 kg

Body weight of adult female: 600 kg

Average slaughter weight: 400 kg, at the age of 16 months

Lactation duration: 270-305 days

Milk yield: 1,800 kg

Milk fat: 7.04 percent

Sources [1, 5, 9]

Breed: EGYPTIAN

Buffaloes were introduced into Egypt from India, Iran and Iraq approximately during the middle of the 7th Century. The distinction between the different types of Egyptian buffaloes is only environmental. It is the most important and popular livestock for milk production in Egypt.

Description: it consists of two main types: Saidi (bred in South Egypt) which is small, almost black, hairy and poor milkers and Beheri (North Egypt) big, gray in color with smooth skin and better milkers. Both are multi-purpose animals, used mainly for milk, meat and additionally as draught power in some regions. They are small to medium size with no distinct conformation. Udder teats are not well conformed to be similar in shape, size or length.

They are blackish grey in color, horn form varies from lyre to sword-shaped. The head is long and narrow, the jaws are long and strong. Ears are long and dropping. The neck is rather long, thin and straight. The forelegs are rather short and heavy boned. Ribs are wide, deep and well sprung. The rump is sloping and the tail setting is low.

Height at withers of adult male: 178 cm, body weight is 600 kg

Height at withers of adult female: 144 cm, body weight is 500 kg

Lactation duration: 210-280 days

Milk yield: 1,200-2,100 kg

Milk fat: 6.5-7.0 percent

Sources [1, 5]

Breed: JAFARABADI

The existence of the Jafarabadi breed in Gujarat (India) goes back to 1938.

Description: One of the high milk yielding buffalo breeds but of late maturity; has an amber-black color with a white tuft on the tail; body is massive, neck is long and tender, head is big and heavy; horns are heavy and wide, declining and falling down on both sides of the neck, curled backwards and upwards; crown and forehead are occupied to a great extent by the bottom of the horns; forehead is largely protruding; body is long but not compact; chest is wide and deep; udder is very well developed with well shaped long teats, with strongly prominent milk veins observed.

Height at withers of adult male: 142 cm, body weight varies from 600 to 1,500 kg

Height at withers of adult female: 140 cm, body weight is about 550 kg, some individuals may weigh as much as 700-800 kg

Lactation duration: 350 days

Milk yield: 1,800-2,700 kg

Milk fat: 8.5 percent

The performance characteristics of the Jafarabadi breed maintained at the Junagarh Centre (India) of the Network Project on Buffalo are presented below (Sethi, 2003).

Age at first calving: 1,925±196 days

All lactation length: 320.1±11.6 days

Average fat: 7.7±1.0 percent

Average dry period: 159.8±10.9 days

Sources [1, 5]

Breed: JERANGI

Description: Black in color, with small horns running backwards. It is a small animal. It is localized along the border of Orissa with Andhra Pradesh.

Source [5]

Breed: KUHZESTANI or IRAQI BUFFALO

Description: Horns are short and grow upward forming a ring at the end. In size, it is very likely the biggest buffalo breed in the world.

Height at withers of adult male: 148 cm, body weight is 800 kg

Height at withers of adult female: 141 cm, body weight is 600 kg

Overall growth rate: 580 g/day

Lactation duration: 200-270 days

Milk yield: 1,300-1,400 kg

Milk fat: 6.6 percent

Sources [1, 5]

Breed: KUNDI

Domestication of draught animals in the Indus valley civilization is referred to

about 4,500 years ago. It is the second most important breed in Pakistan.
Origin: Pakistan
Description: Originates from Murrah; mostly colored black, but some are light brown; horns are thick at the bottom, bent backwards and pointed upwards with a moderate curve at the end; head is small, forehead is slightly prominent, face is hollow and eyes are small; hindquarters are massive; udder is well developed with prominent milk veins and teats are squarely placed; tail is long with a black tuft.
Height at withers of adult male: 135 cm, body weight is 700 kg
Height at withers of adult female: 125 cm, body weight is 600 kg
Lactation duration: 320 days
Milk yield: 2,000 kg
Milk fat: 7.0 percent
Milk protein: 6.0 percent
Sources [1, 5]

Breed: LIME
It is thought that the pure Lime breed may have originated from the wild Arna, and it has been domesticated along the known history of Nepal. This breed amounts to the 35 percent of the total indigenous buffalo population, to be found throughout the hills and mountains of the country.
Description: Light brown color, small body size, characteristic chevrons of grey or white hair below the jaws and around the brisket, small sickle-shaped horns, curved towards the neck.
Height at withers of adult female: 115 cm, body weight is 399 kg
Lactation duration: 351 days
Milk yield: 875 kg
Milk fat: 7.0 percent
Source [5]

Breed: MANDA
This is an improved local breed, resulting from the selection of Indian breeds of buffaloes.
Description: color: grey, brown.
Milk yield: 4 kg/day
Source [5]

Breed: MEDITERRANEAN or EUROPEAN

The Mediterranean buffalo originates from the Indian buffalo. It was introduced into Europe with the advent of Islam and the Arab occupation as well as through other central European conquerors in the 6th and 7th Centuries. The buffalo population in Europe has been dramatically declining since the Second World War, with the advent of Holstein and mechanization.

Description: These buffaloes have similar conformation in different European countries although some separate types have been developed in the course of centuries as a result of the different environmental conditions of the regions and countries. Buffalo in Bulgaria is represented by two varieties, the plain type and the semi-mountainous type. In Romania, this breed also includes two types, the lighter one in the valley of the Danube River and the heavier one in Transylvania while only one type is characterized in Italy. They are mostly black, black and brown and dark gray; have a white tuft on the tail and some have a white mark on the forehead; horns are medium, long, flat in the bottom, pointed backwards and slightly outwards and straightened backwards, the top is pointed inwards; head is comparatively long; compact body conformation, with deep and wide chest and well developed pectoral; back is short and in some cases hollow; rump is wide but short and sometimes dragged and eave-shaped; tail is thin and short; legs are short, thick, with a strong hoof horn; udder is medium with squarely placed quarters and halves, teats are cylindrical and set wide apart but they are often pressed at the bottom. Italian Mediterranean buffaloes have an udder best shaped and suitable for machine milking.

Average mature weight: 569 kg (Bulgarian), 550-650 kg (Italian), 487-565 kg (Romanian)

Lactation duration: 270 days

Milk yield: 900-4,000 kg

Milk fat: 8.0 percent

Milk protein: 4.2-4.6 percent

Sources [1, 5]

Breed: MESHANA

The existence of the Meshana breed in north Gujarat, India, is referred to 1940. This breed is the result of selection of Indian breeds of buffalo.

Description: Characteristics can be described as intermediate between Surti and Murrah. Jet black skin and hair are preferred. Horns are sickle-shaped but more curved than the Surti. The udder is well developed and well set. Milk veins are prominent.
Body weight of adult male: 570 kg
Body weight of adult female: 430 kg
Lactation duration: 305 days
Milk yield: 1,800-2,700 kg
Milk fat: 6.6-8.1 percent
Milk protein: 4.2-4.6 percent
Source [5]

Breed: MURRAH
In the north-west of the sub-Indian continent, buffaloes have long been selected for milk yield and curled horn. It is the most important and well-known buffalo breed in the world.
Description: The color is jet black with white switch in the tail, while the skin texture is soft and fine. The horns are tightly and spirally curved, and the animals are in general massive and very well built. Neck and head are light with short limbs, broad hips and drooping quarter and wedge shaped conformations. Udder and teats are well developed, with teats black, long and stout. The animal is placid.
Height at withers of adult male: 142 cm, body weight is 750 kg
Height at withers of adult female: 133 cm, body weight is 650 kg
Lactation duration: 305 days
Milk yield: 1,800 kg
Milk fat: 7.2 percent
Average body weight: 495 kg
Age at first calving: 50.6±2.0 months
Average fat: 6.70 percent
Sources [1, 3, 9]

Breed: NAGPURI
It is an improved local breed, the result of a selection of Indian breeds of buffaloes.

Description: Black in color, sometimes there are white markings on the face, legs and switch. Horns are 50-65 cm long, flat-curved and carried back near to the shoulders. Nasal flap is mostly absent and even if present is very short.
Height at withers of adult male: 140 cm, body weight is 522 kg
Height at withers of adult female: 130 cm, body weight is 408 kg
Lactation duration: 243 days
Milk yield: 825 kg
Milk fat: 7.0 percent
Sources [1, 5]

Breed: NILI-RAVI
Domestication of draught animals in the Indus valley civilization is referred to have started about 4,500 years ago. Nili and Ravi were two different breeds until 1950, but after this period it became difficult to distinguish the two breeds, possibly due to the adoption of similar selection criteria among breeders. Therefore the name Nili Ravi became popular and such breed is nowadays the most important livestock in Pakistan, although it is also present in India and in the Punjab. The most important difference between Murrah and Nili-Ravi is represented by the white markings on the extremities and walled eyes. The horns are less curled than Murrah, and the udder is well shaped and extends well forward up to the naval flaps.
Origin: Pakistan
Description: Usually black with white markings on the forehead, muzzle, face and legs; white switch and wall eyes; horns are small and lightly coiled; medium-sized deep frame with elongated, coarse and heavy head, bulging at the top, depressed between the eyes and ending in a fine muzzle.
Height at withers of adult male: 135 cm, body weight is 700 kg
Height at withers of adult female: 125 cm, body weight is 600 kg
Lactation duration: 305 days
Milk yield: 2,000 kg
Milk fat: 6.5 percent
Products: Milk, ghee, cream, meat.
First lactation total yield: 1,571 kg
Sources [1, 5, 9]

Breed: PARKOTE

Parkote buffaloes live the mid-hills and river valleys of Nepal. Their pure form is now declining due to the traditional practice of crossbreeding with Lime buffalo and in addition and in more recent times, crossbreeding with the Indian Murrah. At present the purebreed population is estimated to be only 25 percent of the indigenous population within the hills and mountains of Nepal.

Description: The Parkote are dark in coat color and of medium-built body size, with sword-shaped horns directed laterally or towards the back. Black skin, black muzzle, black eyebrows. Usually they have no markings on the legs.

Height at withers of adult female: 114 cm, body weight is 410 kg

Lactation duration: 351 days

Milk yield: 875 kg

Milk fat: 7.0 percent

Source [5]

Breed: SAMBALPURI

Description: Black in color, with white switch on tail, with narrow and short horns, curved in a semi-circle, running backward, then forward at the tip.

Lactation duration: 350 days

Milk yield: 2,400 kg

Source [5]

Breed: SURTI

The existence of the Surti breed in north Gujarat (India) is referred to 1940. It is the result of a selection of Indian breeds of buffalo. It is one of the most important breeds in Gujarat and in Rajasthan.

Origin: India

Description: Black color coat, skin is black or reddish. They have two white chevrons on the chest. Animals are characterized and preferred by white markings on the forehead, legs and tail tips. Horns are flat, of medium length, sickle shaped and are are directed downward and backward, turning then upward at the tip to form a hook. The udder is well developed, finely shaped and squarely placed between the hind legs. The tail is fairly long, thin and flexible ending in a white tuft.

Height at withers of adult male: 131 cm; body weight is 700 kg

Height at withers of adult female: 124 cm; body weight is 550-650 kg
Lactation duration: 350 days
Milk yield: 2,090 kg
Milk fat: 6.6-8.1 percent
Milk protein: 4.2-4.6 percent
Sources [5, 9]

Breed: TARAI
Description: Black to brown color coat; sometimes there is a white blaze on the forehead, tail switch is white. Horns are long and flat with coils bending backwards and upwards.
Height at withers of adult male: 127 cm; body weight is 375 kg
Height at withers of adult female: 120 cm; body weight is 325 kg
Lactation duration: 250 days
Milk yield: 450 kg
Milk fat: 6.6-8.1 percent
Milk protein: 4.2-4.6 percent
Source [5]

Breed: TODA
Population size: 6,000
Description: Unicolor, light or dark grey. Horns are set wide apart with curved tip inwards, outward and forward. They are large and powerful animals.
Height at withers of adult male: 160 cm; body weight is 380 kg
Height at withers of adult female: 150 cm; body weight is 380 kg
Lactation duration: 200 days
Milk yield: 500 kg
Source [5]

DESI

Along with the river and swamp buffalo types, some authors [2, 11] add the third group of buffaloes, known in India and Pakistan as Desi. This group was neglected in the classification for a long time but it includes a great number of buffaloes raised in these countries. They are strong and resilient crosses of unidentified breeds obtained as a result of random and uncontrolled crossing between different buffalo breeds in rural conditions. The Desi buffaloes vary in horn construction, which are usually twisted or sickle-shaped. Most of them are used for draught and others are raised as dairy animals on small farms. They have good meat production.

The African buffalo (Syncerina) mentioned in the classification still exists in the wild in some African countries. As a result of hunting, however, the number of these wild buffaloes has greatly decreased lately [1]. There are over 60 varieties of African wild buffaloes. However, due to the fact that there is not enough evidence of the existence of so many species and sub-species, Shalash [2] identifies three groups of African wild buffaloes:

1. Cape buffalo (*Syncerus caffer caffer*) - also known as the Caffer wild buffalo that lives in the savanna areas of East and South Africa.
2. Wild Congo buffaloes (*Syncerus caffer nanus*) - those that live in the equatorial forests or their outskirts; smaller than the Cape buffaloes.
3. Intermediate forms of wild African Cape and Congo buffaloes (*Syncerus caffer aqeauinoctialis*) - living in the savanna areas.

The wild African buffaloes are extremely resilient in the unfavorable environmental conditions they live in, characterized with periodic droughts and scarce feed, endemic diseases and parasite problems, *etc.* considering the scientific experience with the Asian buffalo domestication in Australia, it can be assumed that the wild African buffalo domestication is also possible.

According to Shalash [2], the total number of wild African and Asian buffaloes is about 5 million. He also points out that river type accounts for the greatest proportion of the total number of the domestic water buffaloes in the world – 70.3% (including the Mediterranean buffalo) and the other 29.7% belong to the swamp type.

5. GENETIC IMPROVEMENT

Crossing between river and swamp buffaloes is mainly carried out in some countries of East and South East Asia to increase the milk yield of swamp buffaloes. For most of them, the crossing is accomplished with Murrah and Nili-Ravi only in a couple of countries. Genetic studies using karyotyping of different genotypes of swamp and river buffaloes further marked their differences. The swamp buffalo has 48 chromosome number while the river type has 50. Crossbreeds between these two types, carry 49 chromosome complement which inevitably may affect the outcome in terms of productive and reproductive performances [8].

China started crossing swamp buffalo with Murrah and Nili-Ravi in 1957, where a national program for the creation of triple-breed crosses was successfully implemented. First, they import 55 Murrah buffaloes which were used for crossing with swamp buffaloes. Then in 1974, artificial insemination with deep-frozen semen was implemented, resulting in an encouraging production of 10,000 crosses. In 1974, a new import of river buffaloes, this time 50 Nili-Ravi from Pakistan, was included as a second breed in the crossing program started in 1977. Crossing of F1 crosses Murrah x swamp buffalo with Nili-Ravi breed started in Guangxi for the creation of a new triple-breed milk-and-meat buffalo type with 50% blood of Nili-Ravi, 25% of Murrah and 25% of the indigenous swamp buffalo. This experimental crossing expanded, including also several Southern provinces. At the end of 1988, there were 800 purebred Murrah buffaloes in the country, 150 Nili-Ravi and about 200,000 crosses [1].

Alexiev [1] comprehensively presented the findings of Xiao and Jianxin in China in 1988 and 1990, respectively. They reported that Murrah crosses were superior to the swamp buffalo by conformation and milk yield with maintained draught ability. Milk yield increased with the increase of the genetic input from Murrah. The F1 crosses (50% Murrah blood) had an average milk yield of 1,097-1,154 kg and those with 75% Murrah blood a milk yield of 1,540 kg with 8.5% fat, 5.15% protein and 5.55% lactose. In fattening, the crosses had a higher average daily gain and lower feed conversion ratio. Compared to Murrah, the crossing of the swamp buffalo with Nili-Ravi produced better results. The F1 Nili-Ravi crosses were superior to those of Murrah by growth rate. For a 308-day lactation period they had an average milk yield of 2,125 kg with 7.9% fat and 4.5% protein. The fat content, however, was at a lower level. Nili-Ravi crosses had an average milk yield for first lactation of 1,825 kg, second lactation 2,087 kg and third lactation

2,096 kg with 7.94% fat, 4.90% protein and 4.53% lactose. The maximum daily milk yield was 19.9 kg.

Compared to the F1 Murrah and Nili-Ravi crosses, the triple-breed crosses produced much better results. Those crosses had an average milk yield of 2,119.7 kg for a 292-day lactation period and its average milk yield was 2,389.9 kg with 8.0% fat at a maximum individual milk yield of 4,342.4 kg. For the period of 1980-1984, the triple-breed crosses had an average milk yield for first lactation of 2,100.7 kg, second lactation 2,574 kg and third lactation 2,704.9 kg with 8.11% fat, 4.71% protein and 5.01% lactose. An average live weight for the triple-breed buffalo cows was of 665 kg, and milk yield of 2,236 kg with 7.8% fat and 4.5% protein. Again, according to Alexiev [1], the live weight and milk yield decreased in within-breeding of triple x triple-breed crosses.

The triple-breed crosses are large animals with a higher hind part, well developed udder, well developed muscles and lighter bone structure. The horns are more curled than those of the Murrah crosses. The hair color is dark gray. Some of the animals have white spots on the forehead. The white chevrons across the chest are rare. The animals have a mild temperament due to the 50% Nili-Ravi blood. As a result of the crossing, the dressing percent improved as well, increasing from 46.9% for the swamp buffalo to 49.0% for the F1 Murrah crosses, 51.9% for Nili-Ravi and 53.5% for the triple-breed crosses. Days of pregnancy were also decreased from 330 days for the swamp buffalo to 305.5-310.3 days for the purebred animals and different crosses. The triple-breed crosses had a 175 days shorter generation interval [1].

The experiments also showed that the F1 crosses of Nili-Ravi x swamp buffalo rank second by milk yield, which is a good reason to expect a positive result from the following upgrading crossing with Nili-Ravi. Chinese experience is a convincing proof of the fact that the milk yield capacity of the indigenous swamp buffalo can be significantly increased only by its crossing with river type breeds, the best results being achieved in the triple breed crosses. As a matter of fact, this is a new synthetic milk buffalo type, created for the first time in the world buffalo practice.

In the Philippines, a large scale national program for crossing the indigenous buffalo Carabao with Murrah river type buffalo is in effect. The beginning was set in 1981, spearheaded then by the Philippine Carabao Research and Development Center (PCRDC), now the Philippine Carabao Center (PCC), with the development of the first breeding program in the country, intended for milk yield increase of the Philippine swamp buffalo Carabao. Initially test crossing with the breeds Murrah and Nili-Ravi was performed in three phases, for the creation of crosses with 50% blood of those two breeds of the river type with improved size, milk and meat productivity but with maintained work ability of the indigenous Carabao. For the purpose of this crossing deep-frozen semen doses of Murrah and Nili-Ravi were even imported from India and Pakistan, respectively.

These obtained crosses have shown a better growth rate than the swamp buffalo, The average live weight at birth of the Carabao calves, was 26 kg, 35 kg for F1 Murrah crosses and F1 Nili-Ravi crosses. At 12 months of age the average live weight of the breed groups was 160, 210 and 215 kg, respectively; at 18 months it was 204, 281 and 283 kg, respectively; at 24 months it was 239, 318 and 332 kg, respectively and at 36 months it was 305, 462 and 460 kg, respectively.

The average milk yield for the first lactation of Carabao buffalo cows from the control group was 259.4 kg, from purebred Murrah was 1,804.4 kg, from F1 Murrah crosses was 705.6 kg, and from the F1 Nili-Ravi crosses was 623.1 kg. In other words, compared to the swamp buffalo, the F1 Murrah and Nili-Ravi crosses have demonstrated higher milk yield 2.4 and 2.7 times, respectively.

Crossbreeding of swamp buffalo with Murrah buffaloes to improve draft ability resulted into a crossbreed characterized by lighter bodyweights than the swamp buffalo at the same age, while the working ability of the crossbreed having the same body weight and heat resistance was comparable to the local buffalo. Crossbred animals were superior to local swamp buffaloes in terms of working ability, *i.e.*, draft power, area plowed per unit time, plowing speed, and duration of work [9].

The studies on reproductive characteristics showed that the F1 crosses of Murrah and Nili-Ravi reach age of puberty, first fertilization and first calving about a year earlier compared to the Carabao. No significant differences were established in the remaining reproductive traits. The crossing of the swamp buffalo with Murrah has also been carried out to a limited extent in Thailand, Malaysia, Indonesia and Vietnam.

In the Thai trials, the average live weight at weaning of the indigenous swamp buffalo calves was 189 kg, for Murrah 201 kg, for crosses with 50% Murrah blood 212 kg and for crosses with 75% Murrah blood 175 kg. At the age of 1 year weights were 241, 242, 240 and 213 kg, respectively. The result on milk yield on the Government Farm at the Livestock Breeding Station in Nongkwang, Rajaburi Province, show that the average lactation milk yield of the swamp buffalo cows is 447 kg, for Murrah 1,105 kg and for their crosses 1,113 kg with an average fat content of 8.8%,7.6% and 8.6% respectively [1]. This type or crossing is also carried out in some Latin American countries, raising swamp buffaloes of different origin.

CONFLICT OF INTEREST

The authors confirm that they have no conflict of interest to declare for this publication.

ACKNOWLEDGEMENTS

Declared none.

REFERENCES

[1] Alexiev AI. The Water Buffalo. St. Kliment Ohridski University Press 1998.

[2] Shalash M. The Present Status of Buffaloes in the World. Proc III World Buffalo's Congress Varna. Bulgaria. 1991; pp. 243-67.

[3] Bhat PN. Genetics of River Buffaloes. Tulloh, NM and Holmes, JHG (eds) "Buffalo Production" Elsevier. 1992; pp. 13-58.

[4] The Water Buffalo: New Prospects for an Underutilized Animal. Washington, D.C.: National Academy Press 1984.

[5] Borghese A. Buffalo Production and Research. FAO Regional Office for Europe Inter Regional Cooperative Research Network on Buffalo. Avaiable from:ftp://ftp.fao.org/docrep/fao/010/ah847e/ah-847e00.pdf. ESCORENA 2005.

[6] Chunxi Z, Zhongquan L. Buffalo genetic resources in China. Buff News 2001; 16: 1-7.

[7] Popovici I. Buffalo Newsletter 1996; 5: 9-10.

[8] Parker BA. Genetic improvement. In: Faylon PS, Ed. Carabao production in the Philippines. Ranjhan, SK: PCARRD and FAO/UNDP 1992; pp. 50-8.

[9] The Philippines Recommends for Carabao Production. Philippine Council for Agriculture, Forestry and Natural Resources Research and Development. Philippines Recommends Series No 37-A

[10] Faarungsang S. Thai Swamp Buffalo General Information. Thailand: Department of Animal Science, Kasetsart University 2003. [http://www.angrin.tlri.gov.tw/apec2003/Chapter1Thai.pdf]

[11] Cockrill RW. Present and future status of buffaloes in the world. Buffalo J 1985; 1: 93-107.

CHAPTER 2

The Cytogenetics of the Water Buffalo

Alessandra Iannuzzi* and **Leopoldo Iannuzzi**

National Research Council (CNR), Institute of Animal Production Systems in Mediterranean Environment (ISPAAM), Laboratory of Animal Cytogenetics and Gene Mapping, Naples, Italy

Abstract: Though world buffalo population is about 1/9 of cattle population, more human beings depend from buffaloes, especially in South-East Asia. Indeed, there are about 168 million water buffaloes in the world, mostly (161 million) raised in Asia. The River buffalo has received great attention from West countries which are particularly interested to both milk and meat production. For this reason, the genetic improvement of buffaloes still remains one of the most important goal in this species. Cytogenetic is one of the biotechnologies which supports the genetic improvement of buffaloes, especially for the selection of reproducers. In this chapter, an update of the latest results obtained in the cytogenetics of buffaloes is reported, starting from its cytotaxonomy and going through clinical and molecular cytogenetics, cytogenetic investigations and breeding objectives.

Keywords: Chromosome abnormality, Cytogenetics, Evolution, Fertility, Water buffalo.

1. INTRODUCTION

Though buffaloes are about 1/9 of cattle, they interest a world human population greater than that raising cattle. For this reason this species attracts the interest of many people, especially in East countries, and is of great economic importance. Among buffaloes, the Asiatic water buffalo, in particular the riverine type, is the most important one. The main findings obtained so far in cytogenetics of this species, are summarized in this chapter.

* **Corresponding author Alessandra Iannuzzi:** National Research Council (CNR), Institute of Animal Production Systems in Mediterranean Environment (ISPAAM), Laboratory of Animal Cytogenetics and Gene Mapping, Naples, Italy; Tel: +39 081 5964977, +39 081 5966006; Fax: +39 081 5965291; E-mail: alessandra.iannuzzi@ispaam.cnr.it

Giorgio A. Presicce (Ed.)

2. ORIGIN AND EVOLUTION

The buffalo belongs to the Bovini tribe, Bovidae family, Ruminantia suborder and Cetartiodactyla order (Table **1**). The African buffalo (*Syncerus caffer*) and the Asiatic buffalo (*Bubalus bubalis*) are the most important species raised in the world. Within the African buffalo (*Syncerus caffer*) three subspecies can be identified: the Cape Buffalo (*Syncerus caffer caffer*), the Forest Buffalo (*Syncerus caffer nanus*) and the Sudan Buffalo from West Africa (*Syncerus caffer brachyceros*) [1, 2]. Karyotypes of these species differ among them and represent the most simple method to distinguish their genotypes, also in their inter-specific hybrids. Cytogenetic investigations have shown that *Syncerus caffer caffer* has 2n = 52 with a fundamental number (FN) equal to 60, while *Syncerus caffer nanus* has 2n = 54 and FN = 60. Crosses between these two species are possible, with F1-hybrid having 2n = 53. This condition may be cause of reduced fertility for the formation of unbalanced gametes due to erroneous meiotic segregations, as it occurs in other species [3, 4]. Four (*Syncerus caffer caffer)* and three (*Syncerus caffer nanus*) biarmed autosome pairs are the cause of the different diploid number found in these two species, being all remaining chromosomes acrocentric, including the X-chromosome (the largest acrocentric one) and the Y-chromosome. The biarmed pairs in *S.c. caffer* have been originated by Robertsonian translocations of cattle (ancestral bovid) chromosomes 1;13, 2;3, 5;20 and 11;29 [5].

Two main species are considered in the Asiatic buffalo or water buffalo (*Bubalus bubalis*): the river buffalo (2n = 50, FN = 60) and the swamp buffalo (2n = 48, FN = 58). Since all chromosomes (chromosome arms) have been conserved in the two species, crosses between them are possible, although the hybrid has 49 chromosomes and may originate reproductive problems due to unbalanced gametes. The river buffalo (2n = 50) is the most important and numerous buffalo species in the world. It has five submetacentric autosomes, being the remaining chromosomes acrocentric, including the X-chromosome (the largest one) and the Y chromosome. The five submetacentric river buffalo chromosomes (BBU) originated by Robertsonian translocations of cattle homologous (cattle ancestor) chromosomes and relative syntenic groups (U): BBU1 (1;27-U10/U25), BBU2 (2;23-U17/U20), BBU3 (8;19-U18/U21), BBU4 (5;28-U3/U29), and BBU5

(16;29-U1/U7) according to the standard karyotypes of both river buffalo [6] and cattle [7].

The swamp buffalo (2n = 48) karyotype differs from the river type for the presence of a large chromosome (chr 1), which was formed by tandem fusion translocation between river buffalo chromosomes 4 (BBU4) and 9 (BBU9). Since BBU4 was formed by translocation (centric fusion) of cattle homologous chromosomes 5 and 28 [6], and BBU9 is homologous to cattle chromosome 7 [6], three cattle (ancestor) homologous chromosomes (and bovine synthenic groups - U) constitute swamp buffalo chromosome 1: BTA5 (U3), BTA28 (U29) and BTA7 (U22) [8].

By comparing the karyotypes of African (*Syncerus*) and Asiatic (*Bubalus*) buffaloes, it appears evident that no biarmed chromosome pairs are common between the two species [6 - 9].

In Table **1** cytogenetic data of different species of buffaloes in the world are summarized.

Table 1. Cytotaxonomy of buffaloes in the world and their chromosome diploid (2n) and fundamental (FN) number.

Order	Cetartiodactyla				
Suborder	Ruminantia				
Family	Bovidae				
Species	African buffalo (*Syncerus caffer*)			Asiatic buffalo (*Bubalus bubalis*)	
Subspecies	Large black savannah or Cape Buffalo (*Syncerus caffer caffer) 2n=52 NF=60*	Intermediate Sudan buffalo from West Africa (*Syncerus caffer brachyceros) 2n=53 NF=60*	Small reddish forest buffalo (*Syncerus caffer nanus) 2n=54 NF=60*	River buffalo 2n=50 NF=60	Swamp buffalo 2n=48 NF=58

3. CYTOGENETIC INVESTIGATIONS

3.1. G- and R-banding

G(Giemsa) and R-(reverse) banding are the usual techniques applied for the identification of both chromosomes and chromosome abnormalities, the latter involving the chromosome number or chromosome rearrangements such as translocations, deletions, inversions or duplications of chromosome segments.

G- and R-banding comparisons between cattle and river buffalo chromosomes have revealed a substantial amount of banding homologies between the two species, both at early-metaphase [8, 10] and prometaphase stages [11]. In particular, each of the five river buffalo biarmed pairs originates from a centric fusion translocation between two of ten homologous cattle autosomes (Fig. **1**), a fact that is highly supportive of the hypothesis that all bovids have a common ancestor [12].

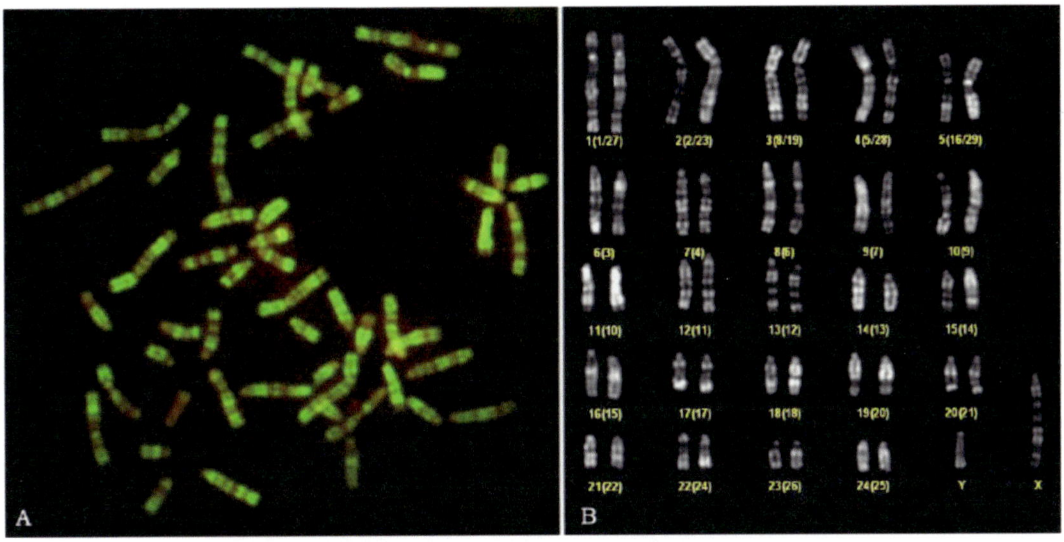

Fig. (1). High resolution RBA-banded male river buffalo metaphase plate (**A**) and corresponding karyotype (2n = 50, XY) (**B**), according to the river buffalo standard. Numbers reported in parenthesis refer to cattle homologous chromosomes.

3.2. C-banding

C-banding technique detects the presence of constitutive heterochromatin (HC = C-bands), which is usually located in centromeric regions of chromosomes in the majority of analyzed species.

The C-banding technique (in particular, the CBA-banding) makes possible to distinguish the gonosomes (in particular, the Y-chromosome) from the autosomes and it is normally applied to study chromosome abnormalities in sex chromosomes of river buffalo [13 - 16]. In the case of the river buffalo, the five centric fusion have been followed by a substantial loss of constitutive heterochromatin when compared with both cattle homologous chromosomes, and remaining river buffalo acrocentric chromosome. The X gonosome shows the largest HC-block at the centromere. Y-chromosome shows variable C-banding pattern according to different treatments during the C-banding technique. Indeed, it is entirely heterochromatic or with a C-band distally located, being the centromere C-banding negative (Fig. **2**). This particular feature allows to distinguish very easily the Y-chromosome from small acrocentric chromosomes. In the swamp buffalo, the C-banding is slightly different from the river buffalo. In fact, in swamp chromosome 1, the C-band material in the region of junction between chromosome 4 and 9, is present as a light-staining area. The fusion occurs between the centromere of river buffalo chromosome BBU9 and the telomere of chromosome BBU4p, and results in loss in the satellite II (SAT II) DNA, being SAT I DNA conserved (Fig. **3**) [17].

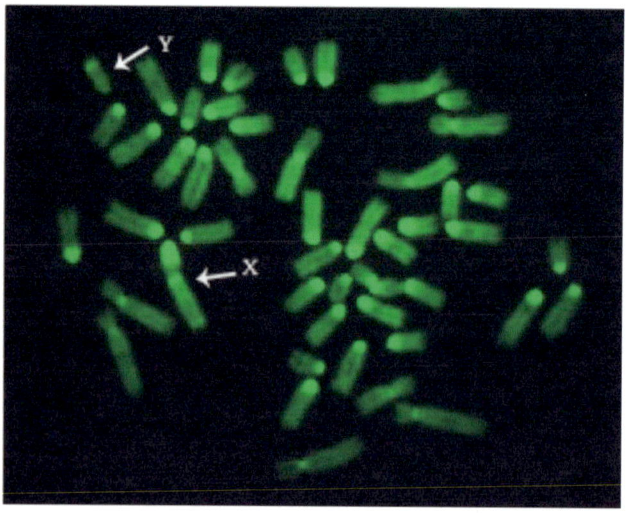

Fig. (2). CBA banding in a male river buffalo metaphase plate. While large C-bands can be seen in all acrocentric chromosomes, including the X, showing the largest C-band with an additional and proximal C-band. The Y gonosome (also acrocentric) has a positive C-band distally located, being the centromeric region C-band negative.

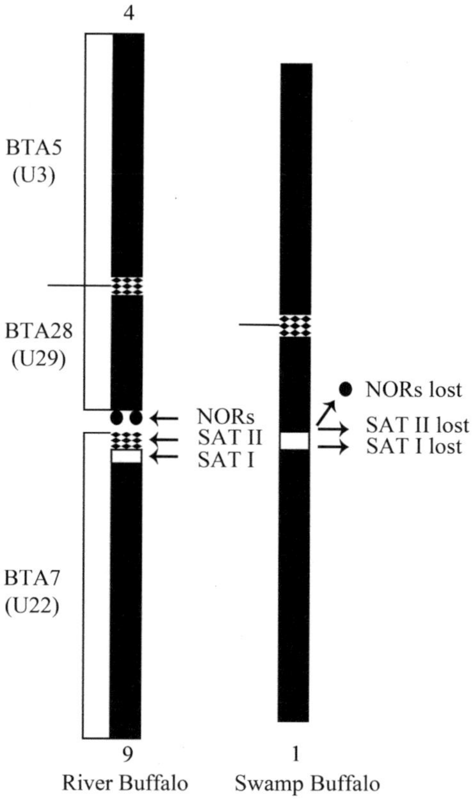

Fig. (3). Genesis of swamp buffalo chromosome 1 by translocation of tandem fusion type involving river buffalo chromosomes 9 (acrocentric) and 4 (biarmed). The fusion was originated along the centromere of BBU9 and the telomere of BBU4p, resulting in losses of both nucleolar organizer regions (NORs) from BBU4p and satellite II (SAT II) DNA from BBU9, being SAT I DNA conserved. The homologous cattle (BTA) chromosomes and relative synthetic groups (U) present in both BBU4/BBU9 and swamp buffalo chromosome 1 are reported.

3.3. Nucleolus Organizer Regions (NORs)

NORs are specific chromosome sites where ribosomal genes are highly transcribed. Each species has a specific number of NORs and nucleolar organizer chromosomes (NOC). In domestic bovids, NORs are located at the telomeres of five or six autosomes [18 - 20]. The use of sequential G- or R-banding/Ag-NORs techniques have demonstrated that NORs in bovids have been only partially conserved in the same homologous chromosomes [21]. NORs can be revealed by using silver nitrate (Ag) staining, which reveals only active NORs (NORs which have organized at least one nucleolus during previous cell inter-phase), or specific ribosomal probes with the fluorescence *in situ* hybridization (FISH) technique that reveals active and not active NORs.

In river buffalo NORs have been localized at the telomeric regions of chromosomes 3p, 4p, 6, 21 and 24 (Fig. **4**) [22]. In swamp buffalo during the tandem fusion translocation forming chromosome 1, the centromere of BBU9 was apparently lost or inactivated while the NORs located at the telomeres of BBU4p [20] were lost (Fig. **3**) [8]. Therefore, they are localized at the telomeric regions of chromosomes 4p, 8, 20, 22 and 23 [8].

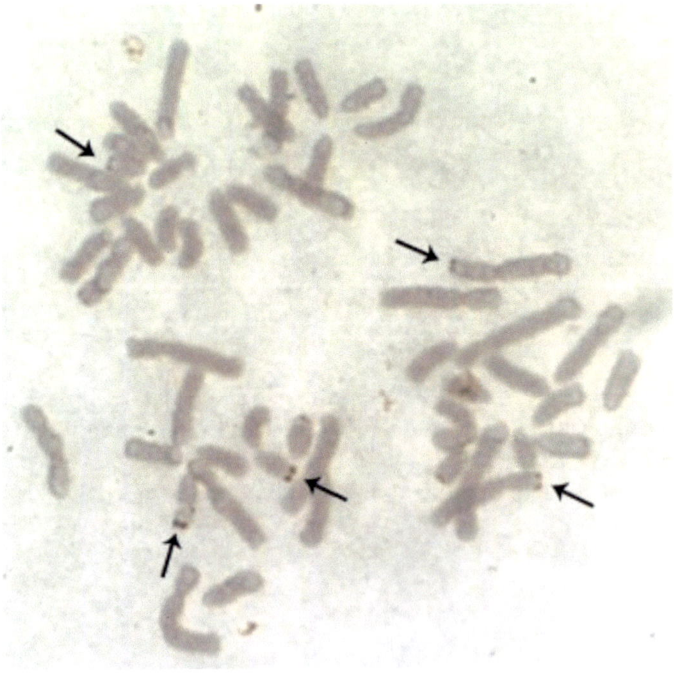

Fig. (4). Nucleolar organizer regions (NORs) revealed by silver nitrate staining (arrows) in a river buffalo metaphase plate.

3.4. Sister Chromatid Exchanges (SCEs)

SCEs consist in exchanges between the chromatids of the same chromosome after breakages at the DNA level occurring during the S-phase and induced by mutagens forming DNA adducts, which interfere with DNA replication. The best method to obtain SCEs is to incorporate a thymidine base analogue (5-Bromo-2-deoxyuridine–BrdU) into replicating DNA during the last two S-phases (*generally the BrdU is incorporated 28-30 h before harvesting*). SCE analysis has often been applied both in human and in farm animals, as a cytogenetic assay for biomonitoring and genotoxicity testing of potentially mutagenic and carcinogenic chemicals [23, 24]. Cytogenetic test are useful to reveal the presence of chromosome damages originated by mutagens present in the environment, including the food chain. Chromosome instability has been found in calf affected by limb malformations [25] by using the SCE test as well as in river buffaloes exposed to dioxins (Fig. **5**) [26].

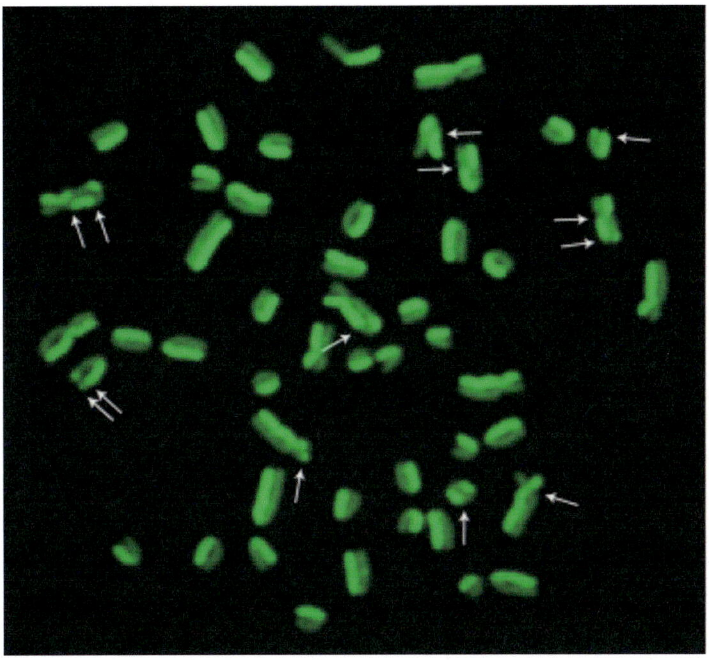

Fig. (5). Sister chromatid exchanges (SCE) in a female river buffalo metaphase plate from a cell naturally exposed to dioxins. Arrows indicate the presence of 12 SCEs.

3.5. Pseudoautosomal Regions (PAR) and Pseudoautosomal Boundary Regions (PAB)

The PAR is a short region of sequence homology between the sex chromosomes, which is involved in sex chromosome pairing, recombination and segregation during meiosis (separation of paired alleles into different gametes). The region has been found in many plant and animal species, including mammals [27, 28] (Fig. **6**).

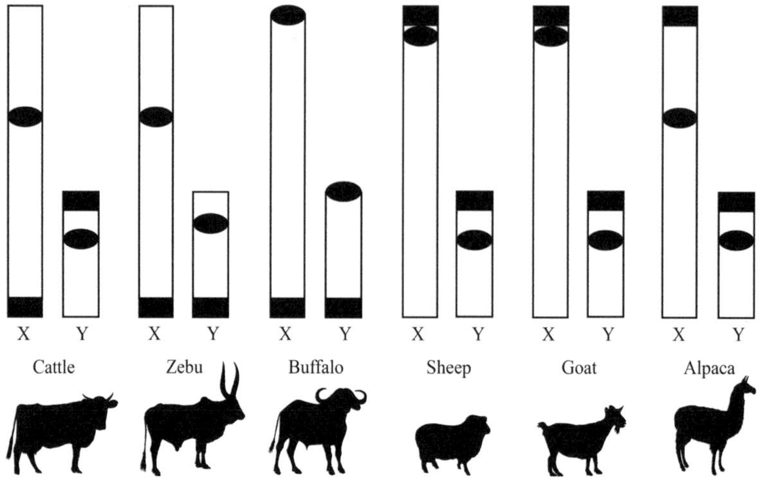

Fig. (6). A schematic representation showing the location of the PAR on the sex chromosomes of cattle, zebu, river buffalo, goat, sheep and alpaca. (From Raudsepp *et al.*, 2012).

The physical domain of the PAR lies between the terminal ends of the sex chromosomes and the pseudoautosomal boundary (PAB) – a border across which the sequence homology between the X and the Y chromosome decreases, and recombination cases and regions specific to individual sex chromosome begin [29, 30]. Loci located within the PAR behave similarly to autosomal loci: they are diploid, undergo recombination in males and females and are not subject to dosage compensation by X inactivation in females [27 - 31]. These features led to naming of the region as pseudoautosomal [32], primarily to indicate the autosome-like properties, despite being on the sex chromosomes. The location of the PAR on the sex chromosomes of river buffalo is telomeric in both X and Y chromosomes, while in cattle is located on telomere of Xq and Yp [33].

4. CLINICAL CYTOGENETIC

4.1. Standard Karyotype

Clinical cytogenetics has been only recently applied in river buffalo, especially in

Italy where both males used for reproduction and many females with reproductive disturbances have been analyzed by using cytogenetic techniques.

A standard karyotype of river buffalo using six banding techniques and G and R banded ideograms has been established by an international committee (Fig. **1**) [6]. A comparison between river buffalo standard karyotype, based on specific chromosome river buffalo genetic markers [14], has been performed when arranging the latest standard karyotype of cattle, sheep and goat [7], allowing the correlation of buffalo chromosomes to the related bovids (Fig. **1B**).

4.2. Autosomal Aberrations

Chromosome abnormalities involving autosomes have rarely been found in river buffalo, probably because few cytogenetic investigations have been performed in this species until now. A translocation involving BBU3 and BBU6 was found in a male river buffalo with normal body conformation, but no indications on fertility were reported [34]. A case of centric fission and fusion in a river buffalo cow, with reduced fertility, has been found in a farm producing milk to obtain mozzarella cheese [35]. A similar case has been found in a very famous Italian river buffalo used in artificial insemination (AI) [36].

4.3. Sex Chromosome Aberrations

Sex chromosome abnormalities occur with relative higher frequency in river buffalo, especially among females, comparing to autosome abnormalities. Cytogenetic analyses revealed that 20% of Italian river buffalo females, with reproductive problems, were found carriers of sex chromosome abnormalities [13-14-15-16-37-4-38].

The following are the most common chromosome abnormalities found so far in river buffaloes:

X-monosomy: This syndrome is rare in domestic animals, although several cases have been reported. Five females 2n = 49, X have been found so far in river buffaloes: three in India [39 - 41] and two in Italy [13 - 37]. These females are generally sterile for damages to internal sex adducts.

X-trisomy: Only three cases have been found so far in river buffaloes, two in India (Murrah breed) [39 - 41] and another in Italy (Razza Bufala Mediterranea Italiana) [15]. Sterility of these females occurs inevitably as a consequence of damage to the internal sex adducts, due to presence and action of all the three Xs before their inactivation (2/3), and/or to genes escaping gene inactivation, especially those of the PAR.

Sex-Reversal Syndrome: This syndrome is present in both males and females showing a karyotype which is opposite to their phenotype (XX or XY, respectively). XX-males are originated by errors occurred during meiosis with translocations of small Y-chromosome regions (where genes affecting sex differentiations are present) to the X-chromosome. XY females arise from deletion or mutations of genes inducing sex determination, especially the SRY-gene. This syndrome is uncommon in domestic animals. The female carries are characterized by gonadal dysgenesis. In river buffalo only two (sterile) females were found in Italy: one was missing its internal sex organs (with closed vagina) and the other one was characterized by atrophic Muller's ducts [14, 15].

XXY-Syndrome: This syndrome is very uncommon in farming animals, compared to humans where it is reported as Klinefelter's syndrome. Only one case was found river buffalo [42]. It was an unusual case, because the male carrier showed a karyotype 2n = 50,Y, t(X;X), being the two Xs fused along their centromeres.

XX/XY Chimerism (Freemartin): This is the most common chromosome abnormality found in sex chromosomes of both cattle and river buffalo. The frequency of this abnormality is strictly related to the frequency of births with twins, although almost all studied cases in Italian river buffaloes were from single birth. This occurred because one of the two co-twins dies during early embryonic life, but only after that placental anastomosis and sex differentiation have occurred, allowing thus serious damages in the living female twins, since sex differentiation occurs earlier in males than in the females [43]. The living twin (generally female), is generally sterile due to pronounced damages to the internal sex organs, which may vary from atrophies of Muller's ducts to the complete lack of internal sex organs (with closed vagina) [16 - 37]. The damages in the internal sex ducts are due to the Y-chromosome. Indeed, placental anastomosis occurs earlier (20-25 days) than sex differentiation (40-45 days) during the embryonic life. In river buffalo, XX/XY-mosaicism is the most common chromosome anomaly present in both Indian [44] and Mediterranean Italian (bufala mediterranea italiana) [16] breeds.

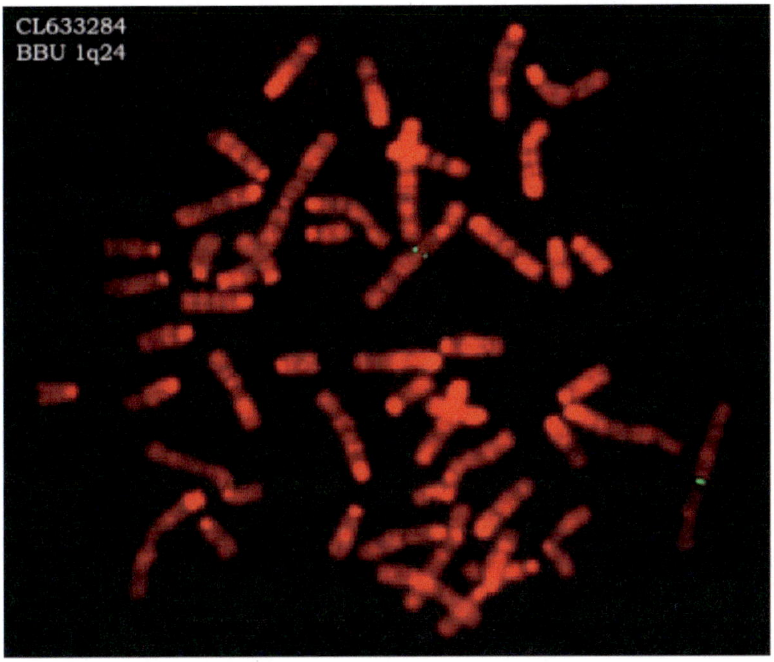

Fig. (7). FISH mapped marker of MINA gene (BAC CH243-1I24) on BBU1 chromosome. FITC signals were superimposed on RBPI-banding (R-banding using early BrdU-incorporation and propidium iodide staining). (From Di Meo *et al.*, 2011).

5. MOLECULAR CYTOGENETIC

The advent of Fuorescence *In Situ* Hybridization (FISH) technique and the availability of probes containing large insert (BAC-clones) or entire chromosome libraries [45], has expanded the field of cytogenetics. Thanks to this technique, it has been possible to study, in details, the physical organization of mammalian genomes, including the river buffalo. In fact, several loci have been assigned to this species by both somatic cell hybrid technique [46, 47] and (mostly about 95%) by FISH-mapping technique with DNA-probes such as cDNA for multi-copy genes, cosmids and BAC-clones for single copy genes [48, 37]. Fig. (**7**) shows an example of the FISH-mapping of MINA gene in BBU1 chromosome

[35]. Cytogenetic maps are very useful and important for many reasons: (a) genes or DNA-sequences can easily be assigned to specific chromosomes regions and bands; (b) specific molecular markers can be used to identify, correctly, the chromosome involved in the chromosome aberrations; (c) detailed comparisons between cytogenetic maps of related (bovids) and unrelated (bovids-humans) species can be performed to establish with more details and resolution, conserved chromosome regions and the rearrangements occurred during chromosome evolution of species.

6. BREEDING OBJECTIVES

River buffaloes are reared for the production of both milk and meat. In east countries (India, Pakistan, Egypt, and Nepal, in particular), approximately 50% of the milk produced is used for daily consumption. In Italy buffalo milk is processed to get cheese, in particular the mozzarella cheese [49]. The production and consumption of buffalo meat is usual in many countries (east and west countries) while in Italy is quite low, although recently in this country the interest on river buffalo meat has increased.

Breeding programs are implemented in order to speed up the genetic improvement for milk production, using both progeny tests and milk trait recording. In Italy, the highest proportion (28.6%) of milking buffaloes are officially registered, followed by Bulgaria (8.5%) and Iran (4.5%) [50]. A breeding program, today present in Italy and performed in collaboration with buffalo breeder associations, includes also the cytogenetic screening of bulls kept in reproductive centers (or males used for reproduction), as well as studies in females showing reproductive disturbances.

CONCLUSION

Cytogenetic is one of the most important biotechnologies recently applied to buffalo studies and analyses, contributing noticeably to the knowledge of its genome and to the genetic selection of reproducers. The certification with banded karyotype should be a requirement for all bulls entering into reproduction centers and to all females with reproductive problems.

The pronounced chromosome homology present between river buffalo and cattle, and the sequencing of both cattle and buffalo genomes, should expand our knowledge on the water buffalo.

CONFLICT OF INTEREST

The authors confirm that they have no conflict of interest to declare for this publication.

ACKNOWLEDGEMENTS

This study has been supported by the projects CISIA-VARIGEAV and CAMPUS-QUARC.

REFERENCES

[1] Buchholtz C. Cattle. In: Parker SP, Ed. Grzimek's Encyclopedia of Mammals. New York, USA: McGraw-Hill 1990; 5: pp. 360-417.

[2] Kingdon J. The Kingdon Field Guide to African Mammals. Academic Press London and New York 1997.

[3] Gustavsson I. Chromosome aberrations and their influence on the reproductive performance of domestic animals – a review. Z Tierzuchtg Zuchtgsbiol 1980; 97: 176-95. [http://dx.doi.org/10.1111/j.1439-0388.1980.tb00925.x]

[4] Villagómez DA, Parma P, Radi O, *et al.* Classical and molecular cytogenetics of disorders of sex development in domestic animals. Cytogenet Genome Res 2009; 126(1-2): 110-31. [http://dx.doi.org/10.1159/000245911] [PMID: 20016161]

[5] Gallagher DS Jr, Womack JE. Chromosome conservation in the Bovidae. J Hered 1992; 83(4): 287-98. [PMID: 1401875]

[6] Iannuzzi L. Standard karyotype of the river buffalo (Bubalus bubalis L., 2n = 50). Report of the committee for the standardization of banded karyotypes of the river buffalo. Cytogenet Cell Genet 1994; 67(2): 102-13. [http://dx.doi.org/10.1159/000133808] [PMID: 8039419]

[7] Di Berardino D, Di Meo GP, Gallagher DS, Hayes H, Iannuzzi L. ISCNDB2000 International system for chromosome nomenclature of domestic bovids. Cytogenet Cell Genet 2001; 92: 283-99.

[8] Di Berardino D, Iannuzzi L. Chromosome banding homologies in Swamp and Murrah buffalo. J Hered 1981; 72(3): 183-8. [PMID: 6168678]

[9] Gallagher DS Jr, Womack JE. Chromosome conservation in the Bovidae. J Hered 1992; 83(4): 287-98. [PMID: 1401875]

[10] Gupta P, Ray-Chaudhuri SP. Robertsonian changes in chromosomes of Indian Murrah buffalo,

Bubalus bubalis. Nucleus 1978; 21: 90-7.

[11] Iannuzzi L, Di Meo GP, Perucatti A, Ferrara L. The high resolution G- and R-banding pattern in chromosomes of river buffalo (*Bubalus bubalis* L.). Hereditas 1990; 112(3): 209-15. [http://dx.doi.org/10.1111/j.1601-5223.1990.tb00059.x] [PMID: 2211179]

[12] Wurster DH, Benirschke K. Chromosome studies in the superfamily Bovoidea. Chromosoma 1968; 25(2): 152-71. [http://dx.doi.org/10.1007/BF00327175] [PMID: 5709393]

[13] Iannuzzi L, Di Meo GP, Perucatti A, Zicarelli L. Sex chromosome monosomy (2n=49,X) in a river buffalo (Bubalus bubalis). Vet Rec 2000; 147(24): 690-1. [PMID: 11132677]

[14] Iannuzzi L, Di Meo GP, Perucatti A, Di Palo R, Zicarelli L. 50,XY gonadal dysgenesis (Swyers syndrome) in a female river buffalo (Bubalus bubalis). Vet Rec 2001; 148(20): 634-5. [http://dx.doi.org/10.1136/vr.148.20.634] [PMID: 11394803]

[15] Iannuzzi L, Di Meo GP, Perucatti A, Incarnato D, Di Palo R, Zicarelli L. Reproductive disturbances and sex chromosome abnormalities in two female river buffaloes. Vet Rec 2004; 154(26): 823-4. [http://dx.doi.org/10.1136/vr.154.26.823] [PMID: 15260445]

[16] Iannuzzi L, Di Meo GP, Perucatti A, *et al.* Freemartinism in river buffalo: clinical and cytogenetic observations. Cytogenet Genome Res 2005; 108(4): 355-8. [http://dx.doi.org/10.1159/000081531] [PMID: 15627757]

[17] Tanaka K, Matsuda Y, Masangkay JS, Solis CD, Anunciado RV, Namikawa T. Characterization and chromosomal distribution of satellite DNA sequences of the water buffalo (*Bubalus bubalis*). J Hered 1999; 90(3): 418-22. [http://dx.doi.org/10.1093/jhered/90.3.418] [PMID: 10355126]

[18] Di Berardino D, Arrighi FE, Kieffer NM. Nucleolus organizer regions in two species of Bovidae. J Hered 1979; 70(1): 47-50. [PMID: 89140]

[19] Di Meo GP, Iannuzzi L, Ferrara L, Rubino R. Identification of nucleolus organizer chromosomes in goat (*Capra hircus*). Caryologia 1991; 44: 309-16. [http://dx.doi.org/10.1080/00087114.1991.10797196]

[20] Di Meo GP, Iannuzzi L, Perucatti A, Ferrara L. Identification of nucleolus organizer chromosomes in sheep (*Ovis aries* L.) by sequential GBG/Ag-NOR and RBG/Ag-NOR techniques. Cytobios 1993; 75(302-303): 183-90. [PMID: 7694824]

[21] Iannuzzi L, Di Meo GP, Perucatti A. Identification of nucleolus organizer chromosomes and frequency of active NORs in river buffalo (*Bubalus bubalis* L.). Caryologia 1996; 49: 27-34. [http://dx.doi.org/10.1080/00087114.1996.10797347]

[22] Iannuzzi L, Di Meo GP, Perucatti A, Ferrara L, Gustavsson I. Sister chromatid exchange in chromosomes of cattle from three different breeds reared under similar conditions. Hereditas 1991; 114(3): 201-5. [http://dx.doi.org/10.1111/j.1601-5223.1991.tb00325.x] [PMID: 1960099]

[23] Natarajan AT. Chromosome aberrations: past, present and future. Mutat Res 2002; 504(1-2): 3-16. [http://dx.doi.org/10.1016/S0027-5107(02)00075-1] [PMID: 12106642]

[24] Perucatti A, Di Meo GP, Albarella S, *et al.* Increased frequencies of both chromosome abnormalities and SCEs in two sheep flocks exposed to high dioxin levels during pasturage. Mutagenesis 2006; 21(1): 67-75.
[http://dx.doi.org/10.1093/mutage/gei076] [PMID: 16434450]

[25] Peretti V, Ciotola F, Albarella S, *et al.* Increased SCE levels in Mediterranean Italian buffaloes affected by limb malformation (transversal hemimelia). Cytogenet Genome Res 2008; 120(1-2): 183-7.
[http://dx.doi.org/10.1159/000118761] [PMID: 18467846]

[26] Genualdo V, Perucatti A, Iannuzzi A, *et al.* Chromosome fragility in river buffalo cows exposed to dioxins. J Appl Genet 2012; 53(2): 221-6.
[http://dx.doi.org/10.1007/s13353-012-0092-2] [PMID: 22415351]

[27] Charlesworth D, Charlesworth B, Marais G. Steps in the evolution of heteromorphic sex chromosomes. Heredity (Edinb) 2005; 95(2): 118-28.
[http://dx.doi.org/10.1038/sj.hdy.6800697] [PMID: 15931241]

[28] Ming R, Moore PH. Genomics of sex chromosomes. Curr Opin Plant Biol 2007; 10(2): 123-30. [http://dx.doi.org/10.1016/j.pbi.2007.01.013] [PMID: 17300986]

[29] Galtier N. Recombination, GC-content and the human pseudoautosomal boundary paradox. Trends Genet 2004; 20(8): 347-9.
[http://dx.doi.org/10.1016/j.tig.2004.06.001] [PMID: 15262406]

[30] Ross MT, Grafham DV, Coffey AJ, *et al.* The DNA sequence of the human X chromosome. Nature 2005; 434(7031): 325-37.
[http://dx.doi.org/10.1038/nature03440] [PMID: 15772651]

[31] Urbach A, Benvenisty N. Studying early lethality of 45,XO (Turners syndrome) embryos using human embryonic stem cells. PLoS One 2009; 4(1): e4175.
[http://dx.doi.org/10.1371/journal.pone.0004175] [PMID: 19137066]

[32] Burgoyne PS. Genetic homology and crossing over in the X and Y chromosomes of Mammals. Hum Genet 1982; 61(2): 85-90.
[http://dx.doi.org/10.1007/BF00274192] [PMID: 7129448]

[33] Raudsepp T, Das PJ, Avila F, Chowdhary BP. The pseudoautosomal region and sex chromosome aneuploidies in domestic species. Sex Dev 2012; 6(1-3): 72-83.
[http://dx.doi.org/10.1159/000330627] [PMID: 21876343]

[34] Vijh RK, Tanita MS, Sahai R. Translocation in Murrah buffalo. Indian J Anim Sci 1994; 64: 534-8.

[35] Di Meo GP, Goldammer T, Perucatti A, *et al.* Extended cytogenetic maps of sheep chromosome 1 and their cattle and river buffalo homoeologues: comparison with the OAR1 RH map and human chromosomes 2, 3, 21 and 1q. Cytogenet Genome Res 2011; 133(1): 16-24. [http://dx.doi.org/10.1159/000323796] [PMID: 21282943]

[36] Albarella S, Ciotola F, Coletta A, Genualdo V, Iannuzzi L, Peretti V. A new translocation t(1p;18) in an Italian Mediterranean river buffalo (*Bubalus bubalis*, 2n = 50) bull: cytogenetic, fertility and

inheritance studies. Cytogenet Genome Res 2013; 139(1): 17-21.
[http://dx.doi.org/10.1159/000342360] [PMID: 22986410]

[37] Di Meo GP, Perucatti A, Di Palo R, *et al.* Sex chromosome abnormalities and sterility in river buffalo. Cytogenet Genome Res 2008; 120(1-2): 127-31.
[http://dx.doi.org/10.1159/000118751] [PMID: 18467836]

[38] Favetta LA, Villagómez DA, Iannuzzi L, *et al.* Disorders of sexual development and abnormal early development in domestic food-producing mammals: the role of chromosome abnormalities, environment and stress factors. Sex Dev 2012; 6(1-3): 18-32.
[http://dx.doi.org/10.1159/000332754] [PMID: 22024933]

[39] Yadav BR, Kumar P, Tomer OS, Kumar S, Balain DS. Monosomy X and gonadal dysgenesis in a buffalo heifer (*Bubalus bubalis*). Theriogenology 1990; 34(1): 99-105.
[http://dx.doi.org/10.1016/0093-691X(90)90580-M] [PMID: 16726819]

[40] Prakash B, Balain DS, Lathwal SS. A 49, XO sterile murrah buffalo (*Bubalus bubalis*). Vet Rec 1992; 130(25): 559-60.
[http://dx.doi.org/10.1136/vr.130.25.559] [PMID: 1496757]

[41] Prakash B, Balain DS, Lathwal SS, Malik RK. Trisomy-X in a sterile river buffalo. Vet Rec 1994; 134(10): 241-2.
[http://dx.doi.org/10.1136/vr.134.10.241] [PMID: 8197685]

[42] Patel RK, Singh KM, Soni KJ, Chauhan JB. Novel cytogenetic finding: an unusual X;X-translocation in Mehsana buffalo (*Bubalus bubalis*). Cytogenet Genome Res 2006; 115(2): 186-8.
[http://dx.doi.org/10.1159/000095241] [PMID: 17065802]

[43] Ruvinsky A, Spicer LJ. The Genetics of Cattle. CABI Publ, Wallingford, Oxon, UK. Dev Genet 1999.

[44] Balakrishnan CR, Yadav BR, Goswami SL. Sex chromosome chimerism in heterosexual Murrah buffalo triplets. Vet Rec 1981; 109: 112.
[http://dx.doi.org/10.1136/vr.109.8.162] [PMID: 7336550]

[45] Iannuzzi L, Di Meo GP, Perucatti A, Bardaro T. ZOO-FISH and R-banding reveal extensive conservation of human chromosome regions in euchromatic regions of river buffalo chromosomes. Cytogenet Cell Genet 1998; 82(3-4): 210-4.
[http://dx.doi.org/10.1159/000015102] [PMID: 9858819]

[46] El Nahas SM, Oraby HA, de Hondt HA, *et al.* Synteny mapping in river buffalo. Mamm Genome 1996; 7(11): 831-4.
[http://dx.doi.org/10.1007/s003359900245] [PMID: 8875891]

[47] El Nahas SM, de Hondt HA, Womack JE. Current status of the river buffalo (*Bubalus bubalis* L.) gene map. J Hered 2001; 92(3): 221-5.
[http://dx.doi.org/10.1093/jhered/92.3.221] [PMID: 11447236]

[48] Iannuzzi L, Di Meo GP, Perucatti A, *et al.* The river buffalo (*Bubalus bubalis*, 2n = 50) cytogenetic map: assignment of 64 loci by fluorescence *in situ* hybridization and R-banding. Cytogenet Genome Res 2003; 102(1-4): 65-75.
[http://dx.doi.org/10.1159/000075727] [PMID: 14970681]

[49] Zicarelli L. Buffalo milk: its properties, dairy yield and mozzarella production. Vet Res Commun

2004; 28 (Suppl. 1): 127-35.
[http://dx.doi.org/10.1023/B:VERC.0000045390.81982.4d] [PMID: 15372941]

[50] Moioli B. Breeding and selection of dairy buffaloes. In: Borghese A, Ed. Buffalo Production and Research REU Tech Sr. FAO Regional Office for Europe 2005; pp. 41-50.

CHAPTER 3

Molecular Genetics and Selection in Dairy Buffaloes: The Italian Situation

Alfredo Pauciullo* and **Leopoldo Iannuzzi**

National Research Council (CNR), Institute of Animal Production Systems in Mediterranean Environment (ISPAAM), Laboratory of Animal Cytogenetics and Gene Mapping, Naples, Italy

Abstract: The Italian river buffalo was characterized by an extensive period of isolation, which did not allow crossbreeding. This has brought to a morpho-functional differentiation of the Mediterranean type, whose population has increased 19 fold in Italy in the past fifty years. This increase is mainly due to the rising interest in the productive characteristics of this rustic animal; actually bred mainly as dairy purpose animal. Marker assisted selection (MAS) might be a promising choice for planning appropriate breeding schemes for Italian river buffaloes. In this respect, the genetic markers significantly associated to milk yield traits may give the right information for the identification of animals with high breeding value. The literature associated with different aspects of the genetic progress in buffalo is abundant, and this chapter is a review of the molecular bases for the improvement of the quali-quantitative characteristics of the Italian dairy buffaloes occurred during the last decade.

Keywords: Casein cluster, Genetic improvement of dairy traits, Milk yield, Molecular selection, River buffalo.

1. INTRODUCTION

The domestic water buffalo was historically split into the swamp and river subspecies, due to their difference in morphology, behaviour, and chromosome number (2n=48 and 2n=50, respectively). Swamp buffalo is predominant in Southeast Asia and China, whereas the river type is mainly found in India,

* **Corresponding author Alfredo Pauciullo:** National Research Council (CNR), Institute of Animal Production Systems in Mediterranean Environment (ISPAAM), Laboratory of Animal Cytogenetics and Gene Mapping, Naples, Italy; Tel: +39 011 6708598; Fax. +39 011 6708506; E-mail: alfredo.pauciullo@ispaam.cnr.it

Giorgio A. Presicce (Ed.)

Southwest Asia and in the Mediterranean area [1]. Despite their phenotypic differences, there is still a great interest on their time of domestication [2], as well as a debate as to consider appropriate their classification into two related subspecies [3]. In fact, molecular evidences based on mitochondrial DNA analysis [4, 5], molecular markers [6, 7] and Y-chromosome gene variations [8] showed that the two types are distinct and the separation of swamp and river type pre-dates domestication. They share several haplotype both at genomic and mitochondrial level, but the swamp and the river buffaloes constitute two distinct subspecies.

In the last years, several research projects have focused on the buffalo genome. In particular, 8 different consortium groups are working to fill the gap with other livestock species. Five out of 8 projects are related to transcriptome sequencing, 2 focused on the genome sequencing and one is relative to radiation hybrid. The NCBI database (http://www.ncbi.nlm.nih.gov/assembly/GCA_000471725.1/#/st) reports the following state of art for the UMD CASPUR WB 2.0 project updated at 30th September 2013:

UMD CASPUR WB 2.0	
Assembly level:	Scaffold
Genome representation:	Full
Total sequence length	2,836,150,610
Total assembly gap length	74,388,041
Gaps between scaffolds	0
Number of scaffolds	366,982
Scaffold N50	1,412,388
Number of contigs	630,367
Contig N50	21,938
Total number of chromosomes	0

Although the sequencing of buffalo genome is complete, currently the annotation of the sequences is not yet available and the knowledge of nuclear genes with known function is still very limited, representing only 1.47% of the sequences present in the database [9].

A list of sequences is available on the website of NCBI: 16692 nucleotide sequences, 1868 EST and 4797 GSS, almost all (11203) belonging to *Bubalus bubalis* species, followed by *Bubalus bubalis* bubalis (107) and other taxa.

The lack of the gene annotation is reflected also in the very limited information for the genetic variability, which represents the first step of the knowledge for the genetic improvement of the species.

The total number of available reference SNP reported on NCBI data base is only 502 for this species (http://www.ncbi.nlm.nih.gov/snp/?term=bubalus+bubalis) and the validation status of these polymorphisms is in most cases missing. Considering the close distance between *Bos taurus* and *Bubalus bubalis*, [10] employed the Illumina Bovine SNP50 BeadChip in buffalo. Although most of SNP were fully scored (41870 *vs* 54001), only 1159 SNP were polymorphic in the species.

The conservation of the SNP sites but not of the polymorphisms between cattle and buffalo indicates that as long as the buffalo genome and its annotation is not complete, the use of already existing tools for the genetic improvement of the species is not useful at all. Therefore, the application of genome wide association studies (GWAS) is still very far to be a reality as for instance happens in cattle, and a classical research approach based on marker assisted selection (MAS) or gene assisted selection (GAS) seems to be still far away for the planning and the application of breeding selection schemes.

2. THE ITALIAN SITUATION

The buffalo reared in Italy belongs to the Mediterranean Italian breed, and it is different from other river types reared in Europe. Although these breeds belong to the same lineage, they are characterized by a different genetic level [11]. Demography data show that the Buffalo population in Italy is a small reality compared to the huge populations of the East Asian countries. Despite that, the Italian buffalo population has increased 19 fold in the past fifty years (http://faostat.fao.org), becoming the livestock that has registered the highest increase (together with Brazil) in the world among the years 1961-2011 (Table **1**).

Table 1. First ten stocks of buffaloes given in thousands of heads and ranked for the incidence of growth rate folds between the years 1961-2011 (FAO, 2013).

Country	Total Buffalo Population		Growth Rate Fold
	1961	2011	
Brazil	63000	1278075	19,28
Italy	18000	365086	19,28
Nepal	795000	4993650	5,28
Pakistan	6700000	31726000	3,74
Syrian Arab Republic	1400	5000	2,57
Myanmar	1048523	3096887	1,95
China	8043000	23378000	1,91
Lao People's Democratic Republic	420000	1197000	1,85
Bangladesh	500000	1394000	1,79
Egypt	1501000	3800000	1,53

The reason for this increase lies in the growing interest in the productive characteristics of this rustic animal, actually bred mainly as dairy purpose animal. In Italy, the produced milk is processed almost completely into mozzarella cheese PDO (Protected Denomination of Origin - Reg. EC 510/2006). The increased demand for this product, both on the national and international market (14% of the Italian production is exported to Germany, France, UK, Switzerland, USA and Japan), together with the cow milk quotas imposed by the EU have favoured the buffalo breeding and productions [9]. The buffalo milk production amounted to 1,924,553 tons in 2012, with an increase of 7,79% compared to 2010 (http://www.aia.it). Also milk composition has been improved. On average the protein and fat content increased from 4,65 and 8,10% in 2003 to 4,70 and 8,30% in 2012, respectively (http://www.anasb.it/home.htm).

The official Herd book has recorded 56075 Italian buffaloes, which are involved in a dairy recording program. However, to some extent and up to very recently, the application of progeny tests and EBV evaluation have been hindered by low AI efficiency. In fact, although about 11,000 semen doses have been used for AI only in 2011 within the herd-book, natural mating is still the most widely used reproductive approach in buffalo farms. This is mainly due to the difficulties in revealing buffalo estrus and additional aspects related to variability in heat expression and signs which finally may cause AI failure [12]. Furthermore, the imprecise identification of paternity gives rise to difficulties in the evaluation of estimated genetic parameters [13]. Problems related to paternity in the buffalo have always existed and even today they are not easy to solve due to logistic and financial constraints, therefore the genetic importance of buffalo females is still much higher than in dairy cattle. Italian breeders association (ANASB) is working hard to increase the reliability of genetic merit predictions, including the evaluation of the genetic merit of natural mating bulls, which are strongly perceived by the managers of larger farms.

3. MOLECULAR SELECTION IN ITALIAN RIVER BUFFALO

Marker assisted selection (MAS) may be a promising choice for planning appropriate breeding schemes for Italian river buffaloes. In this respect, genetic markers significantly associated to milk production traits may give the right information for the identification of animals with high breeding value. Recently, in this direction the Italian government financed a research project named SelMol (currently updated with the Innovagen project) with the aim to start a partnership programme which connects breeders and researchers in order to improve the productive performances of dairy buffaloes with the support of information derived from the application of molecular genetics. Since almost all the buffalo milk produced in Italy is used to produce mozzarella cheese, the most important breeding goal for Italian buffaloes is the estimated mozzarella yield per lactation (PKM), a trait calculated in a single trait animal model according to the following formula:

$$\text{PKM} = \text{Milk (kg)} * \{[(3.5 * \text{protein }\% + 1.23 * \text{fat }\%) - 0.88] / 100\}$$

It is quite clear that the improvement of each of the aforementioned milk components results in higher values of the PKM. Therefore, several candidate genes were chosen for the improvement of quali-quantitative characteristics of buffalo milk. In particular, the following loci *OXT, OXTR, PRL, etc...* were studied for the milk yield; the casein cluster (*CSN1S1, CSN1S2, CSN2, CSN3*) for protein content; *DGAT1, FASN, LEP*, and other genes for fat content, whereas *SCD, ACACA, LPL,* and other loci for the quality of fatty acids. Examples of molecular genetics progresses are reported below for some of these genes.

3.1. Oxytocin Gene (OXT)

The oxytocin gene (OXT) is a candidate locus for the improvement of dairy traits like milk quantity and milk ejection, due to the natural role of oxytocin in the regulation of alveolar contractions responsible for a complete emptying from milk of both cisternal and alveolar cavities of the udder. For the total milk removal, the pituitary gland has to release oxytocin in the bloodstream, and once delivered to the mammary gland it acts on myoepithelial cells to stimulate the contraction [14]. The ejection of milk under a suckling or milking stimulation is realized through a neuro-endocrine reflex [15], which is of great interest in buffalo species. In fact, almost 95% of the buffalo milk is stored in the alveolar cavity instead of the udder cistern, which is usually small or even missing [16, 17]. The size of the OXT gene is 912 bp. It codes for oxytocin-neurophysin, a protein complex 106 aa long. Three single nucleotide polymorphisms have been found in this gene for the Italian river buffalo.

The promoter region is characterized by two SNP (AM234538: g.28C>T and g.204A>G), whereas the third polymorphic site (g.1627G>T) has been detected at the level of the exon 2 and it is responsible for the amino acid replacement Arg97>Leu of the mature protein. As consequence of these polymorphic sites, 2 alleles called A (EMBL ID: AM234538) and B (EMBL ID: AM234539) [18], have been identified, respectively. Recently, an association study involving these SNPs and milk production has been reported by Pauciullo *et al.* [19]. In particular, the genotype TT (transversion g.1627G>T) showed a relevant higher milk production (more than 1,7 kg/d) compared to the heterozygous genotype. Furthermore, this tendency is constant during the entire lactation (Fig. **1a**). Similar data have been reported also in dairy cattle for other genes. In particular, the DGAT1 [20], also considered a candidate locus affecting dairy traits, whose effect can be observed after 40 days in milk.

Additional studies need to confirm on a wider population the data reported in buffalo, which refers to a single herd. However, these data are of great importance because they represent one of the first indications of association between a milk yield and genetic markers in candidate genes in river buffalo.

Results on milk ejection rate are of a lower scale as far the effect of the gene is concerned (Fig. **1b**). The significance of its contribution to the total phenotypic variance in milk flow is lower when compared to the case of milk.

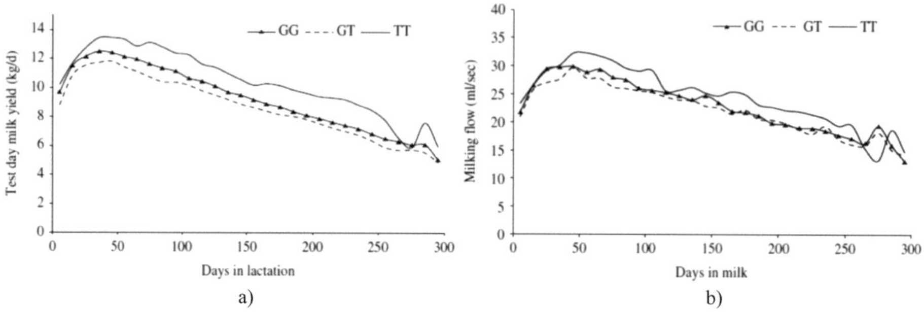

Fig. (1). Curves of lactation for the 3 OXT genotypes of the SNP g.1627G>T for: (**a**) milk production (kg/d) and (**b**) milking flow (ml/s). (Modified from Pauciullo *et al.* [19]).

Such result is surprising if we consider the biological role of the oxytocin hormone and the correlation between milk production and flow rate. Nevertheless, in former studies, it was suggested that milk flow rate is affected by the increase of oxytocin above a threshold level and not by the absolute concentration of the hormone itself [21, 22].

3.2. The Casein Cluster

As for the other ruminants also, the buffalo milk caseins (αs1, β, αs2, and k) are encoded by the following four genes (CSN1S1, CSN2, CSN1S2, and CSN3, respectively) which have been mapped on BBU 7 [23]. The complete amino acid sequences of buffalo casein [24] are accessible. In addition, also the regulatory sequences of the genes encoding for the αs1 [25] and k casein [26], the 5' UTR, and the incomplete cDNA of the CSN1S1 (EMBL IDs: GU593719, AF529305, AY948385, AJ005430), and the CSN1S2, as well as short intron sequences belonging to the same gene, are available [27]. Feligini *et al.* [28] established a technique for the quantization of the casein fractions in river buffalo milk using a reverse phase high-performance liquid chromatography, whereas a recent investigation by Cosenza *et al.* [29] reported, for the first time, a quantitative characterization of the buffalo casein transcripts and showed that the four genes are not transcribed and translated with the same efficiency. The findings of this research are very important to explain the different technological properties of buffalo milk compared to the milk of other domestic ruminants (cattle, sheep and goat).

In particular, the absolute quantification of individual samples revealed the β (53.45%, SD 6.63) and the αs1 (20.61%, SD 4.29), as the most represented casein fractions present in buffalo milk, whereas the αs2 and k (14.28%, SD 4.88, and 11.66%, SD 2.26, respectively) were less abundant. These results disagree with the data reported for for cattle, sheep and goat by Bevilacqua *et al.* [30], where the absolute quantification showed a content of about 38% for both β and αs1 casein fractions.

Such a difference could account for the peculiar technological properties of buffalo milk compared to those characterizing the milk of other ruminant species. The absolute quantization of the related mRNAs showed the following distribution of the casein's transcripts: αs1, 16.48 (SD 4.99); β, 23.18 (SD 5.41), αs2, 55.87 (SD 8.22); and k, 4.47 (SD 0.96). As for the proteins, also the quantification of buffalo transcripts was significantly different from the transcript analysis carried out on the same genes in cattle, sheep and goats, where casein transcript accounted approximately for 25% each of the total casein transcript population [30]. The presence of both phenotypic and transcriptomic data in buffalo allowed the evaluation of the translation efficiency for the casein cluster by the calculation of a ratio: single protein fractions / rate of transcripts produced in the udder.

The CSN1S2 transcripts showed a lower translation efficiency (0.25, SD 0.07), while for the CSN3, CSN2 and CSN1S1 the efficiency was higher. In particular: k, 2.69 (SD 0.74); β, 2.39 (SD 0.49) and αs1, 1.31 (SD 0.30).

The context of the AUG (codon responsible for the translation initiation) plays significant roles in determining the translation level [31, 32], therefore a possible explanation of a such difference in the translation level of buffalo casein cluster genes might be found in the comparative analysis with the Kozak consensus sequence. Usually, higher sequence homology is indication of strong consensus with Kozak sequence, therefore higher will be the efficiency of mRNA translation [33].

The sequence homology for the 4 transcripts in river buffalo Table **2** shows for the CSN1S1, CSN2 and CSN3 mRNAs the highest similarity with the Kozak sequence. In particular, for CSN1S1 and CSN2 three residues directly upstream of the initiation are consecutive (-3, -2 and -1), while CSN3 is characterized only by two consecutive nucleotide (-3 and -2).

Table 2. Comparative homology for the sequences flanking the AUG for the four casein transcripts in the Italian river buffalo. The Kozac consensus sequence representing the optimal situation for the initiation is reported in the first line. The start codon in the four casein transcripts (AUG) is underlined. Conserved nucleotides are shown in shade. (Modified from Cosenza *et al.* [29]).

-6	-5	-4	-3	-2	-1	+1	+2	+3	+4	
G	C	C	R	C	C	A	U	G	G	Kozak consensus sequence
A	G	A	G	C	C	A	U	G	A	*CSN2*
G	U	A	A	A	C	A	U	G	A	*CSN1S2*
A	C	A	A	C	C	A	U	G	A	*CSN1S1*
G	G	U	A	C	A	A	U	G	A	*CSN3*

On the contrary, CSN1S2 shows the worst combination, because despite having three nucleotides matching with the consensus sequence, these are not consecutive (-6, -3 e -1) (Table **2**) and, therefore, can be considered having a weak context.

The k-casein showed higher translation efficiency if compared to the data reported by Bevilacqua *et al.* [30]. The comparative analysis of the homologous mRNA sequences elucidates the result. In fact, buffalo, cattle, sheep, goat, mouse, rabbit and pig CSN3 mRNA have two successive AUG, but excluding the buffalo sequence, all these species show a G in position -3 as the first start codon (Table **3**).

It was proven [33] that the translational activity is influenced by the presence of specific nucleotides in position -3 (taking as reference the AUG). In particular, the presence of an adenine in such position gives rise to a higher efficiency compared with a guanine in the same position. The A characterizes the buffalo CSN3 sequence, likely representing the best translation condition for this species differently from other ruminants.

Table 3. Comparative homology for the sequences flanking the AUG for the k casein transcripts in different species. The first of the two consecutive AUG codons in ruminants, pig, rabbit and rat is in shade and underlined. (Modified from Cosenza *et al.* [29]).

-6	-5	-4	-3	-2	-1	+1	+2	+3	+4	+5	+6	+7		EMBL
G	G	U	A	C	A	A	U	G	A	U	G	A	buffalo	AM900443
G	G	U	G	C	A	A	U	G	A	U	G	A	cattle	AY380229
G	G	U	G	C	A	A	U	G	A	U	G	A	sheep	NM_001009378
G	G	U	G	C	A	A	U	G	A	U	G	A	goat	X60763
G	G	U	G	C	A	A	U	G	A	U	G	A	pig	NM_001004026
G	G	U	G	C	A	A	U	G	A	U	G	A	rabbit	Z18243
G	G	U	G	C	A	A	U	G	A	U	G	A	rat	NM_007786

Compared to other domestic ruminants, the genetic polymorphism detected in the buffalo casein cluster is quite poor. So far, no polymorphic sites have been detected for the CSN2 gene (β-casein). Cosenza *et al.* [27] characterized the CSN1S2 and found a transversion (g.773G>C) responsible for the inactivation of the intron 7 splice donor site (B allele). This polymorphism resulted in the allele-specific splicing out of the complete exon 7 (27 bp) corresponding to 9 amino acids. Although a shorter αs-2 protein should affect the total protein content, this was never verified. However, excluding the aforementioned case, currently no other quantitative alleles have been detected. Two alternative forms of αs1-casein were described by Ferranti *et al.* [34]. The analysis of CSN1S1 exon 17 showed the occurrence of a transversion (c.578C>T) which results in the amino acid substitution Leu178(A) → Ser(B) of the mature polypeptide chain. Similar situation can be reported for the k-casein, where Feligini *et al.* [28] detected a polymorphism through RP-HPLC. Sequencing of CSN3 exon 4 demonstrated, in agreement with Mitra *et al.* [35], a c.467T>C transversion in the complete coding sequence, where the presence of T corresponds to the allele X1, whereas C corresponds to the allele X2. This nucleotide substitution results in the amino acid change Ile135(X1)→Thr(X2) of the mature polypeptide chain. Recently, Bonfatti *et al.* [36, 37] evaluated the combined effect of two loci (αs1 and k) on the composition of milk protein traits and milk coagulation properties (Fig. **2**). Regarding the milk protein composition, the presence of the A allele at the locus CSN1S1 seems to be associated to higher level of this protein fraction in the total casein (TCN). On the contrary, a combination of the following genotypes AB-X1X1 and BB-X1X2 appeared to be associated with a lower content of αS1-casein in the total casein, but also linked to a higher rate of αS2-casein.

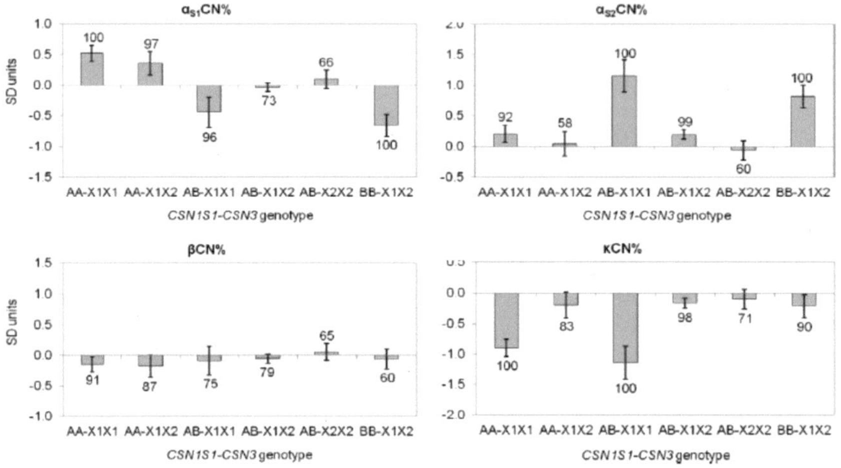

Fig. (2). Effect (mean ± SD of the marginal posterior density) of CSN1S1-CSN3 composite genotype, relative to genotype BB-X2X2 on casein content. Numbers at the top of the bars are marginal posterior probabilities of the effect being greater than 0 (if positive). Effects were measured in standard deviation unit of the trait. Caseins were measured as percentage of total casein content. (Modified from Bonfatti *et al.*, [37]).

Regarding the latter protein fraction, a difference in TCN was also linked to the presence of the X1 and X2 alleles at the k-CN encoding gene (CSN3). In particular, higher αS2-casein content was associated to composite genotypes carrying the X1 allele, differently from what observed for those carrying CSN3 X2. Furthermore, the allele X1 seems to be responsible also for the lower glycosylation level of such protein fraction, which finally is responsible for the general lower content of total κ-CN in milk.

Regarding the milk production traits, the test day milk production is negatively affected (−0.21 SD units of the trait) by the heterozygous genotype at the CSN1S1 (AB) in the combination with X2X2 and compared to the BB-X2X2. The combined genotypes had no effects for the total milk protein content, but it had effects on other traits. In particular, the milk fat content was higher for the genotype AB-X1X1 compared to the BB-X2X2 (+0.28 SD) and the AB-X1X2 (+0.43 SD).

Milk coagulation properties were measured according to the standard parameters, rennet clotting time (RCT), curd-firming time at 20 min (K20), and curd firmness at 30 min (A30). In this case the effect of the combined genotype was consistent for the rennet clotting time, where the main difference (+1.91 min, 0.61 SD) was revealed between AA-X1X2 and AB-X1X1.

In summary, the B allele at αs1-casein was associated with increased RCT and K20 together with weaker curds compared with allele A. Conversely, the allele X2 at the k-casein had contrary effects on milk coagulation properties compared to CSN1S1 B. However, these two alleles seems to have a cis- phase and segregate together for effect of the linkage disequilibrium. Therefore, the X2 allele likely cancels the positive effect of B allele.

From these two studies, it is quite evident that mating of animals with favorable genotypes may move quickly the allele frequency at the loci of economic interest (like the casein genes), representing an active way to change milk protein composition, which can also play an important role in the variation of milk coagulation properties and technological characteristics of buffalo milk.

3.3. The Stearoly CoA Desaturase Gene (SCD)

Stearoyl-CoA desaturase (SCD) belongs to the group of microsomal enzymes and it plays a fundamental role in the metabolism of the fatty acid (FA). This enzyme catalyzes the insertion of the first cis-double bond at the Δ9 carbon for a wide spectrum of fatty acyl-CoA substrates [38]. For this reason, it is known also as delta-9-desaturase. The corresponding SCD gene has been considered as a candidate gene influencing milk FA profile [39]. In river buffalo, the SCD gene and its promoter region have been characterized by Pauciullo *et al.* [40, 41]. Most of the consensus sequences regulating the lipid metabolism have been found in a short DNA fragment (130 bp long between the nucleotides -382/-250 of the promoter region), suggesting an essential function of this region in the gene expression (Fig. **3**). 15 SNPs were detected, and among these, the transversion g.133A>C at position -461 of the promoter falls between two SP1 binding sites, thus creating a new consensus site for this transcription factor. As a consequence, the carriers of the C allele are characterized by three consecutive SP1 binding sites.

```
                       C/EBPα                        NF-1
GAAACTTCCCCAGTGCCCATCCATTTGCGAATTGCCCGGGGCCAGTTCTGGGCTGGCACG        -534

CATCCCCGCGCCACTCCCCGACAGGGTCTTCTCCCTCTCCCCGAGCGCCTCCGAGGCGGC        -474
  SP1             SP1
AGGGTGCCCGGTMGAGGCCCAGCGGCCGGTGTAAGAGAAGCCGAGGAGAAAGGGAGGGGA        -414
                                  SREBP       C/EBP NF-1
GGGGGAGTGAGGAGCTCGCGGCAGAGGGAACAGCAGATTGCGCCGAGCCAATGGCAACGG        -354
           NF-1 C/EBPα            C/EBPα
CAGGACGAGGTGGCACCAAATTCCCTTCGGCCAATGACGCGCCAGAGTCTACAGAAGCCC        -294
        C/EBPβ          C/EBPα     C/EBPα
ATTAGCATTTCCCCAGGGGCAGGGGCAGAGGCAGGGGCTGCGGCGGCTAAGCCGCGGTGT        -234
                C/EBPα
GTCTGCAGCATCCAGTTCTTGCTTCTTCGGCCCCCAGCACGCCTCGGCGCTCTGTCTCCT        -174

CCCCTCTCCCGCCCATGCGGATCTCCCACGGTGAGCCAACTCTGCGCACTTTGCCCCTTG        -114
  NF-1    TATA box     C/EBPα                  SREBP     SP1
TTGGCAACGAATAAAAGGGGTCTGAGGAAATACGGGACACAGTCACCCCCTGCCAGCGCT         -54
TATA BOX            PPARγ                  SP1
ATTAAATCCCCAGCACAGCAGGTCGGGTCCGGACACCGGTCCAGCGCGCACCGtgcagcg           7
   PPARγ
gaaggtcccgagcgcagcgccgcggatcgccacgcaaaagcaggctcaggaactagtcta          67
```

Fig. (3). Key transcription factors binding sites found in the promoter region of the river buffalo SCD gene. The conserved PUFA response region, including the sterol response element (SREBP), CCAAT-box (C/EBP), nuclear factor (NF)-1 and stimulator protein 1 (SP1) binding site, are shown. TATA motifs and peroxisome proliferator activated receptor-γ (PPAR-γ) are also shown proximal to the transcription start site. SNP g.133A>C is indicated with M nucleotide according to international nomenclature. (Modified from Pauciullo *et al.* [41]).

SP1 binding sites are well-known enhancer elements for gene expression and occur frequently in clusters generated by the promoter VNTR (Variable Number Tandem Repeats) [42]. Mutation analysis of SP1-binding sites showed that the number of SP1-binding sites within a cluster could determine the transcription rate of the respective gene [43]. Therefore, the variability found in the buffalo SCD SP1 cluster could be responsible for the variation in SCD expression and consequently SCD activity.

Since SCD is known to be the key enzyme controlling the desaturation rate of FA, the level of SCD activity can be assumed to have a direct effect on desaturated fat content in several tissues. A preliminary association study with the milk fatty acid content confirmed that the C allele significantly affects the total desaturation index ($P<0.01$) [40].

The same SNP was also significantly associated with test day milk ($P=0.02$) with an effect of the genotype AC accounting for more than 2 kg/d in comparison with the genotype CC, which means about 28% more milk per day. Conversely, the genotype AA showed slightly lower milk yield than AC. The lactation curves of the 3 genotypes had a constant behavior during the entire lactation period.

The allele substitution effect of the A into C was estimated in about -1 kg/d ($P<0.01$), whereas the total phenotypic variance was affected for a total of 12% by the variance of the genotype (Table **4**).

Table 4. Mean ± SE of milk yield (kg/d) for the substitution effect g.133A>C in the promoter region of the river buffalo SCD gene and contribution of such polymorphism to the phenotypic variance. (Modified from Pauciullo *et al.* [41]).

Trait	**α**	**P**	**d**	**P**	σ^2_{SCD}	σ^2_c	σ^2_e	r^2_c	r^2_{SCD}
Milk yield	-1.01±0.38	0.007	1.22±0.49	0.013	0.93	4.21	2.72	0.61	0.12

α: Substitution effect

d: dominance effect

σ^2: variance components associated to the genotype (SCD); to the individual buffalo cow (c), to residuals (e)

r^2: contributions of genotype (SCD) and of individual buffalo cow (c) to the total phenotypic variance

A dominance effect was also found in the same population and for the same trait (Table **4**). It accounted for more than 1.2 kg ($P<0.02$) of milk yield. In general, this genetic interaction effect is considered non-significant because numerically much lower than the additive effect, although it can also have an influence on allele substitution effect. However, its detection can explain the higher productive level of the animals (AC) compared to the best phenotype (AA).

It is also well-known that the lipid metabolism and the biosynthesis of *de novo* FAs are characterized by multiple pathways and they are energetically expensive. In dairy cattle [44, 45], cows characterized by higher desaturase activity, also liven up less nutrients to milk yield. This situation seems to be observed also in river buffalo, where the carriers of the genotype CC for the SCD gene are characterized by a higher MUFA content in milk [40], but they also have a lower milk yield.

CONCLUSION

The improvement of the productive level of domestic animals starts with the improvement of environmental condition. This was regularly applied for several years in river buffalo, so that health, feeding and livestock systems has improved remarkably in recent years. Conversely, little has been done in terms of genetic progress in this species. In this chapter, although not exhaustive, knowledge dealing with the molecular bases of genetic selection in river buffalo has been reviewed. Several recent studies showed new genotyping data and haplotype structure of key genes involved in the improvement of quali-quantitavive characteristics of milk. These findings open the way for a future application of selection programs assisted by genetic markers (MAS or GAS), which may represent a promising choice for planning appropriate breeding schemes for Italian river buffaloes. In this respect, genetic markers significantly associated to milk production traits may give the right information for the identification of animals with high breeding value.

CONFLICT OF INTEREST

The authors confirm that they have no conflict of interest to declare for this publication.

ACKNOWLEDGEMENTS

The study has been supported by the project CISIA-VARIGEAV (*Caratterizzazione e valorizzazione delle risorse genetiche animali e vegetali della Campania e della Sardegna finalizzate allo sviluppo della filiera bufalina mediante approcci multidisciplinari ed innovativi*), National Research Council (CNR) of Italy.

REFERENCES

[1] Ajmone-Masan P, Marco Milanesi M. The International Buffalo Consortium Biodiversity among Buffalo genomes. International Plant and Animal Genome Conference Future Dates, XXI Conference; January 12-16, 2013; San Diego.

[2] Kierstein G, Vallinoto M, Silva A, Schneider MP, Iannuzzi L, Brenig B. Analysis of mitochondrial D-loop region casts new light on domestic water buffalo (*Bubalus bubalis*) phylogeny. Mol Phylogenet Evol 2004; 30(2): 308-24.
[http://dx.doi.org/10.1016/S1055-7903(03)00221-5] [PMID: 14715223]

[3] Lau CH, Drinkwater RD, Yusoff K, Tan SG, Hetzel DJ, Barker JS. Genetic diversity of Asian water buffalo (*Bubalus bubalis*): mitochondrial DNA D-loop and cytochrome b sequence variation. Anim Genet 1998; 29(4): 253-64.
[http://dx.doi.org/10.1046/j.1365-2052.1998.00309.x] [PMID: 9745663]

[4] Kumar S, Nagarajan M, Sandhu JS, Kumar N, Behl V, Nishanth G. Mitochondrial DNA analyses of Indian water buffalo support a distinct genetic origin of river and swamp buffalo. Anim Genet 2007; 38(3): 227-32.
[http://dx.doi.org/10.1111/j.1365-2052.2007.01602.x] [PMID: 17459014]

[5] Lei CZ, Zhang W, Chen H, *et al.* Independent maternal origin of Chinese swamp buffalo (*Bubalus bubalis*). Anim Genet 2007; 38(2): 97-102.
[http://dx.doi.org/10.1111/j.1365-2052.2007.01567.x] [PMID: 17313588]

[6] Barker JS, Moore SS, Hetzel DJ, Evans D, Tan SG, Byrne K. Genetic diversity of Asian water buffalo (*Bubalus bubalis*): microsatellite variation and a comparison with protein-coding loci. Anim Genet 1997; 28(2): 103-15.
[http://dx.doi.org/10.1111/j.1365-2052.1997.00085.x] [PMID: 9172308]

[7] Zhang Y, Sun D, Yu Y, Zhang Y. Genetic variation and divergence among swamp buffalo, river buffalo and cattle: a microsatellite survey on five population in China. Asian-Aust. J Anim Sci 2008; 21(9): 1238-43.

[8] Yindee M, Vlamings BH, Wajjwalku W, *et al.* Y-chromosomal variation confirms independent domestications of swamp and river buffalo. Anim Genet 2010; 41(4): 433-5.
[PMID: 20219068]

[9] Michelizzi VN, Dodson MV, Pan Z, *et al.* Water buffalo genome science comes of age. Int J Biol Sci 2010; 6(4): 333-49.
[http://dx.doi.org/10.7150/ijbs.6.333] [PMID: 20582226]

[10] Michelizzi VN, Wu X, Dodson MV, *et al.* A global view of 54,001 single nucleotide polymorphisms (SNPs) on the Illumina BovineSNP50 BeadChip and their transferability to water buffalo. Int J Biol Sci 2010; 7(1): 18-27.
[PMID: 21209788]

[11] Borghese A. Buffalo Cheese and Milk Industry. Buffalo Production and Research. FAO Regional

Office for Europe 2005.

[12] Barile VL. Improving reproductive efficiency in female buffaloes. Livest Prod Sci 2005; 92: 183-94. [http://dx.doi.org/10.1016/j.livprodsci.2004.06.014]

[13] Rosati A, Van Vleck LD. Estimation of genetic parameters for milk, fat, protein and mozzarella cheese production for the Italian river buffalo (*Bubalus bubalis*) population. Livest Prod Sci 2002; 74: 185-90. [http://dx.doi.org/10.1016/S0301-6226(01)00293-7]

[14] Bruckmaier RM, Blum JW. Oxytocin release and milk removal in ruminants. J Dairy Sci 1998; 81(4): 939-49. [http://dx.doi.org/10.3168/jds.S0022-0302(98)75654-1] [PMID: 9594382]

[15] Wakerley JB, Clarke G, Summerlee AJ. Milk ejection and its control. The Physiology of Reproduction Knobil E & Neill JD. New York: Raven Press 1994; pp. 1131-77.

[16] Thomas CS, Svennersten-Sjaunja K, Bhosrekar MR, Bruckmaier RM. Mammary cisternal size, cisternal milk and milk ejection in Murrah buffaloes. J Dairy Res 2004; 71(2): 162-8. [http://dx.doi.org/10.1017/S0022029904000081] [PMID: 15190943]

[17] Caria M, Murgia L, Pazzona A. Effects of the working vacuum level on mechanical milking of buffalo. J Dairy Sci 2011; 94(4): 1755-61. [http://dx.doi.org/10.3168/jds.2010-3134] [PMID: 21426964]

[18] Cosenza G, Pauciullo A, Mancusi A, *et al.* Mediterranean river buffalo oxytocin-neurophysin I (OXT) gene: structure, promoter analysis and allele detection. Ital J Anim Sci 2007; 6: 303-6. [http://dx.doi.org/10.4081/ijas.2007.s2.303]

[19] Pauciullo A, Cosenza G, Steri R, *et al.* An association analysis between OXT genotype and milk yield and flow in Italian Mediterranean river buffalo. J Dairy Res 2012; 79(2): 150-6. [http://dx.doi.org/10.1017/S0022029911000914] [PMID: 22280971]

[20] Strucken EM, de Koning DJ, Rahmatalla SA, Brockmann GA. Lactation curve models for estimating gene effects over a timeline. J Dairy Sci 2011; 94(1): 442-9. [http://dx.doi.org/10.3168/jds.2009-2932] [PMID: 21183055]

[21] Thomas CS, Bruckmaier RM, Östensson K, Svennersten-Sjaunja K. Effect of different milking routines on milking-related release of the hormones oxytocin, prolactin and cortisol, and on milk yield and milking performance in Murrah buffaloes. J Dairy Res 2005; 72(1): 10-8. [http://dx.doi.org/10.1017/S0022029904000457] [PMID: 15747726]

[22] Schams D, Mayer H, Prokopp A, Worstorff H. Oxytocin secretion during milking in dairy cows with regard to the variation and importance of a threshold level for milk removal. J Endocrinol 1984; 102(3): 337-43. [http://dx.doi.org/10.1677/joe.0.1020337] [PMID: 6541240]

[23] Iannuzzi L, Di Meo GP, Perucatti A, *et al.* The river buffalo (*Bubalus bubalis*, 2n = 50) cytogenetic map: assignment of 64 loci by fluorescence *in situ* hybridization and R-banding. Cytogenet Genome Res 2003; 102(1-4): 65-75. [http://dx.doi.org/10.1159/000075727] [PMID: 14970681]

[24] DAmbrosio C, Arena S, Salzano AM, Renzone G, Ledda L, Scaloni A. A proteomic characterization of water buffalo milk fractions describing PTM of major species and the identification of minor

components involved in nutrient delivery and defense against pathogens. Proteomics 2008; 8(17): 3657-66.
[http://dx.doi.org/10.1002/pmic.200701148] [PMID: 18668696]

[25] Cosenza G, Feligini M, Mancusi A, *et al.* Italian Mediterranean river buffalo CSN2 gene structure and promoter analysis. Ital J Anim Sci 2009; 8: 57-9.

[26] Masina P, Rando A, Di Gregorio P, Cosenza G, Mancusi A. Water buffalo kappa-casein gene sequence. Ital J Anim Sci 2007; 6 (Suppl. 2): 353-5.

[27] Cosenza G, Pauciullo A, Feligini M, *et al.* A point mutation in the splice donor site of intron 7 in the alphas2-casein encoding gene of the Mediterranean River buffalo results in an allele-specific exon skipping. Anim Genet 2009; 40(5): 791.
[http://dx.doi.org/10.1111/j.1365-2052.2009.01897.x] [PMID: 19422363]

[28] Feligini M, Bonizzi I, Buffoni JN, Cosenza G, Ramunno L. Identification and quantification of alphaS1, alphaS2, beta, and kappa-caseins in water buffalo milk by reverse phase-high performance liquid chromatography and mass spectrometry. J Agric Food Chem 2009; 57(7): 2988-92.
[http://dx.doi.org/10.1021/jf803653v] [PMID: 19256489]

[29] Cosenza G, Pauciullo A, Coletta A, *et al.* Short communication: Translational efficiency of casein transcripts in Mediterranean river buffalo. J Dairy Sci 2011; 94(11): 5691-4.
[http://dx.doi.org/10.3168/jds.2010-4086] [PMID: 22032393]

[30] Bevilacqua C, Helbling JC, Miranda G, Martin P. Translational efficiency of casein transcripts in the mammary tissue of lactating ruminants. Reprod Nutr Dev 2006; 46(5): 567-78.
[http://dx.doi.org/10.1051/rnd:2006028] [PMID: 17107646]

[31] Kozak M. Effects of long 5 leader sequences on initiation by eukaryotic ribosomes *in vitro*. Gene Expr 1991; 1(2): 117-25.
[PMID: 1820209]

[32] Kozak M. Structural features in eukaryotic mRNAs that modulate the initiation of translation. J Biol Chem 1991; 266(30): 19867-70.
[PMID: 1939050]

[33] Kozak M. Point mutations close to the AUG initiator codon affect the efficiency of translation of rat preproinsulin *in vivo*. Nature 1984; 308(5956): 241-6.
[http://dx.doi.org/10.1038/308241a0] [PMID: 6700727]

[34] Ferranti P, Scaloni A, Caira S, Chianese L, Malorni A, Addeo F. The primary structure of water buffalo alpha(s1)- and beta-casein identification of phosphorylation sites and characterization of a novel beta-casein variant. J Protein Chem 1998; 17(8): 835-44.
[http://dx.doi.org/10.1023/A:1020786503978] [PMID: 9988530]

[35] Mitra A, Schlee P, Krause I, *et al.* Kappa-casein polymorphisms in Indian dairy cattle and buffalo: a new genetic variant in buffalo. Anim Biotechnol 1998; 9(2): 81-7.
[http://dx.doi.org/10.1080/10495399809525896] [PMID: 9713674]

[36] Bonfatti V, Giantin M, Gervaso M, Coletta A, Dacasto M, Carnier P. Effect of CSN1S1-CSN3 (α(S1)-κ-casein) composite genotype on milk production traits and milk coagulation properties in Mediterranean water buffalo. J Dairy Sci 2012; 95(6): 3435-43.

[http://dx.doi.org/10.3168/jds.2011-4901] [PMID: 22612978]

[37] Bonfatti V, Giantin M, Gervaso M, *et al.* Short communication: CSN1S1-CSN3 (α(S1)-κ-casein) composite genotypes affect detailed milk protein composition of Mediterranean water buffalo. J Dairy Sci 2012; 95(11): 6801-5.
[http://dx.doi.org/10.3168/jds.2012-5601] [PMID: 22959943]

[38] Ntambi JM. Regulation of stearoyl-CoA desaturase by polyunsaturated fatty acids and cholesterol. J Lipid Res 1999; 40(9): 1549-58.
[PMID: 10484602]

[39] Gautier M, Barcelona RR, Fritz S, *et al.* Fine mapping and physical characterization of two linked quantitative trait loci affecting milk fat yield in dairy cattle on BTA26. Genetics 2006; 172(1): 425-36.
[http://dx.doi.org/10.1534/genetics.105.046169] [PMID: 16172504]

[40] Pauciullo A, Cosenza G, DAvino A, *et al.* Sequence analysis and genetic variability of stearoyl CoA desaturase (SCD) gene in the Italian Mediterranean river buffalo. Mol Cell Probes 2010; 24(6): 407-10.
[http://dx.doi.org/10.1016/j.mcp.2010.07.009] [PMID: 20691778]

[41] Pauciullo A, Cosenza G, Steri R, *et al.* A single nucleotide polymorphism in the promoter region of river buffalo stearoyl CoA desaturase gene (SCD) is associated with milk yield. J Dairy Res 2012; 79(4): 429-35.
[http://dx.doi.org/10.1017/S0022029912000507] [PMID: 22994977]

[42] Yang X, Fyodorov D, Deneris ES. Transcriptional analysis of acetylcholine receptor a3 gene promoter motifs that bind SP1 and AP2. J Biol Chem 1995; 270(85): 14-20.

[43] Simsek S, Bleeker PM, van der Schoot CE, von dem Borne AE. Association of a variable number of tandem repeats (VNTR) in glycoprotein Ib alpha and HPA-2 alloantigens. Thromb Haemost 1994; 72: 757-61.

[44] Macciotta NP, Mele M, Conte G, *et al.* Association between a polymorphism at the stearoyl CoA desaturase locus and milk production traits in Italian Holsteins. J Dairy Sci 2008; 91(8): 3184-9.
[http://dx.doi.org/10.3168/jds.2007-0947] [PMID: 18650296]

[45] Kay JK, Weber WJ, Moore CE, *et al.* Effects of week of lactation and genetic selection for milk yield on milk fatty acid composition in Holstein cows. J Dairy Sci 2005; 88(11): 3886-93.
[http://dx.doi.org/10.3168/jds.S0022-0302(05)73074-5] [PMID: 16230694]

CHAPTER 4

Animal – Environment Interaction: Buffalo Behavior and Welfare

Fabio Napolitano[1,*], Corrado Pacelli[1], Ada Braghieri[1], Fernando Grasso[2] and Giuseppe De Rosa[2]

[1] *Scuola di Scienze Agrarie, Forestali, Alimentari ed Ambientali, Università della Basilicata, Via dell'Ateneo Lucano 10, 85100 Potenza, Italy*

[2] *Dipartimento di Agraria, Università di Napoli Federico II, Via Università 133, 80055 Portici (NA), Italy*

Abstract: This chapter will focus on the effects of interaction of river buffaloes with the environment both in confinement and in extensive conditions, on their behavior and welfare. Firstly, the time and place of domestication are described. Sections on time budget, foraging and feeding habit, maternal and social behavior, and some aspects of style of interaction with the environment and temperament are then elucidated. Subsequently, focus is shifted on the quality of relationship between stock-people and animals, which is an important aspect affecting animal welfare in modern farms. Finally, the welfare consequences of intensive farming on buffalo welfare are evaluated using a number of animal-based indicators.

Keywords: Animal welfare, Behavior, Dairy buffalo, Housing system.

1. INTRODUCTION

The wild species belonging to the genus Bubalus were widely distributed in Asia and Europe during the Pleistocene. The subsequent climate changes restricted the area of distribution of wild species to the Asian continent, from India to the far South-East. The corresponding domestic animals are generally referred to as

* **Corresponding author Fabio Napolitano:** Scuola di Scienze Agrarie, Forestali, Alimentari ed Ambientali, Università della Basilicata, *Via* dell'Ateneo Lucano 10, 85100 Potenza, Italy; Tel: +39 0971 205078; Fax: +39 0971 205378; E-mail: fabio.napolitano@unibas.it

Giorgio A. Presicce (Ed.)

water buffaloes and grouped in two main classes on the basis of their genetic make-up and phenotype. The river buffaloes present 50 chromosomes, and are currently widespread in Italy, few eastern European countries, middle east and India; the swamp buffaloes present 48 chromosomes and are mainly found in South-East Asia (China, Bangladesh, Vietnam, *etc.*) [1]. The time and place of domestication of buffaloes have been debated for a long time but recently, Kumar *et al.* (2007) proved that river and swamp buffaloes were independently domesticated [2]. In particular, all of the buffaloes belonging to the river type (including both Indian and Mediterranean animals) are likely to be derived from the same stocks [3]. This sub-group was domesticated around 6300 years BP, whereas archaeological studies identified the South-East of India as the place of domestication [3]. Most likely in the period around 2600 BP, water buffaloes were taken by Arabs from Mesopotamia to the Near East. During the Middle Ages, pilgrims and crusaders possibly brought the domestic animals back to Europe. There, buffaloes were reared in extensive conditions for centuries, whereas nowadays they are predominantly kept in intensive conditions. This chapter will deal with the expression of river buffalo behavior, in intensive and in extensive conditions, and will subsequently focus on how different housing systems and management practices can affect the welfare of these animals.

2. BEHAVIOR

2.1. Time Budget in Extensive Conditions

In extensive conditions in ruminants, time is allocated and spent on different behaviours, according to stocking density, nutritional requirements as well as availability and distribution of food together with the perceived threat of possible predators. A significant amount of data is available on time budget of cattle, sheep and goats in extensive temperate and tropical zones [4, 5], whereas little is known about the allocation of the time performed by the buffaloes. The wild African buffalo (*Syncerus caffer*) at the Kruger National Park (South Africa) has been studied with regard to the analysis of its diurnal activity, and it has been shown that these buffaloes spend approximately 40% of the time grazing, followed by 30% resting and 30% ruminating [6]. Accordingly, in Uganda buffaloes of the same species spend 9 h a day grazing and 6.4 h a day ruminating [8]. Conversely, the feeding time of Cape buffalo (*Syncerus caffer caffer*) covers 52% of the daytime with peaks observed in the morning and in the evening, whereas resting has been more often observed at midday [7]. In Italy buffalo farming has been run extensively for a long time. Buffaloes are still characterized by some physiological and morphological features acquired through natural selection, which are then capitalized to reinforce their ability to thrive well in open environments (*e.g.* reproductive seasonality, melanin-pigmented skin). Recently, an experiment on maintenance behavior of buffalo heifers [9] was conducted in a fenced Mediterranean maquis located in Southwest Italy. At the beginning of the experiment, animals were about 8 to 9 months of age. They were free to graze and continuous focal animal sampling was used to collect behavioural data [10] from April to October. The activities displayed by the buffaloes during 6-h observation periods are depicted in Fig. (**1**). The behavioural pattern of other ruminants reared in extensive environmental conditions was similar [4].

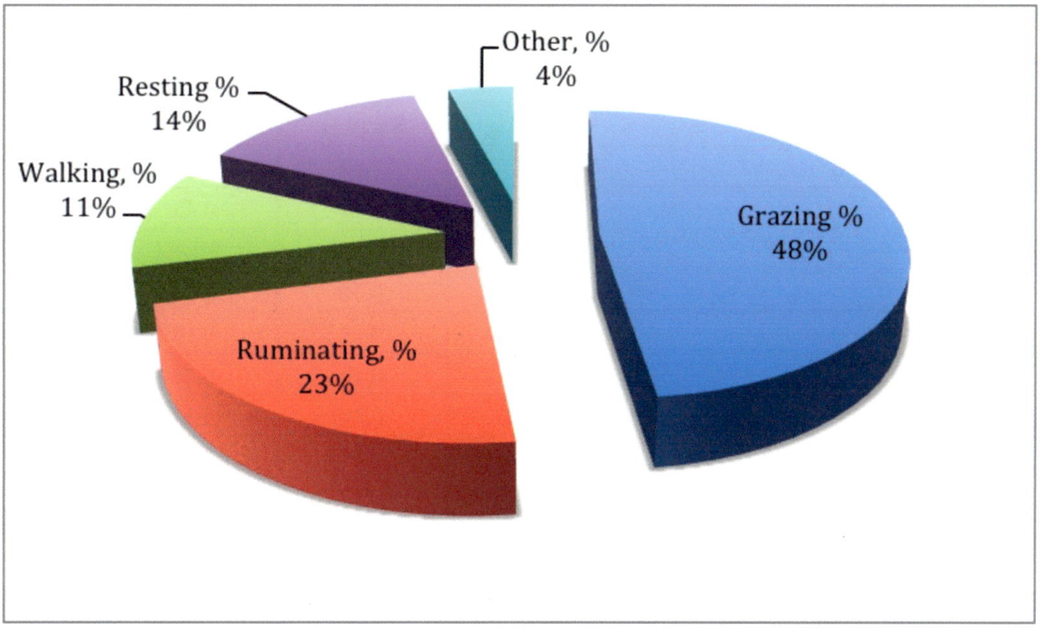

Fig. (1). Behavioral pattern (%) of buffalo heifers observed over 6-h periods in extensive conditions [9].

No significant effect of season on the distance covered by the animals was found by authors, although a longer distance was run in spring time (Table **1**). Ryan and

Jordaan [6] report a distance of 3-4 km covered by the African buffalo in 24-h. Grazing activities were found by the same authors to be performed more frequently during the dry rather than the wet season, whereas the proportion of time spent grazing by Mediterranean buffalo heifers was not influenced by season, with values ranging from 0.60, in spring to 0.41, and 0.43, in summer and autumn, respectively. This may be due to the fact that in the latter study behavioural observations were mainly run in the first half of the day, whereas grazing would be more frequent among animals in the summer during late afternoon and night. Mediterranean buffalo heifers lay less in spring (0.21) than in autumn (0.43) and summer (0.43). Similarly, ruminating was less often displayed in spring (0.11) than in autumn (0.32) and summer (0.26). These results collectively suggest that animals are characterized by high levels of inactivity during the day in response to high environmental temperatures, as witnessed by a more frequent lying down, resting and ruminating behaviours.

Table 1. Season effect on activity budget (least square means and s.e.) of buffalo heifers observed in a 6-h periods.

Variable	Spring	Summer	Autumn	P
Distance travelled, km	2.83	1.59	1.77	0.26
Lying down[1]	0.21	0.43	0.43	0.05
Location in the shade or mud[1]	0.23	0.43	0.248	0.21
Grazing[1]	0.60	0.41	0.43	0.13
Walking[1]	0.10	0.11	0.10	0.99
Resting[1]	0.11	0.19	0.12	0.46
Ruminating[1]	0.11	0.26	0.32	0.02
Other[1]	0.08	0.04	0.02	0.13
Self-grooming[2]	1.17	0.83	1.00	0.91

[1]Data are expressed in terms of proportion of time.
[2]Data are expressed in terms of number of events per animal.

It has been reported that buffaloes tend to spend 39% of their time on ruminating, 34% on resting and 27% on feeding [11]. Napolitano *et al.* [9] and Bud *et al.* [12] reported more time spent on feeding (37-54 and 48%, respectively) and less time on ruminating (28 and 23%, respectively) in buffaloes, whereas the remaining time was spent resting (18-35 and 14%, respectively) and walking. Similar results were obtained by Braghieri *et al.* [13] in Podolian cattle. However, in buffaloes much of resting was performed while wallowing in the mud. Although little data are available on this specific buffalo behavior, these animals wallow frequently when water is available for thermoregulatory purposes, as it is also shown by a higher sebum secretion, which has the function to protect the skin while the animals lay in the mud. [14]. In summer the heifers spent in the mud a proportion of time (Table **1**) much higher than in the other seasons [9], while about 50% of adult female buffaloes wallow when mud or water are available [15]. Insufficient heat dissipation in buffaloes has been associated with reduced dry matter intake and milk production [16], whereas in cattle reduced conception rate and milk production has been observed as a consequence of heat stress [17]. In addition, in buffaloes a lack of free access to water during the hot season determines reduced milk production [15] and fertility [18]. Bathing and wallowing usually induce buffaloes to perform integumentary care, considering that self-grooming is often reported to be associated with body muddiness [19]. Napolitano *et al.* [20] have proposed, as a potential indicator of good welfare, self-grooming behaviours. In fact, animals find difficult to turn their head around, to bend their spine or to spread their legs, if the floor is slippery, because they will, very likely, tend to loose their balance. With animals kept on pasture, the availability of natural flooring may ease their behavioural expression of self-grooming [15].

2.2. Time Budget in Intensive Conditions

Confinement of domestic animals radically changes their life by affecting the habitat, activity and capability of individuals to choose whether to stay or leave.

Buffaloes have evidently less room for movement under confinement conditions, and the promotion of expression of species-specific behaviours may be affected due to lack of proper stimuli. Murrah buffaloes in loose-housing conditions devoted more time on eating, idling and walking during day, whereas at night more time was devoted to ruminating and sleeping [21]. In lactating buffaloes eating behavior was predominantly expressed at 04:00, 09:00, 13:00, 15:00, and 19:00. Conversely, ruminating was more often performed during early morning and late evening, sleeping was more frequent at 3:00 and 23:00 and idling at noon. The main behavioral categories observed in adult dairy buffaloes kept in confinement are reported in Fig. (**2**) [22].

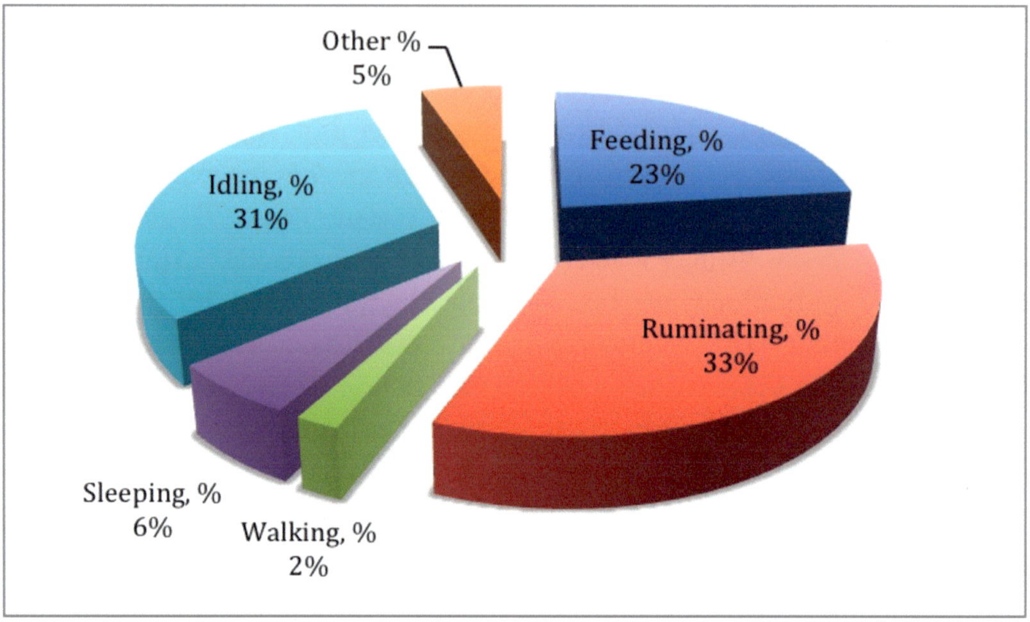

Fig. (2). Behavioral pattern (%) of buffaloes observed in intensive conditions [22].

Buffaloes kept in intensive conditions spend less time feeding and more time idling as compared with buffaloes reared in extensive conditions. The reduced level of activity expressed in confinement is also suggested by the high percentage of animals observed in lying postures.

The concept of boredom has been used to explain the state of animals in these conditions [23]. Other authors have stated that a high level of idling can be considered an abnormal behavioral expression [24 - 26]. A number of farm animals are able to display long periods of inactivity that may reflect the inadequacy of their surrounding environment [27]. Accordingly, in intensive conditions, where facilities such as water for wallowing and pasture are not available, buffalo cows increase the time spent idling [28] and show a reduction in exploration [15]. Buffaloes show a strong motivation to investigate the surrounding environment [29] and reduced explorative activities, as observed in intensive conditions, and this can be regarded as an indicator of poor adaptation to the environment. No direct studies in the buffalo species have been conducted on the real space needed, when the intensification of buffalo farming inevitably leads to a reduction of space allowance. Such a reduction may have a number of negative effects on buffalo welfare. In particular, health may be impaired due to possible increased incidence of injuries and lesions and increased expression of agonistic behaviors. An evident stress reported in several categories of buffaloes such as un-weaned and weaned calves, heifers and cows, results from a lack of space [28 - 31].

It has been found that space allowance affects the lying positions of young buffaloes [29, 30]. Animals kept in a restricted space are more subjected to being trodden on by their pen-mates, thus they increase the number of bent legs, lying preferentially in a sternal recumbency. Calves at higher space allowance are more often observed lying idle, which may be considered as an indicator of animal comfort [29], whereas in a restricted space this posture may be hindered by the activities of the group-mates [30]. In another study on adult buffaloes, lying idle was not influenced by a higher space allowance as these animals also benefited from an outdoor paddock and facilities for wallowing [15, 28], which may elicit more varied behavioral activities.

In addition, it has been found that un-weaned calves, when subjected to space restriction, increase their feeding activity only during the last period of weaning [30], whereas in weaned calves this occurs throughout the experimental period [29]. In both studies weight gain was not influenced by space allowance, thus suggesting that a lower space allowance may have a detrimental effect on feed conversion rates. Similarly, lactating buffaloes did not modify their feeding activity at different space allowances, whereas a lower milk production was observed in the restricted buffaloes as a possible effect of reduced feed conversion rates [15].

2.3. Ingestive Behavior

The quality and availability of forage for ruminants grazing in the Mediterranean areas change spatially and seasonally [32]. For example, as herbaceous plants tend to become senescent during the hot and dry seasons, the concentration of crude protein declines while there is an increase in the fibre level [33]. Intake of any plants seems to be influenced by its physical characteristics, its accessibility and its palatability [34, 35]. The availability and accessibility of the various pasture components is dependent on their relative height, position and density [36, 37]. Palatability depends on feed's taste and its relationship with post-ingestive feedback, determined by both food's chemical characteristics and the physiological state of the animal [38, 40]. Animals discriminate among foods using taste, odor, and sight, which are source of hedonic sensations [40, 41]. They acquire preferences for nutritious foods and dislike foods with low nutrient contents or high toxin levels [39, 40, 42].

According to Macandza *et al.* [43], African wild buffaloes observed in a savannas environment incorporate into their diet plant species initially disliked. In particular, they prefer grass plants such as *Heteropogon contortus, Cenchrus ciliaris, Panicum coloratum* and *Panicum maximum* during the entire dry season, whereas other grass species initially disliked such as *Digitaria eriantha*, *Urochloa mosabicensis* and *Urochloa oligotricha* are significantly included into their diet from late August onward, and *Eragrostis superba* and *Bothriochloa* spp. are only eaten in October (end of the dry season). Therefore, African wild buffaloes cannot be regarded as unselective bulk grazers, as they changed grass selection and grazing places according to forage quality and availability throughout the dry season, which represents the most critical period. For instance, when the availability of both preferred *Panicum* declined, nutritious but with medium height (less available) plants such as *Digitaria* and *Urochloa*, took over as main foods during the dry season. Nevertheless, fecal samples indicated that wild buffaloes are not browsers, as they rarely ingested woody plants or shrubs.

In an experiment conducted in the Mediterranean basin [9], where woods and shrubs occupied 10% of the vegetation and the remaining consisted of grass, the intake of woods and shrubs was not observed, thus suggesting that dairy buffaloes, as also shown for the wild buffaloes by Macandza *et al.* [43], cannot be considered highly selective animals (*i.e.* browsers), rather they can be classified as grazers [44]. The same authors showed that bite rate and body weight were negatively correlated with increasing body size, and animals could take larger bites and therefore needing more time to be chewed and swallowed [9]. Heifers, in addition to natural pasture, also received meadow hay and dehydrated beetpulps from December to March. These animals showed lower weight gains and puberty weights as compared to buffalo heifers kept in confinement. However, puberty age was similar in the two experimental groups. In addition, grazing animals needed a lower input of feeds in competition with humans (*e.g.* cereals) and a lower use of fossil fuel, chemical fertilizers, water for irrigation and pesticides. Therefore, farming buffalo heifers in extensive conditions may reduce their environmental impact with negligible effects on production efficiency. As observed for African wild buffaloes living in the savannas, the domestic buffaloes originating from tropical areas (see paragraph 1) are well fit to an environment which is characterized by a large variety of food availability and related quality. In fact, during floods in the Brazilian Amazon, when cattle become isolated on small patches of high ground, many may suffer from foot rot and fasting, buffaloes are able to swim out to islands of floating aquatic plants and eat them. They can also dive to graze beneath the floodwaters. In other parts of the world buffaloes voluntarily consume vegetation unpalatable to other ruminants [45]. It has been reported that buffaloes have higher digestive efficiency in terms of crude protein and fiber fractions as compared to sheep and cattle. These findings may be related to the fact that these animals receive less energetic rations [46]. In addition, dairy buffaloes have a rumen with the following anatomic and physiological features: high bacterial activity, small outflow rate, slow movements and large volume [47 - 50]. However, these higher digestive performances are less evident, when high-energy diets are used [51].

Large variations in diet composition and feeding habits have also produced a higher resistance to dietetic unbalances, such as protein in excess. In cattle the provision of diets with high nitrogen contents induce high concentrations of NH_3 in the rumen, which is converted into urea in the liver and found in the blood; technopathies such as lameness have been often related to these conditions. By contrast, in buffaloes protein surplus can be more easily excreted under the form of urea and even re-ingested through the saliva and re-utilized, with no effects on animal health (Fig. **3**). On average in lactating buffaloes, the intake of dry matter (16 kg DM/animal/d) is 30% lower than in dairy cattle (22 kg DM/animal/d) [52].

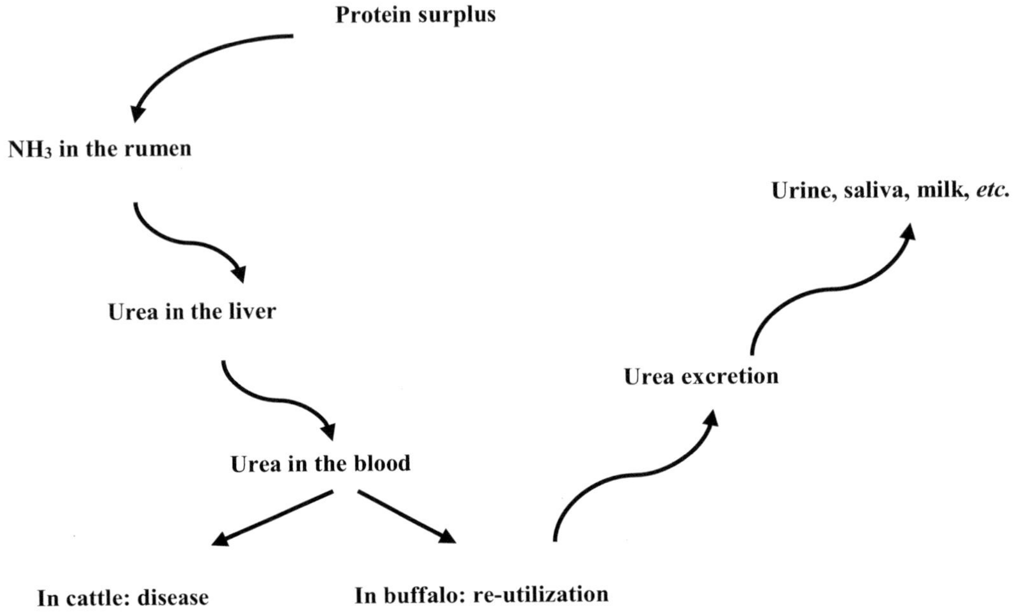

Fig. (3). Re-utilization of nitrogen consequent to protein surplus in buffaloes.

2.4. Mother-Young Relationship

As in other domestic mammals, buffaloes develop a strong mother-calf relationship soon after parturition during a sensitive period, which allows the dam to acquire a selective behavior [53, 54]. In fact, after this period the buffalo cows accept their own young and actively reject alien calves. However, in this species Murphey *et al.* [55] frequently observed a form of behavior defined as allo-nursing and consisting in female lactating cows suckling a group of alien calves. In terms of fitness this behavior represent an advantage for the sucking calves and a disadvantage for the suckling cows, whereas from a technical point of view allo-nursing may determine uneven growth of the calves, as dominant animals can have more frequent access to the udder and ingest more milk than subordinates [56]. A subsequent research showed that this behavior was not associated with either kinship or affiliative social behavior between cows, rather it was attributed to inexperience of young cows combined with high motivation to feed in calves receiving insufficient amount of milk from less productive cows [57]. No studies have been conducted on the exact age of natural weaning in buffaloes. However, many factors can affect it. In particular, the onset of a new pregnancy may reduce milk production and motivate the calf to search for alternative source of foods, whereas a low availability of palatable forage may induce the calf to rely on maternal milk for longer.

In modern buffalo farming most of the male calves exceeding the replacement needs are unwanted due to their low growth rates, which makes male calves' rearing uneconomical. This may raise concerns about their welfare if inappropriately treated when euthanized or sold at such an early age. Conversely, most of the female calves are kept as replacement animals, although they are soon after birth separated from their mothers in order to make more milk available for mozzarella cheese production. The consequent application of a milk replacer based feeding regimen represent a marked emotional and nutritional stress for the calves, which can lead to immune suppression and increased mortality rates. A mortality of 10 to 20% has been reported as the normal range, with even twofold values in farms providing inadequate technical standards [58]. One of the most common causes of increased mortality is scour, which is particularly frequent in calf less than a month old [59].

2.5. Social Behavior

As other domestic ruminants, buffaloes show a strong motivation to live in social groups. Fig. (**4**) displays the voluntary aggregation of a group of free-ranging heifers in a Mediterranean environment. The expression of a marked social behavior has been explained on the basis of the increased fitness possibly induced by augmented protection against predators (advantages deriving from improved detection of predators, increased dilution of prays, more efficient active defence) and increased efficiency in food detection (local enhancement), which have to prevail over the costs of living in groups such as resource sharing. The tendency of buffaloes to maintain close proximity makes handling easier with beneficial effects both on animal welfare and stock-people safety (Fig. **5**).

A study conducted in Central African Republic (Dzanga-Ndoki National Park) on a group of forest buffaloes (*Syncerus caffer nanus*), showed that the spatial distribution of animals within a group can be heavily affected by the habitat characteristics and the social behavior. In particular, the group when in open habitats, displayed a more aggregated spatial distribution than when it was in the forest, and age and sex were relevant factors with regard to their individual positions within the herd. In particular, usually the adult male would be always located in the centre of the herd. In contrast, females and juveniles occupied intermediate and peripheral positions within the group [60].

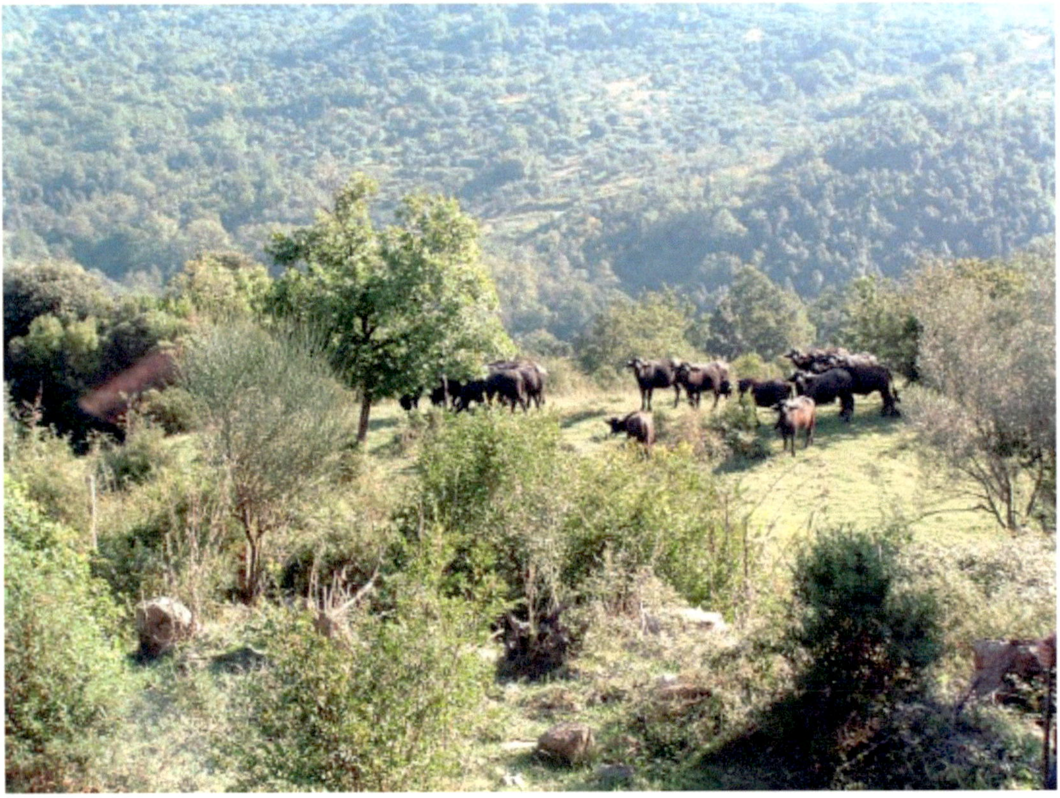

Fig. (4). Buffalo living in extensive conditions and keeping proximity to one another.

Animals living in long lasting social groups show social facilitations of behavior and are often involved in synchronized activities: lack of synchronization may be interpreted as a sign of discomfort. Conversely, a positive state of welfare, and in particular for subordinate animals, may be shown by a high degree of activity synchronization within the herd [61]. Supposedly, the basic feeding and resting requirements of low ranking animals engaged in such behaviours can be met, when there is a low competition for any resources of interest, like night feeding and resting while most animals are occupied by ingestive activities. Their welfare though would be improved if such animals, together with the other members of the group, could choose where and when to perform those behaviours. In such a way, each high or low ranking animal would be allowed to be fully integrated as a herd member.

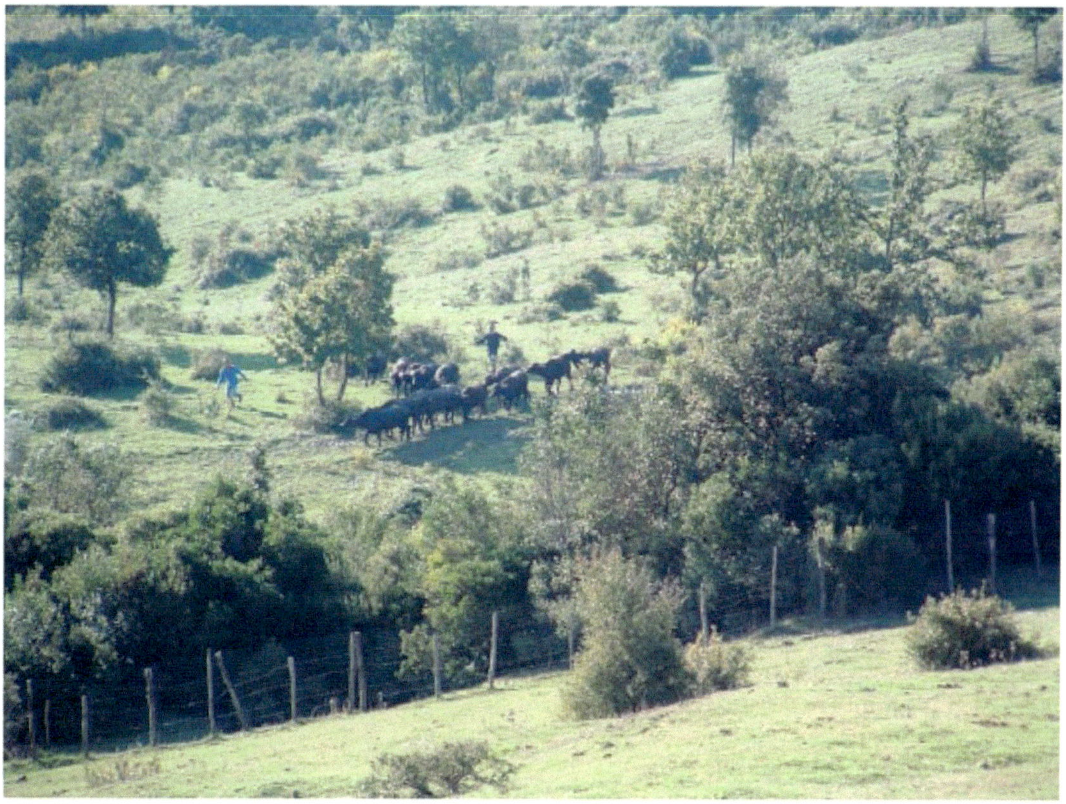

Fig. (5). Buffaloes walking close together when being moved by stock-people.

Associations among some animals may be more frequent than among others. Social interactions can be roughly divided into agonistic (aggressive encounters and threats) and non-agonistic (*e.g.* social licking). In more associated animals socio-positive behaviors are more often observed. In particular, social licking is associated to familiarity (*i.e.* time spent together), and such behavior can therefore be inhibited when frequent grouping occurs, or when a large group size is involved, as a consequence of disturbed social structure [62].

Agonistic interactions in buffaloes, as well as in other domestic animals, are essential for the formation and the maintenance of the social structure of the group. These interactions, after the formation of the social structure of the group, are replaced by threats performed by dominant animals determining a flight reaction by subordinate animals without any physical contact. The frequency and the intensity of agonistic interactions are influenced by different factors (*e.g.* housing system, space allowance, group size). Although the expression of agonistic interactions is considered a normal behavior, in pigs and cattle increased frequency of these interactions have negative effects on their welfare [63, 64]. In addition, dehorning in buffaloes is not practiced and, in horned cattle, it was found that the higher was the level of agonistic interactions the higher was the number of skin injuries [65].

The main social activities of two groups of lactating buffaloes are reported in Table **2**. The animals benefiting from high space allowance and having access to a water for wallowing more often performed socio-positive encounters, such as nuzzling and sniffing conspecifics and social lickings, than animals housed at lower space and without a pool [15]. Behavioral and physiological systems are able to induce beneficial and health–promoting effects as a consequence of socio-positive interactions. Hormones such as endogenous opioids, oxytocin and vasopressin support active systems sustaining the positive components of the homeostatic physiology [66]. In particular, social licking has been defined as a cohesive interaction because it can have a role in stabilizing and strengthening social relationships [67 - 69]. In animals with a higher space availability, the access to a pool stimulated the performance of positive social interactions, thus promoting group cohesion [15]. Unexpectedly, these animals also performed more agonistic interactions. In general, reduced space allowance can determine an increase in agonistic interactions as a consequence of lack of space, which determines a difficulty in withdrawing of subordinate subjects from dominant animals. In weaned buffalo calves a reduced space allowance caused increased agonistic interactions (7.77/animal) in comparison to animals benefiting from a higher space availability (2.06/animal) when observed over a period of six hours [29]. However, in a lactating buffaloes study (Table **2**) the agonistic interactions were much less expressed (0.16 *vs.* 0.08/ animal for animals with and without access to a pool, respectively) than in a previous study, possibly because of the different space allowances used in these two mentioned studies: 3.4 m^2/animal in weaned calves [29] and over 10 m^2 in adult buffaloes [15].

Table 2. Main social interactions (n. of events per animal) expressed by buffalo cows during 5-h periods of observation.

Behavioral Categories	WP[1]	NP[2]	P
Social licking	0.15	0.09	<0.05
Other socio-positive interactions	0.12	0.07	<0.01
Agonistic interactions	0.16	0.08	<0.01

[1]WP = cubicle open barn + outdoor paddock + concrete pool
[2]NP = cubicle open barn

Values reported by De Rosa *et al.* [15] are, in fact, similar to those observed by Sabia *et al.* [9] in heifers kept on pasture. These animals showed a number of agonistic interactions ranging from 0.8 to 2.0 events over six hours of observation and a number of non-agonistic interactions ranging from 2.5 to 3.2 events expressed by the focal animals in six hours of observation.

As already stated, agonistic interactions may be considered normal behaviors and high as well as very low occurrences may suggest that the social environment is not optimal [69].

These studies indicate that in herds kept with appropriate space allowance, the agonistic social interactions do not negatively affect the welfare of buffalo. Grasso *et al.* showed that, soon after group formation, a linear hierarchy is established [70]. Males are often integrated in the female group, where they are dominant. Although generally, once hierarchy has been established, few agonistic interactions can be observed, problems can occur when bulls interact in aggressive manner towards subordinate subjects, thus causing harms to young animals or cows by hitting, horning and head butting.

2.6. Demeanor

A characteristic of buffalo demeanor is the expression of high levels of explorative activities as compared to cattle [71]. Such activities, along with vocalization and locomotion are increased when these animals are subjected to open field tests involving exposure to an unknown environment and isolation. In particular, after a period of space restriction, buffaloes tend to increase the expression of locomotion and other dynamic behaviors, which were somehow suppressed during confinement [29], as a possible consequence of increased motivation to perform physical activity. Exposure to novelty and the consequent increased explorative activities are instead more related to the need of the buffaloes to gain information about an unknown environment. In another experiment the exposure to a novel object represented by a traffic cone induced the buffalo heifers kept in loose housed conditions to spend more time in explorative activities directed towards the new stimulus as compared to animals kept on pasture [9]. This differential response may be due to the fact that in confinement the animals were exposed to a reduced number of stimuli and were therefore more motivated in initiating explorative activities, particularly when new stimuli were available; conversely, free-range animals were used to interact with a more variable environment, thus showing little interest in a novel but irrelevant object. Increased levels of vocalization are generally related to fear responses [72]. However, this behavior is also a form of communication expressing a motivation to re-join the group and it is used to stay in contact with the social partners [73]. The animals kept indoors and living in strict contact were possibly more socially dependent and vocalized more when separated from the other members of the group. Conversely, free-ranging buffalo heifers were possibly more used to separation from their companions due to the presence of physical barriers in the natural pasture (vegetation, rocks, *etc.*), thus showing a reduced vocal response to isolation [9].

Buffaloes, when moved to the milking parlour, show a consistent order of entrance and a strong preference for one side, thus suggesting that management practices disturbing their choices should be avoided in order to minimise stress during farming routines [74]. In addition, habituation to farming routines is recommended when young animals, such as primiparous cows, start to be subjected to new management practices. In fact, the exposure of these animals to a pre-partum habituation programme can reduce the level of restlessness during their first milkings [75].

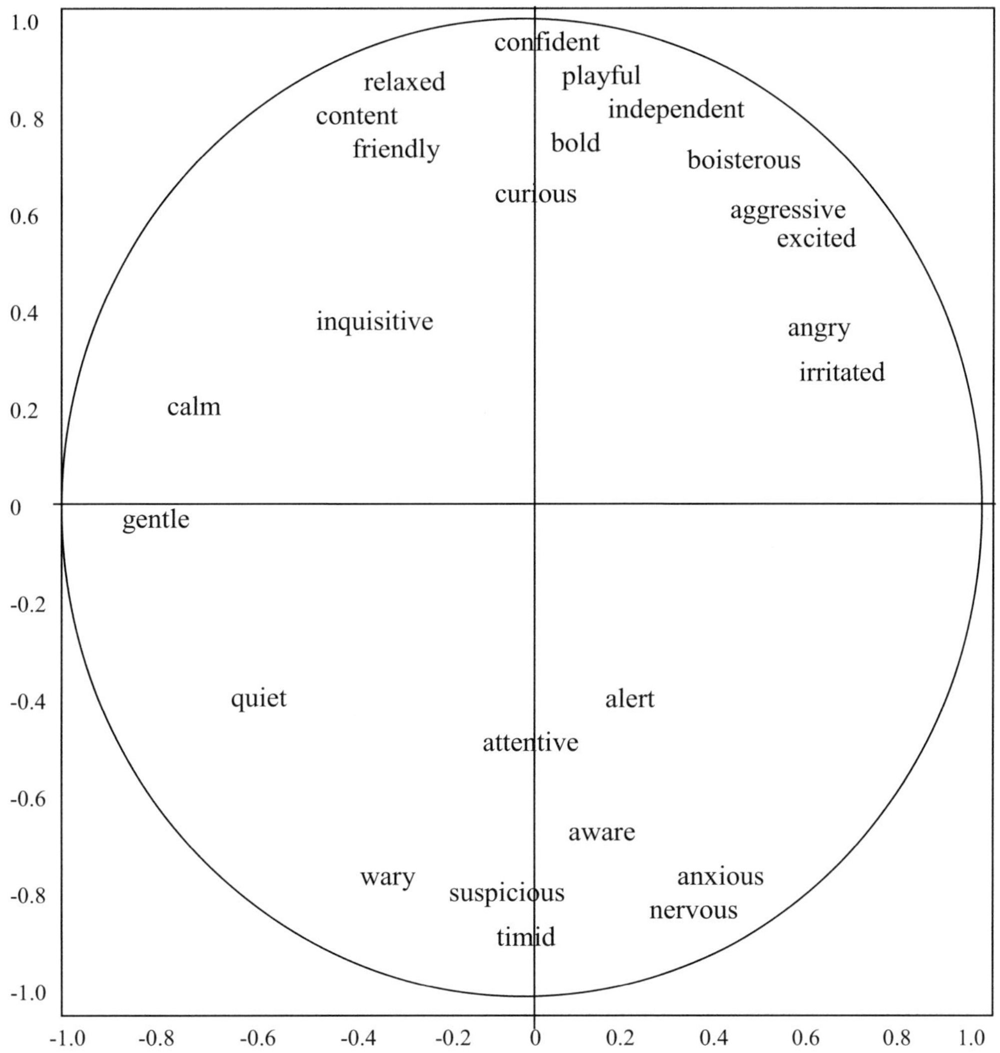

Fig. (6). Word map of observer 1.

A methodology initially developed on pigs by Wemelsfelder *et al.* [76] has been subsequently applied to buffalo heifers [77]: the qualitative behavior assessment (QBA). This approach does not rely on what an animal does: whether it eats, bites, or lies down, but on how the animal behaves; it is based on the integration of several pieces of information, which are usually ignored or separately recorded in the quantitative approaches. These pieces of information are gathered through the free choice profile techniques, which allows the observers constructing their own descriptive vocabularies using terms such as calm, curious, bold, agitated, *etc.*, to assess animal behavior and, in such a way, detecting how the animals interact with the environment. Fig. (**6**) shows the word chart of one out of twelve observers used in this study where his vocabulary and the semantic characterisation of the two dimensions of the consensus space can be seen.

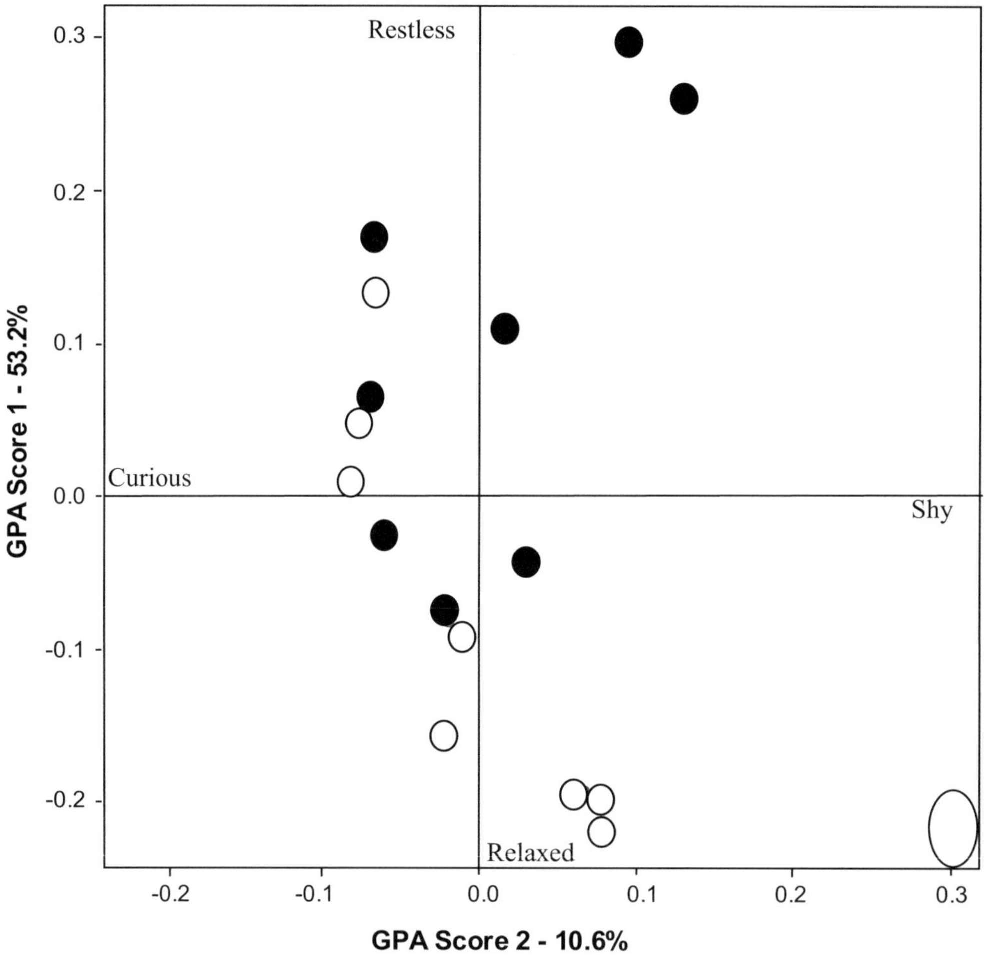

Fig. (7). Plot of buffalo heifers tested in the home indoor pen (empty dots) or in a novel outdoor pen (full dots) in the consensus space.

Data are subsequently analyzed through a multivariate method such as generalized Procrustes analysis. Buffalo heifers were isolated in two experimental conditions: one in the home indoor pen, the other in a novel outdoor pen. In the second condition heifers were more restless and explorative, whereas in the first one the animals were more relaxed and calm (Fig. 7).

Quantitative data confirmed these results in terms of higher levels of galloping, sniffing and flight attempts observed when subjects were tested outdoor [77].

2.7. Human-Animal Relationship

The quality of human-animal relationship is an important factor when considering farm animal welfare. A large mass of experimental data (see Hemsworth for a review) [78] has proven that the theoretical framework proposed by Hemsworth and Coleman in 1998 [79] on the functioning of human-animal relationship was applicable to farm animals. This model sustains that a negative behavior of stock-people may provoke fear reactions from the animals with possible detrimental effects on their welfare, production and handling. In addition, agitated animals may reinforce the negative attitude of stock-people, thus determining more negative interactions towards animals. This model works also in other way around, as positive interactions between stock-people and animals may improve animal welfare [80].

Animal responses to humans are largely influenced by previous experiences [78]. Animals subjected to repeated exposures to humans may undergo to a process called habituation. In addition, they may learn to relate humans with positive or negative events [79]. A number of experiments conducted on sheep explored the possibility to employ humans as social support [81, 82]. Dairy cows during milking in the presence of aversive stock-people showed fear and stress responses as indicated by the increased cortisol level, heart rate and residual milk [83], Empirical observations on dairy buffalo, supported by Saltalamacchia *et al.* [84], report that oxytocin is often injected to ease milk removal from the udder. These authors in 17 farms observed that 9.5% of milked buffaloes were injected with oxytocin with 24% of the injected animals being primiparous. On the contrary, in dairy cattle exogenous oxytocin during milking is rarely used [85]. In the study of

Saltalamacchia *et al.* [84] the frequency of oxytocin injections was positively correlated with number of steps and kicks performed by the animals during milking, whereas a negative association between kicking and positive stockperson behavior (*e.g.* talking quietly, petting) was detected. In addition, negative and neutral stockperson behaviors were not linked with the behaviour of buffaloes during milking. Although it has been reported that for dairy cattle both interactions (positive and negative) are related to animal restlessness at milking [86, 87], Saltalamacchia *et al.* result indicate that also in buffalo the quality of stockperson interactions may affect the behavior of animals during milking. Stepping and kicking performed by the animals during milking may be regarded as a sign of agitation and aggressiveness, respectively [86, 88]. They may be influenced by different factors (*e.g.* poor maintenance of milking machine, presence of insects). However, a clear link between stockperson demeanor and animal agitation during milking was observed in cattle [86, 89]. In particular, these studies showed that the use of positive interactions (*e.g.* low intensity vocalizations, slow movements) increased animal calmness, whereas an increased animal restlessness was observed when negative interactions (*e.g.* hitting, shouting) were performed. Hemsworth *et al.* [90] envisaged that training programs aimed to improve human-animal relationship through the modification of stockperson attitude and behavior may have beneficial effects on dairy cow productivity.

The quality of the human-animal relationship has been assessed through different tests [80]. They range from avoidance tests executed in the home pen or at the manger, to the observation of animal behavior during handling. It has been widely recognized that a valid assessment of human-animal relationship is given by the avoidance distance test [87]. In buffaloes, this variable measured in the pen showed a high short term test-retest repeatability, as its assessment performed on three different occasions at 15-20 d intervals was highly consistent across the measurements [73]. In the same study, this variable was higher in cattle than in buffaloes (242 *vs.* 64 cm), which is higher than goats (69 cm) [91] and similar to that reported for sheep (238 cm) [92]. This may be due to the fact that buffaloes in a novel situation, as can be regarded the execution of an avoidance test, display high level of inquisitive behavior [77]. However, this test may pose at risk the safety of the observers, as buffaloes, when approached in a pen, may run towards the observers and hit them, if there is no space to flee, An additional risk may be due to the presence of bulls, which are often kept with buffalo cows. Therefore, for the observers' safety it is recommended to perform the measurement of avoidance distances at the manger.

Also in the case of avoidance distance measured at manger, buffaloes showed a shorter avoidance distance (mean = 37 cm) [93] than sheep (mean = 68) [91], but higher than fattening bulls (mean = 12-15 cm) [94]. In addition, buffaloes are more willing to be touched (median = 20%) [93] than sheep (mean = 14%) [92]. In buffaloes, these two variables (avoidance distance and proportion of touched animals at the manger) showed a high inter-observer reliability, as indicated by the good agreement between two observers in assessing these measures [93].

3. WELFARE ISSUES

For centuries, buffaloes have been reared with extensive systems in the wetland regions of central-southern Italy. The application of modern husbandry practices (*e.g.* machine milking, artificial rearing, loose housing.) resulting in increased milk production, has determined an intensification of buffalo farming. However, this intensification has jeopardized buffalo welfare. For instance, a reduced space allowance had a detrimental effect on behavioral and physiological responses of calves [29 - 31], whereas in lactating animals the lack of a pool or potholes, during the hot season, prevented the expression of wallowing, a typical buffalo natural behavior [15, 28], and reduced fertility [18, 95]. Inappropriate feeding management applied to dry cows and to female calves has led to increased incidence of vaginal and uterine prolapses [96]. The use of machine milking may determine milk let down difficulties if the functioning of the machine and stockperson behavior are improper. Evidences on buffaloes show that exogenous oxytocin is frequently used to ease milk ejection [84], whereas it is rarely utilized in dairy cattle [85]. Such injections can often cause iatrogenic abscesses. In buffalo calves the artificial rearing performed in intensive farming has also led to increased morbidity (*e.g.* diarrhea), as a result of an impaired immune responses and inappropriate housing conditions [59, 97].

In addition, European consumers are currently becoming more and more concerned with the issue of animal welfare. In fact, animal welfare, together with food safety, is considered an important component of an overall food quality concept. Therefore, it is crucial to develop a monitoring tool for the assessment of buffalo welfare. Welfare has been defined by several researchers [98, 99]. In simple terms good welfare is regarded by many as good physical and mental health of the animal. It is also agreed that the welfare of an animal depends on how it experiences the situation in which it lives. This may include negative feelings, such as hunger, thirst, pain and fear, physical discomfort, injuries or diseases; and positive experiences, such as those produced by the expression of reproductive, maternal and affiliative behaviors. A comprehensive welfare monitoring scheme must consider all these aspects. During the last decade several welfare monitoring schemes have been developed in Europe [100, 101], taking in account various parameters. These schemes have shifted their emphasis from resource-based measures (*e.g.* housing system, space allowance) and management (*e.g.* feeding practices, grouping, milking routine) to animal-based measures (*e.g.* behavior, health) [102 - 104]. This shift reflects the perception that many of the welfare outcomes that vary between farms, do so as a result of the interaction between the animals (breed, age, and temperament), the standard of housing and husbandry, and the attitudes of stock handlers and farm owners. As a result of this interaction it is now agreed that provision of a defined physical environment is not sufficient to ensure good welfare. Therefore, it has been suggested that welfare assessment should essentially be based on variable measured on animals, while including management and resource measures to help identifying causes of poor welfare and advice farmers on possible improvements. All measures should have proven to be valid (measuring the actual welfare status of animals), reliable (acceptable agreement between and within observers) and feasible (practically applicable) [105, 106]. This kind of measures are being integrated into a welfare monitoring scheme specific for buffaloes as a result of the Welfare Quality project (www.welfarequalitynetwork.net).

3.1. Health Indicators

In many farm species, including dairy buffaloes, the variation in energy reserves is usually evaluated through the assessment of the body condition of animals.

Although the development of more appropriate rearing techniques, acquisition of improved management skills and improvement of animal genetic have led to a remarkable increase in milk production, buffalo morphology and metabolism remain closer to that of beef cattle [107]. Generally, lack of food is not a major cause of poor body condition. More often buffaloes become emaciated as a consequence of other health problems (*e.g.* prolapses, injuries). Monitoring buffalo body condition can therefore be a tool to gain information on the general health status of the herd. The body condition scoring for buffalo cows has been adapted from that devised for beef cattle by Lowman *et al.* [108]: The score of this system ranges from 0 (very thin) to 5 (very fat) with 0.5 increments. The system should be utilized to evaluate evident under-nutrition (BCS< 2.5), with a high proportion of animals in poor condition indicating a reduced level of welfare. Unlike cattle, over-condition in buffaloes (BCS> 4) does not represent a risk factor for ketosis [109, 110], whereas after calving may have a detrimental effects on fertility [111].

Coat cleanliness is a measure included in most monitoring schemes. In both the Welfare Quality protocol for cattle and the AWIN protocol for sheep body cleanliness is assessed as it is deemed a reliable indicator of animal comfort. In addition, dirtiness is a predisposing factor for skin inflammatory processes by inhibiting skin anti-microbial ability [112]. Udder and hind-limbs dirtiness may also favor the onset of subclinical and clinical mastitis [113, 114], as uncleanliness of these body regions promote the entrance of pathogens in the teat and udder. In addition, an association between udder cleanliness and clinical mastitis has been reported by Munoz *et al.* [115]. However, in buffaloes the presence of mud covering all or part of the body indicates that these animals have access to facilities such as pools or ponds where they can exhibit the natural behavior of wallowing, which is fundamental for thermoregulation. Conversely, when buffaloes are kept in confinement with no access to water, their skin can become soiled with dung, which represents a potential risk factor for their health.

One of the major health issues in dairy cattle is represented by lameness, which is a relevant cause of pain in these animals. Several locomotion score systems have been developed to assess lameness in cattle [89, 116, 117]. Some of these are more suited to experimental work, being very detailed, while others are simpler and more appropriate for welfare monitoring purposes at herd level. The presence of clinical foot lesions is another indicator of lameness in cattle, but the detection of these lesions requires intensive expert handling of the animals, including lifting their feet, and therefore it is not applicable for welfare monitoring at farm level. Lameness may be due to various factors, including unbalanced rations, bad quality of floor surface, social interactions and related standing time [117, 118]. In particular, subordinate subjects stand more time in the alleys, in the slurry and on concrete surfaces with the hooves being more prone to soft tissue lesions [118]. In dairy buffaloes lameness seems to affect a much lower number of animals. In a recent study the authors report the absence of this pathology in most of the visited farms [93], and explained their results on the basis of the different metabolism and feeding regimen used in buffaloes as compared to cattle [119]. Conversely, hoof overgrowth is often reported in buffaloes [120]. Floor conditions and genetic predisposition have been identified as risk factors. Both Whay *et al.* [102] in dairy cattle and Napolitano *et al.* [93] in dairy buffaloes suggest including the prevalence of affected animals in on- farm welfare monitoring schemes.

Injuries are a significant indicator of animal welfare both in intensive and extensive conditions, as indoors lesions and swellings can derive from slippery floors, inappropriate dimensions of cubicles and feeding rack, inappropriate height of the manger, *etc.*, whereas outdoors stony grounds, stingy brushes, and predator attacks are some examples of risk factors potentially causing various body damages. For instance, cows housed in cubicle systems more frequently had injured or swollen knees and hocks than cows housed in straw-pen systems [103, 121]. For cattle different scoring schemes have been developed [122, 123]. Leeb *et al.* [123] proposed to record on animal body any integument alterations such as swelling and lesions (wounds and scabs), hairless patches, coat thinning and callosity. This approach may also be applied to buffalo cows. However, particular attention should be paid when assessing hairless patches, as adults normally present a sparse hair coat. Additional aspects to be taken into account include withers hygroma and dewlap edema, associated with too low feed neck rail and too high feed kerb, respectively, and iatrogenic abscess, particularly those located at hindquarter level, associated with frequent injections of exogenous oxytocin performed to obtain a complete ejection of milk.

Disease and mortality records represent valid, reliable and feasible indicators of the health at herd level. Unfortunately, at the moment only few countries can rely on good quality farm records keeping. When these data are unavailable, enteric, respiratory, reproductive disorders (*e.g.* metritis, prolapses), mastitis, culling rate due to accidents and, disease and mortality should be recorded.

3.2. Behavioral Indicators

Although resting is a buffalo fundamental need, there are not many studies on this aspect. Calves kept at low space allowance displayed reduced lying and resting times and an increased number of bent legs in comparison with animals of the same age kept at higher space allowance [124]. In addition, when space allowance is reduced, other animals may disrupt resting patterns by hitting or treading on them [29]. Under these conditions buffaloes reduce the time spent lying idle, which is an important form of resting. In cattle, an inappropriate environment may hinder posture changes from standing to lying by raising the probability of slips and hits against cubicle bars. As a consequence, the time spent to lie down and the proportion of animals colliding with pen partitions while lying down may be used to assess the quality of resting in buffaloes [112].

Aggressive behavior of the bulls towards young and subordinate female cows is becoming a welfare issue in modern buffalo enterprises as a possible consequence of the confinement where flight distances may be reduced. In the past herds were free to wander in wetlands, whereas buffalo are presently kept in barns at 5-10 m2/head with outdoor paddocks offering 8-14 m2/head. In addition, buffaloes are rarely dehorned and one or more males are usually kept into the herd, as the efficiency of artificial insemination is still quite low. Social rank is affected by weight, age, and time of permanence in the group [70]. Primiparous buffalo cows are usually kept in one group with the other lactating animals and, for at least some period of the year, with the bulls; since they occupy the lowest ranks they are more frequently affected by injuries and lesions at the udder.

Oral stereotypies have been described in many species, including heifers and adult dairy cattle. These abnormal behaviors tend to be expressed for longer as a consequence of tethering [125], space restriction and reduced ingestion time [126,

127]. In buffaloes only few data are available and oral stereotypies should be studied more thoroughly. Empirical observations report inflammation, infection and injuries at prepuce, navel and teat levels as a consequence of cross-sucking in young buffalo calves. However, inter-sucking, consisting in sucking milk from the teat of a companion, is frequently observed also in adult lactating animals, as indicated by the application of weaning rings in animals performing this behavior with the aim to discourage it and reduce the consequent milk loss.

Good animal welfare not only include the prevention of disease, pain, and other negative states but also the furnishing of living conditions that are appropriate to animal needs. Therefore, the use of housing systems that prevent the expression of natural behaviors may have a detrimental effect on farm animal welfare. In buffaloes, during the last decades, to enhance milk hygiene, the use of pools and potholes, characteristic of traditional system, has been abandoned and rarely replaced by spray systems located in the feeding area. High levels of wallowing and grazing behaviors were observed in buffaloes provided with potholes and spontaneous vegetation [15, 28]. Accordingly, a higher fertility rate was recorded in buffalo cows, which were allowed to wallow in a pool compared to animals furnished with showers in order to ease heat dissipation [95]. Moreover, a decreased calving interval and higher conception rate was recorded in buffalo cows supplied with a pool [18]. The access to a pool also determined a higher milk yield [15, 16]. Thus, the provision of systems eliciting the expression of species-specific behaviours should be promoted.

4. FUTURE TRENDS

Based on the present knowledge, we conclude that further studies are needed to cover aspects so far unexplored. In particular, the welfare of buffaloes could benefit from additional information concerning dominance relationships, bull aggressiveness, synchronization of behavioral activities, with the first two representing a cause of increased rates of injuries in heifers and subordinate animals and increased culling rates of bulls. Another aspect to be studied in more detail is inter-sucking as it can impair buffalo cow welfare in terms of nose ring application as routine management practice and increased culling rate of sucking animals.

As in many other domestic ruminants kept on pasture, also in buffaloes feeding behavior, including search, selection and ingestion of food, and resting in various lying positions represent the two main behavioral categories occupying most of their time budget. However, when resources are available these animals also display specific natural behaviors, such as wallowing and bathing to facilitate heat dissipation. Unfortunately, most of the modern intensive farms do not possess the facilities to allow some of these behavioral expressions, such as grazing and wallowing, whereas in intensive systems other unwanted behaviors are becoming more common (*i.e.* inter-sucking). The application of a valid and reliable monitoring scheme may be used to identify the welfare consequences on the animals and the related main risk factors although additional tools (*e.g.* benchmarking) should be implemented to promote a virtuous circle of continuous improvement of animal welfare.

CONFLICT OF INTEREST

The authors confirm that they have no conflict of interest to declare for this publication.

ACKNOWLEDGEMENTS

The present study is a part of the Welfare Quality® research project which has been co-financed by the European Commission, within the 6th Framework Programme, contract n. FOOD- CT-2004-506508. Thanks are due to Amelia Maria Riviezzi and Giovanni Migliori for expert technical assistance.

REFERENCES

[1] Cockrill WR. The water buffalo: a review. Br Vet J 1981; 137(1): 8-16. [PMID: 7013899]

[2] Kumar S, Nagarajan M, Sandhu JS, Kumar N, Behl V, Nishanth G. Mitochondrial DNA analyses of Indian water buffalo support a distinct genetic origin of river and swamp buffalo. Anim Genet 2007; 38(3): 227-32. [http://dx.doi.org/10.1111/j.1365-2052.2007.01602.x] [PMID: 17459014]

[3] Kumar S, Nagarajan M, Sandhu JS, Kumar N, Behl V. Phylogeography and domestication of Indian river buffalo. BMC Evol Biol 2007; 7: 186. [http://dx.doi.org/10.1186/1471-2148-7-186] [PMID: 17915036]

[4] Schlecht E, Hiernaux P, Kadaourè I, Hulsebusch C, Mahler F. A spatio-temporal analysis of forage

availability and grazing and excretion behavior of herded and free grazing cattle, sheep and goats in Western Niger. Ecosystems and Environment 2006; 113: 226-42. [http://dx.doi.org/10.1016/j.agee.2005.09.008]

[5] Krohn CC, Munksgaard L, Jonasen B. Behavior of dairy cows kept in extensive (loose housing/pasture) or intensive (tie stall) environments I. Experimental procedure, facilities, time budgets - diurnal and seasonal conditions. Appl Anim Behav Sci 1992; 34: 37-47. [http://dx.doi.org/10.1016/S0168-1591(05)80055-3]

[6] Ryan SJ, Jordaan W. Activity patterns of African buffalo *Syncerus caffer* in the Lower Sabie Region, Kruger National Park, South Africa. Koedoe 2005; 48: 117-24. [http://dx.doi.org/10.4102/koedoe.v48i2.98]

[7] Lewis JG. Game domestication for animal production in Kenya: activity pattern of eland, oryx, buffalo and zebu cattle. J Agric Sci 1977; 89: 551-63. [http://dx.doi.org/10.1017/S0021859600061323]

[8] Grimsdel JJ, Field CR. Grazing pattern of buffaloes in the Rwenzori National Park, Uganda. E Afr Wildl J 1976; 14: 339-44. [http://dx.doi.org/10.1111/j.1365-2028.1976.tb00247.x]

[9] Sabia E, Napolitano F, De Rosa G, *et al.* Efficiency to reach age of puberty and behaviour of buffalo heifers (*Bubalus bubalis*) kept on pasture or in confinement. Animal 2014; 8(11): 1907-16. [http://dx.doi.org/10.1017/S1751731114001876] [PMID: 25076110]

[10] Martin P, Bateson P. Measuring behavior. Cambridge: Cambridge University Press 2007. [http://dx.doi.org/10.1017/CBO9780511810893]

[11] Schultz E, Schultz TA, Garmendia JC, Chico CF. Comparison of cattle and domestic buffaloes fed on tropical forage at three vegetative stages. 1. Behavior, intake and rumination. Agronom Trop 1977; 27: 319-30.

[12] Bud I, Velea C, Marcu N, Muresan G, Vomir M, David V. Behavior of dairy buffaloes on pasture. Nutr Abstr Rev 1985; 55: 185.

[13] Braghieri A, Pacelli C, De Rosa G, Girolami A, De Palo P, Napolitano F. Podolian beef production on pasture and in confinement. Animal 2011; 5(6): 927-37. [http://dx.doi.org/10.1017/S1751731110002685] [PMID: 22440032]

[14] Hafez ES, Badreldin AL, Shafie MM. Skin structure of Egyptian buffaloes and cattle with particular reference to sweat glands. J Agric Sci 1955; 46: 19-30. [http://dx.doi.org/10.1017/S0021859600039587]

[15] De Rosa G, Grasso F, Braghieri A, Bilancione A, Di Francia A, Napolitano F. Behavior and milk production of buffalo cows as affected by housing system. J Dairy Sci 2009; 92(3): 907-12. [http://dx.doi.org/10.3168/jds.2008-1157] [PMID: 19233783]

[16] Zicarelli F, Campanile G, Gasparrini B, Di Palo R, Zicarelli L. Influence of the period and of the space on the milk production and on the consumption of dry matter in the Italian Mediterranean Buffalo. Proceedings III Congresso Nazionale sull'Allevamento del Bufalo. In: 1st Buffalo Symposium of Europe and the Americas; Paestum, Italy. 2005; pp. 75-6.

[17] Kadzere CT, Murphy MR, Silanikove N, Maltz E. Heat stress in lactating dairy cows: a review. Livest

Prod Sci 2002; 77: 59-91.
[http://dx.doi.org/10.1016/S0301-6226(01)00330-X]

[18] Di Palo R, Midea D, Campanile G, Rossi N, Zicarelli L. Influence of management system on reproductive activity of dairy buffaloes during the hot season. Proceedings 6th World Buffalo Congress. Maracaibo, Venezuela. 2001; pp. 130-6.

[19] Sato S, Sako S, Maeda A. Social licking patterns in cattle (*Bos taurus*): influence of environmental and social factors. Appl Anim Behav Sci 1991; 32: 3-12.
[http://dx.doi.org/10.1016/S0168-1591(05)80158-3]

[20] Napolitano F, Knierim U, Grasso F, De Rosa G. Positive indicators of cattle welfare and their applicability to on-farm protocols. Ital J Anim Sci 2009; 8: 355-65.
[http://dx.doi.org/10.4081/ijas.2009.s1.355]

[21] Odyuo LT, Jana DN, Das N. Maintenance behavior of Murrah buffalo under an intensive management system. Appl Anim Behav 1995; 45: 293-9.
[http://dx.doi.org/10.1016/0168-1591(95)00573-B]

[22] Thomas CS, Nordstrom J, Svennersten-Sjaunja K, Wiktorsson H. Maintenance and milking behaviors of Murrah buffaloes during two feeding regimes. Appl Anim Behav Sci 2005; 91: 261-76.
[http://dx.doi.org/10.1016/j.applanim.2004.11.002]

[23] Wemelsfelder F. The concept of animal boredom and its relationship to stereotyped behavior. In: Lawrence AB, Rushen J, Eds. Stereotypic Behavior: Fundamentals and Applications to Animal Welfare. Wallingford, UK: CAB International 1993; pp. 65-95.

[24] Barnett JL, Hemsworth PH, Cronin GM, Newman EA, McCallum TH, Chilton D. Effects of pen size, partial stalls and method of feeding on welfare-related behavioral and physiological responses of group-housed pigs. Appl Anim Behav 1992; 34: 207-20.
[http://dx.doi.org/10.1016/S0168-1591(05)80116-9]

[25] Hanlon AJ, Rhind SM, Reid HW, *et al.* Relationship between immune response, liveweight gain, behavior and adrenal function in red deer (*Cervus elaphus*) calves derived from wild and farmed stock, maintained at two housing densities. Appl Anim Behav 1994; 41: 243-55.
[http://dx.doi.org/10.1016/0168-1591(94)90026-4]

[26] Chaplin SJ, Tierney G, Stockwell C, Logue DN, Kelly M. An evaluation of mattresses and mats in two dairy units. Appl Anim Behav Sci 2000; 66(4): 263-72.
[http://dx.doi.org/10.1016/S0168-1591(99)00100-8] [PMID: 10700626]

[27] Fraser AF, Broom DM. Farm animal behavior and welfare. London: Bailliere Tindall 1990.

[28] Tripaldi C, De Rosa G, Grasso F, Terzano GM, Napolitano F. Housing system and welfare of buffalo (*Bubalus bubalis*) cows. Anim Sci 2004; 78: 477-83.

[29] Napolitano F, De Rosa G, Grasso F, Bordi A. Influence of space restriction on welfare of weaned buffalo claves (*Bubalus bubalis*). Livest Prod Sci 2004; 86: 117-24.
[http://dx.doi.org/10.1016/S0301-6226(03)00148-9]

[30] Grasso F, Napolitano F, De Rosa G, Quarantelli T, Serpe L, Bordi A. Effect of pen size on behavioral, endocrine, and immune responses of water buffalo (*Bubalus bubalis*) calves. J Anim Sci 1999; 77(8): 2039-46.

[http://dx.doi.org/10.2527/1999.7782039x] [PMID: 10461979]

[31] Grasso F, De Rosa G, Marsico I, Napolitano F, Migliori G, Bordi A. Welfare of buffalo heifers in relation to feeding and space allowance. Ital J Anim Sci 2003; 2: 148-50.

[32] Martiniello P, Berardo N. Residual fertilizer effects on dry-matter yield and nutritive value of Mediterranean pastures. Grass Forage Sci 2007; 62: 87-99. [http://dx.doi.org/10.1111/j.1365-2494.2007.00567.x]

[33] Martiniello P, Terzano GM, Pacelli C, Mazzi M, Sabia E. Qualitative and quantitative biomass production of improved Mediterranean pasture on phytocoenoses and body growing in young buffalo heifers until puberty. Ital J Anim Sci 2007; 6: 1241-4. [http://dx.doi.org/10.4081/ijas.2007.s2.1241]

[34] Kenney PA, Black JL. Factors affecting diet selection by sheep. I. Potential intake rate and acceptability of feed. Aust J Agric Res 1984; 35: 551-63. [http://dx.doi.org/10.1071/AR9840551]

[35] De Rosa G, Fedele V, Napolitano F, Gubitosi L, Bordi A, Rubino R. Dietary preferences in adult and juvenile goats. Anim Sci 1997; 65: 457-63. [http://dx.doi.org/10.1017/S1357729800008651]

[36] Hodgson J. Ingestive behavior. In: Leaver JD, Ed. Herbage intake handbook. Hurley, UK: British Grassland Society 1982; pp. 113-38.

[37] Milne JA. Diet selection by grazing animals. Proc Nutr Soc 1991; 50(1): 77-85. [http://dx.doi.org/10.1079/PNS19910013] [PMID: 1881933]

[38] De Rosa G, Napolitano F, Marino V, Bordi A. Induction of conditioned taste aversion in goats. Small Rumin Res 1995; 6: 7-11. [http://dx.doi.org/10.1016/0921-4488(94)00038-9]

[39] Provenza FD. Post ingestive feedback as an elementary determinant of food preference and intake in ruminants. J Range Manage 1995; 48: 2-17. [http://dx.doi.org/10.2307/4002498]

[40] Provenza FD. Acquired aversions as the basis for varied diets of ruminants foraging on rangelands. J Anim Sci 1996; 74(8): 2010-20. [http://dx.doi.org/10.2527/1996.7482010x] [PMID: 8856457]

[41] De RG, Moio L, Napolitano F, Grasso F, Gubitosi L, Bordi A. Influence of flavor on goat feeding preferences. J Chem Ecol 2002; 28(2): 269-81. [http://dx.doi.org/10.1023/A:1017977906903] [PMID: 11925067]

[42] Kyriazakis I, Papachristou TG, Duncan AJ, Gordon IJ. Mild conditioned food aversions developed by sheep towards flavours associated with plant secondary compounds. J Chem Ecol 1997; 23: 727-46. [http://dx.doi.org/10.1023/B:JOEC.0000006407.68081.26]

[43] Macandza VA, Owen-Smith N, Cross PC. Forage selection by African buffalo in the late dry season in two landscapes. S Afr J Wildl Res 2004; 34: 113-21.

[44] Gordon IJ, Illius AW. Incisor arcade structure and diet selection in ruminants. Funct Ecol 1988; 2: 15-22. [http://dx.doi.org/10.2307/2389455]

[45] The water buffalo: new prospects for an underutilized animal. Washington: National Academy Press 1981.

[46] Ichhponani JS, Sidhu GS. Effect of urea on the voluntary intake of wheat straw in Zebu cattle and the buffalo. Indian Vet J 1966; 43(10): 880-6.
[PMID: 5977577]

[47] Jalaludin S, Ho YW, Abdullah N, Kudo H. Rumen micro-organism of the water buffalo. Buffalo J 1992; 8: 211-20.

[48] Kennedy PM. Intake and digestion in swamp buffaloes and cattle. 4. Particle size and buoyancy in relation to voluntary intake. J Agric Sci 1995; 124: 277-87.
[http://dx.doi.org/10.1017/S0021859600072944]

[49] Di Lella T, Infascelli F, Cutrignelli MI. Rumen degradability and protein value of feed utilized by buffaloes. Bubalus Bubalis 1995; 1: 38-48.

[50] Masucci F, Di Francia A, Proto V. *In vivo* digestibility, rate of particulate passage and dry matter rumen degradability in buffaloes and sheep. Proceedings 5th World Buffalo Congress. Caserta, Italy. 1997; pp. 296-301.

[51] Masucci F, Di Francia A, Gioffrè F, Zullo A, Proto V. Prediction of digestibility in buffalo. Proceedings 13th ASPA Congress. Piacenza, Italy. 1999; pp. 345-7.

[52] Terramoccia S, Bartocci S, Borghese A. Nutritional requirements in buffalo cows and heifers. Buffalo production and research. Rome, Italy: FAO 2005; pp. 145-60.

[53] Brake SC. Suckling infant rats learn a preference for a novel olfactory stimulus paired with milk delivery. Science 1981; 211(4481): 506-8.
[http://dx.doi.org/10.1126/science.7192882] [PMID: 7192882]

[54] Napolitano F, De Rosa G, Sevi A. Welfare implications of artificial rearing and early weaning in sheep. Appl Anim Behav Sci 2008; 110: 58-72.
[http://dx.doi.org/10.1016/j.applanim.2007.03.020]

[55] Murphey RM, Paranhos da Costa MJ, Lima LO, Duarte FA. Communal suckling in water buffalo (*Bubalus bubalis*). Appl Anim Behav Sci 1991; 28: 341-52.
[http://dx.doi.org/10.1016/0168-1591(91)90166-U]

[56] Paranhos da Costa MJ, Andriolo A, Simplicio de Olivera J, Schmidek W. Suckling and allosuckling in river buffalo calves and its relation with weight gain. Appl Anim Behav Sci 2000; 66: 1-10.
[http://dx.doi.org/10.1016/S0168-1591(99)00083-0]

[57] Murphey RM, Paranhos da Costa MJ, Silva RG, Souz RC. Allonursing in river buffalo, *Bubalus bubalis:* nepotism, incompetence, or thievery? Anim Behav 1995; 49: 1611-6.
[http://dx.doi.org/10.1016/0003-3472(95)90083-7]

[58] Correale E, Citro A. Buffalo calves: morbidity and mortality. Bubalus Bubalis 1997; 3: 11-4.

[59] Masucci F, De Rosa G, Grasso F, Napolitano F, Esposito G, Di Francia A. Performance and immune response of buffalo calves supplemented with probiotic. Livest Sci 2010; 137(1-3): 24-30.
[http://dx.doi.org/10.1016/j.livsci.2010.09.019]

[60] Melletti M, Delgado MM, Penteriani V, Mirabile M, Boitani L. Spatial properties of a forest buffalo

herd and individual positioning as a response to environment cues and social behavior. J Ethol 2010; 28: 421-8.
[http://dx.doi.org/10.1007/s10164-009-0199-z]

[61] Metz JH. Food competition in cattle. Farm Animal Housing and Welfare. Dordrecht, NL: Martinus Nijhoff Publisher 1983; pp. 164-70.

[62] Keeling LJ, Gonyou HW. Social Behavior in Farm Animals. Wallingford, UK: CAB International 2001.
[http://dx.doi.org/10.1079/9780851993973.0000]

[63] Otten W, Puppe B, Stabenow B, *et al.* Agonistic interactions and physiological reactions of top- and bottom-ranking pigs confronted with a familiar and an unfamiliar group: preliminary results. Appl Anim Behav Sci 1997; 55: 79-90.
[http://dx.doi.org/10.1016/S0168-1591(97)00036-1]

[64] Albright JL, Arave CW. The Behavior of Cattle. Wallingford, UK: CAB International 1997.

[65] Menke C, Waiblinger S, Fölsch DW, Wiepkema PR. Social behavior and injuries of horned cows in loose housing systems. Anim Welf 1999; 8: 243-58.

[66] Carter CS. Neuroendocrine perspectives on social attachment and love. Psychoneuroendocrinology 1998; 23(8): 779-818.
[http://dx.doi.org/10.1016/S0306-4530(98)00055-9] [PMID: 9924738]

[67] Winckler C, Buehnemann A, Seidel K. Social behavior of commercial dairy herds as a parameter for on-farm welfare assessment. Proceedings 36th International Congress ISAE. Egmond aan Zee, The Netherlands. 2002; p. 86.

[68] Wasilewski A. Friendship in ungulates? Sociopositive relationships between non-related herd members of the same species. Dissertation 2003. http://archiv.ub.uni-marburg.de/diss/z2003/0639.

[69] Laister S, Stockinger B, Regner AM, Zenger K, Knierim U, Winckler C. Social licking in dairy cattle - Effects on heart rate in performers and receivers. Appl Anim Behav Sci 2011; 130: 81-90.
[http://dx.doi.org/10.1016/j.applanim.2010.12.003]

[70] Grasso F, Napolitano F, De Rosa G, Braghieri A, Migliori G, Bordi A. Social hierarchy in unweaned buffalo calves. Proceedings 55th Annual Meeting EAAP. Bled, Slovenia. 2004; p. 147.

[71] Napolitano F, Grasso F, Bordi A, *et al.* On-farm welfare assessment in dairy cattle and buffaloes: evaluation of some animal-based parameters. Ital J Anim Sci 2005; 4: 223-31.
[http://dx.doi.org/10.4081/ijas.2005.223]

[72] De Passillé AM, Rushen J, Martin F. Interpreting the behavior of calves in an open field test: a factor analysis. Appl Anim Behav Sci 1995; 45: 201-13.
[http://dx.doi.org/10.1016/0168-1591(95)00622-Y]

[73] Watts JM, Stookey JM. Vocal behaviour in cattle: the animals commentary on its biological processes and welfare. Appl Anim Behav Sci 2000; 67(1-2): 15-33.
[http://dx.doi.org/10.1016/S0168-1591(99)00108-2] [PMID: 10719186]

[74] Polikarpus A, Grasso F, Pacelli C, Napolitano F, De Rosa G. Milking behaviour of buffalo cows: entrance order and side preference in the milking parlour. J Dairy Res 2014; 81(1): 24-9.
[http://dx.doi.org/10.1017/S0022029913000587] [PMID: 24308320]

[75] Polikarpus A, Napolitano F, Grasso F, *et al.* Effect of pre-partum habituation to milking routine on behavior and lactation performance of buffalo heifers. Appl Anim Behav Sci in press [http://dx.doi.org/10.1016/j.applanim.2014.10.003]

[76] Wemelsfelder F, Hunter TE, Mendl MT, Lawrence AB. Assessing the whole animal: a free choice profiling approach. Anim Behav 2001; 62: 209-20. [http://dx.doi.org/10.1006/anbe.2001.1741]

[77] Napolitano F, De Rosa G, Grasso F, Wemelsfelder F. Qualitative behavior assessment of dairy buffaloes (*Bubalus bubalis*). Appl Anim Behav Sci 2012; 141: 91-100. [http://dx.doi.org/10.1016/j.applanim.2012.08.002]

[78] Hemsworth PH. Human-animal interactions in livestock production. Appl Anim Behav Sci 2003; 81: 185-98. [http://dx.doi.org/10.1016/S0168-1591(02)00280-0]

[79] Hemsworth PH, Coleman GJ. Human-livestock interactions The stockperson and the productivity and welfare of intensively farmed animals. Wallingford, U.K: CAB International 1998.

[80] Waiblinger S, Boivin X, Pedersen V, *et al.* Assessing the human-animal relationship in farmed species: a critical review. Appl Anim Behav Sci 2006; 101: 185-242. [http://dx.doi.org/10.1016/j.applanim.2006.02.001]

[81] Boivin X, Tournadre H, Le Neindre P. Hand-feeding and gentling influence early-weaned lambs attachment responses to their stockperson. J Anim Sci 2000; 78(4): 879-84. [http://dx.doi.org/10.2527/2000.784879x] [PMID: 10784177]

[82] Tallet C, Veissier I, Boivin X. Temporal association between food distribution and human caregiver presence and the development of affinity to humans in lambs. Dev Psychobiol 2008; 50(2): 147-59. [http://dx.doi.org/10.1002/dev.20254] [PMID: 18286582]

[83] Rushen J, De Passillé AM, Munksgaard L. Fear of people by cows and effects on milk yield, behavior, and heart rate at milking. J Dairy Sci 1999; 82(4): 720-7. [http://dx.doi.org/10.3168/jds.S0022-0302(99)75289-6] [PMID: 10212458]

[84] Saltalamacchia F, Tripaldi C, Castellano A, Napolitano F, Musto M, De Rosa G. Human and animal behavior in dairy buffalo at milking. Anim Welf 2007; 16: 139-42.

[85] Bruckmaier RM. Normal and disturbed milk ejection in dairy cows. Domest Anim Endocrinol 2005; 29(2): 268-73. [http://dx.doi.org/10.1016/j.domaniend.2005.02.023] [PMID: 15998500]

[86] Hemsworth PH, Coleman GJ, Barnett JL, Borg S. Relationships between human-animal interactions and productivity of commercial dairy cows. J Anim Sci 2000; 78(11): 2821-31. [http://dx.doi.org/10.2527/2000.78112821x] [PMID: 11063304]

[87] Waiblinger S, Menke C, Coleman G. The relationship between attitudes, personal characteristics and behavior of stockpeople and subsequent behavior and production of dairy cows. Appl Anim Behav Sci 2002; 79: 195-219. [http://dx.doi.org/10.1016/S0168-1591(02)00155-7]

[88] Munksgaard L, DePassillé AM, Rushen J, Herskin MS, Kristensen AM. Dairy cows fear of people: social learning, milk yield and behaviour at milking. Appl Anim Behav Sci 2001; 73(1): 15-26.

[http://dx.doi.org/10.1016/S0168-1591(01)00119-8] [PMID: 11356287]

[89] Breuer K, Hemsworth PH, Barnett JL, Matthews LR, Coleman GJ. Behavioural response to humans and the productivity of commercial dairy cows. Appl Anim Behav Sci 2000; 66(4): 273-88. [http://dx.doi.org/10.1016/S0168-1591(99)00097-0] [PMID: 10700627]

[90] Hemsworth PH, Coleman GJ, Barnett JL, Borg S, Dowling S. The effects of cognitive behavioral intervention on the attitude and behavior of stockpersons and the behavior and productivity of commercial dairy cows. J Anim Sci 2002; 80(1): 68-78. [http://dx.doi.org/10.2527/2002.80168x] [PMID: 11831530]

[91] Mattiello S, Battini M, Andreoli E, Minero M, Barbieri S, Canali E. Avoidance distance test in goats: a comparison with its application in cows. Small Rumin Res 2010; 91: 215-8. [http://dx.doi.org/10.1016/j.smallrumres.2010.03.002]

[92] Napolitano F, De Rosa G, Girolami A, Scavone M, Braghieri A. Avoidance distance in sheep: test-retest reliability and relationship with stockmen attitude. Small Rumin Res 2011; 99: 81-6. [http://dx.doi.org/10.1016/j.smallrumres.2011.03.044]

[93] Napolitano F, Pacelli C, Grasso F, Braghieri A, De Rosa G. The behaviour and welfare of buffaloes (*Bubalus bubalis*) in modern dairy enterprises. Animal 2013; 7(10): 1704-13. [http://dx.doi.org/10.1017/S1751731113001109] [PMID: 23803231]

[94] Windschnurer I, Boivin X, Waiblinger S. Reliability of an avoidance distance test for the assessment of animals responsiveness to humans and a preliminary investigation of its association with farmers' attitudes on bull fattening farms. Appl Anim Behav Sci 2009; 117: 117-27. [http://dx.doi.org/10.1016/j.applanim.2008.12.013]

[95] Zicarelli L, Midea D, Piccolo G, Di Palo R, Neglia G, Campanile G. Influenza della presenza di una vasca con acqua e fertilità nella bufala. Proceedings 1st National Congress on Buffalo management. Eboli, Italy. 2001; pp. 327-31.

[96] Zicarelli L. Considerations about the prophylaxis of the uterine and vaginal prolapse in Italian Mediterranean buffalo cows. Bubalus Bubalis 2000; 6: 71-90.

[97] Di Francia A, Masucci F, De Rosa G, Varricchio ML, Proto V. Effects of *Aspergillus oryzae* extract and a *Saccharomyces cerevisiae* fermentation product on intake, body weight gain and digestibility in buffalo calves. Anim Feed Sci Technol 2008; 140: 67-77. [http://dx.doi.org/10.1016/j.anifeedsci.2007.02.010]

[98] Broom DM. Animal Welfare defined in terms of attempt to cope with the environment. Acta Agriculturae Scandinavica, Section A -. Anim Sci 1996; 27: 22-9.

[99] Duncan IJ. Animal Welfare defined in terms of feelings. Acta Agriculturae Scandinavica, Section A -. Anim Sci 1996; 27: 29-36.

[100] Bartussek H. An historical account of the development of the animal needs index ANI-35L as part of the attempt to promote and regulate farm animal welfare in Austria: an example of the interaction between animal welfare science and society. Anim Sci 2001; 30: 34-41.

[101] Main DC, Whay HR, Leeb C, Webster AJ. Formal animal-based welfare assessment in UK certification schemes. Anim Welf 2007; 16: 233-6.

[102] Whay HR, Main DC, Green LE, Webster AJ. Assessment of the welfare of dairy cattle using animal-based measurements: direct observations and investigation of farm records. Vet Rec 2003; 153(7): 197-202.
[http://dx.doi.org/10.1136/vr.153.7.197] [PMID: 12956296]

[103] Haskell MJ, Rennie LJ, Bowell VA, Bell MJ, Lawrence AB. Housing system, milk production, and zero-grazing effects on lameness and leg injury in dairy cows. J Dairy Sci 2006; 89(11): 4259-66.
[http://dx.doi.org/10.3168/jds.S0022-0302(06)72472-9] [PMID: 17033013]

[104] De Rosa G, Napolitano F, Grasso F, *et al.* Welfare Quality®: a pan-European integrating project including buffalo. Ital J Anim Sci 2007; 6: 1360-3.
[http://dx.doi.org/10.4081/ijas.2007.s2.1360]

[105] Winckler C, Brinkman J, Glatz J. Long-term consistency of selected animal-related welfare parameters in dairy farms. Anim Welf 2007; 16: 197-9.

[106] Windschnurer I, Schmied C, Boivin X, Waiblinger S. Reliability and inter-test relationships of tests for on-farm assessment of dairy cows' relationship to humans. Appl Anim Behav Sci 2008; 114: 37-53.
[http://dx.doi.org/10.1016/j.applanim.2008.01.017]

[107] Campanile G, De Filippo C, Di Palo R, Taccone W, Zicarelli L. Influence of dietary protein on urea levels in blood and milk of buffalo cows. Livest Prod Sci 1998; 55: 135-43. a
[http://dx.doi.org/10.1016/S0301-6226(98)00123-7]

[108] Lowman BG, Scott N, Sommerville S. Condition scoring of cattle, Revised edition. Edinburgh: Bulletin No. 6, East of Scotland College of Agriculture 1976.

[109] Morrow DA. Fat cow syndrome. J Dairy Sci 1976; 59(9): 1625-9.
[http://dx.doi.org/10.3168/jds.S0022-0302(76)84415-3] [PMID: 965540]

[110] Gillund P, Reksen O, Gröhn YT, Karlberg K. Body condition related to ketosis and reproductive performance in Norwegian dairy cows. J Dairy Sci 2001; 84(6): 1390-6.
[http://dx.doi.org/10.3168/jds.S0022-0302(01)70170-1] [PMID: 11417697]

[111] Campanile G. Relationship between nutrition and reproduction in buffalo. Proceedings 3rd Course on biotechnology of reproduction in buffaloes; Caserta, Italy. 1998; pp. 217-35.

[112] Winckler C, Capdeville J, Gebresenbet G, *et al.* Selection of parameters of on-farm welfare-assessment protocols in cattle and buffalo. Anim Welf 2003; 12: 619-24.

[113] Schreiner DA, Ruegg PL. Relationship between udder and leg hygiene scores and subclinical mastitis. J Dairy Sci 2003; 86(11): 3460-5.
[http://dx.doi.org/10.3168/jds.S0022-0302(03)73950-2] [PMID: 14672175]

[114] Reneau JK, Seykora AJ, Heins BJ, Endres MI, Farnsworth RJ, Bey RF. Association between hygiene scores and somatic cell scores in dairy cattle. J Am Vet Med Assoc 2005; 227(8): 1297-301.
[http://dx.doi.org/10.2460/javma.2005.227.1297] [PMID: 16266020]

[115] Munoz MA, Bennett GJ, Ahlström C, Griffiths HM, Schukken YH, Zadoks RN. Cleanliness scores as indicator of Klebsiella exposure in dairy cows. J Dairy Sci 2008; 91(10): 3908-16.
[http://dx.doi.org/10.3168/jds.2008-1090] [PMID: 18832213]

[116] Sprecher DJ, Hostetler DE, Kaneene JB. A lameness scoring system that uses posture and gait to

predict dairy cattle reproductive performance. Theriogenology 1997; 47(6): 1179-87. [http://dx.doi.org/10.1016/S0093-691X(97)00098-8] [PMID: 16728067]

[117] Winckler C, Willen S. The reliability and repeatability of a lameness scoring system for use as an indicator of welfare in dairy cattle. Anim Sci 2001; 30: 103-7.

[118] Galindo F, Broom DM, Jackson PG. A note on possible link between behaviour and the occurrence of lameness in dairy cows. Appl Anim Behav Sci 2000; 67(4): 335-41. [http://dx.doi.org/10.1016/S0168-1591(99)00114-8] [PMID: 10760612]

[119] Campanile G, Di Palo R, d'Angelo A. Haematological profile in buffalo. Proceedings 3rd Course on biotechnology of reproduction in buffaloes; Caserta, Italy. 1998; pp. 236-49.

[120] Cammarano A, Marino AL. Theorical-practical course of phonology. Bubalus Bubalis 2003; 9: 13-7.

[121] Livesey CT, Marsh C, Metcalf JA, Laven RA. Hock injuries in cattle kept in straw yards or cubicles with rubber mats or mattresses. Vet Rec 2002; 150(22): 677-9. [http://dx.doi.org/10.1136/vr.150.22.677] [PMID: 12074235]

[122] Wechsler B, Schaub J, Friedli K, Hauser R. Behaviour and leg injuries in dairy cows kept in cubicle systems with straw bedding or soft lying mats. Appl Anim Behav Sci 2000; 69(3): 189-97. [http://dx.doi.org/10.1016/S0168-1591(00)00134-9] [PMID: 10906403]

[123] Leeb CH, Main DC, Whay HR, Webster AJ. Bristol welfare assurance programme, Cattle assessment. University of Bristol. Available from: http://www.vetschool.bris.ac.uk 2004.

[124] Grasso F, Napolitano F, De Rosa G, Migliori G, Bordi A. Valutazione dell'effetto del cromo sul benessere in vitelle bufaline. Zoot Nutr Anim 2001; 27: 55-63.

[125] Redbo I. Changes in duration and frequency of stereotypies and their adjoining behaviors in heifers before, during and after the grazing period. Appl Anim Behav Sci 1990; 26: 57-67. [http://dx.doi.org/10.1016/0168-1591(90)90087-T]

[126] Redbo I, Jacobsson KG, van Doorn C, Pettersen G. A note on the relationship between oral stereotypies in dairy cows and milk production, health and age. Anim Prod 1996; 54: 166-8. [http://dx.doi.org/10.1017/S0003356100020730]

[127] Redbo I, Nordblad A. Stereotypies in heifers are affected by feeding regime. Appl Anim Behav Sci 1997; 53: 193-202. [http://dx.doi.org/10.1016/S0168-1591(96)01145-8]

CHAPTER 5

Thermal Balance in the Buffalo Species

Ramesh C. Upadhyay[1,*] and **Narongsak Chaiyabutr**[2]

[1] *Dairy Cattle Physiology Division, National Dairy Research Institute, Karnal-13200, Haryana, India*

[2] *Department of Physiology, Faculty of Veterinary Science, Chulalongkorn University, Bangkok 10330, Thailand*

Abstract: Buffalo maintain thermal balance by physiological and behavioural processes. During heat stress, on exposure to direct solar radiation or during work, buffaloes exhibit signs of distress. Under extreme hot dry or hot-humid environmental conditions ability of buffaloes to regulate temperature is compromised, and body heat balance that is dissipated at later stage or during cool periods by heat exchange processes, is increased. The responses of body functions under either acute or short term heat are discussed in relation to the initiation of panting by thermal stimulation of peripheral receptors and to the control of respiratory activity by deep body temperature. During heat exposure, an increase in water turnover reflects adaptation to maintain fluids for evaporative cooling. Acute exposure or short term exposure to heat evokes several responses of plasma volume and its composition, including changes in potassium metabolism. Acute heat exposure gives rise to a change in renal hemodynamics and electrolytes excretion. Changes in renal electrolyte excretion during heat stress are discussed in relation to the alteration of hormonal level and to the acid-base status of the blood. The effect of heat exposure on various other reactions is also summarized in thyroid activity, the levels of hormones in the pituitary and adrenal glands.

Keywords: Buffaloes, Heat exchange, Responses of body functions, Thermoregulation.

* **Corresponding author Ramesh C. Upadhyay:** Dairy cattle physiology division, National dairy research institute, Karnal-13200, Haryana, India; Tel: +91 184 225 9023; Fax: +91 184 225 0042; E-mail: ramesh5304@rediffmail.com

Giorgio A. Presicce (Ed.)

I. FACTORS AFFECTING THERMAL BALANCE OF BUFFALOES

1. INTRODUCTION

Buffaloes, though well suited to hot and humid climates and muddy terrain because of their morphological and anatomical characteristics, yet exhibit signs of great distress on exposure to direct solar radiation or during work in the sun. Buffaloes maintain their homeothermy *via* various physiological and behavioural mechanisms under normal comfortable environmental conditions. Under extreme hot dry or hot-humid environmental conditions, thermoregulatory ability of buffaloes is compromised and they are unable to maintain core body - HYPERLINK http://en.wikipedia.org/wiki/Core_temperature\o Core temperature - temperature within physiological limits. This process is one aspect of - HYPERLINK http://en.wikipedia.org/wiki/Homeostasis\o Homeostasis - homeostasis in buffaloes and a dynamic state of stability between an animal's internal environment and its external environment.

2. TYPES OF THERMOREGULATION

Buffaloes have been observed to use two types of thermoregulation:

i. Physiological Regulation**:** Physiological regulation of body temperature in buffaloes induces sweating to cool body down and exposure to cold induce shivering in young and adult buffaloes. Young buffalo calves and neonates shiver to keep warm and generate heat.
ii. Behavioural Regulation**:** Buffalo changes its behaviour to regulate body temperature particularly during extreme hot and cold climatic conditions. Under hot dry conditions, buffaloes avoid direct solar exposure and seek shade. Under hot and hot- humid weather, when body starts to get hot because of the intense solar radiations, buffaloes may want to seek a shade to reduce direct exposure and cool down or prefer wallowing. Buffaloes have unique ability to regulate body temperature by wallowing.

A. Core and Skin Surface Temperature

The core body temperature of buffaloes is 36.5° C and remains within ± 1° C of such value during normal comfortable ambient conditions, but it may increase by several degrees under stressful hot climatic condition.

Buffalo exhibit a diurnal variation in body temperature. In general body temperature is minimum in the early morning and maximum in the late afternoon. Diurnal variations occur in core temperature of buffaloes, and the evening temperature is about 0.5-1.0 ^{0} C higher than early morning body temperature. The rectal temperature of buffaloes increase by 2-3^{0}C under direct solar exposure, and magnitude of rise may be higher in working buffaloes during hot conditions. This variation largely reflects activity and feeding during the day and rest during the night.

B. Skin Characters

In general buffalo skin colour is dark black; however, skin colour may vary with the condition of management. It has been observed that housing buffaloes may cause a loss of their skin pigmentation which may be regained following further exposure to solar radiation. Pigment is brown or black in colour and is restricted to the cytoplasm of the epidermal cells. The density of the pigment is proportional to the exposure of the skin to sunlight and due to this reason dorsal and ventral areas, which are more exposed to sunlight, exhibit greater pigmentation than ventral and less exposed parts [1]. The most striking feature of buffalo skin is the thickness of the epidermis, which may be 1.5-2% of the total skin thickness. The horny layer (*Stratum corneum*) is very conspicuous and may be twice thick as in cattle. The typical black color of the buffalo skin surface is given by the melanin particles contained in the basal cells of the epidermis [2]. The melanin particles are more numerous in skin from the dorsal region of the buffalo and less numerous on the belly and the inner surface of the thigh [1]. The ultraviolet rays are trapped by the melanin particles, interrupting thus penetration of the same rays through the dermis and into deeper tissues. The tropics and subtropics are characterized by abundant ultraviolet rays, and a detrimental effect can be foreseen if an excessive exposure to those rays is not avoided, with the result of even skin tumors. The thick epidermis and *stratum corneum* may be beneficial to the buffalo as they protects the sparsely covered or nearly bare skin surface of buffaloes from harmful mechanical and chemical agents. The skin of buffaloes also acts as thermal insulator against hot air both due to thickness and subcutaneous fat that also protect from ecto-parasites.

The skin thickness of buffaloes is about twice that of cattle and there is also a significant difference between the two species in the distribution of skin blood vessels. In buffaloes, branching of the arteries is seen more frequently with the result of producing more arterioles and capillaries. In addition, lymphatics are more frequent in buffalo than in the skin of the cattle [3].

C. Hair

Hair density in buffalo is low ranging from 100–200 hairs per cm^2 as compared to 1000 hairs/cm^2 in cattle. In buffalo hair grow singly, not in group and each is associated with one sweat gland and one sebaceous gland. The adult buffaloes have two types of hair fibre; about 80% are short and fine and the rest are long and coarse. Low hair density on dorsal areas of body, particularly back and other regions of buffaloes, facilitates heat dissipation by convection and radiation during the hot environment condition.

D. Sweat Gland

Buffaloes have lower number of sweat glands as compared to cattle [4]. Egyptian buffaloes have sweat glands with a glandular surface per single sweat gland of 0.247 cm^2, which are about twice the size found for a group of contemporary cattle (0.124 cm^2), and there is a high correlation between sweat glands and the number of hair follicles in each species. Glandular surface of sweat gland per cm^2 of skin surface is less in buffaloes as compared to cattle [3]. The sweat glands of buffalo are of apocrine type and in shape they are a simple oval sac or a wide convoluted tube. Sweat glands of buffalo are associated with the hair and they secrete sebum, spreading on the surface of the skin and covering it with a fatty lubricant, with the result of slipping away both water and mud from the skin surface. Therefore, the absorption of water and its contained solutes from the skin is prevented by such fatty sebum and the thick top layer of the skin. The buffaloes then, to some extent, are protected by such skin arrangement from any harmful chemical compound present in the water. The fatty sebum melts in the course of hot weather, so that the skin is made glossier and more apt to reflect solar rays.

The sweat gland density is related to the heat tolerance capacity of the animal. It has been reported by Nagarcenkar and Sethi [5] that buffaloes are characterized by a higher sweat gland density and sweating volume coefficient, make these animals more heat tolerant.

3. HEAT EXCHANGE

A. Laws of Thermodynamics

The laws of thermodynamic are equally applicable to biological processes, and the physical basis to all thermoregulation is the first law of thermodynamics. It asserts that the total amount of energy in an isolated system remains constant. From this law one can derive the ubiquitous energy budget equation for the body of buffalo:

$$M \pm W \pm K \pm R \pm C \pm E = S \qquad \textbf{Eq. (1)}$$

The equation 1 links the rate of metabolic energy turnover (M) and the physical work rate (W) with the rate of heat exchange. The exchange of heat with the environment occurs by conduction (K), radiation (R), convection (C), and evaporation (E). The metabolic heat production including work (W) is represented by the (M+W). S represents the rate of heat storage within the body of the buffalo and is equal to zero during thermal equilibrium. In order to survive, buffaloes must achieve thermal equilibrium without an excessive deviation in body temperature. If over a given period, the rate of heat storage is not zero, then, for a buffalo of fixed mass, the average temperature of the body tissue must have risen or fallen over that period, and duration of this period usually remain unknown. For a buffalo of fixed mass and specific heat, the rate of heat storage is directly proportional to the rate of change in mean body temperature *i.e.* the average temperature of the body. However, it is very difficult to measure the accurate mean body temperature. In general heat storage of buffalo is calculated from body size *i.e.* mass or weight, changes in body temperature (rectal and skin surface) and specific heat of tissue (3.47 kJ. $Kg^{-1.}$ ^{o} C^{-1}). On average, a buffalo with a body weight of 500 Kg exposed to direct solar radiation for 4 hours increase body temperature and store 2500 kJ heat. This heat load is about 2/3 of total metabolic heat produced during a day, therefore such high heat loads are detrimental to buffalo productivity and health.

B. Physical Basis of Heat Exchange

In the process of body's temperature regulation, heat is transferred from its internal body to the external environment or to the skin *via* the blood. Four different physiological processes such as conduction, convection and radiation (known as sensible heat loss), as well as skin and pulmonary evaporation (known as insensible heat loss), are the ways the heat is transferred to the external environment from the skin.

i) **Conduction**: When molecular contact is responsible for the heat transfer from one material to the other. In this way the heat reaches the outer surface of the skin and is released into the outside environment, through transfer from the body's interior and passing through one adjacent tissue to the other. Of course, this mechanism of heat transfer works the way around: in fact, if a hot object touches the skin, heat is transferred similarly to the body interior through the skin.

ii) **Convection:** When the transfer of heat from one place to another is accomplished by the motion of air, or gas or liquid across the heated surface. Animals live in open environment and therefore the air flows constantly over the animal skin, so that the air molecules come in contact with the skin, and once they have been warmed up, are displaced in the open. The greater the velocity of air (or liquid, such as water), the greater is the amount of heat removed by convection. The body can gain heat by convection when this is combined to conduction. This is true particularly in hot environment when the skin surface temperature is lower than the environment temperature. In addition, the body will always gain heat by both conduction and convection, whenever the surrounding air or water has a higher temperature than the skin of the animal. Although both the conduction and convection mechanisms are the main mechanisms of heat dissipation, their contribution to the body's total heat loss is relatively small being only about 10% to 20%. On a different condition, buffaloes submerged in cold water tend to dissipate heat in greater amount than if they were exposed to air at similar colder temperature. It can be stated conclusively, that the contribution of heat loss or gain by both conduction and convection, is dependent very much on the ambient temperature exceeding or not the body temperature of the animal. The temperature gradient works in both directions.

iii) **Radiation**: In the process of heat transfer, the heat is given off in the form of infrared rays, which are a type of electromagnetic wave. In a resting state, the animal body discharges extra internal heat by radiation and therefore heat is radiated by the skin in all direction to nearby objects. At normal ambient temperatures (21-25°C), the body loses about 60% of its heat *via* radiation. The body also receives heat from warmer objects around it *via* radiation. In fact, radiation is responsible for heat transfer and gain from surrounding warmer objects to the skin. One such heat gain, is the radiational heat received from exposure to the sun and some heat is also gained from hot objects located in surroundings of animals.

iv) **Evaporation**: Evaporation from the skin and pulmonary surface accounts for the main heat dissipation in animals. The heat passes into the external environment in the course of water evaporation, and this mechanism is responsible for about 80% of the total heat loss in the course of various activities, and only 20% when the animal is at rest. When the external environment comes into contact with the body fluids, like in the lungs, at the mucosa level and at the skin, undetectable water loss is taking place. Insensible water loss occurs without any conscious recognition of the animal from the body to the external environment, although this mechanism, which is relatively constant even in the course of the various activities, is responsible for only 10% of the total metabolic heat produced by the body. Therefore, heat has to be more quickly lost by the body whenever the animal is exposed to intense heat or muscular work, as the mechanism of insensible water loss is not at all efficient. In addition, whenever the internal body temperature increases, an increase in sweat production is also recorded from skin surface. In the process of sweating, just before reaching the skin surface, sweat is converted into vapour by the heat of the skin surface itself. Evaporation of 100 gm of sweat results in the loss of 58.0 kcal. The water vaporization loss in buffaloes has been observed to vary from 6 to 18 kg/day [6] and the sweat losses are lower during winter (5.3 lit/day) than summer (19.2lit/day) months [7]. Diurnal variations have also been observed in sweat loss.

4. THERMAL BALANCE AND HOMEOSTASIS

The maintenance of thermal balance by a buffalo depends on a dynamic equilibrium between heat loss (sensible and insensible) and heat production/gain (metabolic and activity). Over short periods either heat production or heat loss is in excess leading to transient changes in the thermal balance. In its simplest form thermal balance of buffalo is expressed as:

Heat production = Heat loss + Heat storage

Radiation (R)± Conduction(Cn) ± Convection(Cv) ± Skin Evaporation (Ev_{sk}) ± Pulmonary Evaporation (Ev_{pulm}) = 0

A variety of metabolic activities taking place in the heart, liver and muscles is responsible for the production of heat, and the latter may also be taken up from the environment. During work, more than 80% of the total amount of heat, is produced by the skeletal muscles, whereas on the contrary, such amount is greatly reduced when the body is at rest. Radiation, conduction and convection are responsible for heat loss from the animal body, together with water evaporation from the skin, the respiratory process itself and the excretion of urine and feces. When the acquisition of heat and its loss reaches an equilibrium, then the body has come to a thermal steady state.

Thermal homeostasis therefore is reached when the body acquires the ability to regulate physiologically its inner body temperature, so that the body, responding to fluctuation occurring in the outside environment, is able to ensure its stability. One of the fundamental principles of organic life was disclosed by the French physiologist Claude Bernard, according to his understanding which is still valid to our days. Such principle refers to the concept of homeostasis, considered as a chemical / physical stability of the internal environment of cells and tissues. The concept proposed: the fixity of the internal environment is the condition for free life had the following explanation by quoting Claude Bernard: The living body, though it has need of the surrounding environment, is nevertheless relatively independent of it. This independence which the organism has from its external environment, derives from the fact that in the living being, the tissues are in fact withdrawn from direct external influences and are protected by a veritable internal environment which is constituted, in particular, by the fluids circulating in the body.

A. Thermo Receptors

The changes in surface or core temperature are picked up by two different sets of thermo-receptors: peripheral receptors and central receptors. The information perceived by these receptors is summed up and transmitted to the coordinating and integrating hypothalamus or other parts of Central Nervous System, in order to reach homeothermy.

B. Peripheral Receptors

Peripheral receptors as the name indicates, are located in the peripheral region of the body, like skin surface and mucosal membranes. The exact structure of the receptors sensitive to increasing temperature of the skin and in other mucosal areas is partially known. There are two kinds of thermoreceptors: warmth receptors for sensation of heat and cold receptors for cold. These receptors perceive information and this is passed to the hypothalamus and the cerebral cortex, so that the temperature is consciously perceived by the animal which can directly and voluntarily control the exposure to either cold or warm environments. The sudden temperature rise causes a transient increase in frequency of discharge at receptors *i.e.* a phasic response from a steady discharge rate *i.e.* a static response of receptors. However, exposure to cold elicits an opposite response, and temperature drop causes a transient increase in discharge at receptors (phasic response). During water splashing or high sweat evaporation or submerged state as in wallowing, it is possible that a condition in which the body interior is hyperthermic (overheated) while cold is perceived by the skin, can occur. In this case it is likely that the hypothalamus and the cerebral cortex are incorrectly notified by the peripheral receptors of perceived cold, whereas on the contrary the body is experiencing a condition of heat.

C. Central Receptors

Within the hypothalamus central thermoreceptors are located, and therefore they have to be considered the core of the thermoregulatory system. Blood temperature are monitored by such central thermoreceptors, when blood itself circulates within the brain. Minor changes in temperature can be perceived by these central receptors, when they take place within animal body and may be as little as .018°F.

D. Role of Hypothalamus in Temperature Sensing

The hypothalamus plays an important role in the thermoregulation and maintains thermal equilibrium under thermal challenge. The anterior portion of the hypothalamus is integrated with the control of heat loss, and posterior hypothalamus controls heat production. The neurones of hypothalamus behave like receptors in their response to change in blood temperature in the brain. Local heating of anterior hypothalamus causes activation of heat loss mechanisms and local cooling evokes marked peripheral vasoconstriction and shivering.

In general neuronal signals coming from the peripheral receptors (like hot skin) passes further upwards to the thalamus. In the central nuclei of this complex of connector neurons, it is likely that perception of heat takes place. Study in *Bos taurus* have showed that heating in medial preoptic area in the region of the anterior commissure by thermode (heat stimulation) initiate panting, sweating and dilation of arterioles [8]. Hypothalamic neurones increase their rate of signal when the hypothalamus is heated so that body temperature is lowered by panting and sweating. The relative importance of peripheral, spinal and hypothalamic thermo receptors in determining the set point of the body thermostat in buffaloes is not known. All mammals, though living under similar conditions, maintain their body temperature at different set points. The physiological processes that operate in buffaloes with specific reference to their low set point are inadequately understood. However, the physiological and behavioural mechanisms that operate in buffaloes for temperature regulation are most likely coordinated and controlled similarly to cattle or other mammals.

5. PHYSIOLOGICAL RESPONSES TO HEAT

The compensatory physiological responses of an animal to the thermal or heat stress include a) circulatory adjustment or vasomotor adjustment which regulates the rate of heat exchange between the core and peripheral tissue, and subsequently between surface of the body and the environment, b) evaporative heat loss mechanism, and c) heat loss by sweating and panting *etc.*

A. Circulatory Adjustment

Heat balance is maintained by animals by vasomotor control and regulation of blood flowing by either vasodilation or vasoconstriction of cutaneous vessels. The promoter center is stimulated by vasodilation, so that the hair cover is flattened and a better heat dissipation is allowed through conduction, convection and radiation. A rise in skin temperature is achieved when cutaneous vasodilation occurs, in turn the gradient of thermal exchange for external temperature below skin temperature is increased, and finally this events increase heat dissipation from the skin.

The skin acts as a thermal insulator, and its effectiveness decreases with increased blood flow and *vice versa*. Change in skin blood flow not only affects the rate of heat exchange between animal and the environment, but also determines the rate of heat transfer from the deep body tissues to the periphery. In particular, blood volume and its flow to the skin surface in buffaloes is increased in the course of hot conditions, so that a high skin temperature is maintained in order to ease heat dissipation when the animal is in the water or mud [9]. Thick layer of fat under buffalo skin helps to keep heat in, and under thermal stress reduces heat exchange. The exchange of heat at countercurrent heat exchange vessels, helps in cooling blood and the side-by-side contact of vessels let heat travel from warm blood to cool blood.

Vasodilation of skin blood vessels in buffaloes occurs during hot conditions, so that body heat is transferred to the skin to allow exchange and dissipation through the processes of convection and radiation [10]. Heat exchange occurs readily in buffaloes with relatively cooler external air or water when wallowing, thanks to the sub epidermis plexus of capillaries structurally supplying the skin [2, 11 - 13]. Buffaloes, both young and adult, on exposure to direct solar radiations during summer raise their body temperature by several degree Celsius. The rise in body temperature of buffaloes by several degrees occurs as an adaptive process similar to deferred dissipation mechanisms employed by camel and other adult mammals under thermal stress [14]. This mechanism helps buffaloes and other animals to reduce thermal exchange particularly at high ambient temperatures and high skin surface temperature during summer. Buffaloes allowed to wallowing, exchange stored heat to water very quickly and cool body. The buffaloes maintained in open, exchange stored heat to environment. Air velocity and humidity play an important role in heat dissipation from skin. Summer stress imposes severe restrictions on the productivity of buffaloes due to disturbances to internal milieu besides homeothermy. The studies on buffaloes have revealed that higher number of erythrocytes and haemoglobin observed during hot dry summer help in combating heat stress. The hot humid conditions as observed during rainy season reduce erythrocyte count and haemoglobin in buffaloes. Wallowing and water shower alleviate thermal stress of buffaloes but erythrocyte count and haemoglobin is lowered. During heat stress the level of haemoglobin, oxyhemoglobin and packed cell volume decrease, while blood leucocytes increase moderately due to increase in circulating neutrophils. Plasma volume, blood volume and blood pH increase significantly while packed cell volume decreases due to acute heat exposure to the sun in buffalo [15].

B. Evaporative Heat Loss

Thermal stress in buffalo is a major problem for improving livestock productivity due to influence on reproduction and milk production. Evaporative heat loss from skin and pulmonary surface is an insensible mean of heat loss and it is the most effective means of thermal regulation in the profusely sweating animals but is of limited importance in buffalo. Evaporative losses from the skin and lungs of buffalo increase gradually as ambient temperature increases. In buffaloes evaporative cooling is less due to low number of sweat glands per unit surface area and the sweating ability. Skin water loss from buffalo skin at 37 °C is about 460g/m2/h, which increases to more than 800g/m2/h after exposure to direct solar radiation and when ambient temperature is about 42°C. Pulmonary surface evaporative loss increases about two fold (65g/m2/h to 128 gm/m2/h) after 4 h of direct solar exposure in buffaloes. The proportion of heat loss from pulmonary surface increases with rise in ambient temperature [16] and loss from skin is decreased.

In buffaloes, pulmonary activity increases with rise in ambient temperature. Under mild hot conditions, low respiratory frequency of buffaloes and high volume of O_2 consumption and high pulmonary volume, contribute partially to an improved efficiency of energy utilization. Respiratory evaporation has been found to be more important in maintaining thermal homeostasis than sweating under hot conditions in buffaloes [16]. Buffaloes unable to dissipate, increase their body heat balance and defer heat dissipation. Relative humidity at high ambient temperature has a direct effect on respiratory vaporization. A decrease in respiratory vaporization is recorded when the relative humidity rises coupled to high environmental temperature [17].

In particular, a very little or absent heat loss by evaporation characterizes the buffalo calf, and therefore whenever a high external temperature is accompanied to high relative humidity, internal body temperatures are found similar and rise in progression to time. On the contrary, when high external temperature is coupled to low relative humidity, some water evaporates from the mucosa in the course of inspiration, with the final outcome of cooling the mucosa itself. Therefore, air humidity governs the evaporative cooling of the mucosa and determines the extent of water which is regained by condensation on cold mucosa upon exhalation.

C. Water Vaporization

The water evaporation is increased in response to rise in ambient temperature in buffaloes similar to other livestock species. The water vaporization loss was 5- 6 kg/ day during winter and 18 -20 kg/day during summer [6, 7]. The insensible perspiration has been observed to increase from 5.4 to 14.5 L/day with rise in ambient temperature from winter to summer in buffaloes [18]. The insensible water loss increases many folds (up to six times) in summer when compared to winter [7, 19]. The temperature of the epidermis surface and the air vapour pressure are partly responsible for the passive transfer of water through the skin.

Water intake of buffalo increases due to increase in turnover rate during hot weather. Water turnover has also been used in order to compare different species and heat adaptability of breeds. In general, during the summer season, volume of water intake (free water ± water through feedstuffs), metabolic water, water voided (faeces ± urine) and water vaporization are increased [20, 21].

6. REACTIONS TO EXTREME ENVIRONMENTAL TEMPERATURES

A. Tolerance to Heat and Solar Exposure

The remarkable ability of buffaloes to withstand heat and solar exposure has been established by different studies. In buffaloes, the rectal temperature starts rising above normal at an air temperature of 34ºC and open mouth panting begins at a rectal temperature of 40ºC. The open mouth panting in buffaloes may be observed in working buffaloes even at lower body temperatures. In buffaloes both sweating and panting are important thermoregulatory mechanisms. The sweating rate increases with a rise in ambient temperature above 30ºC. As the environmental temperature rises, the rate of breathing increases and polypnea is observed at rectal temperatures above 40ºC. The change in tidal volume (decrease/increase) also occurs with frequency of breathing during heat exposure which helps protection against reduction of carbon dioxide and maintenance of acid base balance. The protrusion of tongue with excessive salivation during heat and work is not uncommon in buffaloes.

B. Heat Stress

Similar to other livestock species buffaloes also have a range of comfortable ambient temperatures that is termed the thermo-neutral zone, and temperature below or above this range causes heat stress. Heat stress is the state at which physiological response gets activated to maintain thermal balance under thermal challenges. Heat stress associated to various environmental elements affect the physiological systems which govern thermal regulation, and the control of positive heat loss is mainly given by factors such as environmental temperature, relative humidity as well as radiant energy.

C. Panting

Panting is a rapid shallow breathing and consists of a controlled increase in the frequency of the respiratory acts, coupled to a decrease in tidal volume. Panting primarily offers the possibility to increase ventilation of the upper respiratory tract, together with preserving the ventilation of the alveolar structure and increase heat loss by evaporation from the pulmonary surface. Thermal polypnea, heat tachypnea and thermally induced hyperpnea are used as synonyms for the panting. Polypneic panting is characterized by a breathing frequency between 200 and 400 breaths/min with an open mouth and tongue protruding. Usually panting comes together with increased salivary secretion and a significant increase in respiratory evaporative cooling. An increased temperature of the external environment, skin surface or inner body can be the main reasons to the beginning of panting, prior to an increase in temperature of blood supplying the brain. Panting is an efficient way to increase the evaporative heat loss in buffaloes, cattle and dog.

D. Water Wallowing

Buffaloes are traditionally adapted to various environmental and temperature changes by building their resilience to the tropical environment. Wallowing means rolling or floundering in mud or in water. Buffaloes wallow in ponds of water and muddy pools. In extreme hot conditions they prefer wallowing and move to colder waters and wallow for several hours. Buffaloes decrease their activity and submerge their whole body in water to avoid solar exposure. The high specific heat of water than that of air helps in transfer of body heat to water even under warm conditions, therefore each unit of water adjacent to the skin surface of buffalo during wallowing help in absorbing more heat than that of air can receive.

The heat transfer to water is about 200 times more than to air at 28°C from buffaloes considering uniform air and water velocity. It is known that the time needed for water to heat up or cool down is much longer when compared to air, due to a higher specific heat. Therefore in buffaloes exposed to hot environments, the body can be maintained at normal temperature by wallowing or by a constant exposure to water, especially if coupled to a wind responsible for drying it off [22].

Rather than seeking shade, buffaloes prefer and tend to cool off by wallowing, and this is explained by the greater capacity of water to absorb and exchange heat [23]. Buffalo may wallow for several hours during hot summer and can be easily seen immersed in water or covered by mud while they chew with semi-closed eyes. When temperature and humidity are high, buffaloes wallow or roll in mud during hot or even cold seasons. This process complements sweating process in buffalo and help in transfer of heat to mud/ water. Wallowing is then for buffaloes an efficient thermoregulation system, and this is ensured by a high amount of sebum secretion responsible for skin protection while covered with mud [3]. In buffaloes while wallowing, heat is dissipated by conduction and water evaporation, through direct contact of the skin with either water or mud. Typically, when exposed to hot environments, buffaloes increase their blood volume and flow to the surface of the skin, so that a high skin temperature is kept which facilitates dissipation of heat while immersed in water or mud [9]. Buffaloes during wallowing lose heat many times faster in water than in air at the same temperature. Buffaloes, similarly to rhinoceros or pigs, also roll in cool mud and coat their skin to lose heat and protect from direct solar heat and sunburn. The heat loss to mud on body of buffaloes is an effective means of cooling due to higher specific heat and conductivity of mud.

E. Sprinkler System

In sprinkler system water is showered at a fixed rate on the skin surface of buffalo and it helps in reducing the thermal load on the buffalo. The use of sprinklers without a mechanical ventilation system is likely to increase humidity at high temperature, and can cause severe stress to livestock, and therefore it should be restricted. The sprinkler system is relatively an expensive and water consuming cooling device, therefore it should be used judiciously for livestock cooling in areas which suffer from scarcity of water.

Sprinkling adult females for 2 h reduces 0.9 °C in body temperature [24]. A drastic decrease in physiological parameters such as rectal temperature reduction and respiratory rate, can be observed in young female buffaloes when they are sprinkled for 15 min [25]. Water sprinkling in buffalo reduced rectal temperature by 0.1°C as compared to wallowing by 0.5°C, and therefore the utility of water sprinkling for buffaloes may be of limited use besides economics of sprinkler system [26]. The differences may be due to limited opportunity for heat dissipation from thick skin of buffalo into the air as compared to water, indicating greater utility of water wallowing in buffaloes.

7. ENDOCRINE FUNCTIONS AND HORMONAL CHANGE DURING HEAT AND COLD

Thyroxine (T4) and Triiodothyronine (T3)

Thyroid hormones are essential for maintenance of basal metabolic rate and play a role in growth activity and regulation. The thyroid hormones are influenced by seasonal changes and physiological functions. The acute heat exposure decreases plasma level of T3 and T4 in young (aged 6 months) and old buffalo calves [20]. In lactating buffaloes, plasma T3 concentration decreased significantly with the increase of ambient temperature from 17.5 to 37.1 °C [27]. The T3 takes at least 72 h to reach its minimum level after heat exposure. In buffaloes, the T3 levels are observed to reach the highest peak in winter, and decrease in spring while continuing such decline of values and reaching the lowest values in summer [28].

Cortisol

Stressful climatic conditions can be confronted with two of the most important physiological responses, such as cortisol activation through the hypothalamic-pituitary-adrenal axis and the subsequent increase in the concentration of plasma glucocorticoids. Cortisol, the main component of adrenal corticoids, is responsible for physiological corrections and adjustments which enable the animals to face such stressful conditions. Concentration of cortisol is altered by acute and chronic heat exposure [29]. Acute heat exposure of young and old buffalo calves induced significant increases in plasma cortisol concentration [20]. Seasonally, blood cortisol levels increase significantly due to increase in ambient temperature from February to July. Exposure of non-pregnant female buffaloes for 2–3 h to direct solar radiation at high temperature, increases plasma cortisol concentration rapidly [30].

Insulin

A decrease in plasma insulin level is generally reported following exposure to high temperature, while an increase of the insulin level in the course of high temperature has a strict correlation to a marked increase in plasma glucose level.

Estrogen

The level of estrogen are significantly reduced in summer season as compared to winter season.

8. PHYSIOLOGICAL RESPONSES TO COLD

The physiological responses to cold exposure allow an animal to maintain homoeothermy by two ways: i) a reduction of heat loss which is brought about by peripheral cutaneous vasoconstriction and piloerection; and ii) an increase in metabolism through shivering and other means of increased thermogenesis, broadly classified as nonshivering thermogenesis.

A. Reduction in Heat Loss

In general, in order to prevent heat loss, the blood flow to the skin is reduced by vasoconstriction and this allows the skin to get cool and establish an equilibrium with ambient conditions to prevent or minimize the heat loss from skin surface.

B. Increase in Heat Production

One of the important physiological responses to cold is the increase in the metabolic heat production. The rate at which heat is produced by cellular thermogenesis process is directly related to the total metabolic rate.

C. Shivering and Non Shivering Thermogenesis (NST)

Shivering is a largely uncontrolled rapid contraction of certain skeletal muscles and is controlled, at least in part, by the somatic nervous system.

Non shivering thermogenesis, is an increased heat production without the contraction of skeletal muscle and is under the control of autonomous nervous system.

II. PHYSIOLOGICAL EFFECTS OF ACUTE AND SHORT TERM HEAT EXPOSURE ON CHANGES IN BODILY FUNCTIONS OF SWAMP BUFFALO

9. INTRODUCTION

Many animal studies have concentrated on the effects of acute (30 to 300 min) and intense high temperatures (41 to 42ºC) on physiological parameters. However, in general, animals are often exposed to chronic environmental conditions (days to months). In the livestock industry, the economic losses associated with heat stress (HS) are mainly due to the negative effects on feed intake, activity, daily gain, male and female reproductive performance, embryo development, *etc.* [31]. Whenever the capacity of an animal for heat dissipation is somewhat exceeded by the amount of heat acquired through direct exposure to high environmental temperature, then an adaptive response termed as heat stress occurs. Heat exchange occurs between an individual and the environment by conduction, convection, radiation and evaporation. The former three modalities are limited by high environmental temperature; while the latter in environments of humidity are limited by an individual's capacity to maintain an adequate fluid balance during a sustained period of intense perspiration. Thus, the influence of thermal environment on animal production must be realized as a function of heat production and heat loss of animals. Livestock performance is affected by high temperatures both directly and indirectly. Exposure to stressful conditions initially results in impaired cellular performance [32]. The genetic expression from livestock animal is an important factor during exposure to high temperature. The effect of heat stress may affect some animals more than others; for example, animals with low active secretion of sweat gland rely primarily on respiration for heat dissipation, by means of evaporative cooling. Heat dissipation mechanisms in different species also show dissimilarities in relation to the body size and evaporative cooling by panting or sweating. This implies that the environment affects different animals to different extents [33]. Therefore, the environmental influences on the adaptive responses to environmental conditions for satisfactory animal performance, must be considered.

Water buffaloes are found in the humid tropics, and approximately 90% of the world's water buffalo population is found in Asia. They are important sources of draft, meat, hides, fresh milk, and milk products. Compared to other domestic ruminants, the buffalo is a large animal with a large body size. The effect of heat stress on body fluid compartments may be more pronounced in this animal species. It is known that body water is the vehicle used for evaporative cooling during heat dissipation mechanism. Different mechanisms of heat dissipation as a response to high external temperature, may affect the the animal's water status and balance. Buffalo has low active secretion of sweat gland; evaporative heat loss from the body surface plays a minor role. Buffalo has a highly developed panting mechanism that permits a high rate of evaporative cooling from the respiratory tract. These adaptive responses have important physiological consequences in terms of greatly increased water turnover, modified avenues of water exchanges and bodily functions. Metabolism and utilization of water by buffalo combating environmental stress may vary considerably and more so than in other homeothermic animals both in magnitude and direction. As a result of direct heat stress effects, numerous changes occur in many body systems, for example, digestive tract, acid-base chemistry, and hormone activity [34]. These imbalances develop secondary to circulatory adjustments, water and electrolyte losses induced by profuse sweating and evaporative losses from the respiratory system. It is important to thoroughly understand how buffalo is able to physiologically thermoregulate in its environment. Understanding this mechanism will allow new insights into increasing efficiency, productivity, and longevity through approaches in handling and management.

From the above considerations, during heat exposure in animals, there are two types of physiological responses: fast and slow responses. Fast response is a specific action which deals with homeostasis including cardio-respiratory and behavioural responses. Slow response is a series of non-specific actions dependent on integrative capacities of metabolic, nervous and endocrine systems. Although the physiological responses to acute or short-term heat exposure of resting or non-active buffalo have been reported by Chaiyabutr and Johnson [35], precise information regarding changes in bodily functions in response to the combined stress factors related to high ambient temperature, has not been available until recently. This review deals with thermal effects during exposure to high temperatures on the physiological changes involving water balance, distribution of volumes and compositions of body fluids and related various organ functions in the maintenance of homeostasis under acute and short-term heat exposure.

10. EVAPORATION AND CUTANEOUS HEAT LOSS

In thermoregulation, heat loss from the skin usually occurs by radiation, convection and evaporation. Heat loss by evaporation is the most efficient means of dissipating heat from the animal body. The use of sweating for evaporative heat loss is a mechanism of adjustment of the body to dissipate the body heat load. Heat production within body is transported partly by conduction through the tissues. Heat transfer from the central core of the body to the surface, is achieved mainly by internal convection through the blood circulation *via* cardiac output. Buffalo possess sweat glands of the apocrine type, reaching almost all the hair follicles with a poor blood supply [3, 36], similarly to temperate cattle breeds [37]. The number of sweat glands per unit area of skin is relatively low, about one-third, and the thickness of the corneum layer and epidermis is about double, when compared to cattle [3]. The thickness and the black pigment of the buffalo skin probably are responsible for a higher absorption of heat, and to a disproportionate heat loss from the extremities by convection and radiation when exposed to solar radiation. This evidence indicates a lower efficiency of sweating in buffaloes, which plays little or no part in heat regulation. If skin water loss diffusion between water-vapor pressure in the air occurs, even in the absence of sweat gland activity in buffalo is still a matter of speculation. The study of Ranawana and co-workers [38] indicated that the cutaneous water loss of buffalo exposed to high temperature is not due to true sweating but partly due to insensible loss of moisture by passive diffusion through the epidermis. This suggestion indicates that diffusion moisture alone cannot serve to regulate body temperature during heat exposure.

11. CARDIORESPIRATORY RESPONSES TO HEAT EXPOSURE

It is known that increased vasodilation of blood vessels in the skin occurs during heat exposure. Heat is brought to the skin *via* the blood supply and then lost by radiation and convection into the animal's surroundings. The structure of the blood supply to the skin of buffalo has been elucidated by Shafie [2], who demonstrated that their vascular architecture is similar to cattle [39]. There are three networks or plexuses of arteries and veins in buffalo skin. In the extremities and appendages, arteries are always closely accompanied by veins (*venae comitantes*). This arrangement allows heat to be interchanged between an artery carrying warm blood to the surface and a vein carrying cooled blood back to the heart. Consequently, pre-cooling of arterial blood can occur followed by the reduction of the temperature gradient at the surface of the skin. This is a useful feature for the conservation of heat in a cold climate but not an adequate process of heat loss in a hot climate. Therefore the counter-current heat exchange system for thermoregulatory mechanisms between superficial blood vessels is inadequate for buffalo exposed to high ambient temperature [40].

A high environmental temperature causes changes in cardiovascular and respiratory function. In some mammal species with fewer sweat glands, panting is quantitatively more important for heat dissipation *via* respiratory evaporation during exposure to high temperatures. In swamp buffalo, heart and respiratory rates and rectal temperature are only minimally affected by an outside air temperature of 30°C [41, 42], indicating that the buffalo easily manages to balance its heat production against its heat loss. The change in respiratory frequency is marked when air temperatures of 30ºC is exceeded, and the animal immediately begins to pant. The peripheral receptors of the thermal regulation system are held responsible for initiation of panting, without any reported rise in rectal temperature [42]. The most obvious effects of acute heat stress on the cardiorespiratory system are increased heart rate and respiratory rate. A comparison of the effect of heat stress under high environmental temperatures and direct exposure to the sun shows different patterns of physiological responses (Table **1**). There is evidence from experiments on buffaloes that the proportional rises in heart rate and respiratory rate during acute exposure to solar radiation for 4 hr were much more marked than for animals after 4 hr exposure in a hot room at an ambient temperature of 41 °C [41, 43]. The heart rate is little affected, but the animal's respiration rate rises rapidly at about three to four times normal values under this condition. Changes in cardiorespiratory frequency in animals exposed to solar radiation were associated with elevation of rectal temperature. These changes suggest that sensitivity to thermal stimulation is higher in buffaloes exposed to the sun. The result is, in part, due to the nature of the skin of the buffalo, *i.e.* the black pigment and the thickness of the skin [3]. These factors will enhance absorption of more solar radiation from the sun and interfere with heat loss, resulting in a higher heat storage. In a study of the effects of coat color on heat exchange in goats and buffaloes, black coats absorbed more heat than white coats [44, 45].

Table 1. Effects of acute and short term heat exposure of swamp buffalo after acute heat exposure either direct to the sun or in the hot room, mean values of changes in respiratory rate, heart rate and rectal temperature at 14:00 h. (Adapted from [41, 43]).

			Non-shaded period		
	Control	Hot room 4h	4h	5d	10d
Ambient temperature (°C)	31	41	39	40	40
Relative humidity (%)	51	42	62	59	55
Rectal temperature (°C)	38.0	39.5	41.9	41.9	41.7
Respiratory rate (breaths/min.)	58	79	112	180	175
Heart rate (beats/min.)	48	55	59	76	72

The effect of short-term heat exposure of non-shaded buffaloes on heart rate, respiratory rate, and rectal temperature has been studied by Chaiyabutr *et al.* [46]. It is apparent that under radiant heat load, buffaloes are unable to keep their body temperature constant. When the buffalo is exposed to the sun for 8 hours daily over a period of 10 days without wallowing, the maximum respiratory rate, heart rate and rectal temperature recording at 14:00 hours are still as high on the tenth as on the fifth day of exposure, indicating that buffalo has low efficiency for acclimatization during intermittent heat exposure. The minimal time for acclimation in buffaloes during exposure to high environmental temperature is still unknown, although the experiments in cattle showed that 3 weeks of daily exposure to high temperature would induce some degree of acclimation [10]. It is reasonable to speculate on the minimum time for acclimatization in buffalo as heat becomes more intense. Changes in respiratory rate by shift from thermal polypnoea (panting) to thermal hyperpnoea (slow, deeper breath) during exposure to high temperature may be less likely to cause respiratory alkalosis.

12. WATER TURNOVER AND TOTAL BODY WATER

When considering the various mechanisms adopted to ensure heat dissipation, body water is of paramount importance for the effectiveness of evaporative cooling. It has been reported that the buffalo is somewhat higher in body water turnover than other domestic ruminants [47]. The body-water turnover shows marked increases during 21 days without wallowing [48] and while in open pastures [49]. The effects of acute heat exposure on total body water and water turnover rate of swamp buffaloes were measured using the ^{3}H-radioisotope dilution technique. A single does of 3000 μCi of carrier-free tritiated water per animal was injected intravenously [41]. During acute heat exposure to high ambient temperatures (41°C, 42% RH) for 4-5 hours, the water turnover rate of buffalo has been shown to increase by 86% compared to animals kept at normal ambient temperature (30°C, 51% RH) [41]. During acute heat stress, the increase in the water turnover rate is reflected by the higher water requirement in buffaloes. An increase in water turnover simply reflects a part of the process of adaptation by maintaining fluids for evaporative cooling and helping regulate body temperature during the rise of environmental temperature. No significant alterations have been observed in total body water and body weight when buffaloes are in acute heat exposure.

In short-term heat exposure, the non-shaded buffaloes prevented from wallowing, have a drastically reduced ability to conserve total body water during the first five days after spending up to 8 hours of the day in an unshaded pen. The total body water markedly decreases on the fifth day of the nonshaded period while body water turnover rate increases with time of exposure [46]. It is contrary to what has been reported for swamp buffaloes which are not allowed to wallow and kept largely in shaded conditions [38]. The results of this investigation have demonstrated that lactating, pregnant and heifer buffalo showed a marked increase in water turnover rate with no alteration of total body water when prevented from wallowing over two weeks in an ambient temperature range of 27.7-32.8°C and relative humidity of 62.9%. It has been suggested that an increase in water intake during this period is an attempt to compensate for the lack of wallowing. This is the best indication of the importance of wallowing for the swamp buffaloes as a means of cooling themselves. A decrease in body water during prolonged heat exposure without wallowing, is harmful to buffaloes in a hot climate, because it decreases their ability to dissipate the heat through water vaporization and to slow down the elevation in body temperature by virtue of the high specific heat of water. The significance of these results, however, emphasises the importance of having water available for buffaloes at all times.

Table 2. Changes in water turnover rate and total body water of swamp buffalo during acute heat exposure (4h) and short-term heat exposure to the sun. (Adapted from [41, 46]).

Shaded	**Non-Shaded**			
	Control	**5h**	**day 5**	**day 10**
Water turnover ($ml/kg^{0.82}.d$)	361	506	665	665
Total body water (L/100kg)	63.0	62.6	51.8	51.5
Biological T1/2 ^3H_2O (h)	87	49	55	42
Body weight(Kg)	343	345	339	339

13. PLASMA, BLOOD VOLUME AND COMPOSITIONS

Whenever high temperatures characterize external air, a change in the total content of body water in animals is recorded, and such change can be considered an adaptive reaction to fight heat stress. Important physiological consequences are followed by such reaction, as witnessed by a significant increase in water turnover, as related also to water exchange and cardiovascular function. Changes in blood volume and plasma volume as well as their compositions have been reviewed in buffaloes exposed to high temperatures [35]. A study in swamp buffaloes using T-1824 showed that blood volume and plasma volume increased by approximately 7% while packed cell volume slightly decreased when buffaloes were acutely exposed to high temperature (41°C 42% RH) for 5 hours [41] (Table 3). It has been shown that a plasma volume increase cannot be held solely responsible for an increase in blood volume. Considering that the increase is greater in the plasma volume as compared to the cell volume, the decrease in packed cell volume cannot be held accountable for an increase in plasma volume; it has also been shown that the volume of circulating blood cells increases by approximately 4.5%, in heat-stressed animals. The increase in circulating cell volume observed in buffaloes exposed to severe heat could be explained by the action of noradrenalin, which has been reported to increase in heat-stressed animals [50]. However, the increase in plasma volume is not only a dilution accompanied by a reduction in plasma solids, since the concentration of plasma solids which consist mainly of protein increases significantly when exposed to severe high temperature [43]. It has been postulated that during intravascular volume expansion in heat-stressed buffalo, an increase in plasma water could come from extravascular tissue space. An increased concentration of plasma protein is a causative factor responsible for an increase in colloidal osmotic pressure, and in turn water passage from the extravascular to the intravascular compartment is increased. Alternatively, the increase in plasma water may derive from the digestive tract as a result of the increased liquid flow rate from the rumen [41]. The increase in the plasma water content is an adaptive mechanism which enables the animal in gaining a higher heat tolerance thanks to the higher specific heat of water, by slowing down the elevation of body temperature.

Table 3. Changes in blood volume and plasma volume and compositions of swamp buffaloes during acute heat exposure for 5 hours and short-term heat exposure of non-shaded period (Adapted from [41, 46]).

Shaded	**Non-Shaded**			
	Control	**5 h**	**day 5**	**day 10**
Blood volume (ml/kg)	63.9	68.1	62.5	56.7
Plasma volume (ml/kg)	47.4	50.8	46.4	42.3
Cell volume (ml/kg)	16.5	17.2	15.7	14.3
Total plasma water (ml/kg)	43.0	45.8	42.6	38.7
Total plasma solid (g/kg)	4.4	5.0	5.1	5.1
Plasma protein (g%)	8.9	9.4	9.5	9.9
Plasma glucose(g%)	79	100	102	100
Packed cell volume (%)	27.6	25.9	25.3	25.2

Under short term heat exposure to the sun for 10 days accompanied by denial of wallowing, changes of body fluid compartments of buffalo are considered in two different phases [46]. The first phase occurs within the first five days with initial increases in plasma volume and total plasma water which slightly expand 'isotonically' as a result of addition of fluid which is used for heat dissipation. Total circulating protein increases, but total body water decreases on the forth day of heat exposure. This is not reflected in the behaviour of blood volume because water is supplied to the blood at a similar rate as it is lost. However, by the tenth day both plasma and blood volume do not follow the same pattern of the first phase but drop by 9% in a second phase of the responses to short-term heat exposure (Table **3**). These changes may be attributed to adaptive mechanisms. Packed cell volume and circulating cell volume on the tenth day of the non-shaded period change little from those of the fourth day. Total body water decreases to a point which does not differ from that of the fourth day, while water turnover rate of non-shaded buffalo increases stepwise, indicating higher water requirements for evaporative cooling and lower efficiency in the water retention mechanism during 5-10 days of heat exposure.

14. EFFECTS OF HEAT STRESS ASSOCIATED WITH POTASSIUM METABOLISM

It has been known that the body water is distributed between three major compartments: i) the intracellular space; ii) the extracellular (interstitium), and iii) the vascular space. The intracellular volume and the fine balance of its volume is essential for physiological cellular functions, and this is accomplished by regulating plasma osmolality *via* changes in water balance. Potassium ion account for almost all the intracellular osmoles and acts to hold water within the cells. When animals are exposed to high temperatures, intracellular and extracellular compositions are affected. These changes will affect thermodynamic equilibrium of water across the plasma membrane. A change in intracellular or extracellular solute concentrations generate a transmembrane osmotic gradient resulting in the immediate flow of water in or out of the cell until osmotic equilibrium is restored. Potassium ion is the major ion having a role in the maintenance of cellular osmosis and water balance. The response to high environmental temperature *via* many mechanisms such as decreased feed consumption, sweating, panting, water intake and alterations in fluid volume distribution, will affect the animal's potassium balance.

In short term heat exposure in buffaloes, the decrease in plasma potassium concentration coincided with an increase in urinary fractional excretion of potassium [46]. Increased urinary excretion of potassium during heat stress may be due to increases in plasma aldosterone production and urinary aldosterone in dairy cattle [51]. However, it has been suggested that heat stress does not necessarily affect plasma concentration of aldosterone, which has been observed as a response in man. The plasma glucose concentration increased and this correlated with an increase in the plasma insulin level in acute and chronic heat stress. An increase in plasma glucose concentration during heat stress may relate to the action of either glucocorticoids [52] or catecholamines [53]. These have been shown to be elevated during heat stress. An increase in plasma insulin level during heat stress may be controlled by elevation of plasma glucose [15]. One of the physiological responses of the cell to heat stress is a marked increase in the red blood cell potassium concentration (Table **4**). This change coincided with an increase in the activity of the red blood cell Na-K ATPase, whereas the red blood cell sodium and chloride concentrations decreases. This mechanism could be due to a hormone-induced increase in activity of the Na-K ATPase pump which mediated active transport of sodium out of the cell and potassium into the cell [54, 55]. A variety of factors, including glucocorticoids [56] and mineralocorticoid [57] are also known to modulate Na-K ATPase activity. An increase in the activity of the red blood cell Na-K ATPase may be associated with the role of insulin in promoting the entry of K^+ into the cell [15].

Table 4. Changes in plasma concentrations of glucose, insulin, activity of red blood cell Na, K-ATPase, the concentrations of electrolytes in plasma and red blood cell (RBC) of swamp buffaloes during shaded and non-shaded periods (mean±S.D.) (Adapted from [15]).

Shaded	Non-Shaded			
	Control	5 h	day 5	day 10
Plasma glucose (mg%)	52.7±4.3	72.8±10.8*	87.4±24.6*	65.2±7.0***
Plasma insulin (µ I.U/ml)	4.98±2.24	9.74±2.23*	11.68±4.10*	10.98±3.78**
Red blood cells: RBC- Na, K-ATPase (nmol Pi/mg Pr/h)	132.4±35.1	155.6±40.7*	143.6±30.9	163.8±50.5
Plasma Na^+ (mEq/L)	133.4±2.4	134.4±2.2	133.2±1.6	133.6±0.9
Plasma K^+ (mEq/L)	4.3±0.4	4.5±0.4	3.7±0.3*	3.9±0.2
Plasma Cl^- (mEq/L)	104.4±6.2	105.0±12.8	103.8±4.6	101.0±4.4

(Table 4) contd.....

Shaded	Non-Shaded			
	Control	**5 h**	**day 5**	**day 10**
RBC Na^+ (mEq/L_{Rbc})	39.7±9.6	21.9±17.4	28.8±12.2	35.6±8.8
RBC K^+ (mEq/L_{Rbc})	60.5±1.0	81.4±12.8**	79.6±5.5**	83.7±6.0***
RBC Cl^- (mEq/L_{Rbc})	95.0±18.7	66.3±25.4	58.9±35.7	59.6±15.4**
Plasma pH	7.38±0.03	7.43±0.01**	7.45±0.05*	7.39±0.01

Values with respect to shaded period: * P<0.05, **P<0.01, ***P<0.001.

15. RUMEN LIQUID FLOW RATE

It is clear that the digestive canal of ruminating animals provides fluid for the body. In proportion, buffaloes are characterized by having a larger rumen capacity when compared to other domestic ruminants. The study of the digestive physiology of heat-stressed buffalo was carried out using chromium-51 ethylenedia-minetetra-acetate (^{51}Cr-EDTA) to determine liquid flow from the rumen [41]. The rate of liquid flow from the rumen increased significantly by 29% during acute heat exposure in a hot room, while the biological half-life of ^{51}Cr-EDTA decreased from the control value from 13 hr to 9 hr. The retention time in the rumen, of water and particles, has been calculated as the mean retention time of 51Cr-EDTA, which has been found to be reduced in heat-stressed buffaloes from 18.7 ± 3.6 to 13.5 ± 3.1/hr. These changes would have contributed to a reserve of water for an evaporative cooling system by water replacement from the lower digestive tract, as Kamal and Shebaita (1968) [58] have shown that an increase in blood volume of water buffaloes in hot climates is due to an increase in the absorption of water in the intestine.

Short-term heat exposure of non-shaded buffaloes also influenced the fluid dynamics in the rumen. On day 10, rumen fluid volume decreased significantly. The decrease in rumen fluid volume was associated with a 19% increased rate of liquid flow from the rumen. The mean retention time of marker (polyethylene glycol, PEG) residues in the rumen of non-shaded buffaloes decreased from 12.5 hr to 7.9 hr on day 10 of short-term exposure. These findings are to be expected, in view of the increased liquid flow from the rumen to the lower digestive tract, which would have contributed to a reserve of water for the evaporative cooling system. The pattern of changes is similar to the results with acute heat-stressed buffaloes. The mechanism involved in the regulation of the rate of passage of digesta in the rumen during exposure to heat is probably complex. It is regulated by both neural and hormonal mechanisms [59]. It seems unlikely that the increased liquid flow from the rumen was due to enhanced rumen motility. Experiments in cattle kept in high environmental temperatures showed that as voluntary food intake declined, rumen contractions became smaller in amplitude and slightly less frequent [60]. The reduction in rumen movement is still present in animals when food is added to or taken out of the rumen through a fistula [61]. In non-shaded buffaloes, the rumen fluid volume decreased while water intake tended to increase. The decrease in rumen fluid volume was associated with an increased concentration of fluid marker PEG, and an increased rate of fluid flow from the rumen. A rapid absorption of water across the rumen wall probably occurs in heat-stressed buffaloes in accordance with the theory of ruminal absorption proposed for many desert-living animals [62].

16. RESPONSES OF RENAL FUNCTIONS

A. Renal Hemodynamics

Dissipation of heat is the primary problem confronting animals during exposure to high temperature. Therefore, it can be concluded that in heat stressed animals alimentary water is the source of water, while the kidneys are responsible for retaining as much water as possible. Studies of the renal physiology of buffaloes during acute heat exposure were carried out either in a hot room (41°C DB) or exposed to the sun (39°C DB). A slight decrease in the rate of urine flow was apparent during exposure both to the hot room and to the sun. The renal clearances were measured using either endogenous creatinine or inulin for determinations of glomerular filtration rate (GFR) and para-aminohippuric acid (PAH) to determine renal plasma flow (RPF) [63]. The effects of acute heat exposure for 4 hr showed no effect on GFR in both hot environments, while RPF and renal blood flow (RBF) had a tendency to increase. An increase in RPF and RBF concomitant with the decrease in filtration fraction was noted during exposure to solar radiation. These findings indicate that a number of factors could be responsible for the increase in RBF in acute heat-stressed buffaloes. An increase in RBF is probably involved in the elevation of perfusion pressure to the kidneys. This would be related to an increase in cardiac output. It has been reported that heat-stressed oxen showed a marked increase in cardiac output [64]. If the increase of cardiac output occurs in heat-exposed buffaloes, it should be accompanied by increases in both heart rate and blood volume [41]. The question remains whether an increased RBF in heat-stressed buffaloes is affected by an increase in cardiac output, because these changes could not be demonstrated in either heat-stressed sheep [65] or goats [66]. The increase in RBF in heat-stressed buffaloes could be attributed both to a decrease in renal vascular resistance and local vasodilatation. The GFR of the buffaloes is not affected by acute heat exposure, thus, an autoregulatory mechanism could be exerted entirely by intrarenal factors. An unchanged GFR while the RPF increases, may be due to a decrease in resistance of both afferent and efferent arterioles in kidneys. However, in man both GFR and RPF fall during the first few hours of heating [67], as a result of blood being diverted from the kidneys to the skin as cooling takes place. This is not so in the buffaloes, which rely on respiratory evaporation for heat dissipation. Whether this represents a mechanism to maintain a core temperature, a shift in blood distribution away from other parts of the body to kidneys, and thereby to reduce body heat through urine excretion, is open to speculation. During short-term heat exposure, non-shaded buffalo have been shown to increase their rate of urine flow by 50% on day 10 of exposure [68]. Whether this represents a mechanism to maintain a core temperature, a shift in blood flow distribution away from other parts of the body to the active tissue like kidneys and thereby non-evaporative cooling through urine excretion is open to speculation.

B. Renal Electrolyte Excretion

The rate of urinary excretion and fractional excretion of sodium increased, while those of potassium and chloride ions showed a tendency to decrease, during 4 hr of sun exposure. However, the changes in urinary electrolyte excretion are not caused by changes in filtered load (GFR X plasma electrolyte concentration), which remained constant during heat exposure. This is thought to be related in part to changes in the activity of renal tubular cells. An increase in urinary sodium excretion, but a decrease in potassium excretion in buffaloes exposed to the solar radiation, may be caused by decreased aldosterone, which has also been reported in heat-stressed cattle [69]. This is in contrast to the observation in man, where exposure to a hot environment leads to an increase in aldosterone, resulting in a reduction of Na^+ loss in urine [70]. More salt is normally lost from sweating in man than in other animals during heat exposure. This may cause a reduction of plasma Na^+ concentration, which may stimulate aldosterone secretion [33].

During short-term heat exposure for 10 days [68], non-shaded buffaloes showed an increase in the rate of urine flow by 50% on day 10 of exposure. This change coincided with increases in renal osmolar clearance, urinary excretion of potassium, and urine pH. The urinary and fractional excretion of inorganic phosphorus and chloride ion decreased throughout the non-shaded period, while the urinary and fractional excretion of sodium markedly increased in the first 5 days of heat exposure, and fell thereafter. The urinary excretion of calcium and magnesium showed no alteration throughout the experimental period. According to these findings, the kidneys of non-shaded buffaloes are responsible for retaining both water and electrolytes. Throughout all the experiments, the buffalo received the same diet. herefore, changes in electrolyte excretion during heat stress in swamp buffalo have been shown to be due to change in bodily status.

On day 5 in the non-shaded buffaloes, urinary sodium excretion markedly increased nearly three-fold, concomitant with an increase in plasma volume. The renal loss of sodium seemed to be carefully controlled to maintain optimal sodium concentration in the extracellular fluid. In this period both plasma sodium concentration and plasma osmolality remained constant. There is evidence, obtained by El-Nouty and coworkers from their study in cattle, that prolonged heat exposure can reduce plasma aldosterone level [69]. Therefore, if a reduction of plasma aldosterone occurs in non-shaded buffaloes, sodium will be excreted *via* the kidney rather than retained. This may be an important adaptive mechanism; buffalo cannot excrete sodium *via* sweating, unlike man exposed to heat [70, 71].

On day 10 of the non-shaded buffaloes, the urinary and fractional excretion of sodium markedly decreased, while a marked increase was noted for potassium. These changes were related to a marked reduction of total body water and plasma volume. The dislocation of body fluids during heat stress may stimulate the kidneys to conserve salt and water until plasma volume is increased to a steady state. The kidney is much less able to conserve potassium than sodium, which probably relates to increased aldosterone levels in plasma during the period of dehydration. A possible secretion of aldosterone may be accompanied by an elevation of plasma cortisol, as has been demonstrated in non-shaded buffaloes exposed to heat for 10 days [72].

When non-shaded buffaloes were exposed to intense environmental heat, signs of distress like rapid and shallow breathing, usually resulting in alkalosis, were reported. It is possible that increases in urine pH and plasma chloride concentration in non-shaded buffaloes could be due to respiratory alkalosis. A likely explanation might be that compensation for this disturbance occurs by increased renal excretion of base instead of chloride, resulting in an increase in plasma chloride concentration to replace base lost from the body [73]. An increase in either urinary or fractional excretion of potassium could be explained by the fact that during alkalosis, the kidney plays a significant role in acid-base regulation by an increased exchange of potassium ions for hydrogen ions in the renal tubular fluid [73]. However, an increase in urinary potassium excretion in non-shaded buffalo may also be superimposed on the effect of either aldosterone or antidiuretic hormone (ADH) [74].

During short term heat exposure, non-shaded buffaloes showed a marked reduction of the plasma concentration of inorganic phosphorus. This reduction is similar to the effect of acute heat exposure. The process of cellular trapping of phosphorus for elevation of the metabolic rate and ATP production during heat stress may be responsible for the decrease in the plasma level of inorganic phosphorus. Therefore, the reduction of the urinary excretion of inorganic phosphorus might be attributed to a reduction of filtered load. However, renal handling of inorganic phosphorus was not similar to that of calcium and magnesium ions, which were not altered in the non-shaded period, although all of these ions are under control of circulation PTH. It seems likely that prolonged heat exposure did not influence the renal handling of both calcium and magnesium ions, which probably share a common intratubular transport mechanism.

On day 10, an increase in the rate of urine flow in buffaloes exposed to heat was not due to a shortage of ADH, as free water clearance (C_{H2O}) showed a decrease under this condition. An increase in electrolyte excretion, particularly potassium ions, can create an osmotic diuretic effect (increased osmolar clearance), which may contribute to an increase in urine output in buffaloes. In ruminants exposed to hot environments, there is also an elevation of plasma vasopressin. The kidney responds to this polypeptide differently from man or dog. A rise in plasma vasopressin in sheep, camel or cattle [75], and buffalo [68] increases renal potassium secretion to a level higher than normal. There is then an increase in the rate of excretion of water by osmotic diuresis (Fig. **1**).

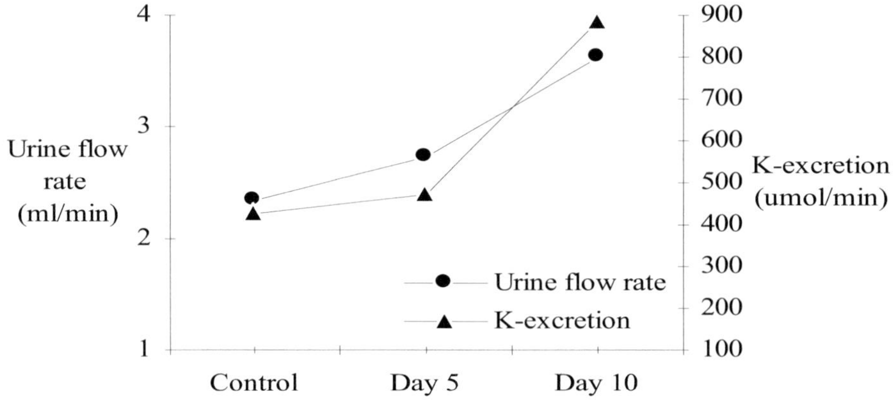

Fig. (1). Changes in the rate of urine flow and urinary potassium excretion of swamp buffalo exposed to the sun for days and 10 days (adapted from [68]).

17. HORMONAL RESPONSES

Hormones from endocrine glands, *e.g.* pituitary gland, thyroid gland and adrenal gland, are known to control many vital physiological and biochemical events to maintain homeostasis under different environmental stresses. It is known that high environmental temperature has an effect on the function of the endocrine system of most animals [76]. However, little is known of the effect of a hot environment and work on the endocrine activity of buffalo. Loypetjra and co-workers [72] have studied the effect of short- term heat exposure on hormonal response in resting swamp buffalo. Changes of serum concentrations of thyroid hormone have been reported in buffaloes exposed to the sun for 10 days. In the first day of acute sun exposure, the concentration of Triidothyronine (T3) in the blood serum slightly increased. Serum T3 concentration became reduced below normal if buffaloes remained continuously exposed to the sun. These responses are similar to observations in sheep and cattle exposed to hot environments [77, 78]. There is no significant change in the serum growth hormone (GH) of non-shaded buffaloes while serum concentrations of prolactin (PRL) and cortisol markedly increase, particularly in the afternoon throughout the non-shaded period [72]. There is no correlation between the temperature humidity index (THI) and T3 or GH levels in either shaded or non-shaded periods. The correlation is apparent between THI and prolactin (PRL) or cortisol in non-shaded buffaloes but not in the shaded buffaloes. However, knowledge of the role of these hormones in regulation of bodily functions in response to high temperatures is incomplete and further research is required in buffalo.

CONFLICT OF INTEREST

The authors confirm that they have no conflict of interest to declare for this publication.

ACKNOWLEDGEMENTS

Declared none.

REFERENCES

[1] Singh A. Skin pigmentation in buffalo calves. Can Vet J 1962; 3(11): 343-6. [PMID: 17421544]

[2] Shafie MM. Physiological responses and adaptation of water buffalo. In: Yousef MK, Ed. Stress Physiology in Livestock. Boca Raton, FL: CRC Press Inc. 1985; pp. 68-80.

[3] Hafez ES, Badreldin AL, Shafei MM. Skin structure of Egyptian buffaloes and cattle with particular reference of sweat glands. J Agric Sci (Camb) 1955; 46: 19-30. [http://dx.doi.org/10.1017/S0021859600039587]

[4] Shafie MM, Abou El-Khair MM. Activity of the sebaceous glands of bovines in hot climate (Egypt). J Anim Prod., Cairo. UA R 1970; 10: 81-98.

[5] Nagarcenkar R, Sethi RK. Association of adaptive traits with performance traits in buffaloes. Indian J Anim Sci 1981; 51: 1121-3.

[6] Raghavan GV, Mullick DN. Effects of air temperature and humidity on the metabolism of nutrients in the buffalo. Ann Biochem Exp Med 1961; 21: 277-82. [PMID: 14489874]

[7] Ghosh TK, Singh WB, Verma DN, Saxena KK, Ranjhan SK. Measurement of water turnover and water requirements in different species of animals in two seasons. Indian J Anim Sci 1980; 50: 615-9.

[8] Findlay JD, Ingram DL. Brain temperature as a factor in the control of thermal polypnoea in the ox (Bos taurus). J Physiol 1961; 155: 72-85. [http://dx.doi.org/10.1113/jphysiol.1961.sp006614] [PMID: 13699550]

[9] Koga A. Internal changes of blood compartments and heat distribution in swamp buffaloes in hot condition: Comparative study of thermoregulation in buffaloes and Freisian cows. Asian-australas J Anim Sci 1999; 12: 886-90. [http://dx.doi.org/10.5713/ajas.1999.886]

[10] Bianca W. The effect of repeated short exposures to heat on the volume and hydration of the blood of the calf. Br Vet J 1957; 113: 227-41.

[11] Shafie MM, Badreldin AL. The role of blood in regulating body heat in bovines. J Animal prod UAR 1962; 11(1): 61-74.

[12] Shafie MM, Badreldin AL. Skin temperature and temperature gradient in bovines. Proceedings of the Animal Production Conference. Vol II: 375-84.

[13] Ashour G, Shafie MM. Water balance in riverine buffaloes. I- Mobilization of body fluids under heat and dehydration stresses. International symposium on prospects of buffalo production in the Mediterranean and the middle east, EAAP Publication No 62 1993; 194-7.

[14] Taylor CR. Responses of large animals to heat and exercise. 1981.

[15] Chaiyabutr N, Komolvanich S, Sawangkoon S, Chanpongsang S. Alterations in potassium homeostasis during heat stress in swamp buffaloes (*Bubalus bubalis*). J Themal Biol 1997; 22(3): 207-12. [http://dx.doi.org/10.1016/S0306-4565(97)00013-2]

[16] Aggarwal A, Upadhyay RC. Studies on evaporative heat loss from skin and pulmonary surfaces in male buffaloes exposed to solar radiations. Buffalo J 1998; 2: 179-87.

[17] Kibler HH, Brody S. Influence of humidity on heat exchange and body temperature regulation in Jersey, Holstein, Brahman and Brown Swiss cattle. Missouri Agric Exp Sta Bull No 522 Columbia USA. 1953.

[18] Mullick DN. A study on the metabolism of food nutrients in cattle and buffaloes under climatic stress. Arid Zone Res 1964; 14: 137.

[19] Ashour GA. Water balance in bovine as related to heat regulation 1990.

[20] Nessim MG. Heat-induced biological changes as heat tolerance indices related to growth performance in buffaloes. Ph.D. Thesis, Faculty of Agriculture. Ain Shams University, Cairo, Egypt 2004; 30(5)

[21] Pal S, Pal RN, Thomas CK. Effect of restricted access to water supply and shelter on the physiological norms and production of Murrah buffaloes. Indian J Dairy Sci 1975; 28: 41-8.

[22] Cockrell W. 1974.

[23] Pant HC, Roy A. The water buffalo and its future. In: McDowell RE, Ed. Improvement of Livestock Production in Warm Climates. San Francisco: W.H. Freeman and Company 1972; pp. 563-99.

[24] Ragab MT, Asker AA, Ghazy MS. Effect of age on milk yield and length of lactation period in Egyptian buffaloes. Indian J Dairy Sci 1953; 6: 181-8.

[25] Titto EA, Russo HG, Lima CG. Efeito do banho de água sobre o conforto térmico de bubalinos.

[26] Aggarwal A, Singh M. Changes in skin and rectal temperature in lactating buffaloes provided with showers and wallowing during hot-dry season. Trop Anim Health Prod 2008; 40(3): 223-8. [http://dx.doi.org/10.1007/s11250-007-9084-3] [PMID: 18484125]

[27] Habeeb AA, Ibrahim MKh, Yousef HM. Blood and milk contents of triiodothyronine (T3) and cortisol in lactating buffaloes and changes in milk yield and composition as a function of lactation number and ambient temperature. Arab J Nuclear Sci Applic 2000; 33: 313-22.

[28] Kamal TH, Ibrahim II. The effect of the natural climate of the Sahara and controlled climate on thyroid gland activity in Friesian cattle and water buffaloes. Int J Biometeorol 1969; 13(3): 287-94. [http://dx.doi.org/10.1007/BF01553036] [PMID: 5385715]

[29] Christison GI, Johnson HD. Cortisol turnover in heat-stressed cow. J Anim Sci 1972; 35(5): 1005-10. [http://dx.doi.org/10.2527/jas1972.3551005x] [PMID: 5085291]

[30] Zhengkang H, Zhenzhong C, Shaohua Z, Vale WG, Barnabe VH, Mattos JC. Rumen metabolism, blood cortisol and T3, T4 levels and other physiological parameters of swamp buffalo subjected to solar radiation. Proas World Buffalo Cong. vol. 2San Paulo, Brazil. 1994; pp. : 39-40.

[31] Collier RJ, Dahl GE, VanBaale MJ. Major advances associated with environmental effects on dairy cattle. J Dairy Sci 2006; 89(4): 1244-53. [http://dx.doi.org/10.3168/jds.S0022-0302(06)72193-2] [PMID: 16537957]

[32] Schwimmer H, Eli-Berchoer L, Horowitz M. Acclimatory-phase specificity of gene expression during the course of heat acclimation and superimposed hypohydration in the rat hypothalamus. J Appl Physiol 2006; 100(6): 1992-2003. [http://dx.doi.org/10.1152/japplphysiol.00850.2005] [PMID: 16469936]

[33] Ingram LD, Mount LE. Man and animal in hot environments. In: Schaefer KE, Ed. Topics in Environmental Physiology and Medicine. New York: Springer-Verlag 1975; pp. 64-80.

[34] West JW. Environmental effects on production of lactating dairy cows. J Dairy Sci 2003; 86: 2131-44. [http://dx.doi.org/10.3168/jds.S0022-0302(03)73803-X] [PMID: 12836950]

[35] Chaiyabutr N, Johnson HD. The regulation of body fluids and electrolytes of the buffalo. In: Tsuda T, Sasaki Y, Kawashima R, Eds. Physiological Aspects of Digestion and Metabolism. Academic Press, Inc. 1991; pp. 297-319. [http://dx.doi.org/10.1016/B978-0-12-702290-1.50021-7]

[36] Nair PG, Benjamin BR. Studies on sweat glands in the water buffalo. Indian J Vet Sci 1963; 33(2): 102-6.

[37] Findlay JD, Yang SH. The sweat glands in Ayrshire cattle. J Agric Sci 1950; 40: 126-33. [http://dx.doi.org/10.1017/S0021859600045573]

[38] Ranawana SS, Tilakaratne M, Srikandakumar A. Utilization of water by buffalo in adapting to wet-tropical environment. The use of Nuclear Techniques to Improve Domestic Buffalo Production in Asia. Vienna: IAEA 1984; pp. 171-87.

[39] Goodall AM, Yang SH. Myoepithelial cells in bovine sweat gland. J Agric Sci 1952; 42: 159-61. [http://dx.doi.org/10.1017/S0021859600058755]

[40] Benjamin BR. The thermoregulatory mechanism and its regulation to exocrine glands and skin

structures (histological) in buffalo. In: Buffalo Seminar on Reproduction and Meat Production, Tanaku Andhra Pradesh, India. 1982; pp. 15-7.

[41] Chaiyabutr N, Buranakarl C, Muangcharoen V, Loypetjra P, Pichaicharnarong A. Effects of acute heat stress on changes in the rate of liquid flow from the rumen and turnover of body water of swamp buffalo. J Agric Sci (Camb) 1987; 108: 549-53. [http://dx.doi.org/10.1017/S0021859600079934]

[42] Chikamune T. Effects of environmental temperature on thermoregulatory responses and oxygen consumption in swamp buffalo and Holstein cattle. Buffalo J 1986; l2: 151-60.

[43] Chaiyabutr N, Chanpongsang S, Loypetjra P, Pichaicharnarong A. Effect of heat stress on renal urea excretion of swamp buffalo. In: Shimizu H, Ed. Current Development and Problems in Swamp Buffalo Production. Tsukuba, Japan 1983; pp. 184-90.

[44] Finch VA, Doniel R, Boxman R, Shkolnik A, Taylor CR. Why black goat in hot deserts? Effects of coat color on heat exchange of wild and domestic goat. Physiol Zool 1980; 53: 19-25. [http://dx.doi.org/10.1086/physzool.53.1.30155771]

[45] Rajaratne AA, Ranawana SS, Tilakaratne N, Srikandakumar A. Comparative tolerance of hot-humid climatic conditions by three species (*Bos Taurus, Bos indicus and Bubalus bubalis)* of Bovidae. Sri Lanka Vet J 1983; 31: 21-6.

[46] Chaiyabutr N, Buranakarl C, Loypetjra P, Chanpongsang S. Effects of prolonged exposure to the sun on body water turnover and volume of the blood of the non-shaded swamp buffalo. Asian Aust J Anim Sci 1990; 3(1): 47-52. [http://dx.doi.org/10.5713/ajas.1990.47]

[47] MacFarlane WV. Isotopes and the ecophysiology of tropical livestock. Proceedings of the International Symposium on Use of Isotopes and Radiation in Agriculture and Animal Husbandry. New Delhi. 1971; pp. 805-27.

[48] Ranawana SS, Tilakaratna N, Srikandakumar A. Daily turnover of body water in growing, pregnant, and lactating buffaloes subjected to restriction of water for drinking and wallowing. J Agric Sci (Camb) 1983; 100: 741-3. [http://dx.doi.org/10.1017/S0021859600035553]

[49] Dollah MA, Marsom S, Kamaruddin M, Liang JB. Water balance of swamp buffaloes under different environments open pasture and plantation. Proc of the 5th International Conference on Livestock Production and Diseases in the Tropics. Kuala Lumpur. 1986; pp. 118-20.

[50] Alvarez MB, Johnson HD. Urinary excretion of adrenaline and noradrenaline in cattle during heat and cold exposure. J Dairy Sci 1970; 53(7): 928-30. [http://dx.doi.org/10.3168/jds.S0022-0302(70)86320-2] [PMID: 5426642]

[51] Bardwell RD, Roussel JD, Gomila BF, Shaffer LM. Effect of temperature on aldosterone levels of synchronized Holstein heifers. J Dairy Sci 1977; 60: 1-15. [PMID: 320235]

[52] Thompson RD, Johnston JE, Breidenstein CP, Guidry AJ, Burnett WT. Effect of hot conditions on adrenal cortical, thyroidal and other metabolic responses of dairy heifers. J Dairy Sci 1963; 46: 227-30.

[http://dx.doi.org/10.3168/jds.S0022-0302(63)89011-6]

[53] Kamal TH, Seif SM. Effect of natural and controlled climates of the Sahara on virtual tritium space in Friesians and water buffaloes. J Dairy Sci 1969; 52(10): 1657-63. [http://dx.doi.org/10.3168/jds.S0022-0302(69)86809-8] [PMID: 5372812]

[54] Brown RS. Extrarenal potassium homeostasis. Kidney Int 1986; 30(1): 116-27. [http://dx.doi.org/10.1038/ki.1986.160] [PMID: 3528616]

[55] Clausen T, Flatman JA. Effects of insulin and epinephrine on Na+-K+ and glucose transport in soleus muscle. Am J Physiol 1987; 252(4 Pt 1): E492-9. [PMID: 3031991]

[56] Kaji DM, Thakkar U, Kahn T. Glucocorticoid-induced alterations in the sodium potassium pump of the human erythrocyte. J Clin Invest 1981; 68(2): 422-30. [http://dx.doi.org/10.1172/JCI110271] [PMID: 6267104]

[57] Petty KJ, Kokko JP, Marver D. Secondary effect of aldosterone on Na-KATPase activity in the rabbit cortical collecting tubule. J Clin Invest 1981; 68(6): 1514-21. [http://dx.doi.org/10.1172/JCI110405] [PMID: 6274911]

[58] Kamal TH, Shebaita MK. Climatic effect on Friesians and buffaloes. I. Blood volume using $Na_2^{51} CrO_4$. J Dairy Sci 1968; 51: 970.

[59] Christopherson RJ. The thermal environment and the ruminant digestive system. In: Yousef MK, Ed. Stress Physiology in Livestock. Boca Raton, Florida: CRC Press 1985; Vol. 1: pp. 163-77.

[60] Worstell DM, Brody S. Environmental physiology and shelter engineering with species reference to domestic animals XX Comparative physiological reactions of European and Indian cattle to changing temperature. Mo Agric Exp Sta Res Bull 1953; p. 515.

[61] Attebery JT, Johnson HD. Effects of environmental temperature, controlled feeding and fasting on rumen motility. J Anim Sci 1969; 29(5): 734-7. [http://dx.doi.org/10.2527/jas1969.295734x] [PMID: 5391972]

[62] Engelhardt W, Rubsamen K. Review of the digestive physiology in camelids. IFS Int Symp Camels. Sudan. 1979; pp. 307-19.

[63] Chaiyabutr N, Chanpongsang S, Loypetjra P, Pichaicharnarong A. Renal function studies in normal and heat-stressed swamp buffalo. Proc. 5th WCAP. Tokyo. 1983; pp. 763-4.

[64] Whittow GC. Cardiovascular response to localized heating of the anterior hypothalamus. J Physiol 1968; 198(3): 541-8. [http://dx.doi.org/10.1113/jphysiol.1968.sp008624] [PMID: 5685287]

[65] Hales JR. Effects of exposure to hot environments on the regional distribution of blood flow and on cardiorespiratory function in sheep. Pflugers Arch 1973; 344(2): 133-48. [http://dx.doi.org/10.1007/BF00586547] [PMID: 4797948]

[66] Feistkorn G, Ritter P, Jessen C. Overall cardiovascular adjustments to thermal stress in conscious goats. Pflugers Arch 1981; 391 (Suppl.): R46.

[67] Kanter GS. Heat and excretion in man. J Appl Physiol 1955; 7(5): 533-6. [PMID: 14367242]

[68] Chaiyabutr N, Buranakarl C, Chanpongsang S, Loypetjra P. Changes in renal functions of swamp buffalo during short term exposure to the sun. Inter J Anim Sci 1990; 5: 175-80.

[69] El-Nouty FD, Elbanna IM, Davis TP, Johnson HD. Aldosterone and ADH response to heat and dehydration in cattle. J Appl Physiol 1980; 48(2): 249-55.
[PMID: 7364609]

[70] Collins KJ, Hellmann K, Jones RM, Lunnon JB. Aldosterone activity in the urine of men exposed to heat. J Endocrinol 1955; 13: 80.

[71] Collins KJ, Weiner JS. Endocrinological aspects of exposure to high environmental temperatures. Physiol Rev 1968; 48(4): 785-839.
[PMID: 4881390]

[72] Loypetjra P, Chaiyabutr N, Chanpongsang S, Pichaicharnarong A, Katti P, Johnson HD. Effect of high ambient temperature on serum cortisol, triiodothyronine, prolactin, and growth hormone in swamp buffaloes. Thai J Vet Med 1987; 17: 287-305.

[73] Johnson PC, Selkurt EE. Respiratory and renal regulation of acid-base balance. In: Selkurt EE, Ed. Physiology. Boston, Mass.: Little, Brown 1966; pp. 537-8.

[74] Macfarlane WV, Kinne R, Walmsley CM, Siebert BD, Peter D. Vasopressins and the increase of water and electrolyte excretion by sheep, cattle and camels. Nature 1967; 214(5092): 979-81.
[http://dx.doi.org/10.1038/214979a0] [PMID: 6055413]

[75] Hafez ES. Environmental effect on animal productivity. In: Hafez ESE, (ed), Adaptation of Domestic Animals Philadelphia: Lea & Febiger 1968.

[76] Yousef MK, Johnson HD. Endocrine system and thermal environment. In: Yousef, MK, (ed), Stress Physiology in Livestock, Vol1 Basic Principle Florida, CRC Press Inc 1985; 133-41.

[77] Guerrini VH, Bertchinger H. Effect of exposure to a hot-humid and a hot-dry environment on thyroid hormone values in sheep. Br Vet J 1983; 139(2): 119-28.
[PMID: 6839122]

[78] Voltorta SE, Bober MA, Becker BA, Hahn L, Johnson HD. Hormonal responses in lactating dairy cows during acclimation to and compensation from heat exposure. J Dairy Sci 1980; 63: 83-4.

CHAPTER 6

Feed Resources, Rumen Fermentation, Manipulation and Production in Swamp Buffalo: A Review

Metha Wanapat*, **V. Chanthakhoun**, **R. Pilajun** and **P. Khejornsart**

TROFREC, Faculty of Agriculture Khon Kaen University Khon Kaen 40002, Thailand

Abstract: Swamp buffaloes (*Bubalus bubalis*) are multipurposes and resourceful animals in agriculture of incredible importance among farmers. Within a smallholding farming system, typical of many Asian countries, seasonal feed resources used on swamp buffaloes, are of paramount importance for an efficient production. In fact, during the dry season, when conventional feed resources are usually scarce, their contribution is incredibly relevant. In addition, the utilization of such feed resources may represent an efficient way to reduce methane production through better use of secondary compounds in tropical plants and herbs (tannins, saponins, *etc.*), and consequently improve the overall rumen ecology and finally buffalo productivity. Currently, the development of food-feed systems (FFS) have been successfully implemented and therefore should be fully integrated into the ordinary use by smallholder farmers. However, in order to improve and make more efficient feeding methodologies, both treatments and/or supplementations should be considered, such as the development of simple and practical feeding and the use of concentrate mixtures based on on-farm resources (home-made concentrates, HMC) in order to reduce production costs and enhance profitability and sustainability of the buffalo production. The manipulation of rumen fermentation by treating roughage and/or by supplementing the available feed resources with plants characterized by high quality feed block, tannin/ saponins, especially cassava hay and other local feed resources, could improve rumen efficiency by maintaining a constant higher pH, optimum NH_3-N, and increasing microbial protein synthesis and essential VFAs, and therefore enhancing ruminant productivity in the tropics. Moreover, buffaloes have been shown to be more efficient in feeds utilization, when compared to cattle. Lately, the application of molecular

* **Corresponding author Metha Wanapat:** TROFREC, Faculty of Agriculture Khon Kaen University Khon Kaen 40002, Thailand; Tel: +66 819324180; Fax: +66 202362; E-mail: metha@kku.ac.th

Giorgio A. Presicce (Ed.)

technology to rumen studies, such as the use of PCR-DGGE and real-time PCR, has been instrumental in offering a wide range of information and data on rumen microbial diversity and the likelihood of a possible functional role in reducing rumen methane as well as enhancing productivity in swamp buffaloes.

Keywords: Buffaloes, Feed resources, Feeding, Integrated livestock system, Methane production, Rumen ecology manipulation.

1. INTRODUCTION

Swamp buffaloes are closer to wild ruminants than their bovine counterparts and have played a very important role in providing draught power, manure as fertilizer and meat for people. An important aspect for ruminants within the rumen ecology, that is well established and understood among researchers, is the function of fermentation within the rumen itself that allows the preparation of end-products, and particularly volatile fatty acids (VFAs) as well as microbial proteins, to be used as a major energy and protein drive for the ruminant host. However, crop residues are definitely the main feed resources available to ruminants, usually by-products derived from the agro-industrial productive systems utilizing native grasses from fertile lands, which, in general, support only low levels of production. This is particularly true in the tropics where, both buffaloes and cattle are raised as an integral part of crop production, and where rice is the most important available commodity, from which the related by-products are employed as feeds [1]. Some local feed resources though, like cassava root/hay/silage, corn stover, leucaena leaves, sweet potatoes vines, sugarcane tops, *etc*., can be considered potential additional feed resources for ruminants which are capable to enhance production efficiency. Usually ruminants are fed roughages, like crop residues, such as rice straw, wheat straw, and maize stalk, and from this use, a significant amount of methane is produced and emitted [2]. In the tropical environment, a large amount of plants contain secondary compounds such as saponins, condensed tannins, essential oil, and plant extracts, which are known to effectively inhibit ruminal methanogenesis [3 - 5]. On the other hands, these same forages have been shown to increase protein availability in the small intestine of ruminants [6]. In addition, cassava and legumes usually contain secondary compounds which could have an effect on rumen fermentation and productivity, whereas rumen bacteria can further detoxify these compounds. It has been reported by Hegarty [7] that a significant reduction of methane production per gram of live weight gain is achieved when animals are shifted from a low to a high digestible pasture.

Due to the lowering of world prices for plant commodities and the projected future increase of animal products caused by higher demands [8], it is possible that a realistic objective may be given by the contribution of food-feed system (FFS) to ruminant production, particularly when in need to review their overall high nutritive values, the positive effects on rumen, as well as the expansion and intensification of these systems. It has to be emphasized that FFS has received over time more and more attention and interest by farmers working within a smallholding system. Historically, the majority of knowledge on rumen microbial composition has been acquired by employing traditional methods such as roll tube technique [9] or most probable-number (MPN) estimates [10]. Some microorganisms though, cannot be cultivated under current technology, although their artificial culture represents only a small fraction of natural microbial communities, and as a consequence, the microbial diversity is grossly under-estimated [11].

Nowadays, microbial diversity found in complex ecosystems like the rumen, has been studied using new gene-based technologies [12]. Both DGGE and real time PCR are culture independent techniques that target that part of DNA encoding the synthesis of small subunit ribosomal RNA (SSU rDNA), which allow a direct analysis and quantification of microorganisms of interest [13]. Such data can offer very useful information and provide the possible functional roles of microorganism themselves in the rumen of swamp buffaloes.

2. SEASONAL FEEDING SYSTEMS FOR RUMINANTS

A seasonal approach to ruminant feeding in a tropical environment can be split into a dry and a rainy seasons, although a reduced productivity can be reported due to an improper feeding supply and regimen with regard to both quantity and quality [14]. Despite its low nutritive value, rice straw has been typically used during the dry season as an ordinary feeding approach, generally practiced by smallholder farmers when green forages are often scarce [15]. Available local feed resources have been recommended for use under smallholder farming [16]. In tropical areas, ruminants feed largely on unrestricted grazing, which is usually free under herder control in countries with available grasslands and fallow. On the contrary, wherever land and cropping are of limited availability, tethering and stall-feeding are usually practiced, due to a limitation in roughage under many circumstances. There have been situations, like on some dairy farms in northeast Thailand, where an excess in concentrate feeding has been practiced as a compensation for the relatively low availability of roughages [17, 18]. To improve the low quality of some feeds, containing poor essential nutritive elements, like some roughages and crop residues, some treatment methods and/or supplementation have to be taken under consideration. In this regard, three different methodologies have to be considered: physical, chemical and biological. Inevitably, the use and suitability of each of the three methodologies is dependent on the geographical and environmental location linked to the typology of animal production, length of crop availability and its economical viability, its technological feasibility, together with farmers perception and acceptance. In this context, some experiments were carried out in order to compare energy value and digestibility of rice straw when subjected to different treatments [19, 20].

Some significant differences were reported in buffaloes when rice straw was treated with urea and used as roughage, and particularly when supplemented concentrate was employed and compared to untreated rice straw [21].

3. SWAMP BUFFALO PRODUCTION AND FOOD-FEED SYSTEM (FFS)

Foods for the human species and feeds for animal production have been derived from the food-feed system. It is interesting to note that intercropping with legumes has the benefit to enrich the soil with nitrogen, as some interventions have proved. Some examples follow:

3.1. Cassava (*Manihot esculenta*, Crantz) and Cowpea (*Vigna unculata*)

Wanapat *et al.* [22] reported that the yield of cassava foliage, when intercropped with legume as intercropping crops, gives an average of 4.35 ton DM/ha of cassava foliage to produce hay (cassava hay) by harvesting 4 times throughout the year. Cowpea residue and intercropped legume produced 5.96 ton/ha of green cowpea pod and 1.51 ton/DM/ha. It was found that productivities of intercrops were improved with biomass of 6.83 ton DM/ha of cassava foliage, and 0.89 ton DM/ha of cowpea residues. In addition, a legume, Stylosanthes, was also intercropped in the cassava plot, and it produced 3.51 to DM/ha. The intercropping methodology of cassava/legumes can improve farm productivity and enhance an autonomous on-farm feed resources availability. Some farmers though, have been facing some problems when drying hay during the rainy season, and therefore some additional and possibly alternative strategies have to be suggested to farmers and implemented such as the construction of solar-drying houses by utilizing easily found material like plastic sheet and bamboo. One of the results of the food-feed system, highlighting its feasibility and efficiency, can be seen in the use of green cowpea for human consumption, as a gift for the neighbours or sold for additional income, whereas cowpea residues and Stylosanthes fodder may be used as feeds for animals. (FFS) [23].

3.2. Cassava and Stylo (*Stylosanthes guyanensis*)

Stylosanthes guyanensis is a perennial legume, characterized by being semi-erect to erect to prostrate, introduced in the lower midland three (LM3) agro-ecological zone as a fodder legume, which can be continuously or rotationally grazed. Kiyothong and Wanapat [24] have reported a potential additional strategy for small-holder dairy farming in the tropics, by feeding cassava hay solely or in combination to *Stylosanthes guyanensis* CIAT 184 hay, as a supplemental protein source. This strategic supplementation has significantly reduced the use of concentrate, resulting in improved milk yields and quality. In addition, lowering the ratio of concentrate to milk yield from 1:2 to 1:3, has increased productivity and higher economical return.

3.3. Cassava and *Phaseolus calcaratus* (TUA-MUN)

Legumes have been considered to be suitable crops to enrich soil nitrogen and for producing high protein foods and feeds for human beings and animals, respectively. In fact [25]. *Phaseolus calcaratus* (PC) has been found to be a potential plant to improve foliage biomass, CT and crude protein yield [26]. It is well established that legumes are important crops to be used for intercropping and producing hay as feed for animals, whereas at the same time seeds can be considered a valuable protein source for human consumption (FFS). A high protein content can be found in *Phaseolus calcaratus* (PC: 17-20.4% in DM), to be used for ruminant nutrition, with a biomass yield of 1.9 tonnes DM/ha and a CP which is 18.1% of DM; an NDF of 42% and an ADF which is 36.1% of DM, and the capacity of growing in poor soils and dry areas. Preliminary studies on PC have reported a growth up to a height of about 60 cm at fully blooming, and can produce pods at about 3 to 4 months. Hay from PC can be produced from the entire PC crop following sun-drying in about 2 to 3 days, and usually the first hay harvest from the foliage is made three months after planting. Soil fertility is enriched if inter-cropping of leguminous fodder as food-feed with PC is made, providing in addition supplemental fodder. Some trials on the use of PC for nutrition in buffaloes have been carried out, and they have revealed a high level of DM intake (2.4% of BW), high DM digestibility (71%) and apparent digestibility OM (75.2%). Condensed tannins (2-3% CT) were generally found in lower concentrations in matured PC leaf, although levels were higher in PC harvested at a younger stage. A study by Reed [27] has revealed that if condensed tannins in the feed exceed 6% of DM, a reduction in feed intake and digestibility will be witnessed. Moreover, protein will be protected from rumen digestion if the CT level is found between 2 to 4% of DM, increasing thus the amount of by pass protein. As intercrop, PC should be planted with cassava in the FFS: in fact, this is very likely the best method to improve soil enrichment and in addition enhance crop biomass and protein value. Furthermore, to underline the importance of PC as a valuable intercrop legume, this plant has a high crude protein in DM and an even high proportion of by pass protein [28, 29]. It is possible that such a high level of by pass protein found in this legume may be linked to the content of tannins, having the characteristic to bind to the proteins and making them unavailable to the rumen microorganisms. An increase in maize grain yield has been reported by Agboola and Fayami [30] when compared to control group of plant, when *Phaseolus aureus* (mungbean) was inter planted with the maize. Nitrogen transfer from legumes to maize was found to be equivalent to 45 kg N/ha. The apparent digestibility coefficients of dry matter were 42 and 51% for wheat straw and legume hay, respectively. From these data, it can be estimated that if an adequate amount of hay from such legumes can be produced, then ruminant nutrition will be greatly improved. From the amount of legume produced under a given intercropping system, will depend the increase in digestibility of cereal residue.

4. RUMEN ECOLOGY, FERMENTATION AND CONTRIBUTING FACTORS

The main source of protein supply in ruminants is given by the amount of synthesized microbial protein in the rumen, representing 50 to 80% of the total protein absorbed [31]. The limiting nutritional factors of microbial growth within the rumen are given by the rumen availability of energy and nitrogen [32]. The energy for the synthesis of microbial protein and microbial growth is mainly derived from dietary carbohydrate. Whenever non structural carbohydrates (NSC) are in high proportion in the diet and the ruminal pH is favorable, microorganisms fermenting this substrate will grow rapidly, resulting in increased microbial production. On the other hand, if the accumulation of lactic acid reaches a threshold, a drastic reduction in pH occurs, and with it a change in microbial ecology and dry matter intake [33]. Rumen fermentation and the growth of living bacteria inside it, may be affected by two other major factors, namely: the rumen pH, which may depress the growth of rumen bacteria, especially cellulolytic bacteria and methanogenic Archaea, when it is found below 6.2, and the passage rate, as a differentiation is seen in microbial diversity and growth of microbial cells. When the dilution rate is increased and due to the high renewal rate, some microorganisms with shorter generation will be selected, causing an output of rumen microorganisms characterized by lower growth rates, and therefore increasing microbial efficiency on readily available carbohydrates. In turn, such path is affected on the level of consumption of animal feed, particle size, proportion and quality of the type of forage and the processing of carbohydrates [32, 34 - 36]. According to Waldo and Glen [37], since rumen microorganisms reach the highest efficiency in terms of protein synthesis, then dietary proteins should be supplied as to meet the corresponding microbial needs, once no limitation on energy source and other factors is in force. In order to reach the most efficient use of proteins within the tissues, protein request and demands from the tissues themselves have to be the sum of both dietary non degraded rumen proteins and microbial proteins, qualitatively and quantitatively. With regard to the quantification of microbial protein synthesis in the rumen from microbial fermentation, this has to take into account both population growth and microbial biomass [38]. However, intracellular ammonia of rumen bacteria was highly correlated with rumen NH_3-N and microbial protein synthesis as shown in Fig. (**1**), and declined when NH_3-N was less than 5 mg/dl and unfermented carbohydrates increased. It was also found that intracellular NH_3-N was at least 1.6 mg/dl higher than the extracellular concentration [39]. Song and Kennelly [40] demonstrated that in non lactating Holstein cows on a silage diet, increasing levels of rumen NH_3-N, up to 15.7 mg/dl, significantly increased mixed bacterial numbers and their fermentation patterns, but not the extent of ruminal degradation of feeds. In sheep fed on citrus pulp and Italian ryegrass hay (33% NDF), increasing rumen NH_3-N did not improve OM digestion, VFA concentrations and profiles and microbial protein synthesis [41]. Lactating Holstein cows receiving alfalfa silage, maintaining rumen NH_3-N at a high level (18.7-22.9 mg/dl) and plasma urea N (15.0-20.4 mg/dl), could achieve high milk yield (31.1-32.7 kg/hd/d) [42]. Furthermore, Wanapat and Pimpa [43] reported rumen NH_3-N at 15–30 mg %, which resulted in optimal rumen fermentation and decreasing protozoa population.

The amount of microbial proteins synthesized in the rumen, has been estimated up to 13% of the digestion of the total digestible nutrients (TDN), in beef cattle by NRC (2001). With regard to lactating cattle, Reynal and Broderick [44], given an RDP from 10.6 to 13.2% from DM, have reported a positive linear effect on protein synthesis, with the highest yield observed at 12.3% of RDP. Such data collected in cattle, have yet to be determined effectively in buffaloes, although the minimum concentration of NH_3-N not affecting microbial synthesis has been measured as being 5 mg/100 mL in the rumen fluid [45]. Erdman *et al.* [46] suggested that in order to have the maximum digestion and microbial growth, the minimum concentration of ammonia nitrogen, increases with the fermentability of the diet. In fact, the rapid disappearance of ammonia will be caused by the absorption by the rumen wall or its use by microorganisms. Variable ammonia concentration in the rumen has been measured. The peak NH_3- N concentration in the buffalo rumen has been observed to occur within two hours after the diet [47] with different levels of NDF and obtained an overall average of 21. 5 mg rumen ammonia concentration, whereas two hours after feeding was 31.76 mg. Wanapat and Pimpa [43] have suggested that in swamp buffaloes a value of 14 mg of ruminal ammonia as being optimal, and several studies have confirmed the relationship between protein production and excretion of purine derivatives in urine [48]. A simple and non invasive method to estimate microbial protein production in the rumen is by assessing excretion of purine derivatives (PD) in the urine. This methodology implicitly gives the assumption that the nucleic acids within the duodenum are predominantly of microbial origin, and therefore following intestinal digestion of purine nucleotides, absorbed purines are inevitably catabolized and recovered proportionally in the urine as derivatives of purines.

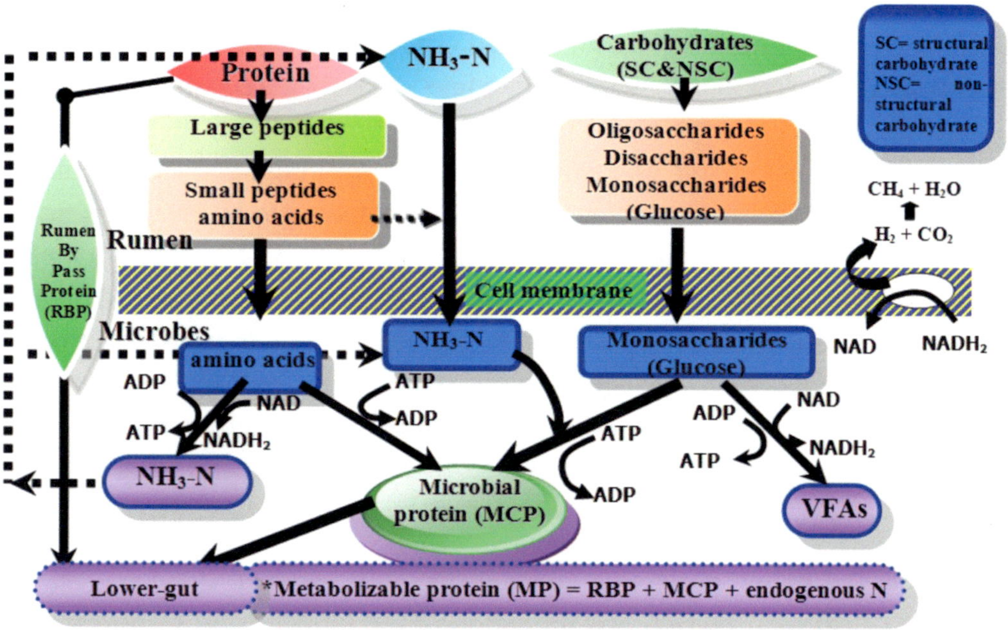

Fig. (1). Energy and protein metabolism in the rumen microbial protein synthesis Source: Modified from [54].

The possibility to predict microbial protein production in cattle, goats, sheep and camels is a reliable procedure, as PD excretion is closely related to protein production following digestion of microbial nucleic acids in the small intestine.

On the contrary, in buffaloes such methodology is not as efficient, because PD excretion is lower than in other species [49 - 52]. Pimpa *et al.* [53] observed that the daily urinary excretion in buffaloes allantoin, uric acid and total purine derivatives were 215.9 mol/ kg BW0.75, 63.4 mol/kg BW0.75 and 279.4 mol/kg BW0.75, respectively.

5. URINARY PURINE DERIVATIVES IN SWAMP BUFFALOES

Recent studies were conducted to investigate the effect of roughage to concentrate ratio [55] in swamp buffaloes using PCR-DGGE and Real-time PCR technique. Under this study, methanogenic bacterial diversity were found and population of predominant cellulolytic bacteria were found with higher population of *F.succinogenes*, *R. flavefaciens* and *R. albus* in both rumen digesta and fluid, respectively. Chen *et al.* [56] carried out a comprehensive study regarding a specific comparison between buffaloes and cattle on urinary excretion of purine derivatives (PD) and tissue xanthine oxidase. From these studies, xanthine oxidases were found in plasma, liver and intestinal tissues, respectively and patterns of PD (allantoin and uric acid) excreted were similar between buffalo and cattle. It was also reported by Liang *et al.* [57] that swamp buffalo significantly excreted less urinary allantoin and total purine derivative as compared to those of Malaysian Kedah cattle. In connection with this regard, it was clearly shown that difference in purine derivative excretion in buffalo was due to a lower glomerular filtration rate (GFR). As a consequence, such compounds will spend more time in the blood and will be recycled more into the rumen and therefore metabolized by microorganisms, or alternatively the blood-to-rumen permeability is greater in buffalo than cattle, in contrast with earlier work by Pimpa *et al.* [53].

For animals fed below maintenance level, the link between duodenal input of purine and urinary PD output, is a reflection of the biochemical feedback on the *de novo* synthesis process by the salvage of absorbed exogenous purine by tissues [59] rather than exogenous absorption. However, the excretion of urinary purine derivatives (PD; *i.e.*, allantoin and uric acid) may constitute an alternative noninvasive technique based on the principle that the bulk urinary PD is derived from microbial nucleic acid flowing out from rumen. Several authors [56, 60 - 62] have confirmed the relationship between the duodenal supply of RNA and the urinary excretion of PD, although such a relationship is usually obscured by an endogenous fraction coming from the turnover of nucleic acid in tissues and the incomplete urinary recovery of infused purines.

6. COMPARATIVE NUTRITIONAL STUDIES BETWEEN BUFFALOES AND CATTLE

Wanapat *et al.* [63] reported that swamp buffaloes and a crossbreed (Brahman native) were fistulated and randomly assigned to receiving rice straw ad libitum together with or without supplementation of concentrate at 0.3% of body weight, and some significant differences between the two species were reported. In fact, in buffaloes, rumen pH, bacteria and fungal zoospores were higher in content, whereas protozoa were found lower ($P < 0.05$). In addition, in buffaloes, diurnal ruminal NH_3-N concentrations were consistently higher than cattle, and this affected nutrient digestibility, in particular of CP and fibrous digestibility (NDF, ADF). In the same experiment, it was shown that a real-time polymerase chain reaction approach was able to determine the population of cellulolytic bacteria (*Fibrobacter succinogenes, Ruminococcus albus,* and *Ruminococcus flavefaciens*) in digesta and rumen fluid of swamp buffalo (*Bubalus bubalis*) and beef cattle. It was found that the applicability of real-time PCR techniques for the quantification of cellulolytic bacterial numbers (*R. albus*, and *R. flavefaciens*) in the digesta of swamp were higher than cattle. However, at 4h *R.albus* were significantly higher in buffalo than cattle in rumen fluid, but *R. flavefaciens* and *F.succinogenes* tended to be higher in cattle than in buffalo in the rumen fluid. However, the digesta sample had higher cellulolytic bacteria than those found in the rumen fluid. This finding indicates higher ability of buffalo in digesting low-quality roughages. In the tropics, the majority of ruminants are fed on low quality forage, agricultural crop residues and industrial byproducts containing reduced availability of good quality proteins, high level of cellulosic components, low level of fermentable carbohydrate. Moreover, harsh environments characterize long dry seasons, with high temperature, low soil fertility together with reduced feed availability throughout the year. All this will impact negatively on rumen microorganisms and fermentation processes [64, 65]. Furthermore, Wanapat [66] highlighted the importance of local feed resources to be used as animal feed and enhancing rumen fermentation, and as a consequence ruminant productivity in the tropics. It was also reported that in swamp buffaloes, nitrogen utilization is more efficient than in Malaysian cattle [67], especially in particular environmental conditions when feed supply is low in quantity and/or quality. The reasons behind a higher capacity of buffaloes over cattle has not been fully elucidated, although it is likely that such difference may be attributed to the nature of rumen microbial population which in turn is responsible for the efficiency and type of fermentation. Therefore, the difference in digestive efficiency derived by the fermentation of end-products available for absorption and follow up utilization, is a reflection of the variations found in cattle and buffaloes in the proportions of ruminal bacteria, protozoa and fungi. Wora-anu *et al.* [68], on the same line, reported a significant higher amount of ruminal cellulolytic, proteolytic and amylolytic bacteria in swamp buffaloes in comparison to cattle fed similar diets. Another study focusing on a direct comparison among native beef cattle, dairy cattle and swamp buffaloes, revealed significant differences related to a higher content of bacteria (1.61 $x10^{10}$, 1.54 $x10^{10}$ and 2.15 $x10^{10}$ respectively), fungal zoospores (7.80 $x10^{6}$, 4.54 $x10^{6}$ and 15.13 $x10^{6}$ respectively) and lower protozoa (5.15 $x10^{5}$, 5.61 $x10^{5}$ and 2.00 $x10^{5}$ respectively) population in swamp buffaloes when compared to other species [69]. This results confirmed efficient rumen ecology of swamp buffaloes characterized by enhanced and better feed utilization. Bacteria, like *F.succinogenes*, *R. albus* and *R. flavefaciens* are the most important cellulolytic ruminal bacteria, and bacteria in general can be considered the predominant form of microorganisms in the rumen, playing an instrumental role in the degradation of dietary fiber [70, 71]. Some recently developed molecular biology procedures, allow the analysis of the above mentioned bacteria without the need of cultivating them, and giving thus the possibility to identify a number of functional bacteria to be used as target for basic and applied research.

A brief report concluded that when swamp buffaloes receive various rations of roughage to concentrate (R:C), *F.succinogenes* is the highest in population followed by *R. flavefaciens* and *R. albus* measured in rumen digesta and fluid, using Real-time PCR, respectively [72]. Under this study, *F.succinogenes* was found highest in the digesta, and the three cellulolytic bacterial values were 3.21 $x10^{9}$, 4.55 $x10^{7}$, and 4.44 $x10^{6}$ copies/ml for *F.succinogenes*, *R. flavefaciens*, and *R. albus*, respectively.

7. TREATMENT METHODS OF CROP-RESIDUES AND LOW-QUALITY ROUGHAGES

There are many feed resources and low-quality roughage, crop-residues and industrial by-products available in many regions, and especially in the tropics. However, their nutritive values are relatively low, thus any treatment methods are generally required for utilization improvements. In Fig. (**2**), details of the treatment methods are shown. There are a number of development strategies pertinent to feeding and nutrition. Increasing the total feed supply base is of the highest priority since lactating animals require high quality feeds in adequate amounts. This need to be coupled to more complete utilization of existing feeds, and more efforts to be done to cultivate forage on existing land, including waysides and rice bunds. Such fodders as Napier grass; *Pennisetum purpureum*, Guinea grass; *Panicum maximum* and Signal grass; *Brachiaria decumbens*, Ruzi grass, *Brachiaria ruziziensis* and pigeon pea; *Cajanus cajan,* are valuable. In many part of Asia, inadequate production and utilization of the feed resources from the land, rather than limitation in the availability of land *per se*, represents the principal obstacle to high productivity from farm animal and viability of small farm systems. Considerable opportunity exists for increased production of feed from land that has been inadequately cultivated, including the utilization of dry matter yield in the undergrowth of tree crops. More complete use of the available on-farm crop-by-products, an agroindustrial by products is also important [73]. Systems proposed to increase the feed for small holder farmer include backyard pasture establishment and a three-strata-forage (grass-shrub-tree plant) system in an attempts to ensure continuous supply of feeds throughout the year.

In recent years, consideration and attention has been given to improving the feeding value of fibrous agricultural residues and by-product as well as supplementation strategies. A schematic outline of the treatment is illustrated in Fig. (**2**). Quantity and quality of feed resources in the tropics have been limited by seasonality and their nutritive values [14, 73, 74]. Minson [75] has presented a comprehensive coverage of the differences of nutritive value between the tropical and temperate areas in regards to carrying lower protein, metabolizable energy and inertial content, higher fibrous fraction and containing various toxic compounds [76]. However, due to the enormous amount of crop residues available in developing countries, the potential use of these resources have been presented [74, 77 - 79]. Fibrous agricultural residues contain a large pool of structural carbohydrate which can be potentially degraded by rumen microbes into volatile fatty acids. These are the most important disadvantages encountered in the utilization of these resources as feeds. Therefore, proper treatments and/or supplementation are needed to overcome the shortfalls and to improve feeding efficiency [14, 77, 80].

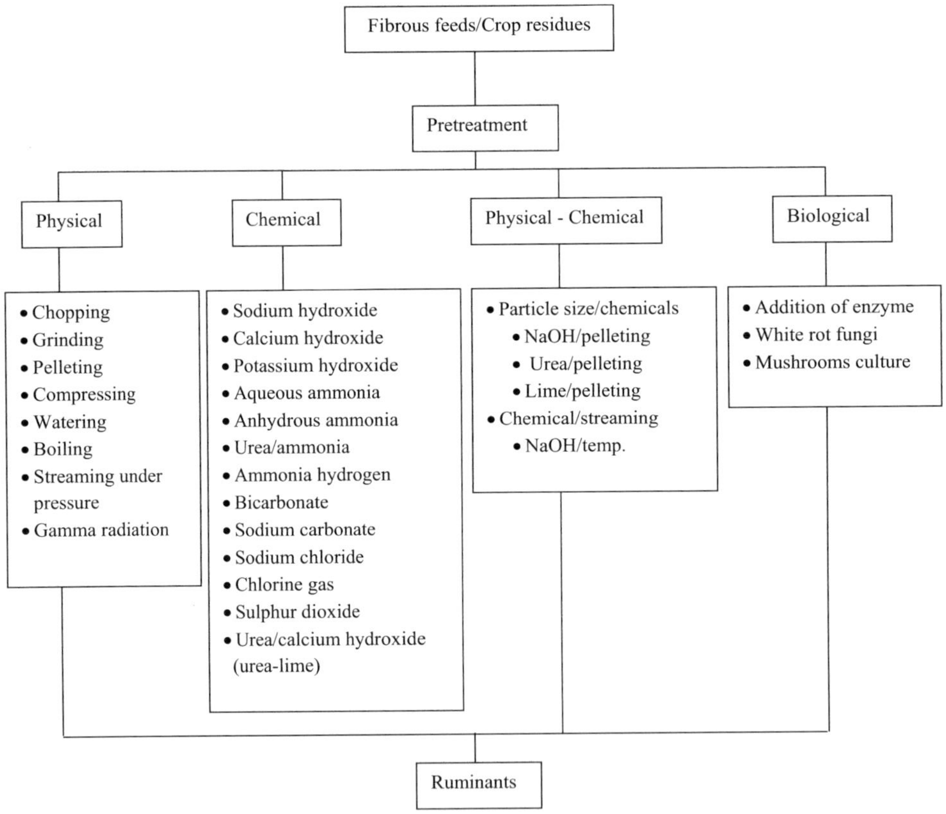

Fig. (2). Treatment methods of crop-residues and low-quality roughages.

8. ROLE OF TANNINS AND SAPONINS ON RUMEN FERMENTATION (FIG. 3)

Plant secondary metabolites such as saponins and tannins (hydrolyzable and condensed) have been extensively assessed for their antimicrobial effects and their potential to modulate ruminal fermentation and improve nutrient utilization in ruminants [81]. Tannins are a complex group of polyphenolic compounds found in a wide range of plant species commonly consumed by ruminants, and are usually classified into two major groups: the hydrolysable and the condensed tannins. For a long time, tannins have been considered to be detrimental to ruminants, although their beneficial or harmful effect may be linked to a number of factors like the type of tannin consumed, its chemical structure and molecular weight, the amount ingested, and the animal species involved. It has been shown that voluntary feed intake and nutrient digestibility are reduced by high concentration of tannins in the diet, whereas the digestive utilization of feed is enhanced by the assumption of low to moderate concentrations of tannins, possibly due to a reduction in protein degradation in the rumen and a subsequent increase in amino acid flow to the small intestine [82]. With regard to saponins, only a limited amount of information is available on their effect on rumen bacteria (Fig. **3**), although an effect on rumen bacteria from condensed tannins/saponins is in place, according to evidence from *in vitro* and *in vivo* cultures. Newbold *et al.* [83] showed that *S. sesban* foliage and *Y.sichidigera* extract, respectively, increased total number of bacteria. This effect seems to be dependent upon the type of saponin and the bacteria species. A significant increase in rumen cellulolytic and total bacteria in sheep fed with *S. saponaria* was reported by Diaz *et al.* in an *in vivo* study [84]. Differently, following 14 h of exposure to saponin, *Y. schidigera*, *Ruminococcus albus* and *Ruminococcus flavefaciens*, but not *Fibrobacter succinogenes*, were found unable to digest cellulose in a study by Wang *et al.* [85]. In another study by Wina *et al.* [86] cellulolytic activity decreased, suggesting that not all the cellulolytic species of bacteria had been taken into consideration, or else that saponins had the effect of decreasing the activity without though a drop in the number of bacteria themselves.

Lately, some interest has been evidenced on the potential effect of saponins on methanogenic archaea and rumen methane production, considering the detrimental effect of saponins on protozoa and that around 25% of ruminal methanogens live in association with protozoa [83], Moreover, Poungchompu *et al.* [87] reported the use of two different strategics consisting in a i) two roughage-to-concentrate ratio (R:C, 70:30 and 30:70), and two different levels of supplementation with soapberry fruit-mangosteen peel (SM) pellet (0 and 4% tannins-saponins of the total diets). As a roughage source, rice straw was chosen, and the diet was given to animals ad libitum as a total mixed ration. SM pellets contained crude tannins and saponins at 12.1 and 15.7% of DM, respectively. It was found that at R:C 30:70 the DM intake and the digestibility of DM, CP and NDF were increased, while SM pellet supplementation reduced the DM digestibility, and ruminal pH was decreased. Following a high increase of SM pellet supplementation, total VFA and propionate increased, whereas simultaneously the acetate concentration and the acetate-to-propionate ratios decreased. Methane production decreased at R:C 30:70, and even more when SM pellets were supplemented. This was in agreement with the percentage of methanogens in total ruminal DNA.

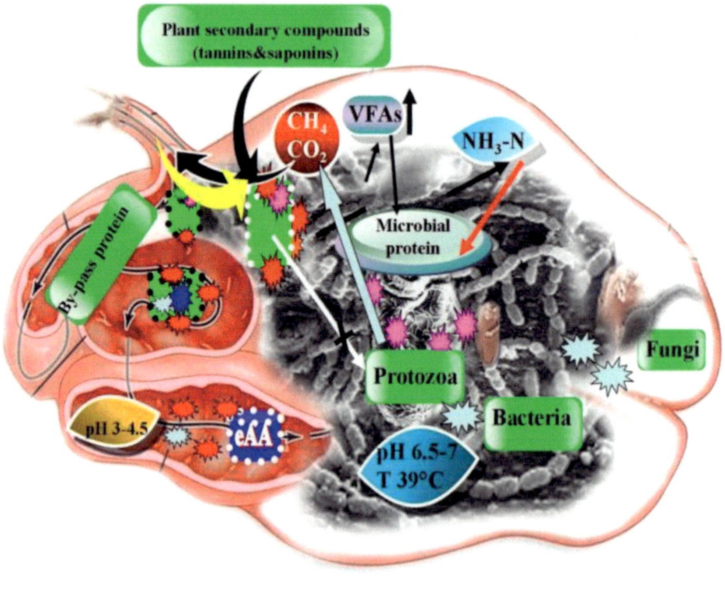

Fig. (3). Plant secondary compounds (tannins & saponins) and rumen fermentation.

In addition, when the same high concentrate proportion was given (R:C 30:70) as well as with SM pellet supplementation, fungal zoospores were reduced, and with SM pellet supplementation also protozoal populations lowered. It can be concluded that in this study, both the roughage-to-concentrate ratio and SM pellet supplementation, may cause changes in ruminal microorganisms and their fermentation end products.

On a different note, it has been shown that meat and milk derived from ruminants contain a number of fatty acids, like CLA which are characterized by exerting beneficial biological properties in mammals. In fact, the cis-9, trans-11 CLA (rumenic acid, RA) has been shown to reduce the incidence of cancer [88], diabetes [89], and atherosclerosis [90]. The CLA content of meat and milk is strongly linked to the ruminal biohydrogenation (BH) of cis-9, cis-12 C18:2 (linoleic acid, LA) and cis-9, cis-12, cis-15 C18:3 (linolenic acid, LNA). During BH, LA and LNA are gradually isomerized and saturated to form several 18 carbon diene and monoene isomer intermediates; the final product of this pathway is C18:0 (stearic acid, SA [91]. The rate and the extent of this pathway are strongly dependent on the diet of the animal [92]. Moreover, RA can also be formed endogenously in the muscle or in the mammary gland from trans-11 C18:1 (vaccenic acid, VA) through the action of Δ9-desaturase enzyme [93].

Another effect that dietary tannins may exert on feeds, is the interference with digestive activities by binding to dietary proteins and by reducing the activity of ruminal microorganisms [94], in addition to reduce ruminal BH *in vitro* [95, 96] and increase muscle Δ9-desaturase protein expression [96] in sheep.

9. USING TROPICAL PLANTS AND HERBS TO IMPROVE RUMEN FERMENTATION AND REDUCE METHANE PRODUCTION

In Tables **1** and **2**, chemical compositions of local feedstuffs and effects of plant secondary compounds and plant oil on rumen fermentation end products are shown, respectively. Total VFAs was affected only by garlic powder and mangosteen peel powder, and a significantly lower ($P<0.05$) total VFAs with respect to a control group was reported following supplementation with 16 mg of garlic powder in an *in vitro* study, although an *in vivo* study was not affected similarly [97, 98]. Newbold *et al.* [99] and Benchaar *et al.* [81], reported a similar outcome in an *in vivo* study on essential oil and rumen fermentation. On the same topic, Whilst [97] reported a linear reduction on total VFAs ($P = 0.08$) following increased supplementation with garlic at 40, 80 and 120 g/h/d. Similarly, in an *in vivo* study a significant increase ($P<0.05$) on total VFAs concentration following mangosteen peel powder was reported, differently from what shown by Ngamsaeng *et al.* [100] in a similar study performed in beef cattle. However, the effects of condensed tannins supplementation were reported to decrease total

VFAs [101], whereas, the effect of condensed tannins plus saponin showed that total VFAs was significantly (P <0.05) increased when supplemented with both compounds [87]. A significant reduction in total VFAs concentration (P<0.05) was reported following use of plant oil supplementation, but not when using 16 mg of supplementation of coconut oil in an *in vitro* study, similarly to results derived from a combined supplementation of plant oil and garlic powder [98, 102].

Table 1. Chemical composition of local feed resources.

Substrate	DM	CP	NDF	ADF	CT*	CS*	References
Mangosteen peel	93.0	18.3	56.8	51.3	16.8	10.0	Ngamsaeng *et al.* (2006)
Guava leaf	91.0	10.1	54.0	29.1	15.8	2.8	
Siam neem leaf	89.0	14.9	52.1	30.0	11.4	2.8	
Sesbania leaf	89.5	28.0	27.4	14.6	4.6	2.0	
Sugar apple leaf	90.1	18.6	49.9	23.1	3.8	nd	
Star gooseberry leaf	89.3	17.4	54.1	28.9	3.4	nd	
Coral leaf	87.2	19.2	50.5	31.1	2.6	1.8	
Bai yanang	90.5	16.4	62.3	37.1	2.3	1.3	
Cassava hay	88.9	21.7	54.0	31.2	2.2	1.7	
Bitter cucumber	85.8	1.3	50.9	30.1	2.1	4.1	
Banana leaf	89.4	13.8	78.2	35.6	1.7	1.3	
Mulberry leaf	87.1	15.2	56.6	18.6	1.6	2.3	
Pak kayaeng	87.6	14.9	63.1	53.8	0.7	1.3	
Fresh banana fruit	83.4	2.3	45.4	11.3	nd	1.9	
Indian mulberry fruit	88.8	7.1	49.8	39.9	nd	3.1	
Banana flower	89.2	12.4	68.5	52.8	nd	nd	
Rice straw	90.6	3.0	85.6	53.2	nd	nd	
Lemongrass powder	93.5	1.3	66.3	42.7	no	no	Wanapat *et al.* (2008a)
Garlic powder	93.0	19.2	6.5	5.1	no	no	Kongmun *et al.* (2010b)
Soap berry tree fruit	no	no	no	no	no	20.1	Poungchompu *et al.* (2009)

* CT = Condensed tannins, CS = Crude saponins, nd = not detectable and no = not observed.

Table 2. Effects of plant secondary compounds and plant oil on ruminal volatile fatty acid production in various studies.

Substrates	Level	Total VFAs	Acetate	Propionate	Butyrate	C2:C3	Animal	References
		(mM)	(mol/100 mol)					
***In vitro* study**								
Bitter cucumber	200 mg	88.0	57.6	34.6	77.7	1.6	Steer (rumen fluid)	Ngamsaeng *et al.* (2006)
Banana leaf	200 mg	72.8	58.6	34.1	7.2	1.7	Steer (rumen fluid)	Ngamsaeng *et al.* (2006)
Guava leaf	200 mg	59.5	52.1	31.3	16.4	1.6	Steer (rumen fluid)	Ngamsaeng *et al.* (2006)
Mangosteen peel powder	200 mg	80.6	59.9	33.8	6.1	1.7	Steer (rumen fluid)	Ngamsaeng *et al.* (2006)
Garlic powder	16 mg	(-) 160.9	(-) 54.0	(+) 33.1	(+) 12.9	(-) 1.6	Buffalo (rumen fluid)	Kongmun *et al.* (2010)
Coconut oil	16 mg	(+)195.4	60.3	28.8	10.8	(+) 2.1	Buffalo (rumen fluid)	Kongmun *et al.* (2010)
***In vivo* study**								
Mangosteen peel powder	100g/h/d	90.3	60.9	24.5	14.4	2.6	Beef cattle	Ngamsaeng *et al.* (2006)
Mangosteen peel powder	100g/h/d	(+) 106.1	(-) 65.2	(+) 23.0	11.8	(-) 2.8	Native beef cattle	Kongmun *et al.* (2009)
Soapberry tree fruit	100g/h/d	102.9	(-) 64.2	(+) 23.5	12.3	(-) 2.7	Native beef cattle	Kongmun *et al.* (2009)
Lemongrass powder	100 g/h/d	114.1	67.7	24.1	8.3	2.8	Beef cattle	Wanapat *et al.* (2008a)
Garlic powder	80g/h/d	98.0	63.3	(+) 23.4	13.3	(-) 2.8	Steer	Wanapat *et al.* (2008b)
Coconut oil	7%	(-) 96.6	66.1	21.4	(+) 12.5	3.1	Native beef cattle	Kongmun *et al.* (2009)
Coconut oil	7%	(-) 93.1	(+) 65.4	(+) 27.2	6.9	(-) 2.4	Buffalo	Kongmun *et al.* (2010a)
Sunflower oil	6%	(-) 99.6	66.7	22.8	10.5	2.9	Buffalo	Wanapat *et al.* (2009)

(Table 2) contd.....

Substrates	Level	Total VFAs	Acetate	Propionate	Butyrate	C2:C3	Animal	References
		(mM)	(mol/100 mol)					
Combination								
Coconut oil + Sunflower oil	6%	(-) 102.9	(+) 68.4	(-) 20.0	11.7	(+) 3.5	Buffalo	Wanapat *et al.* (2009)
Coconut oil: Garlic powder	8:4 (mg)	(-) 167.6	55.1	32.5	12.4	(-) 1.7	Buffalo (rumen fluid)	Kongmun *et al.* (2010b)
Coconut oil + Garlic powder	7% + 100g	(-) 89.9	(-) 65.7	(+) 27.1	7.2	(-) 2.4	Buffalo	Kongmun *et al.* (2010a)

(+) = The value is significantly higher (p <0.05) than control group.
(-) = The value is significantly lower (p <0.05) than control group.

A significant decrease (P<0.05) in the proportion of acetate production was reported when garlic powder, mangosteen peel powder and soapberry fruit powder were used, differently from the use solely of plant oil supplementation. Furthermore, acetate production was again significantly reduced (P<0.05) following a combined of 7% coconut oil and 100 g of garlic powder, as well as plant powder supplementation.

The proportion of propionate production was also affected by a supplementation of garlic powder, mangosteen peel powder, soap berry fruit powder, coconut oil, as well as a combined supplementation with coconut oil and garlic powder. On the same topic, a significant decrease (P<0.05) in propionate production was reported following a combined use of 6% coconut oil and sunflower oil, whereas only the supplementation of coconut oil and garlic powder determined the increase in the proportion of butyrate [103, 104].

A significant decrease in the C2:C3 ratio was seen when either garlic powder, mangosteen peel powder, soapberry fruit powder as well as a combination of coconut oil and garlic powder were used [97, 103, 104]. Methane emission was inhibited by supplementation with garlic essential oil [105], although the same inhibition produced equivalent compounds in need to be disposed, propionate and butyrate being the main alternative [106]. Busquet *et al.* [105] have suggested that acetate and methane proportions are reduced whereas propionate and butyrate are increased to the same extent following action of garlic oil, diallyl disulfide and allyl mercaptan.

This may suggest the idea that both diallyl disulfide and allyl mercaptan are responsible for the majority of the effects reported, more than diallyl sulfide and allicin. Supplementation with plant oils may significantly decrease ($P<0.05$) OM digestibility, and in fact, 7% supplemented coconut oil can be accounted for a digestibility reduction from 2 to 8.7% *in vivo* and up to 12.1% *in vitro*, as shown in Table **3** [103, 104]. Differently, it has been shown that OM digestibility can be increased by the use of garlic powder (*in vitro*) and lemongrass powder, from 15.6% to 48.4% [55, 104]. Supplementation of garlic powder alone could significantly reduce ($P<0.05$) methane gas production up to 22%, although a different supplementation using either 7% coconut oil alone and a combined supplementation of the same 7% coconut oil with 100 g garlic powder can also significantly ($P<0.05$) reduce methane gas production from 9.1% to 10.2%, respectively [104]. Calsamiglia *et al.* [107] reported in methanogenic Archaea, that the synthesis of the isoprenoid units is catalyzed by the hydroxymethylglutaryl coenzyme-A (HMG-CoA) reductase, an enzyme that has also been described in the liver and that participates in the synthesis of cholesterol.

Garlic oil and some derived organosulfur compounds are strong inhibitors of HMG-CoA reductase [108] and as a result, by inhibiting isoprenoid synthesis, instability of Archaea membrane results, followed by cell death. A positive correlation has been highlighted by many studies between methane gas production and ruminal digestibility, although in this study a supplementation with coconut oil alone or in combination with garlic powder has been reported to reduce methane production, without any effect on nutrient digestibility [109] (Table **5**).

Table 3. Effects of plant secondary compounds and plant oil on digestibility and methane gas production in various studies.

Substrates	Level	Digestibility,%	Methane, %	Animal	References
***In vitro* study**					
Bitter cucumber	200 mg	no	no	Steer (rumen fluid)	Ngamsaeng *et al.* (2006)

(Table 3) contd.....

Substrates	Level	Digestibility,%	Methane, %	Animal	References
Banana leaf	200 mg	no	no	Steer (rumen fluid)	Ngamsaeng *et al.* (2006)
Guava leaf	200 mg	no	no	Steer (rumen fluid)	Ngamsaeng *et al.* (2006)
Mangosteen peel powder	200 mg	no	no	Steer (rumen fluid)	Ngamsaeng *et al.* (2006)
Garlic powder	16 mg	(+) 48.4*	(-) 22.0*	Buffalo (rumen fluid)	Kongmun *et al.* (2010b)
Coconut oil	16 mg	(-) 12.1*	(+) 6.4*	Buffalo (rumen fluid)	Kongmun *et al.* (2010b)
***In vivo* study**					
Mangosteen peel powder	100g/h/d	(-) 2.3	no	Beef cattle	Ngamsaeng *et al.* (2006)
Mangosteen peel powder	100g/h/d	(+) 0.9	(-) 10.5	Native beef cattle	Kongmun *et al.* (2009)
Soapberry tree fruit	100g/h/d	(-) 2.1	0.0	Native beef cattle	Kongmun *et al.* (2009)
Lemongrass powder	100 g/h/d	(+) 15.6*	no	Beef cattle	Wanapat *et al.* (2008a)
Garlic powder	80g/h/d	(-) 1.6	no	Steer	Wanapat *et al.* (2008b)
Coconut oil	7%	(-) 28.7*	(+) 39.5*	Native beef cattle	Kongmun *et al.* (2009)
Coconut oil	7%	(-) 2.6	(-) 10.2*	Buffalo	Kongmun *et al.* (2010a)
Sunflower oil	6%	(-) 9.0*	no	Buffalo	Wanapat *et al.* (2009)
Combination					
Coconut oil + Sunflower oil	6%	(-) 2.7	no	Buffalo	Wanapat *et al.* (2009)
Coconut oil: Garlic powder	8:4 (mg)	(+) 4.6	(-) 18.9*	Buffalo (rumen fluid)	Kongmun *et al.* (2010b)
Coconut oil + Garlic powder	7% + 100g	(-) 2.2	(-) 9.1*	Buffalo	Kongmun *et al.* (2010a)

(*) is significantly different ($p<0.05$) from control group. (+,-): increased or decreased values compared to control group. (no) = not observed

10. MOLECULAR BIOLOGY TECHNIQUES AND INVESTIGATION ON RUMEN MICROORGANISM POPULATION AND DIVERSITY

At present, to study rumen ecology and microbial diversity, modern molecular biology techniques based on 16S/18S rRNA/rDNA are always more and more employed, such as real-time PCR and PCR-Denaturing Gradient Gel Electrophoresis (PCR-DGGE). In fact, real time PCR technology has been instrumental in providing useful data on rumen microorganism population, and the influence exerted by supplemented secondary plant compounds, as reported in Table **4**. Population of protozoa has been shown to be reduced following exposure to coconut oil, garlic powder, mangosteen peel powder and lemongrass powder, and a significant reduction ($P<0.05$) following a combination of supplemented garlic powder with coconut oil up to 68.4-75.9% [103]. Protozoa population has been reduced more effectively by garlic powder when compared to mangosteen peel powder, and in fact, garlic powder was able to reduce protozoa population up to 39.4 – 44.1% in an *in vivo* study, whereas the lowest reduction (23.8%) in protozoa population was reported following supplementation with Lemongrass powder [55, 104]. Machmuller *et al.* [110] suggested that supplementation of coconut oil tended to reduce the population of bacteria and ciliate protozoa. The reduction in protozoal population could be due to a decrease in the permeability properties of their cell membrane [111]. In this review, an influence by soapberry tree fruit, coconut oil and sunflower oil has been highlighted on methanogen population of bacteria, with a reduction up to 64.5-93.2% [102, 103]. A similar result was found by Soliva *et al.* [112] reporting a reduction of both methane gas production and the amount of Archaea, following an increase in the proportion of C12 and a proportion of 2:1 of C12/C14, and the highest methane- suppressing activity (96%) was similarly reported as with C12 alone. This confirms the assumptions made by Dohme *et al.* [113] that the methane-suppressing effect of coconut oil is the results of a direct inhibition of ruminal methanogens. Additionally, C12 and C14 seem to inhibit the metabolic activity of the methanogens by absorption onto the microbial cell wall [114]. The effect of supplementation on three predominant cellulolytic bacteria population is shown in Table **4**. It has been shown a significant ($P<0.05$) reduction in cellulolytic bacteria population following a 7% coconut oil supplementation, although such reduction was not evidenced when combined to garlic powder. The reduction of *F.succinogenes* population can be explained by oil supplemented in the feed and with a competition among ruminal microorganisms, and in fact coconut oil may coat rumen digesta and protect digesta attachment of *F.succinogenes*. Population of the *F.succinogenes* was found by Wanapat and Cherdthong [115] more in the rumen digesta than rumen fluid. This is in agreement with Chen and Weimer [116] who found that 67.3% of *F.succinogenes*, 28.8% of *R. albus* and 3.9% of *R. flavefaciens* were adherent to cellulolytic bacteria in continuous condition.

Table 4. Effects of plant secondary compounds and plant oil on ruminal microorganisms population in various studies.

Substrates	Level	Protozoa,%	Methanogenes, %	RF,%	RA, %	FS,%	Animal	References
***In vitro* study**								
Garlic powder	16 mg	(-) 55.2*	no	(+)	(-)	(-)	Buffalo (rumen fluid)	Kongmun *et al.* (2010b)
Coconut oil	16 mg	(-) 28.0*	no	(-)	(-)	(-)*	Buffalo (rumen fluid)	Kongmun *et al.* (2010b)
***In vivo* study**								
Mangosteen peel powder	100g/h/d	(-) 39.4*	no	no	no	no	Beef cattle	Ngamsaeng *et al.* (2006)
Mangosteen peel powder	100g/h/d	no	(+) 6.4	(+)*	(+)*	(+)*	Native beef cattle	Kongmun *et al.* (2009)
Soapberry tree fruit	100g/h/d	no	(-) 93.2*	(-)*	(-)*	(+)	Native beef cattle	Kongmun *et al.* (2009)
Lemongrass powder	100 g/h/d	(-) 23.8*	no	no	no	no	Beef cattle	Wanapat *et al.* (2008a)
Garlic powder	80g/h/d	(-) 44.1*	no	no	no	no	Steer	Wanapat *et al.* (2008b)
Coconut oil	7%	no	(-) 64.5*	(-)*	(-)*	(-)*	Native beef cattle	Kongmun *et al.* (2009)
Coconut oil	7%	(-) 75.9*	(+) 12.3	(+)	(+)	(-)	Buffalo	Kongmun *et al.* (2010a)

(Table 4) contd.....

Substrates	Level	Protozoa,%	Methanogenes, %	RF,%	RA, %	FS,%	Animal	References
Sunflower oil	6%	no	(-) 77.4*	(-)	(+)	(-)*	Buffalo	Wanapat *et al.* (2009)
Combination								
Coconut oil + Sunflower oil	6%	no	(-) 34.6	(-)	(+)	(-)*	Buffalo	Wanapat *et al.* (2009)
Coconut oil: Garlic powder	8:4 (mg)	(-) 59.4*	no	(-)	(+)*	(-)	Buffalo (rumen fluid)	Kongmun *et al.* (2010)
Coconut oil + Garlic powder	7% + 100g	(-) 68.4*	(-) 6.0	(+)	(+)	(-)*	Buffalo	Kongmun *et al.* (2010a)

(*) is significantly different (p<0.05) from control group.
(+,-): increased or decreased values compared to control group.
(no) = not observed

Moreover, Chen and Weimer [116] studied the competition among three predominant ruminal cellulolytic bacteria in the absence or presence of non-cellulolytic bacteria and reported that *Selemonas ruminantium* was inhibiting production and suppressing growth of *R. flavefaciens* and *F.succinogenes*, respectively. However, it was found that mangosteen peel power significantly increased (P<0.05) cellulolytic bacteria population [103].

Currently, supplementation in swamp buffaloes of legumes such as *Phaseolus calcaratus* has resulted in improved rumen microorganisms, and especially cellulolytic bacteria, namely *R. flavefaciens*, *R.albus* and *F.succinogenes*. Chanthakhoun and Wanapat [117], and Wanapat *et al.* [109] reported a comparative study on rumen microorganism population and diversity. The results revealed that swamp buffaloes have higher population of viable bacteria, cellulolytic bacteria and microbial protein synthesis than other species.

Table 5. Effect of carbohydrate sources and cottonseed meal levels on microbial populations and microbial protein synthesis.

	CC[1]		CR3:1		SEM	Significance[2]		
	LCM	HCM	LCM	HCM		CS	CM	I
Total viable bacteria, x10^{10} CFU/ml								

(Table 5) contd.....

	CC[1]		CR3:1		SEM	Significance[2]		
	LCM	HCM	LCM	HCM		CS	CM	I
Young dairy bull	2.7	3.9	5.6	4.9	0.85	*	ns	ns
Beef cattle	3.6	3.1	4.0	3.3	0.72	ns	ns	ns
Swamp buffalo	9.5	9.0	9.4	8.8	1.62	ns	*	ns
Dairy cow	4.5	4.8	4.4	5.0	0.44	ns	ns	ns
Cellulolytic bacteria, x10[8] CFU/ml								
Young dairy bull	3.7	3.9	3.8	3.3	0.88	ns	ns	ns
Beef cattle	2.3	1.9	3.1	1.7	1.09	ns	*	ns
Swamp buffalo	7.4	6.8	7.4	7.0	1.95	ns	*	ns
Dairy cow	3.1	3.5	2.9	3.8	0.52	ns	ns	3.1
Microbial protein synthesis, g N/d								
Young dairy bull	42.4	46.2	53.1	46.0	4.22	ns	ns	*
Beef cattle	74.8	63.9	72.5	64.2	4.58	ns	0.06	ns
Swamp buffalo	79.4	70.6	80.6	68.8	4.27	ns	*	ns

[1] CC=cassava chip, CR3:1=cassava chip + rice bran 3:1, LCM=low cottonseed meal, HCM=high cottonseed meal

[2] CS=energy sources, CM=cottonseed meal levels, I=ES*CM interaction

CFU=colony forming unit

*=P<0.05, ns= non-significant difference, SEM = standard error of the means

Source [114]:

CONCLUSION

Based on the most recent research findings, swamp buffaloes display a unique rumen ecology and a diversity of microorganisms, fermentation processes and ability to effectively degrade low quality roughages, like crop residues and byproducts. Molecular biology techniques allow us to identify rumen microorganisms and providing data on why buffaloes can be more efficient in feed digestion, protein synthesis and microbial enzyme producers. Despite the recent knowledge and acquisition of data, more research effort has to be devoted to swamp buffalo nutrition and feeding, and rumen ecology.

CONFLICT OF INTEREST

The authors confirm that they have no conflict of interest to declare for this publication.

ACKNOWLEDGEMENTS

Declared none.

REFERENCES

[1] Chantalakhana C. Water buffalo: valuable asset of the poor but disappearing. Proc workshop on water buffaloes for food security and sustainable rural development. Surin, Thailand. 2001.

[2] Zhu WY, Liu JX, Chang YF, Ibal MF, Mao SY. Rumen methanogensis and nutritional approaches to the mitigation of ruminant methane. Int Cong Ser 2008; pp. 33-8.

[3] Kamra DN, Agarwal N, Chaudhary LC. Inhibition of ruminal methanogenesis by tropical plants containing secondary compounds. Int Congr Ser 2006; 1293: 156-63. [http://dx.doi.org/10.1016/j.ics.2006.02.002]

[4] Hess HD, Tiemann TT, Noto F, Carulla JE, Kreuzer M. Strategic use of tannin as means to limit methane emission from ruminant livestock. Int Congr Ser 2006; 1293: 164-7. [http://dx.doi.org/10.1016/j.ics.2006.01.010]

[5] Newbold CJ, Roda LM. Dietary additives to control methanogenesis in rumen. Int Congr Ser 2006; 1293: 138-47. [http://dx.doi.org/10.1016/j.ics.2006.03.047]

[6] Niezen JH, Charleston WA, Hodgson J, Mackay AD, Leathwick DM. Controlling internal parasites in grazing ruminants without recourse to anthelmintics: approaches, experiences and prospects. Int J Parasitol 1996; 26(8-9): 983-92. [http://dx.doi.org/10.1016/S0020-7519(96)80076-2] [PMID: 8923145]

[7] Hegarty RS. Mechanisms for competitively reducing ruminal methanogenesis. Aust J Agric Res 1999; 50: 1299-305. [http://dx.doi.org/10.1071/AR99007]

[8] Devendra C. Crop-animal systems in Asia: future perspectives. Agric Syst 2002; 71: 179-86. [http://dx.doi.org/10.1016/S0308-521X(01)00043-9]

[9] Hungate RE. A roll tube method for cultivation of strict anaerobes. 1969.

[10] Dehority BA, Tirabasso PA, Grifo AP Jr. Most-probable-number procedures for enumerating ruminal bacteria, including the simultaneous estimation of total and cellulolytic numbers in one medium. Appl Environ Microbiol 1989; 55(11): 2789-92. [PMID: 2624460]

[11] Amann RI, Ludwig W, Schleifer KH. Phylogenetic identification and *in situ* detection of individual microbial cells without cultivation. Microbiol Rev 1995; 59(1): 143-69. [PMID: 7535888]

[12] Shin EC, Cho KM, Lim WJ, *et al.* Phylogenetic analysis of protozoa in the rumen contents of cow based on the 18S rDNA sequences. J Appl Microbiol 2004; 97(2): 378-83. [http://dx.doi.org/10.1111/j.1365-2672.2004.02304.x] [PMID: 15239705]

[13] Sylvester JT, Karnati SK, Yu Z, Morrison M, Firkins JL. Development of an assay to quantify rumen

ciliate protozoal biomass in cows using real-time PCR. J Nutr 2004; 134(12): 3378-84. [PMID: 15570040]

[14] Wanapat M, Devendra C. Feeding and nutrition of dairy cattle and buffaloes in Asia. Proceedings 6th AAAP Animal Science Congress. Bangkok, Thailand. 1992; pp. 177-94.

[15] Wanapat M. Feeding of Ruminants in the Tropics Based on Local Feed Resources. Khon Kaen, Thailand: Khon Kaen Publishing Comp. Ltd. 1999; p. 236.

[16] Wanapat M. Potential uses of local feed resources for ruminants. Trop Anim Health Prod 2009; 41(7): 1035-49. [http://dx.doi.org/10.1007/s11250-008-9270-y] [PMID: 19015946]

[17] Wanapat M. Improving dairy rice/cassava farming system in Thailand. In: Proc Planning Workshop on Crop-Livestock Systems (C Devendra), held at IRRI, organized by ILRL, Kenya.

[18] Devendra C, Thomas D, Jabbar M, Kudo H. Improvement of livestock production in crop-animal systems in rainfed agro-ecological zones of South-East Asia ILRI. Nariobi, Kenya: International Livestock Research Institute 1997; p. 116.

[19] Wanapat M, Sundstol F, Garmo TH. A comparison of alkali treatment methods to improve the nutritive value of straw. I. Digestibility and metabolizability. Anim Feed Sci Technol 1985; 12: 295-309. [http://dx.doi.org/10.1016/0377-8401(85)90006-9]

[20] Wanapat M. Better utilization of crop-residues for buffalo production. In: Chantalakhana C, Ed. The Buffalo Seminal International Buffalo Information Centre. Bangkok, Thailand: Kasetsart University Library 1986.

[21] Wanapat M, Wachirapakorn C. Utilization on roughage and concentrate by feedlot buffaloes (*Bubalus bubalis*). J Anim Sci 1990; 3: 195-203.

[22] Wanapat M, Petlum N, Wongnen N, Matarat S, Khampa S, Rowlinson P. Improving crop-livestock production systems in rainfed areas of Northeast Thailand. Pakistan Journal of Nutrition 2007; 6(3): 241-6.

[23] Wanapat M. Role of cassava hay as animal feed in the tropics. In: Prestion TR, Ogle B, Wanapat M, Eds. In: Proceedings of International Workshop on Current Research and Development on use of Cassava as Animal Feed; Stockholm. SIDA-SAREC. 2001.

[24] Kiyothong K, Wanapat M. Supplementation of cassava hay and stylo 184 hay to replace concentrate for lactation dairy cows. Cassava-legume intercropping: A potential feed production system for small holder dairy farming. MSc. lactation dairy cows Cassava-legume intercropping: A potential feed production system for small holder dairy farming MSc Thesis in the program "Tropical Livestock System" SLU Dept of Animal Nutrition and Management, Uppasala, Sweden 2004.

[25] Polthanee A, Wanapat M, Wachirapakorn C. Preston TR, Ogle B, Wanapat M. Cassava-Legumes intercropping: A potential food-feed system for dairy farmers. International Workshop Current Research and Development on Use of Cassava as Animal Feed. Thailand: Khon Kaen 2001; pp. 97-107. http://www.mekarn.org/procKK/polt.htm

[26] Chanthakhoun V, Wanapat M, Wanapat S. Study on yield, nutritive value and ruminal degradability of *Phaseolus calcaratus* (Tua-mun) in swamp buffaloes. Proc. 12th AAAP Int. Cong. Hanoi. Vietnam.

2008.

[27] Reed JD. Nutritional toxicology of tannins and related polyphenols in forage legumes. J Anim Sci 1995; 73(5): 1516-28. [http://dx.doi.org/10.2527/1995.7351516x] [PMID: 7665384]

[28] Elizalde JC, Merchen NR, Faulkner DB. Fractionation of fiber and crude protein in fresh forages during the spring growth. J Anim Sci 1999; 77(2): 476-84. [http://dx.doi.org/10.2527/1999.772476x] [PMID: 10100679]

[29] Preston TR, Leng LA. Matching ruminant production system with available resources in the tropics and sub tropics. New South Wales: Penambul Books 1987; pp. 1-200.

[30] Agboola AA, Fayami AA. Fixation and excretion of nitrogen by tropical legumes. Agron J 1972; 64: 409-12. [http://dx.doi.org/10.2134/agronj1972.00021962006400040001x]

[31] Storm E, Orskov ER. The nutritive value of rumen micro-organisms in ruminants. 1. Large-scale isolation and chemical composition of rumen micro-organisms. Br J Nutr 1983; 50(2): 463-70. [http://dx.doi.org/10.1079/BJN19830114] [PMID: 6615774]

[32] Clark JH, Klusmeyer TH, Cameron MR. Microbial protein synthesis and flows of nitrogen fractions to the duodenum of dairy cows. J Dairy Sci 1992; 75(8): 2304-23. [http://dx.doi.org/10.3168/jds.S0022-0302(92)77992-2] [PMID: 1401380]

[33] Sniffen CJ, Robinson PH. Protein and fiber digestion, passage, and utilization in lactating cows. Microbial growth and flow as influenced by dietary manipulations. J Dairy Sci 1987; 70(2): 425-41. [http://dx.doi.org/10.3168/jds.S0022-0302(87)80027-9] [PMID: 3553257]

[34] Huber JT, Higginbotham G, Gomez-Alarcon RA, *et al.* Heat stress interactions with protein, supplemental fat, and fungal cultures. J Dairy Sci 1994; 77(7): 2080-90. [http://dx.doi.org/10.3168/jds.S0022-0302(94)77151-4] [PMID: 7929966]

[35] Owens FN, Goetsch AL. Digesta passage and microbial protein synthesis. In: Milligan LP, Grovum WL, Dobson A, Eds. Control of Digestion and Metabolism in Ruminants. Reston, VA: Reston Publishing Co. 1986; pp. 196-223.

[36] Van Soest PJ. Forage evaluation techniques. Nutritional Ecology of the Ruminant. Ithaca, NY: Cornell University Press 1994; pp. 108-21.

[37] Waldo DR, Glen BP. Foreign systems for meeting the protein requirements of ruminants. II. Meeting protein requirements of cattle. In: OWENS, FN (Ed) Proc Protein requirements for cattle: Symposium. 109: 269-309.

[38] Dove H, Milne JA. Digesta flow and rumen microbial protein production in ewes grazing perennial ryegrass. Aust J Agric Res 1994; 45: 1229-45. [http://dx.doi.org/10.1071/AR9941229]

[39] Russell JB, Strobel HJ. Concentration of ammonia across cell membranes of mixed rumen bacteria. J Dairy Sci 1987; 70(5): 970-6. [http://dx.doi.org/10.3168/jds.S0022-0302(87)80101-7] [PMID: 3597937]

[40] Song MK, Kennelly JJ. Ruminal fermentation pattern, bacterial population and ruminal degradation of feed ingredients as influenced by ruminal ammonia concentration. J Anim Sci 1990; 68(4): 1110-20.

[http://dx.doi.org/10.2527/1990.6841110x] [PMID: 2332386]

[41] Rihani N, Garrett WN, Zinn RA. Influence of level of urea and method of supplementation on characteristics of digestion of high-fibre diets by sheep. J Anim Sci 1993; 71: 1655-67.

[42] Robinson PH, McQueen RE, Burgess PL. Influence of rumen undegradable protein levels on feed intake and milk production of dairy cows. J Dairy Sci 1991; 74(5): 1623-31. [http://dx.doi.org/10.3168/jds.S0022-0302(91)78324-0] [PMID: 1880269]

[43] Wanapat M, Pimpa O. Effect of ruminal NH_3-N levels on ruminal fermentation purine derivatives, digestibility and rice straw intake in swamp buffaloes. Asian-Aus J Anim Sci 1999; 12: 904-7. [http://dx.doi.org/10.5713/ajas.1999.904]

[44] Reynal SM, Broderick GA. Effect of dietary level of rumen-degraded protein on production and nitrogen metabolism in lactating dairy cows. J Dairy Sci 2005; 88(11): 4045-64. [http://dx.doi.org/10.3168/jds.S0022-0302(05)73090-3] [PMID: 16230710]

[45] Satter LD, Slyter LL. Effect of ammonia concentration of rumen microbial protein production *in vitro*. Br J Nutr 1974; 32(2): 199-208. [http://dx.doi.org/10.1079/BJN19740073] [PMID: 4472574]

[46] Erdman RA, Proctor GH, Vandersall JH. Effect of rumen ammonia concentration on *in situ* rate and extent of digestion of feedstuffs. J Dairy Sci 1986; 69(9): 2312-20. [http://dx.doi.org/10.3168/jds.S0022-0302(86)80670-1] [PMID: 3782588]

[47] Souza DG, Coutinho SF, Silveira MR, Cara DC, Teixeira MM. Treatment with a leukotriene B4 receptor antagonist inhibits local and remote reperfusion injury after transient ischemia of the superior mesenteric artery in the rat. Eur J Pharmacol 2000; 403: 121-314. [http://dx.doi.org/10.1016/S0014-2999(00)00574-4] [PMID: 10969152]

[48] Vagnoni DB, Broderick GA, Clayton MK, Hatfield RD. Excretion of purine derivatives by Holstein cows abomasally infused with incremental amounts of purines. J Dairy Sci 1997; 80(8): 1695-702. [http://dx.doi.org/10.3168/jds.S0022-0302(97)76101-0] [PMID: 9276809]

[49] Liang JB, Pimpa O, Abdullah N, Jelan ZA. Estimation of rumen microbial protein production from urinary purine derivatives in zebu cattle and water buffalo. Nuclear Based Technologies For Estimating Microbial Protein Supply In Ruminant Livestock, IAEA-TECDOC 1999; 1093: 35-42.

[50] Moscardini S, Haddi ML, Stefanon B, Susmel P. Measurement of purine derivatives in the urine of some ruminant species. Nuclear based technologies for estimating microbial protein supply in ruminant livestock IAEA-TECDOC-1093. Vienna: IAEA 1999; pp. 111-8.

[51] Makkar HP. Development, standardization and validation of nuclear based technologies for estimating microbial protein supply in ruminant livestock for improving productivity. In: Makkar HP, Chen XB, Eds. 2004; pp. 1-13. [http://dx.doi.org/10.1007/978-1-4020-2844-1_1]

[52] Soejono M, Yusiati LM, Backrudin Z, Budhi SP, Widyobroto BP, Utomo R. Flow of nucleic acids from the rumen and recovery of purine derivatives in the urine of cattle and buffaloes. In Estimation of microbial protein supply in ruminants using urinary purine derivative (ed H P S Makkar and X B Chen), FAO/IAEA, Kluwer Academic Publishers, Dordrecht. Natherland: Springer 2004; pp. 69-74. [http://dx.doi.org/10.1007/978-1-4020-2844-1_8]

[53] Pimpa O, Liang JB, Balcells J. Renal and salivary excretions of plasma purine derivatives in swamp buffaloes and zebu cattle. J Anim Sci 2007; 20(8): 1201-7.

[54] Nocek JE, Russel JB. Protein and energy as an integrated system: Relationship of ruminal protein and carbohydrate availability to microbial synthesis and milk production. J Dairy Sci 1988; 71: 2070-82. [http://dx.doi.org/10.3168/jds.S0022-0302(88)79782-9]

[55] Wanapat M, Cherdthong A, Pakdee P, Wanapat S. Manipulation of rumen ecology by dietary lemongrass (Cymbopogon citratus Stapf.) powder supplementation. J Anim Sci 2008; 86(12): 3497-503. a
[http://dx.doi.org/10.2527/jas.2008-0885] [PMID: 18708607]

[56] Chen XB, Hovell FD, Orskov ER, Brown DS. Excretion of purine derivatives by ruminants: effect of exogenous nucleic acid supply on purine derivative excretion by sheep. Br J Nutr 1990; 63(1): 131-42. b
[http://dx.doi.org/10.1079/BJN19900098] [PMID: 2317474]

[57] Liang JB, Matsumoto M, Young BA. Purine derivative excretion and ruminal microbial yield in Malasyan cattle and swamp buffalo. Anim Feed Sci Technol 1994; 47: 189-99. [http://dx.doi.org/10.1016/0377-8401(94)90123-6]

[58] Chen XB. An Exel Application Program for processing Feed Degradability Data. 1996.

[59] Nolan JV. Prediction of rumen microbial outflow based on urinary excretion of purine derivatives. Nuclear Based Technologies for Estimating Microbial Protein Supply in Ruminant Livestock, IAEA-TECDOC-1093. Vienna: International Atomic Energy Agency 1999; pp. 9-20.

[60] Balcells J, Guada JA, Castrillo C, Gasa J. Urinary excretion of allantoin and allantoin precursors by sheep after different rates of purine infusion into the duodenum. J Agric Sci Camb 1991; 116: 309-17. [http://dx.doi.org/10.1017/S002185960007773X]

[61] Giesecke D, Ehrentreich L, Stangassinger M, Ahrens F. Mammary and renal excretion of purine metabolites in relation to energy intake and milk yield in dairy cows. J Dairy Sci 1994; 77(8): 2376-81. [http://dx.doi.org/10.3168/jds.S0022-0302(94)77180-0] [PMID: 7962859]

[62] Orellana-Boero P, Balcells J, Martín-Orúe SM, Liang JB, Guada JA. Excretion of purine derivatives in cows: Endogenous contribution and recovery of exogenous purine bases. Livest Prod Sci 2001; 68: 243-50.
[http://dx.doi.org/10.1016/S0301-6226(00)00231-1]

[63] Wanapat M, Kongmun P, Chanthakhoun V, Pilajun R. A Comparative study of predominant cellulolytic bacteria of swamp buffalo and Beef cattle using real- time PCR. In: Proc Semi Ann of Agri 26-27 Jan, 2009 Anim Sci session Faculty of Agri KKU Thailand. 2009; pp. 112-4.

[64] Wanapat M, Pimpa O, Petlum A, Wachirapakorn C, Yuanklang C. Participation scheme of smallholder dairy farmers in the northeast Thailand on improving feeding systems. Asian-Aust J Anim Sci 2000; 13: 830-6.
[http://dx.doi.org/10.5713/ajas.2000.830]

[65] Wanapat M. On-farm crop-residues as ruminant feeds: new dimensions and outlook.

[66] Wanapat M. Rumen manipulation to increase the efficient use of local feed resources and productivity of ruminants in the tropics. Asian-Aust J Anim Sci 2000; 13 (Suppl.): 59-67.

[67] Devendra C. Comparative nitrogen utilization in Malaysia Swamp buffaloes and Kedah Kelanton cattle. In: Proc The 7th AFAR Int Workshop (Ed R Dixon), IDPD, Canberra, Australia.

[68] Wora-anu S, Wanapat M, Wachirapakorn C, Nontaso N. Effect of roughage to concentrate ratio on ruminal ecology and voluntary feed intake in cattle and swamp buffaloes fed on urea-treated rice straw. Asian-Aust. J Anim Sci 2000; 3: 75-83.

[69] Ruangprim T, Chantalakhana C, Skunmun P, Prucsasri P, Wanapat M. Rumen microbes and ecology of male dairy beef cattle and buffaloes. Proc Animal Science Annual meeting Khon Kaen, Thailand. 2007; pp. 371-78.

[70] Forster RJ, Gong J, Teather RM. Group-specific 16S rRNA hybridization probes for determinative and community structure studies of Butyrivibrio fibrisolvens in the rumen. Appl Environ Microbiol 1997; 63(4): 1256-60.
[PMID: 9097421]

[71] Shinkai T, Kobayashi Y. Localization of ruminal cellulolytic bacteria on plant fibrous materials as determined by fluorescence in situ hybridization and real-time PCR. Appl Environ Microbiol 2007; 73(5): 1646-52.
[http://dx.doi.org/10.1128/AEM.01896-06] [PMID: 17209077]

[72] Wanapat M, Cherdthong A. Use of real-time PCR technique in studying rumen cellulolytic bacteria population as affected by level of roughage in swamp buffalo. Curr Microbiol 2009; 58(4): 294-9.
[http://dx.doi.org/10.1007/s00284-008-9322-6] [PMID: 19018588]

[73] Wanapat M. Nutritional aspect of ruminant production in Southeast Asia with social reference to Thailand. Bangkok: Funny Pree Pub. Comp. Ltd. 1990; p. 207.

[74] Devendra C. Dairy production system and development in Asia: characteristic and opportunities for their improvement. 1990; 1: pp. 202-07.

[75] Minson DJ. The digestibility and voluntary intake of six Panicum varieties. Aust J Agric Anim Husb 1971; 11: 18-25.
[http://dx.doi.org/10.1071/EA9710018]

[76] Lowvy VB. Toxic factor and problems: methods of alleviating them in animal. In: Devendra C, Ed. Proc International for Farm animals. Ottawa, Canada: IDRC 1989.

[77] Sunstol F, Owen E. Straw and other fibrous by-product as feed. Amsterdam, The Netherlands: Elsevier 1984.

[78] Leng RA. Factors affecting the utilization of poor-quality forages by ruminants particularly under tropical conditions. Nutr Res Rev 1990; 3(1): 277-303.
[http://dx.doi.org/10.1079/NRR19900016] [PMID: 19094342]

[79] Wanapat M. Utilization of forages, crop residues and tree fodder for ruminants in Thailand.

[80] Wanapat M. The use of local feed resources for livestock production in Thailand. In: Guo Tingshuang, Ed. Proceedings of the International Conference on Increasing Animal Production with Local Resources.

[81] Benchaar C, Petit HV, Berthiaume R, Whyte TD, Chouinard PY. Effects of addition of essential oils and monensin premix on digestion, ruminal fermentation, milk production, and milk composition in

dairy cows. J dairy Sci 2006; 89(11): 4352-64.
[http://dx.doi.org/10.3168/jds.S0022-0302(06)72482-1]

[82] Frutos P, Raso M, Hervas G, Mantecon AR, Perez V, Giraldez FJ. Is there any detrimental effect when a chestnut hydrolyzable tannins extract is included in the diet of finishing lambs. Anim Res 2004; 56: 127-36.
[http://dx.doi.org/10.1051/animres:2004001]

[83] Newbold JD, Bott TL, Kaplan LA, Sweeney BW, Vannote RL. Organic matter dynamics in White Clay Creek, Pennsylvania, USA. J N Am Benthol Soc 1997; 16: 46-50.
[http://dx.doi.org/10.2307/1468231]

[84] Diaz A, Avendano M, Escobar A. Evaluation of Sapindus saponaria as a defaunating agent and its effects on different ruminal digestion parameters. Livest Res Rural Dev 1993; 2: 1-6.

[85] Wang Y, McAllister TA, Yanke LJ, Cheeke PR. Effect of steroidal saponin from *Yucca schidigera* extract on ruminal microbes. J Appl Microbiol 2000; 88(5): 887-96.
[http://dx.doi.org/10.1046/j.1365-2672.2000.01054.x] [PMID: 10792550]

[86] Wina E, Muetzel S, Becker K. The dynamics of major fibrolytic microbes and enzyme activity in the rumen in response to short- and long-term feeding of Sapindus rarak saponins. J Appl Microbiol 2006; 100(1): 114-22.
[http://dx.doi.org/10.1111/j.1365-2672.2005.02746.x] [PMID: 16405691]

[87] Poungchompu O, Wanapat M, Wachirapakorn C, Wanapat S, Cherdthong A. Manipulation of ruminal fermentation and methane production by dietary saponins and tannins from mangosteen peel and soapberry fruit. Arch Anim Nutr 2009; 63(5): 389-400.
[http://dx.doi.org/10.1080/17450390903020406] [PMID: 26967797]

[88] Ip C, Singh M, Thompson HJ, Scimeca JA. Conjugated linoleic acid suppresses mammary carcinogenesis and proliferative activity of the mammary gland in the rat. Cancer Res 1994; 54(5): 1212-5.
[PMID: 8118808]

[89] Houseknecht KL, Vanden Heuvel JP, Moya-Camarena SY, *et al.* Dietary conjugated linoleic acid normalizes impaired glucose tolerance in the Zucker diabetic fatty fa/fa rat. Biochem Biophys Res Commun 1998; 244(3): 678-82.
[http://dx.doi.org/10.1006/bbrc.1998.8303] [PMID: 9535724]

[90] Lee JH, Cho KH, Lee KT, Kim MR. Antiatherogenic effects of structured lipid containing conjugated linoleic acid in C57BL/6J mice. J Agric Food Chem 2005; 53(18): 7295-301.
[http://dx.doi.org/10.1021/jf050626e] [PMID: 16131145]

[91] Bessa RJ, Alves SP, Jerònimo E, Alfaia CM, Prates JA, Santos-Silva J. Effect of lipid supplements on ruminal biohydrogenation intermediates and muscle fatty acids in lamb. Eur J Lipid Sci Technol 2007; 109: 868-83.
[http://dx.doi.org/10.1002/ejlt.200600311]

[92] Sackmann JR, Duckett SK, Gillis MH, Realini CE, Parks AH, Eggelston RB. Effects of forage and sunflower oil levels on ruminal biohydrogenation of fatty acids and conjugated linoleic acid formation in beef steers fed finishing diets. J Anim Sci 2003; 81(12): 3174-81.
[http://dx.doi.org/10.2527/2003.81123174x] [PMID: 14677873]

[93] Corl BA, Baumgard LH, Dwyer DA, Griinari JM, Phillips BS, Bauman DE. The role of Delta(9)-desaturase in the production of cis-9, trans-11 CLA. J Nutr Biochem 2001; 12(11): 622-30. [http://dx.doi.org/10.1016/S0955-2863(01)00180-2] [PMID: 12031255]

[94] Priolo A, Waghorn GC, Lanza M, Biondi L, Pennisi P. Polyethylene glycol as a means for reducing the impact of condensed tannins in carob pulp: effects on lamb growth performance and meat quality. J Anim Sci 2000; 78(4): 810-6. [http://dx.doi.org/10.2527/2000.784810x] [PMID: 10784169]

[95] Khiaosa-Ard R, Bryner SF, Scheeder MR, *et al.* Evidence for the inhibition of the terminal step of ruminal alpha-linolenic acid biohydrogenation by condensed tannins. J Dairy Sci 2009; 92(1): 177-88. [http://dx.doi.org/10.3168/jds.2008-1117] [PMID: 19109277]

[96] Vasta V, Priolo A, Scerra M, Hallett KG, Wood JD, Doran O. Δ(9) desaturase protein expression and fatty acid composition of longissimus dorsi muscle in lambs fed green herbage or concentrate with or without added tannins. Meat Sci 2009; 82(3): 357-64. b [http://dx.doi.org/10.1016/j.meatsci.2009.02.007] [PMID: 20416712]

[97] Wanapat M, Khejorsart P, Pakdee P, Wanapat S. Effect of supplementation of garlic powder on rumen ecology and digestibility of nutrients in ruminants. J Sci Food Agric 2008; 88: 2231-7. b [http://dx.doi.org/10.1002/jsfa.3333]

[98] Kongmun K, Wanapat M, Pakdee P, Navanukraw C, Yu Z. Manipulation of rumen fermentation and ecology of swamp buffalo by coconut oil and garlic powder supplementation. Livest Sci 2011; 135(1): 84-92. [http://dx.doi.org/10.1016/j.livsci.2010.06.131]

[99] Newbold CJ, Mcintosh FM, Williams P, Losa R, Wallace RJ. Effects of a species blend of essential oil compounds on rumen fermentation. Anim Feed Sci Technol 2004; 114: 105-12. [http://dx.doi.org/10.1016/j.anifeedsci.2003.12.006]

[100] Ngamsaeng A, Wanapat M, Khampa S. Effects of mangosteen peel (garcinia mangostana) supplementation on rumen ecology, microbial protein synthesis, digestibility and voluntary feed intake in cattle. Pakistan Journal of Nutrition 2006; 5: 445-52. [http://dx.doi.org/10.3923/pjn.2006.445.452]

[101] Puchala R, Min BR, Goetsch AL, Sahlu T. The effect of a condensed tannin-containing forage on methane emission by goats. J Anim Sci 2005; 83(1): 182-6. [http://dx.doi.org/10.2527/2005.831182x] [PMID: 15583058]

[102] Wanapat M, Mapato C, Kongmun P, Pilajun R. Effect of plant oil supplementation on feed intake, digestibility, rumen ecology, rumen fermentation in swamp buffalo. Proc: Animal Science Conference, Animal Science. Khon Kaen, Thailand: Faculty of Agriculture 2009.

[103] Kongmun P, Wanapat M, Nontaso N, Nishida T, Angthong W. Effect of phytochemical and coconut oil supplementation on rumen ecology and methane production in ruminants. Proceedings of FAO/IAEA international symposium on sustainable improvement of animal production and health. 8-11 June 2009; Vienna, Austria. 2009; pp. 246-7.

[104] Kongmun P, Wanapat M, Pakdee P, Nawanukrew C. Effect of coconut oil and garlic powder on *in vitro* fermentation using gas production technique. Livest Sci 2010; 127: 38-44. b

[http://dx.doi.org/10.1016/j.livsci.2009.08.008]

[105] Busquet M, Calsamiglia S, Ferret A, Cardozo PW, Kamel C. Effects of cinnamaldehyde and garlic oil on rumen microbial fermentation in a dual flow continuous culture. J Dairy Sci 2005; 88(7): 2508-16. [http://dx.doi.org/10.3168/jds.S0022-0302(05)72928-3] [PMID: 15956313]

[106] Van Nevel CJ, Demeyer DI, Newbold CJ, Nagaraja TC. Manipulation of rumen fermentation. In: Hobson PN, Demeyer DI, Newbold CJ, Nagaraja TC, Eds. The Rumen Microbial Ecosystem. London: Elsevier Applied Science 1988; pp. 387-443.

[107] Calsamiglia S, Busquet M, Cardozo PW, Castillejos L, Ferret A. Invited review: Essential oils as modifiers of rumen microbial fermentation. J Dairy Sci 2007; 90(6): 2580-95. [http://dx.doi.org/10.3168/jds.2006-644] [PMID: 17517698]

[108] Gebhardt R, Beck H. Differential inhibitory effects of garlic-derived organosulfur compounds on cholesterol biosynthesis in primary rat hepatocyte cultures. Lipids 1996; 31(12): 1269-76. [http://dx.doi.org/10.1007/BF02587912] [PMID: 8972460]

[109] Wanapat M, Pilajun R, Foiklang S. Effect of carbohydrate sources and cotton seed meal in the concentrate: II. Feed intake, nutrient digestibility, rumen fermentation and microbial protein synthesis in beef cattle. 2010.

[110] Machmüller A, Soliva CR, Kreuzer M. Effect of coconut oil and defaunation treatment on methanogenesis in sheep. Reprod Nutr Dev 2003; 43(1): 41-55. [http://dx.doi.org/10.1051/rnd:2003005] [PMID: 12785449]

[111] Demeyer D, Van Nevel C, Teller E, Godeau JM. Manipulation of rumen digestion in relation to the level of production in ruminants. Arch Tierernahr 1986; 36(2-3): 132-43. [http://dx.doi.org/10.1080/17450398609425252] [PMID: 3741109]

[112] Soliva CR, Hindrichsen IK, Meile L, Kreuzer M, Machmüller A. Effects of mixtures of lauric and myristic acid on rumen methanogens and methanogenesis *in vitro*. Lett Appl Microbiol 2003; 37(1): 35-9. [http://dx.doi.org/10.1046/j.1472-765X.2003.01343.x] [PMID: 12803553]

[113] Dohme F, Machmüler A, Wasserfallen A, Kreuzer M. The role of the rumen ciliate protozoa for methane suppression caused by coconut oil. Lett Appl Microbiol 1999; 29: 187-92. [http://dx.doi.org/10.1046/j.1365-2672.1999.00614.x]

[114] Koster IW, Cramer A. Inhibition of methanogenesis from acetate in granular sludge by long-chain Fatty acids. Appl Environ Microbiol 1987; 53(2): 403-9. [PMID: 16347288]

[115] Wanapat M, Cherdthong A. Use of real-time PCR technique in studying rumen cellulolytic bacteria population as affected by level of roughage in swamp buffalo. Curr Microbiol 2009; 58(4): 294-9. [http://dx.doi.org/10.1007/s00284-008-9322-6] [PMID: 19018588]

[116] Chen J, Weimer P. Competition among three predominant ruminal cellulolytic bacteria in the absence or presence of non-cellulolytic bacteria. Microbiology 2001; 147(Pt 1): 21-30. [http://dx.doi.org/10.1099/00221287-147-1-21] [PMID: 11160797]

[117] Chanthakhoun V, Wanapat M. Effect of legume (*Phaseolus calcaratus*) hay supplementation on rumen cellulolytic bacterial populations in swamp buffaloes investigated by the Real-Time PCR technique. J Anim Vet Adv 2010; 9(11): 1654-9. [http://dx.doi.org/10.3923/javaa.2010.1654.1659]

CHAPTER 7

Protein Digestion and Metabolism in Buffalo

Vo Thi Kim Thanh[1,*] and **Egil Robert Orskov**[2]

[1] *Department of Animal Physiology, Hue University of Agriculture and Forestry, Vietnam*

[2] *International Feed Resource Unit, Macaulay Land Use Research Institute*

Abstract: As other ruminants, buffaloes utilize micro-organisms in the rumen to digest the feed. In buffaloes a higher rumen degradability of nitrogen and carbohydrates in concentrates promotes the growth and the synthesis of rumen bacteria, even when fed diets with low protein content. It appears that buffaloes use more efficiently nitrogen coming out from rumen fermentation and metabolism and by recycling it. This efficient accommodation to more limiting feeding condition is enhanced by a higher availability of purine derivatives (PD) of metabolic origin. Many measurements done on buffaloes of various breeds have shown a lower PD nitrogen excretion in urine. In buffaloes, urinary PD excretion is not linked to i) the availability of microbial cells in the rumen or ii) small intestine uptake of purines. Such PD excretion seems to be related more to tissue metabolism differences of which the mechanisms are not yet fully understood. Some explanation is emerging with new studies on swamp buffaloes, summarized in the following two: i) in the first study, weaning of swamp buffalo and cattle calves was accomplished by colostrum administration, and rearing followed by milk bottle feeding. To assess differences in the endogenous secretion of purines, urine samples from the two species were collected. Solid food was not made available in the course of the first month, but access to it was granted in the course of the intervening 2 successive months in order to stimulate rumen development. Then a mixed ration of purines and milk was given to the animals, together with an infusion of intravenous allantoin, so that the effect of the introduced purines in the plasma could be tested. From the results obtained in the course of the suckling period, no differences between the two species in purine excretion was reported. Following rumen development though, purine excretion from buffaloes was less than half when compared to cattle, and likewise, following allantoin infusion, purine recovery in buffaloes was half the

* **Corresponding author Vo Thi Kim Thanh:** Department of Animal Physiology, Hue University of Agriculture and Forestry, Vietnam; Tel: +84 914 192 906; Fax: +84 54 3 524 923; E-mail: votkthanh@gmail.com

Giorgio A. Presicce (Ed.)

amount when compared to cattle ; ii) in the second study in the course of fasting and bottle milk feeding, a determination of urinary PD, basal PD excretion and glomerular filtrate (GFR) rate was made. Following access of the animals to solid feed, an assessment of urinary PD, basal PF excretion and glomerular filtrate rate was also performed. No significant differences were observed between the two species in the course of the milk feeding period in terms of urinary PD excretion, although the same differences were highly significant between the two species at 3 months of age and following 2 months of access to solid feed. In buffaloes, both during the milk feeding and following solid food access, GFR was found lower in buffaloes when compared to cattle. To date it can be stated that some studies report a higher rumen fluid NH_3 concentrate in swamp buffaloes in comparison to yellow cattle. Other studies have shown that only following rumen development, a difference in PD excretion can be seen, and the difference between buffaloes and cattle is due to differences in GFR, so that more urea and PD are recycled, highlighting the fact that buffaloes can tolerate less N in the feed to satisfy microbial needs.

Keywords: Buffaloes, Feeding, GFR, Microbial protein, Purine derivative, Rumen, Rumen NH_3.

1. INTRODUCTION

Feed for ruminants, forages and fibrous roughages, consist mainly of β-linked polysaccharides such as cellulose, which cannot be broken down by mammalian digestive enzymes. Ruminants have therefore evolved a special system of digestion that involves microbial fermentation of feed prior to its exposure to their own digestive enzymes [1]. The rumen microbes can use simple compounds such as ammonia and urea, and build up their cells from them. In fact, they can use any compound which will be degraded into ammonia – even urine. Microbial proteins then provide most of the animal protein need. So in effect, it is not necessary to feed the ruminant animal any protein at all since the microbes in the rumen can provide for them. And almost all the protein in feeds can be degraded by the bacteria. A bigger problem arose when it was shown that nearly all protein in the dung consisted of indigestible microbial cells, whereas only very little protein from the diet was truly indigestible protein. Therefore, if microbial growth occurred in the hind gut of animals, the microbes were not digested at all but passed out in the dung. This of course meant that the measured digestibility had very little meaning as far as actual digestibility of feed protein was concerned [2].

Therefore, the most important source of protein supply for ruminants is constituted by microbial population within the rumen. Nucleic acids are abundant in such microbes, and they possess roughly 18% of the total amount of nitrogen, whereas purines are characterized by a total nitrogen content of about 11%. Rumen microbial population metabolize purines, followed by urine excretion of their end products such as hypoxanthine, xanthine, allantoin and uric acid.That is why the research work has been carried out actively for the past 20-30 years into the urinary excretion of these purine metabolites, with an objective to use the excretion of these metabolites as a parameter to quantitatively estimate the supply of rumen microbial protein to the ruminant.

2. BUFFALO FEEDING AND PROTEIN DIGESTION

Feeding

Buffaloes are ruminants, and ingested feed, which is essentially made of vegetables of various kind, is metabolized in the rumen by micro-organisms, which efficiently convert cellulose and other fibres into high quality milk and meat. Furthermore, it seems that buffaloes are more efficient in using poor quality feed such as rice straw, crop residue or other by-products. Management practices in Asia, such as in Vietnam, Thailand, Lao, Cambodia, China, are run through the adoption of extensive systems in which buffaloes freely graze on natural grasses and marginal lands (roadside, canal banks, rice field following harvesting and dikes), as well as forests, among other conditions.

Rumen Digestion

Although rumen transit of the liquid phase is similar in cattle and buffaloes, the transit of the solid fraction is significantly slower in buffaloes. This difference though is compensated during the post ruminal tract so that, if referred to the overall digestive tract, the feed transit is faster. One must take into account that rumen volume in buffaloes is higher (about 10%) than cattle at the same live weight [3]. The feed transit accounts for the differences observed of rumen degradability of feed fractions. The protein rumen degradability of forages and concentrates is significantly higher in buffaloes than in cattle [3] and sheep [4]. The higher nitrogen degradability affects the ammonia N content of the rumen, which in buffaloes is constantly higher, as it emerges from the studies by Sangwan *et al.* [5], Kennedy *et al.* [6] and Bartocci *et al.* [3]. In buffaloes the higher rumen degradability of nitrogen and of carbohydrates in concentrates promotes the growth and the synthesis of rumen bacteria, even with diet characterized by low protein content. As discussed later, this is also influenced by more recycling of urea to the rumen in buffaloes compared to cattle, and this is also in agreement with bacterial count which shows a higher concentration of micro-organism in buffaloes fed with concentrate feeds [3]. From these results it appears that buffaloes use more efficiently nitrogen coming out from rumen fermentation and metabolism, and recycling. This efficient accommodation to more limiting feeding condition is enhanced by a higher availability of purine derivatives (allantoin, uric acid, xanthine and hypoxanthine, although in urinary excretion in cattle and buffaloes mainly allantoin and uric acid are present) of metabolic origin. In fact many measurements done in buffaloes show a lower purine derivative nitrogen excretion in urine, which corresponds to about 40% of what ordinarily observed in cattle [7].

Smith and McAllan [8] carried out extensive studies on nucleic acid metabolism in the gut of ruminants and demonstrated that exogenous source of nucleic acids were completely broken down in the rumen fluid; and so were the intermediate degradation products, nucleotides and nucleoside. The indication was that nucleic acids in the feed would not contribute significantly to the nucleic acid content in the rumen, and the nucleic acids entering the duodenum of ruminants were essentially of microbial origin. This has provided the basis for using RNA as a marker of microbial biomass synthesis in the rumen. The small intestine is responsible for the digestion of microbial nucleic acids leaving the rumen, whereas the abomasum apparently does not take part in the digestion process. In the small intestine the nucleic acids are hydrolysed by ribonucleases and diesterases to oligonucleotides and then to mononucleotides, nucleosides and free bases. Both forms can be absorbed from the intestine. The digestibility of microbial nucleic acids is about 85% [4 - 11].

Microbial Protein Metabolism in Buffaloes

From 1995 to 2002, following a joint FAO/IAEA project on quote: *Development, standardization and validation of nuclear based technologies for estimating microbial protein supply in ruminant livestock for improving productivity*, it was reported that urinary excretion of PD per unit DOMI is much lower and more variable in buffaloes in comparison to cattle. In addition it was reported that there is no relationship between a lower amount of microbial cells in the rumen or the absorption from the small intestine of purines, to urinary PD excretion in buffaloes. Differently, there must be differences in tissue metabolism for which though there is not yet a full comprehension of the precise mechanism behind it. This is the reason why, presently, it is difficult to adopt any PD prediction methodology.

Vercoe [12] showed that a positive correlation exists, in buffaloes (*Bubalus bubalis*), between allantoin excretion and digestible dry matter intake, although the excretion was low when compared to cattle. Subsequent studies of Chen *et al.* [10], Liang *et al.* [13], Soejono *et al.* [14] and Thanh *et al.* [15], confirmed the same observation. Differently, the profile of xanthine oxidase in the intestine, blood and other tissues was found similar to cattle [10], and therefore it can be safely expected that a similarity to cattle, in the pattern of PD excretion should be similar, *i.e.* the PD excretion is a linear function of purine uptake, and in fact urinary PD only consists of allantoin and uric acid.

Published data showed that PD excretion per unit of digestible organic matter intake (DOMI) was about 3-4 times lower in buffaloes than in cattle (5 *vs* 18 mmol/kg DOMI) [10], suggesting that it is possibly the partitioning of plasma PD occurring between renal excretion and non-renal disposal, to determine a possible difference. In addition, a part of such difference in buffaloes can be further explained by a physiological lower glomerular filtration rate (GFR).

In a recent study of Liang *et al.* [13] purine bases were infused into the duodenum of buffaloes and zebu cattle as a comparison. The relationships between urinary PD excretion (Y, mmol/d) and purine supply (X, mmol/d) were $Y = 0.12X + 0.20\ W^{0.75}$ for buffaloes and $Y = 0.85X + 0.15\ W^{0.75}$ for zebu cattle. There was a 4 times difference in the excretion rate. However, the rate of purine absorption from the small intestine was similar in the two species. An aspect though, that can be considered certain and conclusive, is the low urinary excretion per unit of DOMI, together with the variable values of PD excretion. Urinary PD excretion as an index of microbial N supply is less sensitive when applied to other species of ruminants, and its application should be carried out with caution. (Statements from Joint FAO/IAEA division [11])

So why is the excretion of purine derivatives lower in buffaloes? Some explanation are emerging following some study on swamp buffaloes in Vietnam.

Urinary Excretion of Purine Derivatives: Causes and Differences in Buffaloes and Cattle

In 2004, a study in Vietnam [16, 17] was carried out in order to understand what is the cause of low urinary excretion of purine derivatives in buffaloes. Three experiments were performed prior and following rumen development in cattle and buffalo calves. Then, after rumen development, additional purines were administered to calves by bottle feeding so that they may either pass directly into the abomasum, or by intravenous infusion.

In experiment 1 Vietnamese cattle calves with live weight of 16 kg and three male Vietnamese swamp buffalo calves with live weight of 28 kg, were first given colostrum, reared by milk-bottle feeding, and then weaned. Solid feed was not made available to animals in the course of the first month, and possible differences in the endogenous excretion of purine between the two species was determined following urine collection.

Subsequently and for 2 months, all animals of the two species had access to equal amount of solid feed in order to stimulate rumen development, (buffalo and cattle live weight was on average 51 kg and 37, respectively). Again, differences in purine excretion was determined following urine collection. The results are shown in Table **1**.

Table 1. Purine derivative (PD) excretion in buffalo and cattle calves before and after access to solid feed.

Species	PD excretion in milk-fed calves*(mmol/kg$W^{0.75}$)*	PD excretion in solid-fed calves*(mmol/kg$W^{0.75}$)*
Buffalo	0.69	0.26
Cattle	0.65^{NS}	0.69**

(Table 1) contd.....

Species	PD excretion in milk-fed calves *(mmol/kg$W^{0.75}$)*	PD excretion in solid-fed calves *(mmol/kg$W^{0.75}$)*
s.e	0.06	0.07

**P<0.01; ^{NS}P>0.05

The results showed that in the first part of experiment, 1 purine excretion was not significantly different between the two species, but in the second part of the experiment and following rumen development, purine excretion was significantly different between the two species.

Conclusively, after the animals had access to solid feed, the excretion of PD from buffaloes was highly significant and less than half of cattle.

In experiment 2, purines and milk were mixed and given to the same animals in the course of three different treatments (0, 1.7 and 3.4 g/day). During the experiment, the average live weight of cattle and buffalo calves was 52 and 64 Kg, respectively. In this study the oesophageal groove was instrumental to determine recovery of PD given with milk to the small intestine.

The results are presented in Table **2**. The regression of purine excretion mmol/day (y) was y = 0.6279x + 9.1496 for cattle calves and y = 0.2618x + 5.8594 for buffalo calves where 'x' was the purine administered. It is evident that in cattle a higher PD daily excretion, up to two to three times, was reported in cattle when compared to buffalo calves, and values remained relatively constant independently from the amount of added purine. In cattle calves, the calculated recovery of PD mixed to the milk was also from two to three times higher, when compared to buffalo calves. Moreover the percentage PD recoveries remained almost the same independently from the amount of purine added to milk both in cattle and buffalo calves.

Table 2. The daily urinary excretion of purine derivatives (PD) and of purine supplied *via* nursed milk (mmol/day).

†Level	PD*(mmol/day)*	Buffaloes	Cattle	s.e
L0	Excretion	5.98	9.23*	1.49
L1	Excretion	8.44	15.76**	0.87
L1	Recovery	0.2292	0.6072**	0.085

(Table 2) contd.....

†Level	PD*(mmol/day)*	Buffaloes	Cattle	s.e
L2	Excretion	11.61	22.44**	2.14
L2	Recovery	0.2618	0.6279**	0.0552

† L0 = control: only fresh milk and urea treated rice straw (0.70) mixed with 0.30 molasses given at 50 g dry matter per kg $M^{0.75}$ (L0); L1 = as L0 but milk mixed with 10.8 mmol/day of purines and fed *via* the bottle; L2 = as L1 but milk mixed with 21.5 mmol/day of purines. *P<0.05;**P<0.01; ***P<0.001

In experiment 3, in order to test the effect of purines introduced into the plasma, an allantoin intravenous infusion was administered to the same animals. Within the course of experiment 3, the average live weight of cattle and buffalo calves was 55 and 68 (s.e. 1.8) kg, respectively. In Table **3** are reported the results following allantoin infusion and recovery. Once again, it can be seen that a significant difference between calves of the two species was recorded, recovery being more two times higher in cattle. Regression analysis was also used, and a linear relationship between infusion and excretion was observed. In cattle, the allantoin excretion in mmol/day was y = 0.7177x + 8.438 (r = 0.98), whereas in buffalo allantoin exertion was y = 0.3758x + 4.861 (r = 0.82) where 'x' was allantoin infused in mmol/day. The recovery was two times higher in cattle than buffalo calves.

Table 3. Allantoin infused and excreted during control (L0), level 1 (L1) and level 2 (L2).

†Level	Allantoin (mmol/day)	Buffaloes	Cattle	s.e
L0	Infusion	0	0	
L0	Excretion	4.68	8.59*	0.94
L1	Infusion	18.0	15.0	
L1	Excretion	10.39	18.98**	1.29
L1	Recovery	0.3155	0.6955**	0.0402
L2	Infusion	36.0	30.0	
L2	Excretion	16.43	30.05**	2.36
L2	Recovery	0.3236	0.7199**	0.056

† L0 = control: only fresh milk and urea treated rice straw (0.70) mixed with 0.30 molasses given at 50 g dry matter per kg $W^{0.75}$ (L0); L1 = as L0 but milk mixed with 10.8 mmol/day of purines and fed *via* the bottle; L2 = as L1 but milk mixed with 21.5 mmol/day of purines. *P<0.05;**P<0.01

Previous results showing significant differences between the two species [13 - 15, 18], between cattle and buffaloes, are evident only following rumen development, as clearly illustrated in experiment 1. Such results on recovery rate following rumen development in the two species are also similar to other reports, without any difference detected on the methodology of PD administration used, either through the milk into the abomasum or through intravenous infusion, Liang *et al.* [13] though, found even larger differences between cattle and buffaloes with intravenous infusion, with a higher recovery more than twice when compared to buffaloes.

On the contrary, Liang *et al.* [13] reported a significantly higher recovery in cattle when compared to cattle, when the intravenous infusion was used as the administration route of choice.

Additional reports by Liang *et al.* [18], have also shown that, when PD excretion is used as a measure of endogenous excretion, this is higher in cattle when compared to buffaloes, following fasting. From the above results, it can be stated that fasting excretion cannot be reliably used to determine endogenous excretion in ruminants in general, due to the fact that the rumen is always functioning. Although it is not possible to run a statistical test between the period of feeding PD by either intravenous infusion or milk substitutes, there is a tendency for the slope to be greater than 0.72 and 0.63 for cattle and 0.32 and 0.23 for buffaloes in the period of infusion and milk feeding, respectively. If such effects are real, it is possible that this may be due to some spillage of milk for the excitement of calves when suckling, than to an inefficient closure of the oesophageal groove when the milk enters the rumen [19]. It is interesting to pose the question as to why the detected differences between the two species occur only following rumen development. One possible speculation has to do with the detected difference in glomerular filtration rate (GFR), and in fact, if the latter is physiologically lower in buffaloes, then PD would be found for longer time in the blood and would be exposed to transfer into the rumen for longer time. Nevertheless, Pimpa *et al.* [20], have reported a higher GFR in buffaloes when compared to cattle, and, on the contrary, Norton *et al.* [21], found it lower in the buffalo species. Such discrepancy could be related also to some difference in permeability between rumen and the blood, although, to fully comprehend the exact mechanisms involved, more studies need to be carried out. The available results in our hands so far have clearly established that the differences detected are caused by the development of rumen.

The Physiological Mechanism of Low Purine Derivative Excretion in Urine of Buffaloes

In 2007, a new study was performed in Vietnam [22], using again three cattle calves (*Bos indicus*) and three buffalo calves (*Bubalus bubalis*). As previously described, weaning was done following colostrum feeding and rearing by milk-bottle feeding, and similarly to a previous study, animals did not have access to solid feed for the first month of the experiment. A determination of urinary purine derivative (PD) concentration, basal PD excretion and glomerular filtration rate (GFR) during fasting and feeding, was made. At the end of the first month, in order to stimulate rumen development, animals had access to solid feed (80% of urea-treated rice straw and 20% of molasses). At three months of age, when solid feed were made available, urinary PD, basal PD excretion and GFR were again determined.

Experiment 1: determination of basal urinary purine excretion

The results in Table **4** show that in the course of fasting as well as during milk feeding, no significant differences were reported between the two species with regard to PD excretion (P>0.05).

Table 4. Urinary purine derivative (PD) excretion (mmol/day) in milk-fed calves and in fasting calves during the milk feeding period.

	Buffalo	**Cattle**	**s.e.**
Milk-fed calves			
Excretion (mmol/day)			
PD excretion (mmol/$W^{0.75}$)	0.42	0.45^{NS}	0.02
Live weight (kg)	27	17	4.4
Fasting calves			
Excretion (mmol/day)			
PD excretion (mmol/$W^{0.75}$)	0.53	0.47^{NS}	0.03
Live weight (kg)	35	24	3.9

^{NS}: P>0.05

Experiment 2: determination of urinary purine excretion from calves with access to solid feed

Purine Excretion After 2 Months' Access to Solid Feed

Following 2 months of rumen development in calves, granted by access to solid feed (urea-treated rice straw and molasses), a significantly lower (P<0.01) urinary PD excretion (mmol/kg W0.75) was reported in buffaloes when compared to cattle (Table **5**). The mean daily consumption of feed (g DM/day) was 609 for cattle and 825 for buffalo calves.

Table 5. Urinary purine derivative (PD) excretion in buffaloes and cattle calves in feeding and fasting periods after receiving solid feed at 3 months of age.

	Buffaloes	Cattle	s.e
Solid feed-fed calves			
PD excretion (mmol/$W^{0.75}$)	0.21	0.49***	0.03
Live weight (kg)	42	31	5.18
Fasting calves			
PD excretion (mmol/$W^{0.75}$)	0.23	0.56**	0.07
Live weight (kg)	39	22	1.6

**P<0.01; ***P<0.001

Purine Excretion From Fasting Solid Feed-Fed Calves

The results from Table **5** show that urinary PD excretion was significantly different ($P < 0.05$) between the types of animal. Fasting mature buffaloes were found by Liang *et al.* [18], to have a lower endogenous PD excretion, when compared to cattle, and this difference is clearly linked to the development of the rumen.

Comparison of Feeding and Fasting PD Excretion from Cattle and Buffaloes in Milk-Fed and Solid Feed-Fed Periods

Reported differences between fasting and feeding were small, although slightly higher during fasting. The possible reason behind it may be related to the fact that during fasting, animals are both protein and glucose deficient, as already reported by Orskov [2]. Glucose is derived from the protein turnover pathway, resulting in a much higher N excretion when compared to basal excretion, and this mechanism will have the effect of increasing purine excretion. From the above it can be derived that purine excretion following fasting cannot be used to determine endogenous purine excretion, in consideration of the true increased excretion. Furthermore, the reported differences between the two species may also be related to the recycling of endogenous purines in the rumen in the course of fasting (Table **5** and Fig. **1**).

The differences between buffalo and cattle calves are best illustrated in Fig. (**1**).

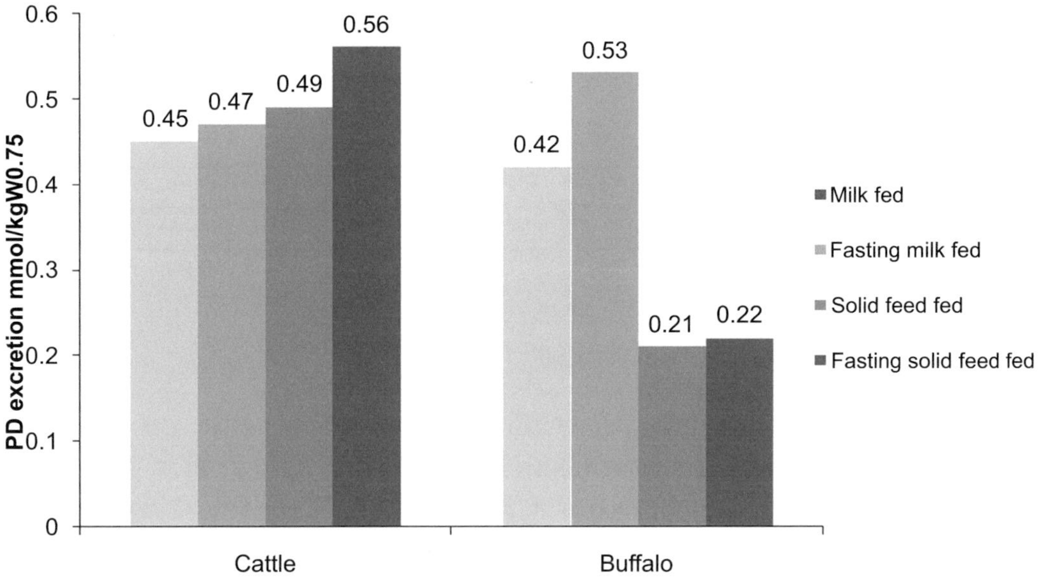

Fig. (1). Comparison of feeding and fasting PD excretion from cattle and buffaloes.

Glomerular Filtration Rate

In order to estimate the GFR [11], a determination of both daily urine creatinine output and creatinine concentration in plasma are required, although, as mentioned in the same report, insulin values may give a more accurate estimate of GFR. Creatine and creatinine phosphate in muscles are necessary to produce creatinine, which is then excreted *via* the urine. Therefore, the muscle mass is a determining factor and strongly correlated to creatinine excretion. Creatinine is filtered from the blood by renal glomerulus and is not affected by either absorption or excretion in the renal tubule, and its daily excretion is relatively constant when the latter is expressed as mmol per kg W0,75. In the following animal species: sheep, cattle, cats and dogs, creatinine is not reabsorbed from or secreted into the renal tubule from the primary urine. Therefore in those animals, creatinine can be used as an endogenous internal marker for determination of GFR. Concentration of creatinine was assessed from blood and urine samples of calves of both species, in the course of milk-feeding and solid-feeding treatment. In Table **6**, it can be clearly seen that buffalo GFR, both prior and following rumen development, was significantly lower (P<0.01) when compared to cattle, and this could be ascribed to differences in the GFR itself [7, 16, 17]. The present study clearly demonstrates a lower GFR in buffaloes compared with cattle.

Table 6. GFR of buffalo and cattle calves before and after rumen development.

	Buffalo	**Cattle**	**s.e.**
Before rumen development (l/Kg$W^{0.75}$/day)	2.3	3.2**	0.1
After rumen development (l/Kg$W^{0.75}$/day)	1.6	2.1***	0.1

**P<0.01; ***P<0.001

Rumen Ammonia

More recently, rumen fluid NH_3 in swamp buffaloes yellow cattle was compared. The experiment was carried on farm with buffaloes and yellow cattle from 2 to 9 years of age, and a body weight from 150 kg to 350 kg. Rumen fluid was obtained by stomach tubes. The results in Table **7** show a significant difference in NH_3 value between types of animal.

Table 7. Rumen fluid NH_3 value in buffaloes and cattle.

Buffaloes (n=43)	Cattle (n=43)	s.e
127.01	75.73***	5.932

***P<0.001. (Vo Thi Kim Thanh. 2009. Unpublished)

CONCLUSION

In both species and prior to the development of the rumen, urine PD excretion was similar during milk-feeding and also in the course of fasting diet, although such

PD excretion in buffaloes was reduced to one-third following rumen development. Therefore, it can be safely speculated that PD metabolism in the two species may be affected by and related to rumen development. In addition, the same study clearly gives indication that in buffaloes GFR is lower when compared to cattle, irrespective of rumen functionality, and this is in agreement with the data previously described and provided by studies of Norton *et al.* [21] and Chen *et al.* [10].

Furthermore, from the evidence presented, it can be said that basal PD excretion is similar between the two species during milk feeding, and no explanation can be derived for a lower PD excretion following rumen development. An inherently lower GFR in buffaloes may accounts for a longer time of PD in the blood flow, and following the activation of rumen functionality and the PD passage from the blood to the rumen, where PD degradation occurs, may help in explaining the reported lower PD excretion in buffalo urine. No evidence is provided if the permeability of transfer from blood to rumen, can be considered an additional factor. Definitely, any difference in PD excretion in the two species can be reported only following rumen development.

The differences in PD excretion reported in the two species are possibly caused by differences in GFR, with the net result of a longer stay of PD in the blood and consequently a greater possibility to be recycled into the rumen. Therefore, more urea will be recycled with the result of higher rumen ammonia concentration, confirming the aspect that buffaloes can tolerate less N in the feed to sustain microbial need.

CONFLICT OF INTEREST

The authors confirm that they have no conflict of interest to declare for this publication.

ACKNOWLEDGEMENTS

Declared none.

REFERENCES

[1] McDonald P, Edwards RA. Greenhalgh and Morgan CA Animal nutrition. UK: Longman Publisher 1995; p. 431.

[2] Ørskov ER. The feeding of Ruminants Principles and Practice. 2nd ed. UK: Chalcombe Publications 2001; pp. 3-15.

[3] Bartocci S, Amici A, Verna M, Terramoccia S, Martillotti F. Solid and fluid passage rate in buffalo, cattle and sheep fed diets with different forage to concentrate ratios. Livest Prod Sci 1997; 52(3): 201-8.
[http://dx.doi.org/10.1016/S0301-6226(97)00132-2]

[4] Infascelli F, Di Lella T, Piccolo V. Dry matter, organic matter and crude protein degradability of high protein feeds in buffaloes and sheep. Zoot Nut Anim 1995; 21 (Suppl.): 89-94.

[5] Sangwan DC, Pradhan K, Bhatia SK, Sagar V, Sadhana S. Associative effect of wheat straw or oat hay with protein supplements on rumen metabolites and nutrient digestibility, in cattle and buffalo. Indian J Anim Sci 1990; 60: 472-9.

[6] Kennedy PM, Boniface AN, Liang ZJ, Muller D, Murray RM. Intake and digestion in swamp buffaloes and cattle. 2. The comparative response to urea supplements in animals fed tropical grasses. J Agr Sci Cambridge 1992; 119: 243-54.
[http://dx.doi.org/10.1017/S0021859600014179]

[7] Chen XB, Ørskov ER. Research on urinary excretion of purine derivatives in ruminants: past, present and future. In: Makkar HS, Ed. Estimation of Microbial Protein Supply in Ruminants Using Urinary Purine derivative. Netherlands: Springer 2004; pp. 180-210.
[http://dx.doi.org/10.1007/978-1-4020-2844-1_21]

[8] Smith RH, McAllan AB. Nucleic acid metabolism in the ruminant. 2. Formation of microbial nucleic acids in the rumen in relation to the digestion of food nitrogen, and the fate of dietary nucleic acids. Br J Nutr 1970; 24(2): 545-56.
[http://dx.doi.org/10.1079/BJN19700052] [PMID: 5452704]

[9] Chen XB, Gomes MJ. Estimation of microbial protein supply to sheep and cattle based on urinary excretion of purine derivatives -an overview of the technical details. International Feed Resources Unit Rowett Research Institute, Bucksburn Aberdeen Ab2 9SB, UK Occasional Publication 1992. http://www.macaulay.ac.uk/IFRU/pdf/chema.pdf

[10] Chen XB, Samaraweera L, Kyle DJ, Ørskov ER, Abeygunawardene H. Urinary excretion of purine derivatives and tissue xanthine oxidase (EC 1.2.3.2) activity in buffaloes (*Bubalis bubalis*) with special reference to differences between buffaloes and Bos taurus cattle. Br J Nutr 1996; 75(3): 397-407.
[http://dx.doi.org/10.1079/BJN19960142] [PMID: 8785213]

[11] A training package: the technique for estimating microbial protein supply in ruminants based on determination of purine derivatives in urine (CD-ROM). Vienna 2003.

[12] Vercoe JE. Urinary allantoin excretion and digestible dry-matter intake in cattle and buffalo. J Agric Sci Camb 1976; pp. 613-5.

[13] Liang JB, Pimpa O, Balcells J, Abdullah N, Jeland ZA. An overview on the use of urinary purine derivatives excretion as a method for estimation of rumen microbial protein production in swamp

buffaloes and zebu cattle Estimation of Microbial Protein Supply in Ruminants Using Urinary Purine derivative Harinder P S Makkar and X B Chen FAO/IAEA Kluwer Academic Publishers. Dordrecht, Boston, London: Printed in the Netherlands 2004; pp. 42-51. [http://dx.doi.org/10.1007/978-1-4020-2844-1_5]

[14] Soejono M, Yusiati L M, Backrudin Z, Budhi SPS, Widyobroto BP, Utomo R. Flow of nucleic acids from the rumen and recovery of purine derivatives in the urine of cattle and buffaloes. In: Makkar H.P.S, Chen X.B. Eds. Estimation of Microbial Protein Supply in Ruminants Using Urinary Purine derivative. 1st ed.. Netherland: Springer 2004; pp. 69-74. [http://dx.doi.org/10.1007/978-1-4020-2844-1_8]

[15] Thi Kim Thanh Vo, Orskov ER. Why is purine derivative excretion in swamp buffaloes, lower than in cattle? Some studies from Vietnam. Proceedings of the 5Th Asian Buffalo Congress on Social Economic Contribution of Buffalo to Rural Area Volume 1. 495-503.

[16] Thi Kim Thanh Vo, Ørskov ER. Causes of differences in urinary excretion of purine derivatives in buffaloes and cattle. Anim Sci 2006; 82(3): 355-58. [http://dx.doi.org/10.1079/ASC200637]

[17] Vo Thi Kim Thanh. Dao Thi Phuong, Tran Thi Thu Hong, Phung Thi Luu, Ngo Mau Dzung, Hoang Quoc Hung, Ørskov ER Comparison of Purine Derivative and Creatinine in plasma and urine between cattle and buffaloes in Vietnam Harinder P S Makkar and X B Chen FAO/IAEA Kluwer Academic Publishers. Dordrecht, Boston, London: Printed in the Netherlands 2004; pp. 75-85.

[18] Liang JB, Pimpa O, Abdullah N, Jeland ZA. Estimation of rumen microbial protein production from urinary purine derivatives in zebu cattle and water buffalo In Nuclear based technologies for estimating microbial protein supply in ruminant livestock IAEA-TECDOC-1093. Austria: Printed by IAEA, Vienna 1999; pp. 35-42.

[19] Ørskov ER, Benzie D, Kay RN. The effects of feeding procedure on closure of the oesophageal groove in young sheep. Br J Nutr 1970; 24(3): 785-95. [http://dx.doi.org/10.1079/BJN19700080] [PMID: 5470779]

[20] Pimpa O, Liang JB, Balcells J, Jelan ZA, Abdullah N. Urinary PD excretion in swamp buffaloes after duodenal purine base infusion. Anim Feed Sci Technol 2003; 104: 191-9. [http://dx.doi.org/10.1016/S0377-8401(02)00329-2]

[21] Norton BW, Moran JB, Nolan JV. Nitrogen metabolism in Brahman cross, buffaloes, Benteng and Shorthorn steers fed on low quality roughages. Aust J Agric Res 1979; 30: 341-51. [http://dx.doi.org/10.1071/AR9790341]

[22] Thi Kim Thanh Vo, Orskov ER, Susmel P. The physiological mechanism of low purine derivative excretion in urine of buffaloes compared to Bos Taurus cattle. Anim Prod Sci 2009; 49: 994-7. [http://dx.doi.org/10.1071/EA08287]

CHAPTER 8

Influence of Seasonality on Buffalo Production

Luigi Zicarelli*

Dipartimento di Medicina Veterinaria e Produzioni Animali - Università "Federico II" – Napoli, Via Delpino, 1 - 80137 Napoli, Italy

Abstract: This review aims at elucidating some of the factors that affect seasonality in the buffalo species, together with the possibility to enhance reproductive performance in buffaloes through the adoption of newly developed technologies. It is known that reproduction in buffaloes is influenced by the season, and an improvement in reproductive performances is reported in the period of the year when the length of the day decreases. If conception is not established in buffaloes in the course of few ovarian cycle, ovarian function is interrupted and a period of ovarian quiescence (anestrus) begins. The transitional period in the buffalo is an important one for reproductive functions, and throughout this period a proper management of the animals has to be taken into consideration, especially in order to properly maintain the hygienic status of the uterus. Buffaloes reared in tropical countries north of the equator may be characterized by a reduced fertility in the summer when hit mainly by restricted feeding and heat stress. In some countries like Pakistan, the breeding season starts in a period of the year characterized by decreasing daylight (autumn), together with an increase in body condition score. Differently, despite a constant feed availability in the course of the year and a moderate daily temperature ranging from 13 to 23 °C, anestrus can be witnessed also in Italy. These two countries are similarly characterized by an increase in daylight from April to June and reaching more than 12 hours of light hours at summer peak. In order to improve fertility in Italian buffalo herds, an increasing number of farms adopt the Out of Breeding Mating Strategy (OBMS) together with the availability of water pools. This is a clear evidence that reproductive performance as a whole can be improved, together with a reduction in the incidence of embryonic mortality and ovarian inactivity, when environmental conditions are also improved.

* **Corresponding author Luigi Zicarelli:** Dipartimento di Medicina Veterinaria e Produzioni Animali - Università "Federico II" – Napoli, *via* Delpino, 1 - 80137 Napoli, Italy; Tel: +39 081 2536800; Fax: +39 081 292981; E-mail: zicarell@unina.it

Giorgio A. Presicce (Ed.)

Keywords: Buffalo, Reproduction, Reproductive technologies.

1. INTRODUCTION

The official FAO data refers that buffaloes are present in 43 countries and are hence bred in 20% (43 *vs.* 212) of the countries in which cattle is bred. On the contrary, countries that currently breed buffaloes are 129 [1] and hence it is likely that this species is bred in 61% of the countries around the world (129/212). Cattle world population (Faostat.fao.org/faostat) moved steadily from 942 millions in 1961 to 1.494 billions (+ 59%) in 2013, and within the same time interval, buffaloes increased from 89 millions to 199 billions (+ 125%). Between 1990 and 2013, the percentual increment in those countries where the two species are bred, has always been higher for the buffalo species (Table **1**). It has to be emphasized though, that most of the countries where the two species are bred, are in Asia, where the human population has considerably increased, and such aspect justifies the increment.

Table 1. Buffalo and cattle population trend (%) between 1961 and 2013.

	Cattle		Buffalo	
World	2013	1961	2013	1961
buffalo and cattle population trend (%) between 1961 and 2013 (x 10^6)	1494 (59)	942	199 (125)	89
buffalo and cattle population trend (%) between 1990 and 2013 (x 10^6)	1494 (15)	1297	199 (35)	148
countries where two species are bred	2013	1961	2013	1961
buffalo and cattle population trend (%) between 1961 and 2013 (x 10^6)	705 (87)	378	199 (127) *	88
buffalo and cattle population trend (%) between 1990 and 2013 (x 10^6)	705 (29)	547	199 (35*)	148

*This increase is mainly due to the increase of River buffalo (50 n; milk production), while the Swamp (48 n; draught animal power), decreased by 27% [2].

The buffalo represents a fundamental and irreplaceable resource for tropical countries. The increase in the number of buffalo heads is mainly due to the increase of River buffaloes (50 n), utilized for milk and meat production, while the Swamp buffaloes (48 n), mainly used as draught animal power, has decreased by 26.69% [2], especially in South-Eastern Asia. The Swamp buffalo in many countries is crossbred with the river type, due to an increase in milk demand. In fact, it is true that the dairy cow is not always able to totally exploit its genetic merit for many months in the tropical areas, due to the high temperatures and high humidity rate. On the contrary, under the same conditions, the River buffalo can still support an optimal production, although, it retains a sensitivity to such environmental conditions. In fact, if nutritive requirements are satisfied, buffaloes are characterized by similar milk productions in both tropical and temperate areas. In the last years, world's buffalo milk percentage has increased from 5 to 14.8%, but such values can bounce from 8.3 to 21.6%, when we consider that buffalo milk is 58% higher in energy than its cattle counterpart.

In Southern Asia, where 78% of the world's buffalo population is bred, in cattle, and compared to the year 1961, a higher milk increase has been observed (+ 657% *vs.* + 581%). This phenomenon can be explained by the use of imported superior genetic gametes and embryos from industrialized countries in order to obtain an improvement in animal production. However, the increase in milk production alone is not sufficient to justify the decision to increase the number of an animal species, or to consider it more economically viable and efficient. Other factors have to be considered, such as: lower susceptibility to diseases, higher adaptability to the tropical environment, higher herd life, and hence, a lower culling rate. These conditions will favour an increase in the number of heads within the herd also for beef production, matching perfectly production and forage availability. In fact, in South Asia, lactation in buffaloes coincides with an abundance of forage availability, while the dry period will match the quiescence of the vegetative cycle. These are fundamental aspects that reduce the advantage in cattle linked to their higher production performance. In particular, and with regard to ordinary culling rate between the two species, if we consider a breeding farm of 100 females in production, it is necessary to breed around 90 (26% culling rate) and 42 (12% culling rate) heads (adult animals), in cattle and buffalo, respectively. Consequently, the same number of cattle heads will need a much larger land when compared to buffaloes, and in those countries where farms are characterized by low size, this difference is economically important.

In India in 1991, buffalo milk consumption was 55% of the total milk produced in the country. In a conference held in Egypt, Krostitz [3] reported that in 1991, the "Technology Mission on Dairy Development", predicted that before the third millennium, this consumption would have decreased to 45% because of the replacement with cattle milk. Currently 51.1%, 45.4% and 3.5% of consumption is given by buffalo, bovine and goat milk, respectively. Not always the right importance is given to factors that allow any farmer to choose the animal species to breed, while the consumer would prefer by tradition and personal taste the buffalo milk which is more pleasing because intrinsically sweeter. If we put aside Nepal (+1.2%) and India (-3%), where milk consumption has not decreased in the last 50 years, a clear deflection has been reported in Egypt (-12.7%) and Pakistan (-8%) (Table **2**). In these last two countries, it is possible that such decrease has been caused by the urbanization that notoriously pushes away the consumer from traditional food. In addition, a further element that contributes to the decrease in buffalo milk consumption, is its seasonal availability, as a consequence of the reproductive characteristics of this species.

Table 2. Buffalo milk consumption in India, Nepal, Egypt and Pakistan.

Consumption (%) of buffalo milk between 1961 and 2014 in India, Nepal, Egypt and Pakistan								
	India		Nepal		Egypt		Pakistan	
	Kg	calories	kg	calories	kg	calories	kg	calories
1961	55,9	66,7	67,5	76,6	66,1	75,5	71,4	79,3
1970	56,7	67,4	69,6	78,3	63,7	73,5	71,3	79,2
1980	56,7	67,4	72,5	80.6	65,8	75,2	74,5	82,2
1990	56,6	67,4	70,2	78,9	56,2	67,0	75,2	82,7
2000	56,8	67,5	69,2	78,0	55,3	66,2	67,8	76,9
2010	53,2	64,2	71,3	79,7	47,0	58,3	64,2	73,9
2014	52,9	64,0	68,7	77,6	53,4	64,4	63,4	73,3

In countries with temperate/continental climate such as Europe, where the cattle is able to express its genetic production potential, we observe that the number of buffaloes and cattle has decreased by 46% and 37%, respectively, while the amount of buffalo milk has increased by 117% and cattle milk by 14%. On the same line, in 1961 the percentage of Italian buffalo milk in Europe was 14.9%, and in 2014 was 95.6%.

In tropical areas south of the Equator, where buffaloes usually calve between February and March and weaning occurs between September to October, this seasonality does not adversely affect the growth of calves thanks to forage availability in November, following beginning of the rainy season.

Differently, the zebu gives birth between September and October and weaning occurs in winter between April and May, a period characterized by a shortage of forage availability, which is responsible of post weaning stress, and growth is also penalized. This difference explains why the buffalo reaches a marketing weight roughly one year before the Zebu. South of the Equator, where most buffaloes calve within 3 to 4 months, the milk is unsuitable for processing into mozzarella cheese due to a low protein content and high titratable acidity.

In Italy and under Italian law, where buffalo milk is mainly used for mozzarella cheese production, only fresh milk can be used for processing (within 60 h from the milking) and cheese production. These aspects are of paramount importance in order to better understand buffalo management as connected to seasonality and buffalo production.

In Asian countries, buffalo milk is used for both drinking purposes and cheese production: generally buffalo milk production throughout the year is inversely correlated to cattle milk.

Hassan *et al.* [4] in Pakistan reported a different seasonality among Nili-Ravi Buffaloes (9,174 lactations), purebred Sahiwal (22,499 lactations) and cross-bred cattle (656 lactations). In this study, the difference between Nili-Ravi Buffaloes (characterized by negative photoperiod) and purebred Sahiwal (characterized by positive photoperiod) has been highlighted. Data similar to those recorded in buffaloes have been observed in cross-bred cattle (Holstein or Jersey x native bred). This finding suggests that crossbreeding with European *Bos taurus* may modify the seasonality of native cattle (Sahiwal), as evidenced by a higher incidence of deliveries during the first 5 months of the year and, hence, highest rate of conception during the hottest months (April-August). An increase of such cross-bred cattle would lead as a consequence to a higher storage of dehydrated, frozen or concentrated milk, and the availability of lower amount of fresh buffalo and cattle milk.

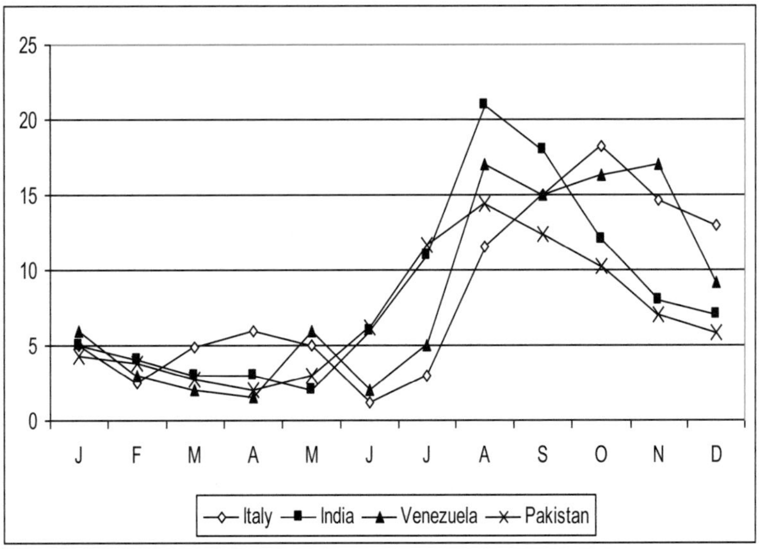

Fig. (1). Monthly calving percentage for Italy, India, Venezuela, and Pakistan.

In Europe, buffalo milk is mainly used for cheese and yogurt production, in order to increase its value. In Italy, buffalo milk is remunerated more than three times in comparison to cattle. In other European countries buffalo milk is remunerated around two times when compared to cattle milk, and this difference may explain the increase of buffalo heads in the South of Italy and the decrease in other European countries. In Latin America, the buffalo shows high fertility and is mainly used for meat production, although in the last years several farms utilize milk for the production of "caso blanco" and other cheeses.

In all the countries where the buffalo is bred, an ovarian cyclic activity is reported throughout the year, although it is accentuated during periods characterized by decreasing daylight length: from August to February (in January and February daylight length increases but the number of dayligth hours is less than 12 h) and from April to July at the North and the South of the Equator, respectively. This tendency to seasonality is emphasized proportionally to the distance from the Equator [5]. Around the equatorial belt, where light/dark ratio varies little throughout the year, the reproductive season is highly conditioned by forage availability instead [6, 7].

Therefore, it can be affirmed [8, 9] that reproductive seasonality is responsible for a lactation to be linked to forage abundance, whereas the dry period is linked to the quiescence of the vegetative cycle of crops and spontaneous plants in tropical areas at north of the Equator, whereas the contrary occurs in zebu. Differently, in tropical areas south of the Equator, forage abundance coincides with the dry period and the first part of lactation. It follows that usually, buffaloes calve being thin and in good nutrition conditions, in tropical areas north and south of the Equator, respectively.

The majority of the authors believe that the main reproductive characteristics of buffaloes are delayed puberty, prolonged postpartum ovarian inactivity, long inter-calving intervals and a tendency toward seasonality [10 - 12]. The reproductive problems though are different depending on the region of the world. In tropical countries north of the equator (TCNE), for example, the majority of the authors assert that summer anestrus is caused by heat stress and forage scarcity. In Italy, however, anestrus is observed in the same period of the year as TCNE, as demonstrated by the calving distribution shown in (Fig. **1**), although feeding in Italy is constant throughout the year and the environmental temperatures are milder.

The aim of this review is to examine the main factors affecting fertility in buffaloes and the strategies that may be adopted to enhance the reproductive performance of this species.

2. OPTIMIZATION OF THE AGE AT FIRST CALVING

Most authors believe that delayed puberty is one of the reproductive features of the buffalo. This is not a characteristic of the species, but rather the consequence of some mistakes occurring in the course of food selection and rationing. It is known that buffalo milk is richer than cattle, and that the buffalo shows a weight gain lower than cattle but higher than zebu. Whenever the buffalo is used for milk production, calf weaning is performed by different techniques (wet-nurse cow, milk replacer) or by utilizing low quantity of buffalo milk, sufficient to the survival of the calf, but insufficient for guaranteeing an optimal growing [13].

In countries where the buffalo is used for meat production (South America), the natural weaning occurs usually at 7-8 months of age. In this case, the age at first calving is earlier than 30 months, similar to what recorded in *Bos taurus* but earlier than *Bos indicus*. When milk replacer is utilized, like in Italy, calves usually weigh 90 kg at 100 days of age. Following weaning, it is necessary to adopt diets characterized by high energy density, ensuring rumen functionality. On the contrary, natural weaning performed at 7-8 months of age guarantees that pasture feeding will substitute progressively maternal milk. The energy density of the mixed dry matter (milk and pasture) from 3 to 7 months is higher than the same energy obtained with hay and concentrate. A higher energetic density is required in buffaloes to obtain performances significantly lower than cattle when "artificial" feeding replaces milking and natural weaning.

Furthermore, it is worth considering that the achievement of a body status typical of a particular age requires a certain amount of body lipids that, in animals with delayed growth, have not been accumulated, implying therefore a higher value of feed conversion index. This explains why buffalo meat is characterized by a lower fat content than beef cattle.

These aspects justify the need to use diets characterized by higher energy compared to cattle, in order to anticipate the age at first calving in buffalo [14]. It cannot be ruled out that the compensatory growth in the buffalo species is less efficient than cattle. With a rationing characterized by an energy density of 0.8 MUF (MUF = Milk unit forages = 1700 kcal NE_l) and 12.5-13% protein content on dry matter, together with forage/concentrate ratio of 50-60%, age at first calving can be targeted at around 28-32 months [15].

Fertility of Primiparous Buffaloes

It is likely that the post partum reproductive inactivity occurs more easily in primiparous animals. These animals can usually restore their ability to cycle again by adopting the usual hormonal treatments if a correct rationing is carried out, whereas such treatments are usually inadequate if the rationing is not correctly performed. The fertility of primiparous animals is usually higher than multiparous animals, at least in Italy, where in the course of the lactation period the rationing is characterized by 0.9 MFU/kg DM, and the effect of feed rationing until the first calving is such as to reduce the food requirement necessary to growth during the first lactation. Usually, a young herd is more fertile than one characterized by more than 3.5 lactations. If primiparous animals have a mean production of 2300 kg of milk (13,76 kg/d FCM), a rationing characterized by 0.9 MFU/kg DM allows to obtain a 50-70 kg live weight increase at the end of the lactation. This is possible because, differently from dairy cattle, the ingestion is often higher than what reported in multiparous animals with similar production that do not require a nutrients surplus to complete growth. Especially if the roughage/concentrate ratio of the ration is optimal, primiparous animals can ingest an average of 15.6 kg DM/d, covering the requirements necessary to face a milk production of 2300 kg, the recovery of weight and the weight gain necessary to complete the growth. In conclusion if primiparous animals are characterized by the lowest fertility within the herd, it may be assumed that the diet has been inadequate during lactation or the growth and the first gestation.

In a recent trial carried out on 390 primiparous animals, we have found that the dry matter intake (DM), the percentage of DM/kg L.W. and DM/equivalent corrected milk (ECM) is related to the days in milk (DIM) and the milk production. In fact, it increases from delivery until 121-150 DIM and then diminishes, while the production of ECM decreases after 61 - 90 days. It is possible to distinguish, likewise cattle, a “catabolic” phase (until 55 days) and an “anabolic” phase. Throughout the “catabolic” phase, the energy intake is less than the requirement and the cow utilizes the body reserves for production. During the “anabolic” phase the opposite occurs: the body reserves are reconstituted and the body weight increases [16].

It has to be underlined that the diet is characterized by 0.9, 15.7%, 38.5% and 50.0% of MFU/kg D.M., Crude Protein, N.D.F. and roughages/concentrate ratio, respectively. The above diet causes an energy deficiency until 55 DIM, but allows to recover body weight at 85 days DIM and to reach the adult weight at end of lactation.

In the trials carried out by Campanile *et al.* [17], it was observed that the intake of DM was conditioned negatively by the content in the cellular walls and positively by milk production, and dry matter intake per kg of ECM (kcal = 740) amounts to 275 g in addition to what required for maintenance (91 g per kg of metabolic weight).

Reproductive Seasonality

The place of origin and the duration of gestation have undoubtedly influenced the way in which reproductive seasonality occurs. The seasonality is the response to a process of "adaptation" between the animal and the surrounding environment: such adaptation is in fact responsible for matching birth and weaning with the best time of the year when the weather is more favourable and it is easier to access the nutritional needs for the calves, in addition to witness less aggressive or present infectious agents and parasites [5]. Those calves born under the most favourable conditions are linked to adult animals naturally selected, because they are endowed with an ideal reproductive seasonality that promotes the survival of the species [8]. Spring calving (March to May), which guarantees good availability of forage to offspring in the temperate zones in the north of the equator, occurs when reproduction takes place in autumn (September to November) in the case of a five month gestation (sheep and goats), or in the previous spring in the case of 11 and 12 month gestation (horses and donkeys). The same calving period, therefore, is conditioned by the neuroendocrine system. The reactivation of the reproductive cycle with regard to the length of gestation (short day breeder - negative photoperiod - or long day breeder - positive photoperiod -) is therefore controlled.

In the tropical areas where the domestic buffalo is present (between 31° N and 2° S), the availability of forage is usually sufficient after the rainy season (July to September). In the same species characterized by a pregnancy length of 310 to 316 days, the sensitivity to the decreasing light stimulus and the breeding season occurs between September and January-February.

Around the equatorial belt, where the light/dark ratio varies little throughout the year, the reproductive season is highly conditioned by forage availability [6, 7, 18]. There is a tendency towards seasonality in buffaloes because this species evolved far away from the equator. Moving the buffalo to other regions of the world has not modified the hypothalamic hypophyseal axis sensitivity to a decreasing light/dark ratio.

In Italy, the seasonality makes it necessary to change the calving calendar in order to meet the milk market demand. This is accomplished by using an out-of-breeding-mating-strategy (OBMS) that entails the interruption of natural mating or the use of artificial insemination (AI) between October and late January in adult females and between September and late March in heifers. The above months are the most-favourable periods for reproductive activity [5, 8, 9].

In studies carried out in Italy [19], it has been demonstrated that buffaloes with a tendency towards seasonality show a high plasma melatonin concentrations two hours after sunset even when they are moved to another farm where other females show low plasma melatonin concentrations and less sensitivity towards light stimulation [20]. In another previous study, it was reported that buffaloes who tend to conceive in autumn (months when daylight hours are decreasing), have a greater increase in plasma melatonin 2 hours from sunset than those who conceive when the hours of daily light increase (late winter – spring). Plasma melatonin concentrations showed a repeatability of 0.733 [21]. If the heredity of plasma melatonin turns out to be high, as we expect on the basis of high repeatability, the plasma melatonin level could be included into genetic selection programmes for buffalo [5]. In an effort to validate this idea, we reported that Romanov 58°N, Karakul 41°N and White-faced 51°N sheep [22] showed continuous cyclic activity throughout the year even if living at latitudes where other genotypes were sensitive to the light/dark ratio. On the contrary, the Soay sheep has only 1 or 2 estrous cycles limited to 1 or 2 autumn months.

Between heifers and adult buffalo cows, the difference between night and day concentrations of plasma melatonin was less in heifers (5.0 times) compared to adult buffaloes (28.3 times) in March [23]. Both buffaloes [21] - more adaptable to out-of-breeding-mating-strategy - and heifers [5, 23] - less sensitive to the photoperiod - that calve in spring, show the same behavioural pattern.

Heifer fertility is not compromised by the season [5, 24 - 28]. During summer and when daylight hours are higher than dark hours, there is an increase in the blood prolactin but, contrary to assertions by Madan [10], the buffalo conceives regularly. We believe that hyperprolactinemia is a consequence of the hypothyroidism [29] during the warm months. The hypothyroidism exerts a positive feedback on thyroid stimulating hormone and hence on thyrotropin releasing hormone. Thyrotropin releasing hormone promotes an increase in prolactin [5, 8, 25].

The majority of authors attribute reproductive seasonality to nutritional factors. The breeding period, in areas where 97% of the buffalo population are bred, takes place in the months of greater forage availability [30 - 35]. Greater forage availability is found during the months of July through November characterized by decreasing daylight length in the TCNE.

If heat stress is the main cause of anestrus, then it should adversely affect the reproductive activity of buffaloes compared to *Bos indicus*. In Italy, the opposite pattern is observed. Among out-of-season mated buffaloes, the conception rate increases between July and September, a period during which Holstein cows show a low conception rate.

In Italian herds where the OBMS technique is not used [36], a condition that was typical of the majority of farms 30 to 40 years ago [37], the resumption of the reproductive cycle (RRC) takes place from September (decreasing light period) to January (Fig. **1**). Sensitivity to the negative photoperiod is also found on farms where a constant balanced diet is provided year-round [5]. This type of seasonality, where reproductive events are not synchronised with forage availability, gives indication that buffaloes bred in Italy are not autochthonous, meaning that they will sometime calve during the periods of forage scarceness and low temperature which in turn hinders the survival of the newborn. Italian findings should be sufficient to define the buffalo as a short day breeder. Indeed, a similar seasonality to that found in Italy and Asian tropical areas is also found in Venezuela [38, 39], Egypt [40] (Fig. **1**) and Columbia (personal observations).

In southern Brazil [41, 42] and Argentina (Zicarelli, unpublished observations), the wet season (and consequently, pasture availability) starts around October to November and continues until March to April, whereas pasture scarcity goes from May to June until October to November. The buffalo calving period under these conditions is mainly concentrated from February to May (Fig. **2**). The breeding period is from April to July and the calf weaning under free range and suckling calf conditions is from September to December. These events permit the coincidence of forage availability within the first 2 to 4 months of lactation and most of the dry period (October to April). The breeding period, however, is mainly concentrated during the pasture scarcity period (May to July).

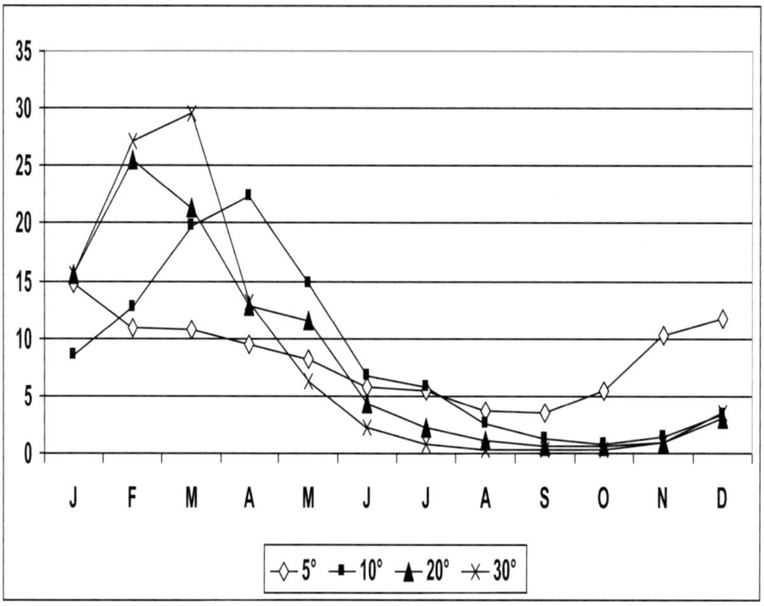

Fig. (2). Monthly calving percentage in Brazil as a function of latitude (°).

Baruselli *et al.* [41], who evaluated data from the Brazilian Breeders Association, observed that the seasonality is more accentuated in the north (0 to 8 degrees latitude) than the south (24 to 32 degrees latitude) of Brazil (Fig. **2**), and hence the calving season is influenced by latitude.

From the findings reported, it can be unequivocally stated that, although the domestic buffalo shows reproductive activity throughout the year, there is a greater tendency to concentrate reproductive activity in the months of decreasing daylight or if increasing, when dark hours prevail.

Reproductive Efficiency

Many scientists affirm that buffaloes show delayed puberty and a long inter-calving interval, both affected by several factors, such as year of calving, season of delivery, genotype and heat stress [15]. The delayed puberty and the consequent older age at first calving has been addressed by many authors. In a study performed on 86 farms (30,735 primiparous buffaloes calving between 1975 and 2005), it was observed that the mean age at first calving decreased by 1 month every 5 years (44.7 ± 6.6 and 35.3 ± 6.5 months, respectively in 1975 and 2005) [15]. The hormonal pattern in cyclic buffalo is similar to *Bos taurus* [43], and the main difference between the two species is the rate of cyclic individuals in the different seasons.

The different reproductive efficiency of buffaloes compared to *Bos taurus* is due to several features. These features must be considered because there is a need to modify the calving calendar in the buffalo in order to meet market demands. There are fewer primordial [44] and antral follicles as well as a lesser ovarian weight (4 *vs.* 8.5 g) and lesser ovarian volume (mean length: 2.5 *vs.* 3.7 cm) in the buffalo species compared to cattle [45]. The number of oocytes in a buffalo calf is one-fifth compared to a cattle calf [44, 46]. After calving, there are a low number of ovarian follicles and follicular waves, and few cycles occur. If conception does not take place, therefore, an anestrus of variable length begins [5]. With regard to this topic, the transition period and the postpartum period have a major importance for fertility in the buffalo compared to cattle. It should be pointed out that in those farms adopting semi-free housing, the presence of mycotoxins in the roughages, *Clostridia*, *Coxiella burnetii*, and the incorrect input of Ca, P and crude protein in the last two months of pregnancy often lead to the occurrence of vaginal or uterine prolapse which impairs the RRC [47]. It is not clear whether the seasonality of the species depends on the reduced follicular population or if this latter effect is the cause of buffalo seasonality.

If the calving calendar is not modified, the delayed RRC after calving can be due to the lack of the "bull effect" [48] and/or to poor nutritional conditions [49]. In small farms in TCNE where the bull is not present, the dry period of the animals (March to June) coincides with the scarcity of forage. South of the equator over the 20th parallel (November to March), the dry period coincides with the abundance of forage and the bull is always present in the herd. In the first case, prolonged inter-calving intervals are observed [32] whereas in the second case inter-calving intervals less than 400 days are recorded [5, 49].

These observations suggest that in those areas, the respect of nutritional requirements and the absence/presence of the bull are the most important factors [48], especially taking into account that the protein content of the pastures is very low (6 to 10% of DM) and leguminosae can be found in irrigated areas or in the course of the rainy season. In Pakistan, Qureshi *et al.* [35, 50] reported that the seasonality is influenced by nutritional and non-nutritional factors. Unless feed deficiencies are serious, however, nutritional factors in general do not play a significant role [16, 51 - 53]. The buffalo cannot yet be considered exactly as having a "*lactiferous habitus*" and therefore a "*catabolicus habitus*" such as that found in the high milk producing cattle, characterized by using body reserves to compensate energy and protein deficiency during early lactation. Actually, within reasonable limits, buffaloes at least with a production of less 3000 kg/lactation, use their reserves with the aim to reproduce, to the detriment of milk production [16].

The effects of the tendency toward seasonal reproduction in the buffalo are particularly evident. Studies conducted in Italy may be useful for countries wishing to increase the consistency of their production of buffalo milk during the year. When primiparous animals are excluded from the survey (heifers are less sensitive to photoperiod), a decrease in calving rate between March and June for farms that are adopting the OBMS technique is observed in Italy whether OBMS is applied or not (Fig. **3**). This confirms that the increase in day light hours (April to June) or number of day light hours >12 h, negatively interferes with reproductive activity. The buffalo that undergoes OBMS can show anestrus, and this phenomenon is emphasized by unfavourable climate conditions.

It is possible to define a "temporary anestrus" (<150 days) and a "deep anestrus" (>150 days) based on the number of days open. It is also possible to distinguish between buffaloes that come into estrus within 70 days from calving, and conceive within or after 90 days, from those which come into estrus after 70 days and conceive within or after 150 days [54].

Anestrus can be identified as a non RRC after parturition or as an interruption of cyclic activity for a number of reasons. Environmental conditions that are responsible for anestrus are accompanied by changes in blood hormones. It is possible that some of these hormones represent the response to stressful factors rather than the cause of the arrest in reproductive activity. Buffaloes calving out of the breeding season, conceive very soon or need several months to conceive. During this period, they are not always acyclic, but are able to conceive and undergo embryonic mortality, in particular between April and May, months characterized by progressively increasing day length. During the year, the embryonic mortality rate is 10% of the pregnancies diagnosed at 40 days and is 22% for conceptions that take place in the month of April [54]. The incidence of this event is considerably affected by the "farm" factor and ranges between 10% and 45%, if calculated on the pregnancies after AI diagnosed by ultrasonography at day 26 [55].

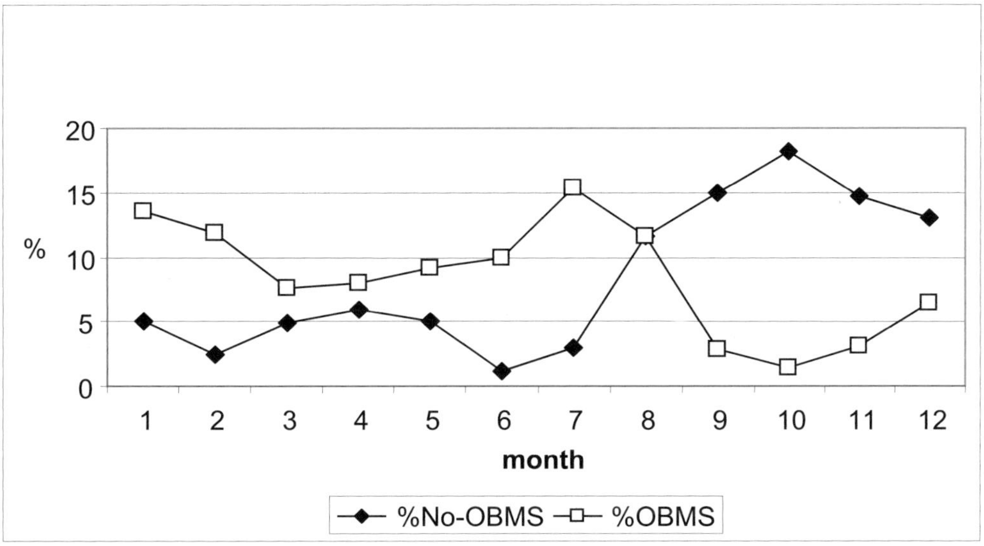

Fig. (3). Calving percentage in farms that use (%OBMS) or do not use (%No-OBMS) the OBMS technique.

A pregnancy is not always detected following observation of a corpus luteum. It can be assumed that the occurrence of an early embryonic mortality or an anestrus condition can be caused by an ovarian cycle with a corpus luteum characterized by inadequate function, because of a short luteal phase or normal luteal phase with low progesterone production [48, 56]. This phenomenon has been found at the onset of anestrus season in sheep, after first ovulation postpartum in cattle and during the prepubertal phase in both species [57].

Some recent papers report an incidence of double ovulations up to 15.5% in dairy cows [58]. A similar value has been previously reported in the buffalo [59]. In the latter, however, only 0.06% of double ovulation may lead to a twin pregnancy. The double ovulations reduce the efficiency of AI in the case of spontaneous estrus, but not in the case of induced estrus [48].

In Italy, the OBMS technique leads to lesser fertility. In fact, when the OBMS technique was not applied, calving intervals of 400 to 445 days were recorded [60]. Recently, a mean inter-calving interval of 487±133 days was reported for 6,052 inter-calving intervals over a period of 5 to 10 years on 5 farms with an annual culling rate lower than 10% [60]. The OBMS technique was adopted and a constant rationing was given throughout the year.

It was shown that the shortest inter-calving periods were recorded in buffaloes that delivered between April and June, and that, therefore, have conceived in the warmest months (between June and August). Short inter-calving intervals were also found in buffaloes that delivered between July and September, the period of the year during which the highest temperatures are recorded in Italy. The longest inter-calving periods were recorded for buffaloes calving between October and December, because of the OBMS technique, which delays mating until February. Long inter-calving intervals were also found in buffaloes that calved between January and March, the coldest period of the year [8, 15, 54, 60]. These buffaloes would conceive in spring, the mildest period of the year, characterized by temperatures between 15 and 22° C. Conception is typically delayed until September, however, except for the 40% of animals that conceive within 90 days from calving. We can conclude, therefore, that in Italy nutrition and the warmest months, especially if a swimming-pool is present on the farm [61, 62], do not affect the inter-calving period. The main factor that has to be taken into account in Italy (latitude of 42 to 45° N) is the light stimulus. Buffaloes that deliver between

January and March would conceive between March and May, a period characterized by increasing day length, or delay their conception until August to September, after three months of decreasing day length. Similarly, buffaloes that deliver in the period of April to September show the shortest inter-calving period considering that at the end of 58 days postpartum (the useful interval in order to reach an inter-calving period of 365 days), decreasing day length begins.

When the OBMS technique is not used, old buffaloes (with more than 7 calvings and still not pregnant after 7 to 9 months from last calving) spontaneously conceive in autumn. The body conditions of buffaloes typically worsens after 12 to 15 years of age and hence farmers are not encouraged to eliminate the animals that are still not pregnant at the end of lactation. This is one of the causes of prolonged inter-calving period [60].

The majority of Indian and Egyptian authors assert that a lower concentration of calving observed between January and May depends on a reduced conception rate between March and July. This phenomenon is influenced by the hot and dry climate (summer anoestrus) of this period of the year. In Italy, in farms that do not use the OBMS, a drop of calving is also observed between January and June (Fig. **1**), a period of the year in which, unlike in India, the climate is either cold or mild and moderately rainy. The fertility markedly improves between July and September, a period that in Italy coincides with the highest temperature (Fig. **4**) and temperature humidity index of the year. This observation makes the buffalo very different from cattle, as the latter species shows a marked decrease in fertility in the hottest months of the year (July to September).

We have already highlighted that in areas located north of the equator a drop in the number of calvings is observed between January and June. The authors from countries located north of the equator attribute buffalo anestrus to heat stress (India, Pakistan) or to the low environmental humidity (Venezuela). In our opinion, the decrease in calving rate between January and June/July (Fig. **1**) depends on the reduced reproductive activity between March and August/ September. In the latter period, the maximum daily temperature (Fig. **4**) ranges between 15°C (March) and 27°C (August) in Naples, Italy; between 25°C and 38°C in Delhi, India; between 27°C (March) and 41°C (June) in Lahore, Pakistan;

and between 25°C (March) and 26°C (August) in Caracas, Venezuela. The maximum daily temperatures that are recorded in Italy and in Venezuela rule out a direct action of environmental temperature on anestrus. If only India and Pakistan are considered, it is not possible to exclude that heat stress, even if it is not the main factor, may contribute to summer anestrus. Furthermore, the RRC (August to September) coincides with a monthly maximum temperature of 28°C (August) and 25°C (September) in Italy, 25°C (August) and 27°C (September) in Venezuela, 34°C (September) in India and 36°C in Pakistan.

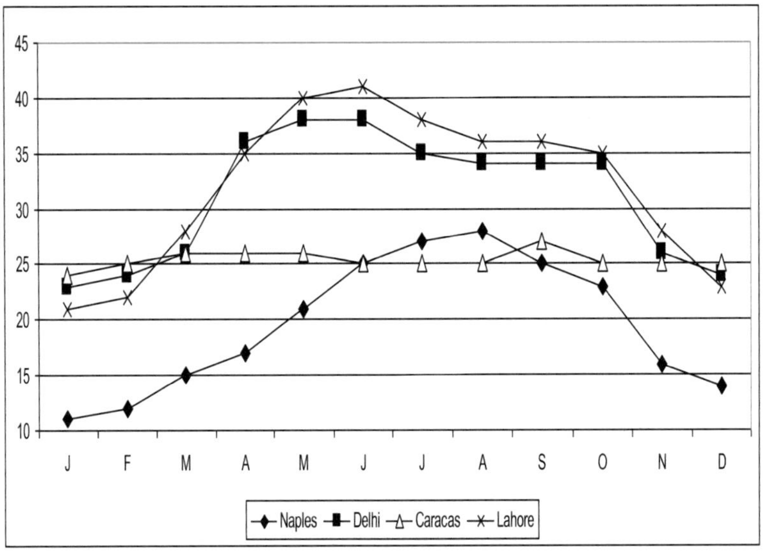

Fig. (4). Monthly maximum temperature in Naples, Dehli, Caracas and Lahore.

The monthly rainfall recorded in Italy and Venezuela between September and October is not different from the same value observed between March and May (Italy) and between June and August (Venezuela) when a lower conception rate is observed (Fig. **5**).

On the contrary, in India and in Pakistan the rainy season takes place between July and September. The cessation of reproductive activity in Italy and Venezuela, therefore, cannot be attributed to the rainfall. In India and Pakistan, the reproductive activity is good in October and November (calving in August and September), when the temperature is lower and the rainfall is already minimal. The trend of day light hours, although with different daily values, is shared by all the breeding areas situated north of the equator (Fig. **6**).

Interestingly, a 4-year retrospective analysis of data, Di Francesco *et al.* [63] obtained in an *in vitro* embryo production laboratory, showed that a significant decrease in blastocyst rate was observed between April to June compared to October to December. Intermediate values were recorded between July and September and between January and March.

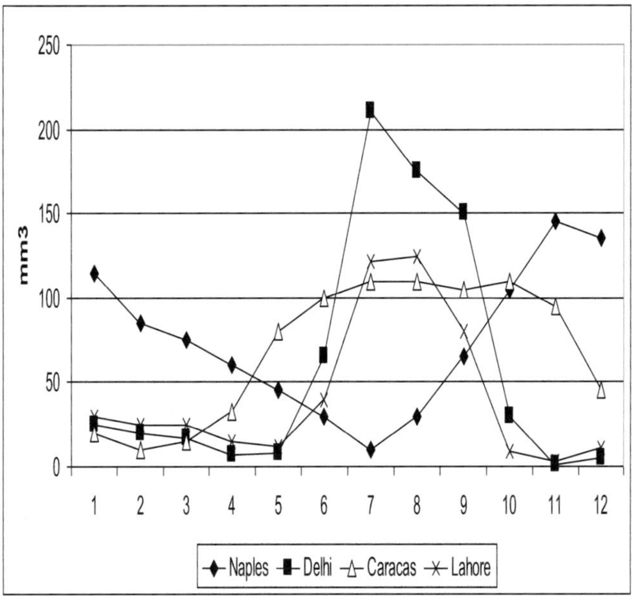

Fig. (5). Monthly rainfall (mm) in Naples, Dehli, Caracas and Lahore.

The drop in oocyte developmental competence coincides with the spring months that at our latitudes are characterized by mild environmental temperatures. This pattern confirms that the light stimulus plays the most critical role in determining seasonality.

South of the equator, Baruselli *et al.* [41] demonstrated that the concentration of calving increases proportionally with increasing distance from the equator (Fig. **2**). It is not possible to show any relationship between daily maximum temperature, rainfall and the calving calendar (Fig. **2**) whereas an evident relationship exists between the calving calendar and the daily light hours at different latitudes (Fig. **7**).

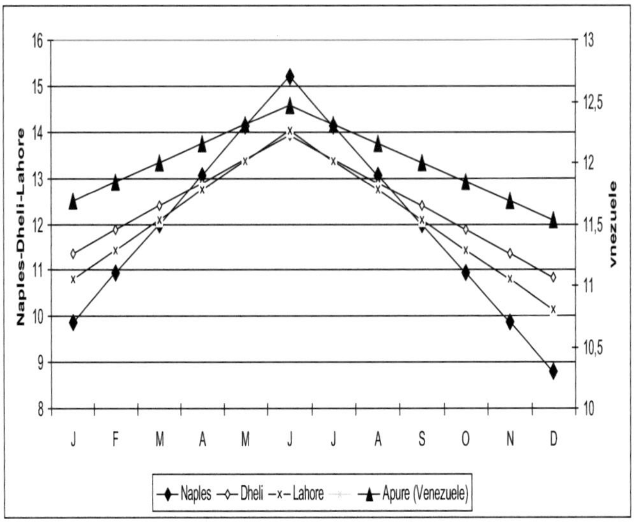

Fig. (6). Day light hours in Naples, Dehli, Appure (Venezuele), Lahore.

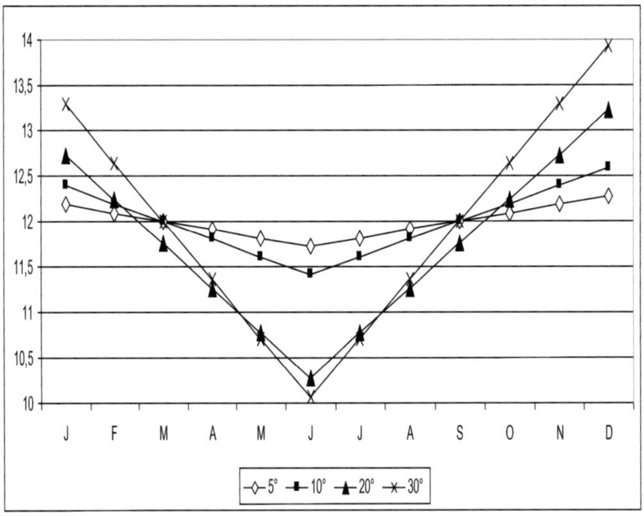

Fig. (7). Day light hours in Brazil as a function of latitude (°).

Throughout this paper, the seasonality of the females has been considered. This phenomenon may affect the males as well. The effects are clear when the animals are used for natural mating. Recently, we observed in the same farm a higher pregnancy rate between January and April in buffaloes inseminated by AI compared to animals that were bred by bull/natural mating. This perhaps occurred because AI avoided the negative effect of the bull. We have in fact recently verified that in April, only 23%, 31% and 29% of the bulls showed values higher than the average value for testosterone, dihydrotestosterone and androstenedione, respectively [64].

Strategies to Enhance Reproductive Performance

Embryonic mortality in buffaloes is primarily due to a reduced secretion of progesterone by the corpus luteum. The importance of progesterone concentration during the first weeks of pregnancy for reducing embryonic mortality has been demonstrated in both cattle [65] and buffalo [9, 55, 66, 67]. In cattle, several treatments have been used typically within 5 days after conception to increase progesterone secretion by the existing corpus luteum or to induce ovulation and formation of an accessory corpus luteum [65]. Treatments on day 5 after insemination do not have any effect on reducing embryonic mortality in the buffalo [66]. Differently, treatment of buffaloes with a GnRH agonist, hCG or progesterone on day 25 after AI, reduced embryonic mortality [67].

Although the light/dark ratio is the main factor affecting reproductive efficiency, another important factor is the satisfaction of the buffalo physiological need of water for bathing. The presence of a swimming-pool reduce the not pregnant buffaloes per corpora lutea ratio (NP/CL) found at rectal examination in buffaloes calving between April and August [61, 62, 68]. The swimming pool apparently acts to reduce heat stress. The NP/CL ratio, as an indicator of an anomalous estrous cycle or embryonic mortality, may be proposed as a specific tool for evaluating buffalo welfare [61].

In absence of water availability, the zebu shows higher resistance to high temperatures, whereas in presence of water the buffalo plunges in it completely and *Bos taurus* and *Bos indicus* plunge only their limbs.

We have already pointed out that the buffalo has a tropical origin and, at least in southern Italy, for the same space (dairy buffalo/m^2), birth order (calving parity) and rationing, the milk production to 135 days from delivery, which corresponds to mid-lactation, is not affected by temperature during summer, differently from winter [14]. During winter [14], a higher DM intake is correlated to lower milk production and hence to a worse conversion index of DM into milk, compared to summer. Furthermore, contrarily to dairy cow, the buffalo does not negatively modify milk quality during summer. The mozzarella cheese produced in this period is more delightful and pleasant to the consumer than that produced during the winter. The higher DM intake during the summer may be caused by, at least when the bull is available in the herd, the motor activity of buffaloes, which is not constant throughout the year. In fact, it varies according to the photoperiod, increasing in relation to the increase of light hours (Fig. **3**), and between July and September when a higher sexual activity is recorded in the herds when the OBMS is applied.

The low temperatures negatively affect milk production and reproduction in buffaloes, at least in Italy. The cold increases thyroid activity [25, 29], loss of body heat and neonatal mortality. High T4 levels negatively influence estrogens and progesterone in follicular fluid, reducing fertility. In farms localized in mountains, with humid and cold climate, the utilization of air heating during the coldest hours of the night for 4 years, increased herd fertility rate from 40 to 70%, decreased the intercalving period from 530 to 475 days and increased milk production of around 7% [69].

High environmental temperature and high THI (temperature humidity index) without adequate stalls, may represent a stress factor, together with cold temperature. In fact, the pigmented skin is able to protect the buffaloes by the damages caused by ultraviolet rays, but hair density in buffalo is 1/8 compared to cattle (394 follicles/cm^2 *vs.* 2893 in bovine). Furthermore, the number of sweat and sebaceous glands is definitely lower than cattle. However, sebum secretion in buffalo is more abundant than in cattle and plays a protective role on the skin when the animals plunge themselves in the mud.

The treatments for anestrus are based on the use of progesterone devices combined with PMSG. The response is influenced by the effects of year and farm and therefore are variable. The above treatments in natural mating conditions do not have an immediate impact, but in primiparous females they have a beneficial effect on the RRC. Unsatisfactory responses are perhaps more useful because they lead to the assessment of the environmental causes that underlie reproductive failures [54]. For instance, we demonstrated that more space and better welfare conditions improved fertility in Italy. On 21 farms in which the OBMS is performed, we observed that 38.1%, 52.4% and 4.8% of the farms increased fertility rate respectively in June, July to August and September (L. Zicarelli, unpublished observations). Out of the 8 farms that resumed fertility in June, 6 (75%) had at their disposal either covered sheds, that shorten the day length on average by 2 h during the year, or wide open spaces in which buffaloes can move for at least 6 h/day, or swimming pools. Out of the 11 farms that resumed fertility in July only 2 (18.2%) had swimming pools available (6/8 *versus* 2/11; $P < 0.05$). Finally, on a farm with a variable number of buffaloes, an increase in reproductive activity was recorded in June and July when more space was made available to the animals. Between January and June, 77% and 68% of births were observed, respectively, for 352 and 451 buffaloes ($P < 0.01$). These results suggest that the effects of the season can be partially alleviated by improving the status of animal welfare.

CONCLUSION

Reproductive problems in the buffalo species are mainly represented by the seasonal anestrus (defined as summer anestrus in tropical countries and spring anestrus in Italy), at least at the actual production level. This phenomenon may be solved by increasing the culling rate (since the tendency to seasonality increases by aging), ensuring space availability to the herd (at least 20 m^2/head), utilizing swimming pools for the animals and providing stalls that supply shadow for both reducing light hours and reducing summer temperatures.

It is particularly important to cull the animals that tend to reproduce during the periods characterized by decreasing daylight length and increase the number of those that are able to reproduce during periods characterized by increasing daylight length. In fact, it has been previously demonstrated that melatonin plasma levels show a high repeatability. Finally, the seasonality in buffalo is influenced by the light/dark ratio throughout the year, and in some countries the seasonality is influenced by nutritional factors.

CONFLICT OF INTEREST

The authors confirm that they have no conflict of interest to declare for this publication.

ACKNOWLEDGEMENTS

Declared none.

REFERENCES

[1] Misra AK, Tyagi S. *In vivo* embryo production in buffalo: present and perspectives. Ital J Anim Sci 2007; 6 (Suppl. 2): 74-91.
[http://dx.doi.org/10.4081/ijas.2007.s2.74]

[2] Cruz LC. Trends in buffalo production in Asia. Ital J Anim Sci 2010; 6 (Suppl. 2): 9-24.
[http://dx.doi.org/10.4081/ijas.2007.s2.9]

[3] Krostitz. Technology Mission on Dairy Development, published in Dairy India 1992. 1993.

[4] Hassan F, Khan MS, Rehman MS, Sarwar M, Bhatti SA. Seasonality of calving in Nili-Ravi Buffaloes, purebred Sahiwal and cross-bred cattle in Pakistan. Ital J Anim Sci 2007; 6 (Suppl. 2): 1298-301.
[http://dx.doi.org/10.4081/ijas.2007.s2.1298]

[5] Zicarelli L. Management in different environmental conditions. Buff J Suppl 1994; 2: 17-38.

[6] Vale WG. Bubalinos: Fisiologia e Patologia da Reprodução. Campinas, SP, Brasil: Fundação Cargill 1988.

[7] Vale WG, Ribeiro HF, Silva AO, Sousa JS, Ohashi OM, Souza HE. 13th Int. Cong. Anim Reprod Proc Sydney. Buffalo. 1996; pp. 19-33.

[8] Zicarelli L. Reproductive seasonality in buffalo. Proc. 3th international course of biotechnology in buffalo reproduction, napoli 6-10/10/97, suppl. bubalus bubalis 1997; 29-52.

[9] Campanile G, Neglia G, Vecchio D, Russo M, Zicarelli L. Pregnancy in buffalo cows. In: Marie O'L, John A, Eds. Pregnancy protein research. New York: Nova Science Publishers, Inc. 2009; pp. 31-91.

[10] Madan ML. Status of reproduction in female buffalo. 2nd world Buf. Cong., New Delhi, compendium of latest research 1988; 89-100.

[11] Misra AK. Application of biotechnologies to buffalo breeding in India. Third course on biotechnology of reproduction in buffaloes CE - Italy supplement to the N° 4 of Bubalus bubalis 1997; 141-66.

[12] Misra AK, Tyagi S. *In vivo* embryo production in buffalo: present and perspectives. Ital J Anim Sci 2007; 6 (Suppl. 2): 74-91.
[http://dx.doi.org/10.4081/ijas.2007.s2.74]

[13] Zicarelli L. Buffalo calf weaning and production. III Simposium Bufalos de las Americas – 2do Simposio de bufalos Europa-America. Colombia: Medellin 2006; pp. 80-6.

[14] Zicarelli L, Ariota B, Gasparrini B, Neglia G, Di Palo R. Buffalo beef production. Ital J Anim Sci 2007; (Suppl. 2 – Part 1)1312 -5. [http://dx.doi.org/10.4081/ijas.2007.s2.1312]

[15] Zicarelli L. Can we consider buffalo a non precocious and hypofertile species? Ital J Anim Sci 2007; 6 (Suppl. 2 – Part 1): 143-54. [http://dx.doi.org/10.4081/ijas.2007.s2.143]

[16] Zicarelli L. Water Buffalo Nutrition, ZOOTEC 2004 – VI Congresso Internacional de Zootecnia, XIV Congresso Nacional de Zootecnia, X Reunião Nacional de Eem Zootecnia e XVII Fórum de Entidades de Zootecnia, Brasília 1-15.

[17] Campanile G, De Filippo C, Di Palo R, Taccone W, Zicarelli L. Influence of dietary protein on urea levels in blood and milk of buffalo cows. Livest Prod Sci 1998; 55: 135-43. [http://dx.doi.org/10.1016/S0301-6226(98)00123-7]

[18] Vale WG, Ohashi OM, Sousa JS, Ribeiro HF. Studies on the reproduction of water buffalo in the Amazon Valley, Brazil Livestock reproduction in Latin America. Vienna: International Atomic Energy Agency 1990; pp. 201-10.

[19] Parmeggiani A, Di Palo R. Melatonina e stagionalità riproduttiva della bufala. Atti Conv. su "Miglioramento dell'efficienza produttiva e riproduttiva della specie bufalina". Agricolture e Ricerca 1994; 153: 41-8.

[20] Di Palo R, Parmeggiani A, Spadetta M, *et al.* Influence of changing farm on the repeatability of melatonin plasma level in Italian Mediterranean buffalo. 5th World Buf. Cong. Proc. Caserta. 758-61.

[21] Di Palo R, Parmeggiani A, Campanile G, Zicarelli L. Repeatability of melatonin plasma levels in buffaloes bred in Italy. Atti XLVII Conv. S.I.S. Vet (Kiev) 1993; 1: 331-3.

[22] Lincoln GA. Photoperiod-pineal-hypothalamic relay in sheep. Anim Reprod Sci 1992; 28: 203-17. [http://dx.doi.org/10.1016/0378-4320(92)90107-O]

[23] Borghese A, Barile VL, Terzano GM, Pilla AM, Parmeggiani A. Melatonin trend during season in heifers and buffalo cow. Bubalus bubalis 1995; 1: 61-4.

[24] Zicarelli L. Recenti acquisizioni sull'attività riproduttiva nella bufala. Atti 4° Meet. Naz. su "Studio dell'efficienza riproduttiva degli animali di interesse zootecnico" 1992; 9-39.

[25] Avallone L, Parmeggiani A, Esposito L, Campanile G. Correlation between prolactin, T3 and T4 levels in buffalo heifers during the whole year. 4th World Buf. Cong. Proc.. vol. IIISão Paulo. 1994; pp. : 477-9.

[26] Borghese A, Terzano GM, Barile VL, *et al.* Pubertà e mantenimento dell'attività ciclica ovarica nella bufala. Agricoltura e Ricerca, XVI 1994; 153: 5-16.

[27] Campanile G, Shehu D, Esposito L, *et al.* Onset of ovarian activity in Italian buffalo heifers. Proceedings III World Buffalo Congress. Varna. 1991; pp. 666-71.

[28] Esposito L, Di Palo R, Campanile G, Boni R, Montemurro N. Onset of ovarian activity in Italian buffalo heifers. Note III. International symposium on prospects of buffalo production in the Mediterranean/middle east. Cairo, Egypt 1993:9-12.

[29] Campanile G, Avallone L, d'Angelo A, Di Palo R, Di Meo C. Influence of the season and of the

number of days after calving on the pattern of thyroid hormones in buffalo cows. 4th World Buf Cong Proc. vol IIISão Paulo. 1994; pp. : 564-6.

[30] Roy A, Raizada BC, Pandey MD, Yadav PC, Sengupta BP. Effect of management on the fertility of buffalo cows bred during summer. Ind J Vet Sci 1968; 38: 554.

[31] Singh V, Desai RN. Calving/breeding season and calving interval of buffaloes in Northern India. Indian J Anim Sci 1979; 49: 256-60.

[32] Shah SN. Prolonged calving intervals in the Nili Ravi buffalo. Utrecht University: PhD Thesis 1990.

[33] Singh M, Chavdhary KC, Takkar OP. Increasing the reproduction performance of buffaloes. 2nd World Buf. Cong. Proc. New Delhi. vol. II: 271-82.

[34] Singh B, Lal K. Effect of season and breed on certain reproductive traits in buffaloes under village condition. Indian J Anim Res 1992; 26: 15-9.

[35] Qureshi MS, Samad HA. Habib, Usman RH, Siddiqui MM. Study on factors leading to seasonality of reproduction in dairy buffaloes. I. Nutritional factors. Asian-Aust J Anim Sci 1999; 12: 1019-24. a [http://dx.doi.org/10.5713/ajas.1999.1019]

[36] Zicarelli L, Di Lella T, de Franciscis G. Osservazioni e rilievi sui parametri riproduttivi e produttivi di bufale in allevamento presso un'azienda della piana del Sele. Acta Med Vet (Napoli) 1977; 23: 183-206.

[37] Ferrara B. Ricerche su alcune statistiche vitali nella popolazione bufalina dell'Italia Meridionale. Nota II: intervallo interparto e distribuzione dei parti. Acta Med Vet (Napoli) 1957; 3: 225-33.

[38] Urdaneta Montiel. Aspectos reproductivos de la búfala. Comportamiento reproductivo en bufalas en un ambiente de bosque muy seco tropical. I simposium internacional de búfalos de Venezuela, Maracaibo 7 – 8 Diciembre 2000; 5-20.

[39] González Rangel AR, González Pérez AR, González Rangel AE. Experiencias en la cria de búfalos y vacunos en la hacienda la concha-agropecuaria Los Angeles c.a. I simposium internacional de búfalos de Venezuela, Maracaibo 7 – 8 Diciembre 2000; 115-27.

[40] Zoheir KM, Abdoon AS, Mahrous KF, Amer MA, Zaher MM. LiGuo Y, El-Nahass EM. Effects of season on the quality and *in vitro* maturation rate of Egyptian buffalo (*Bubalus bubalis*) oocytes. J Cell Anim Biol 2007; 1: 29-33.

[41] Baruselli PS, Bernardes O, Braga DP, Araujo DC, Tonhati H. Calving distribution throughout the year in buffalo raised all over Brazil. VI World Buffalo Congress. Maracaibo, Venezuela. 2001; pp. 234-9.

[42] Da Silva ME, Grodzki L. Study of correlations between climatic factors and seasonal fertility of female buffaloes in the Northeast of the state of Parana. 3rd World Buf. Cong. Proc.. Vol. 4: 689-700.

[43] Seren E, Parmeggiani A, Mongiorgi S, *et al.* Modificazioni endocrine durante il ciclo ovarico nella bufala. *Agricoltura e Ricerca.* XVI 1994; 153: 17-24.

[44] Le Van TY, Chupin D, Driancurt MA. Ovarian follicular populations in buffaloes and cows. Anim Reprod Sci 1989; 19: 171-8. [http://dx.doi.org/10.1016/0378-4320(89)90090-0]

[45] Vittoria A. Third course on biotechnology of reproduction in buffaloes. Supplement, Bubalus bubalis 1997; 4: 15-20.

[46] Gasparrini B. *In vitro* embryo production in buffalo species: state of the art. Theriogenology 2002; 57(1): 237-56.
[http://dx.doi.org/10.1016/S0093-691X(01)00669-0] [PMID: 11775973]

[47] Zicarelli L. Considerations about the prophylaxis of the uterine and vaginal prolapse in Italian Mediterranean buffalo cows. Bubalus bubalis III 2000; 71-90.

[48] Zicarelli L, Esposito L, Campanile G, Di Palo R, Armstrong DT. Effect of using vasectomized bulls in A.I. practice on the reproductive efficiency of Italian buffalo cows. Anim Reprod Sci 1997; 47: 171-80. a
[http://dx.doi.org/10.1016/S0378-4320(97)00008-0] [PMID: 9329858]

[49] Baruselli PS. Comportamento reproductivo, sncronizacão do ciclo estral e da ovulacão e inceminacão artificial em tempo fixo em bufalos I Simposium international de bufalos de Venezuela. Maracaibo 7-8/12 2000; 65-82.

[50] Qureshi MS, Habib RH, Samad HA, Lodhi LA, Usman RH. Study on factors leading to seasonality of reproduction in dairy buffaloes. II. Non-nutritional factors. Asian-Aust J Anim Sci 1999; 12: 1025-30. b
[http://dx.doi.org/10.5713/ajas.1999.1025]

[51] Zicarelli L. Nutrition in dairy buffaloes Perspectives of buffalo husbandry in Brazil and Latin America. Editores Prof. H. Tonhati, Prof. V.H. Barnabe, Prof. P.S., Baruselli, Funep, Jabuticabal 1999; pp. 157-78.

[52] Zicarelli L. Nutrition in dairy buffaloes. Bubalus Bubalis, Tip. Paper Print s.r.l. Montecorvino Pugliano (SA) 2001; 1-66.

[53] Paul SS, Lal D. Nutrient requirement of buffaloes. Satish Serial Publishing House 2010.

[54] Zicarelli L, Campanile G, Esposito L, *et al.* Anaestro e induzione dell' estro in bufale acicliche. (Anoestrus and oestrus induction in acyclic buffaloes). Agricoltura e Ricerca 1994; 153: 25-40.

[55] Campanile G, Neglia G, Gasparrini B, *et al.* Embryonic mortality in buffaloes synchronized and mated by AI during the seasonal decline in reproductive function. Theriogenology 2005; 63(8): 2334-40.
[http://dx.doi.org/10.1016/j.theriogenology.2004.10.012] [PMID: 15826694]

[56] Zicarelli L. Reproductive seasonality in buffalo. Proc. 3th International Course of Biotechnology in Buffalo Reproduction, Napoli 6-10/10/97. Suppl Bubalus Bubalis 1997b; 29-52.

[57] Garverick HA, Zollers VG, Smith MF. Mechanisms associated with corpus luteum lifespan in animals having normal or subnormal luteal function. Anim Reprod Sci 1992; 28: 111-24.
[http://dx.doi.org/10.1016/0378-4320(92)90098-X]

[58] López-Gatius F, López-Béjar M, Fenech M, Hunter RH. Ovulation failure and double ovulation in dairy cattle: risk factors and effects. Theriogenology 2005; 63(5): 1298-307.
[http://dx.doi.org/10.1016/j.theriogenology.2004.06.010] [PMID: 15725438]

[59] Zicarelli L, Campanile G, Infascelli F, Esposito L, Ferrari G. Incidence and fertility of heats with double ovulations in the Mediterranean buffalo cows of Italy. Proceedings of II World Buffalo Congress. vol. IIINew Delhi, India. 1988; pp. : 57-62.

[60] Zicarelli L, Di Palo R, Neglia G, Ariota B, Varricchio E, Campanile G. Estimation of the intercalving

period in Italian Mediterranean buffalo. Ital J Anim Sci 2007; 6 (Suppl. 2): 709-12.
[http://dx.doi.org/10.4081/ijas.2007.s2.709]

[61] Di Palo R, Ariota B, Zicarelli F, De Blasi M, Zicarelli G, Gasparrini B. Incidence of pregnancy failures in buffaloes with different rearing system. Ital J Anim Sci 2009; 8 (Suppl. 2): 619-21.
[http://dx.doi.org/10.4081/ijas.2009.s2.619]

[62] Neglia G, Rendina M, Balestrieri A, *et al.* Influence of a swimming-pool on fertility in buffalo species. Ital J Anim Sci 2009; 8 (Suppl. 2): 637-9.
[http://dx.doi.org/10.4081/ijas.2009.s2.637]

[63] Di Francesco S, Boccia L, Campanile G, *et al.* The effect of season on oocyte quality and developmental competence in Italian Mediterranean buffaloes (*Bubalus bubalis*). Anim Reprod Sci 2011; 123(1-2): 48-53.
[http://dx.doi.org/10.1016/j.anireprosci.2010.11.009] [PMID: 21168984]

[64] Pelagalli A, d'Angelo D, Mastellone V, *et al.* Influence of buffalo dams reproductive status on sexual hormones activity in bulls, *Pakistan Journal Zoology*. Supplementary Series, No 2009; 9: 61-3.

[65] Mann GE. Corpus luteum function and early embryonic death in the bovine. Proceedings of XXII World Buiatrics Congress. Hannover, Germany. 2002; pp. 300-6.

[66] Campanile G, Di Palo R, Neglia G, *et al.* Corpus luteum function and embryonic mortality in buffaloes treated with a GnRH agonist, hCG and progesterone. Theriogenology 2007; 67(8): 1393-8.
[http://dx.doi.org/10.1016/j.theriogenology.2007.03.001] [PMID: 17403533]

[67] Campanile G, Vecchio D, Di Palo R, *et al.* Delayed treatment with GnRH agonist, hCG and progesterone and reduced embryonic mortality in buffaloes. Theriogenology 2008; 70(9): 1544-9.
[http://dx.doi.org/10.1016/j.theriogenology.2008.07.003] [PMID: 18706685]

[68] Zicarelli L. Advanced reproductive technologies for improving buffalo production. Proceedings The First Buffalo Symposium of Americas, September 01 to 08 - Estacao das Docas - Belèm - Parà Brazil. 186-97.

[69] Campanile G, Balestrieri ML. Interaction of environment factors for better production in buffaloes. 1st Buffalo Symposium of Americas. Belém, Brazil. 2002; pp. 287-97.

CHAPTER 9

Buffalo Dairy Production: A Review

Marco A. Zava[1,*] and **Marina Sansinena**[2,3]

[1] *Technical Department of Argentine Buffalo Breeders Association; International Consultant, Arcos 1325, 1426, Buenos Aires, Argentina*

[2] *Animal Biotechnology Laboratory, College of Agriculture, Catholic University of Argentina, Cap. Gral. Ramón Freire 183, 1426 Buenos Aires, Argentina*

[3] *National Council for Research and Technology (CONICET), Buenos Aires, Argentina*

Abstract: Worldwide production of buffalo milk is steadily increasing. In this chapter, the worldwide distribution of buffalo milk production is described, with emphasis on production styles and characteristics by region. Representative buffalo breeds are described, along with production levels and general herd management. Relevant factors such as heat stress, animal nutrition, conversion efficiency, health management, calf rearing systems and sanitary milk production conditions are outlined. Factors influencing buffalo milk performance and production are also outlined in this chapter such as sexual maturity, calving interval, days in lactation, residual milk and performance according to age groups.

Keywords: Breeds, Buffalo, Dairy, Production levels, Worldwide distribution.

1. INTRODUCTION: WORLDWIDE DISTRIBUTION, REGIONAL PRODUCTION AND ECONOMY

Worldwide Distribution

Worldwide production of buffalo cow milk is steadily increasing, and is concentrated in three countries which represent 94% of the total world production: India, Pakistan and Nepal [1]. In addition, significant amounts of

* **Corresponding author Marco A. Zava:** Technical Department of Argentine Buffalo Breeders Association; International Consultant, Arcos 1325, 1426, Buenos Aires, Argentina; Tel: +54 011 4706 2513; Fax: +54 11 4373 9982; E-mail: marcozava@gmail.com

Giorgio A. Presicce (Ed.)

buffalo milk are being produced by China and Egypt (in the latter, bubaline milk production is higher than cattle) [2].

Of the total world buffalo population, 69.73% is found in India and Pakistan and it is mainly dedicated to dairy production [3]. According to FAO 2008 [3], India and Pakistan produce 66.62% and 25.15% of the buffalo cow milk worldwide, respectively. In 2008, India produced 56.960.000 metric tons of buffalo cow milk and Pakistan produced 21.500.000 [3]. India is the largest producer of buffalo heads in the world and also the largest milk producer (cattle + bubaline, approximately 134 million tons). Only 15% of buffalo cow milk is processed by dairy plants, while the rest is consumed as raw milk for human consumption [5].

Buffaloes play a key role in the agricultural economy of the Indo-Pakistani continent. This species is known for being an efficient converter of low-quality forages and by-products into a single valuable commodity: milk. An example to understand the magnitude of the economic importance of bubaline milk production in India: although the 106,63 million buffalo heads [3] represent only 34.35% of total livestock in the country, their milk output accounts for 65% of total dairy and dairy by-products [3, 4, 6].

In the year 2004, bubaline milk accounted for the 12% of the world dairy production (75.833.191 tons of bubaline milk *versus* 608.943.729 total). Between 1996 and 2004, bubaline milk production increased 26%, *versus* only a 10% increase in vaccine milk. According to FAO, in the last three decades worldwide bubaline production increased 200% [4], with an annual growth of 7%. This growth is mainly attributed to the 110% increased milk production of Asia in the last two decades (India 101%, Vietnam 93% and Pakistán 88%) [3], and the continent is now producing 96% of the world bubaline milk. In 2008, Brazil produced 114 million liters and Italy 200 million (600 million euro) [4]. Production of several key countries is shown in Table **1**.

Table 1. Top producers of buffalo cow milk in 2008.

Country	Production (Tons)
India	56,960,000
Pakistan	21.500.000

(Table 1) contd.....

Country	Production (Tons)
China	2,900,000
Egypt	2.300.000
Nepal	930,000
Iran	241.500
Myanmar	205,000
Italy	200.000
Brazil	114,000
Turkey	35.100
Vietnam	31,000
WORLD TOTAL	**84,488,902**

Source: Otavio Bernardes, 2010 [4]

Regional Production and Economy

Europe

In Italy, buffalo industry is an intensive production system that utilizes the latest technology, with more than 60 years of genetic selection and quality control. Average milk production per lactation has increased over 400 kg since the national genetic improvement program started in 1969. In superior herds, lactations of 5000 liters for 250-day lactations with two daily milking sessions can be achieved and for the Mediterranean breed, lactations of 240-270 days with values of 1500, 2700 and 6000 liters have been reported. In 2009, Naples reported 3000 daily kilograms of mozzarella cheese exported to the U.S.A. and Great Britain. Bulgaria has reported productions over 3500 liters, mostly switching from Mediterranean to Murrah breeds.

Seliano Farm, owned by the Bellelli family, in Seliano, Salerno Province, Campania Region, Italy, produces corn, ryegrass, oats and olive trees over 90 hectares of land, 7 of which are occupied by animal facilities. Of a total of 768 buffaloes, 338 are adult females. In the year 2004, they reported a total of 544.200 kg of milk from 220 animals in milking, with an average 2500 kg/lactation, 4.8% crude protein and 8.5% butirose fat. This farm operates non-seasonally (out of season mating). Fifty-six percent of the milk was produced in the summer season and fertility rate was 76%. The farm has implemented genetic selection programs in order to improve milk production. Cows that produce less than 2500 liters are systematically culled, and superior buffalo bulls for genetic improvement are introduced for natural mating [7]. Two of their studs are housed in one of the top artificial inseminations centers of the country, COFA (Cooperativa di Fecondazione Artificiale or Artificial Insemination Cooperative) located in Cremona, near Milan, in Lombardia Region). One of them, Ettore, born in 1999, has a morphological score of 87.5. Its sire has a morphological score of 85 and its dam, 81 [8].

La Cotarda Farm, owned by Benedetti Panici family, is located in Pontinia, Latina Province, Lazio Region, Italy, and has a total of 700 buffalo cows (350 in milking). In 1997, the farm had the second largest production in Italy: 2700 liters for 270-day lactation, with 8.5% butirose fat and 4.5% crude protein. The Farm of Gianni Martini is also located in Latina, near Fossanova. In 100 hectares they produce both beef and milk. They own 800 buffalo heads, 250 are buffalo cows in milking. Their milk production is 12 liters/day for 270-day lactations. Peak productions can reach 25 liters/day. Average milk production/lactation is 3000-3200 liters. They have reported repeated problems with uterine prolapse, attributed to excess body condition (over-conditioning), nutrition (excessive corn) and genetics. Rations consist of 20 kg corn silage, 6 kg of hay and 8 kg of concentrate (unifeed). Forage management rotates alfalfa, ryegrass, oats and corn, according to availability and time of the year [7].

Facchi Farm, located in Cremona, near Milan, Lombardia Region, is the only completely integrated operation in Italy. They own 1150 buffaloes, 400 of which are milking buffalo cows. Average daily milk output is 5 to 12 liters, for 200 to 230-day lactations (average 1900-2000 liters/lactation). The farm has its own cheese production plant where the milk line from milking parlor feeds directly into plant; the whole cheese threading process is done by hand. They produce 2000 liters milk/day with a 27% yield (500 kg mozzarella cheese/day). This operation slaughters and sells steers at 9 months of age with 250 kg of weight. The buffalo production of this farm integrates 3 systems: 1) milk (cheese); 2) meat (steers); and 3) Biogas (fuel), where manure is converted to dry (letame) and fluid (liquame) for energy production [7].

Torre Lupara Farm, in Pastorano, Caserta, Campania Region, Italy [9] produces 12,000 liters daily during winter and 18,000 in the summer (non-seasonal breeding). They milk 1459 heads with 8 workers, including 1400 dams with 520 in twice-daily milking schemes (4,8% protein). Animals are kept on ground corrals which improve overall hoof health. Corrals have manure collection systems, so that manure is pooled in large sediment ponds where liquid and solid fractions are separated. Liquid fractions are used as fertilizers. Animals are allowed 25 m^2 space/head, but if more space is made available, production drops due to excessive walking; if on the contrary less space is available, animals get nervous and uncomfortable due to the restricted space [9].

Aldes Farm (Allevamento De Stefano), Agropoli, Salerno, Campania Region, is one of the top ranked Italian farms based on production [9]. They have 130 cows split into two groups of which 28 fresh (first days of milking). In total they own 500 heads. Artificial rearing is done using powdered milk reconstituted, of the acid type, with mortality rates under 2-3%. Calves are fed colostrum for 3 to 4 days, followed by additional 3-4 days fed with their dam's milk mixed with the acidic milk. Finally, powered reconstituted milk (18-20%) is supplied ad libitum for 25-30 days, near 6 to 8 kg/head. From days 30 to 65, calves are offered 5 liters/day, progressively reduced to 3 liters/day until weaned around 50 days of age. Since 30 days of age they receive solid food. Replacement heifers must develop properly while maintaining adequate body weight without being over-conditioned. Over conditioning is quite common in Italy due to use of corn silage as supplement. This has negative impact on fertility and makes animals more prone to uterine prolapse. Aldes animals have high food intake, but with daily productions of 26-27 liters with 9,4% butirose fat and 4,8-4,9% crude protein, so that their body condition is barely good. Animals are fed 50:50 concentrate to roughage; this includes tomato peels, corn silage and straw. Milk production is typically around 15 liters with peaks up to 30 liters, with 8.86% fat and 4.45% protein for 267-day lactations. Non-seasonal breeding is conducted on about 65% of the herd (spring) in order to achieve production goals during the high demand months of the summer [9].

Riva Bianca Farm, Paestum, Salerno, has an average production of 2400 liters per lactation with 4.8% protein and 8.5% fat, and animals producing less than 2100 are culled. They use scraping blades to remove manure from pens, which is used to produce biogas. Cows are fitted with pedometers: that allows individual identification during milking and also is used as aid in heat detection based on increased overall animal activity. They milk approximately 120 cows per hour. Animals are de-seasonalized by withdrawal of buffalo bulls in early fall (September 20th) and re-introducing them in February [9].

Gaetano Iemma's Farm, Eboli, Salerno, has a total head count of 1000 buffalo, 500 are dairy buffalo cows (300 in milk). Average production is 2500 liters [9].

La Roana Farm, Sezze, Latina, Lazio Region, has 60 hectares and 800 heads. First breeding heifers receive a highly concentrated ration to compensate for their reduced rumen size and thus reduced voluntary intake. Animals are kept in groups of 70. Animals are grouped by calving date and lactation and therefore have similar nutritional requirements. Breeding is also de-seasonalized in order to maintain supply levels throughout the year, genetic improvement is routinely pursued by using only buffalo bulls with 4000-liter record dams. Average daily production is 14.5 liters and total lactation production is 2700 liters [9].

Upper Ninevah Farm, belongs to the Palmer family, west London, UK. They farm 150 acres of excellent pasture with high protein content. In 1998, production levels were 2800 kg per lactation, with 8.59% fat and 4.55% protein and 5.1% lactose. Mechanical milking is conducted twice daily with yearly productions of 200,000 liters. Initially, buffalo milk was destined mainly to satisfy the demand of the Pakistani community in the country, but it is now allocated to the manufacturing of semi-hard cheese. Buffaloes are kept in stables during the winter months and fed hay, wheat straw, beet and forage clippings, and rations are always formulated to meet 14% crude protein, 10.5% fiber and 12.4% metabolizable energy. Buffaloes are bred by AI with semen imported from Italy. Best producing animals yield up to 5229 liters with low microbial count, which allows for milk to be stored and transported to London weekly for yoghurt and cheese manufacturing [9].

In Germany, a herd was reported to produce 2232 kg and 2577 kg for first and second lactations, respectively [14].

Asia

Average milk production in India and Pakistan ranges from 1000 to 1500 liters for 300-day lactations. Superior herds may achieve 2500 liters, with individual buffalo cow yield up to 5000 liters. In the year 2000, 2.5 million dairy buffalo cows were controlled in the state of Gujarat, India. These controls revealed an average yield of 1071 liters (Mehsana breed, 300-day lactation) with 7.01% fat and 1694 liters (Murrah cross) with 6.8% butirose fat [10].

Pakistan produces 38 billion liters of vaccine and bubaline milk per year and has the second largest animal head count: 32 million [11]. Bubaline milk represents 65% of the milk consumed by the 165 million inhabitants [12, 13]. In Pakistan, agricultural waste and forages are converted efficiently by the buffalo. Dairy farms normally operate with one milker every 12 buffalo cows in barns with 200, 1000 and up to 10000 animals. Only 5% of buffalo milk produced in the country is sold to processing plants, the rest is consumed as raw fluid milk. Milk is also used for the manufacture of candy and sweets, both very common staples in Muslim diets. Interestingly, cheese in not considered a traditional foodstuff [13]. Traditionally, small producers (70% of total) have limited access to quality forages, resulting in lactations of 1300 liters for buffalo cow (and 450 for cattle). However, the number of suburban dairies and number of animals milked have been increasing rapidly in recent years; better nutrition and individual animal output is driving production to 3000 liters. Nili-Ravi buffalo cows with productions of 4147 liters during 281-day lactations have been reported. In Punjab Province (Pakistan), production from 6000 buffalo cows from 7 research and military-owned herds and small farms (5-20 animals) was controlled. For the year 2000, average milk production was 1823 liters for 257-day lactations.

The market for dairy products is also steadily increasing in China, with an average 18% growth/year, the second largest growth rate after Brazil. A large number of dairy crossbred buffaloes are being produced in this country, with special emphasis in milk production [15]. Milk production in the south of China is inadequate and cattle production is not sufficient to meet the demand. Therefore, the region is actively directing buffaloes into milk. In recent years, buffalo cow milk production form Guanxi and Guangdong represented 18.8 and 11.5% of the country's total. The Buffalo Research Institute of Nanning, Guanxi, China, monitored milk production of pure and crossbred bubaline breeds, for 278-327-day lactations. They reported 2133 liters for Murrah with 6.73% butirose fat, 4.05% crude protein and 16.73% milk solids; 2262 liters for Nili-Ravi with 6.35% butirose fat, 4.11% crude protein and 16.44% milk solids; 2295 liters for Triple Cross (Nili-Ravi, 50%; x Murrah, 25%; x Swamp, 25%) with 7.43% butirose fat and 4.47% crude protein; 2041 liters for Nili-Ravi (F1) with 8.17% butirose fat and 4.61% crude protein; 2268 liters for Nili-Ravi (F2); 1020 liters for Swamp with 9.50% butirose fat and 4.50% crude protein [16].

The swamp buffalo of Thailand is mostly used for milk production in urban areas. An evaluation of Murrah buffalo cows and their crosses indicated that F1 had an improvement over the swamp variety in average daily gain (900-1080 g/day *versus* 750 g/day) and doubles milk production (Murrah, 1105 liters in 213 days; F1, 1113 liters in 268 days) compared to swamp buffalo (477 liters in 279 days). Fat content and crude protein are also higher [17, 18].

In the Philippines, the Philippine Carabao Center imported 3000 dairy buffaloes of Murrah from Bulgaria and 4000 embryos from India between the years 1995 and 2000 [19, 20]. Carabao (or Swamp Buffalo) produces 400 – 750 liters/lactation (1 - 1.5 liters/day, with 9 – 10% fat). The F1 with Murrah can produce up to 1100 liters and the F2, 1350 liters [21]. Murrah buffaloes imported from Bulgaria produce 1800 liters/lactation [5]. The CLSU Dairy Farm, in Muñoz, Nueva Ecija, Philippines, has 1039 total hectares of land, with 6 hectares occupied by the milking parlor, including 5 hectares dedicated to forages and 1 hectare for other facilities. Of the 200 buffalo heads, 80 are Murrah cows producing 1500 liters (300-day lactation) [20].

Africa

Average milk production in Egypt is 1600 liters for 210 to 280 day lactations, with 6.4-7% fat. Age at first calving is 34 to 41 months. The Ministry of Agriculture is in charge of herd control of the 4 herds owned by the State (around 800 total buffaloes) with an average 2030 liters and 8.2% in 312 days. El Tahir is located east of the Nile delta, with 60 acres under irrigation and 170 buffalo heads. Animals are fed with wheat straw treated with ammonia, forage mix and minerals. Buffalo cows in milk are fed with 3 kg concentrate/day consisting of 40% cotton seed, 35% corn, 15% barley, 10% wheat flour. Egyptian forage consists of Clover (Trifolium alexandrinum sp.) and Elephant Grass [22].

South America

In Venezuela and Brazil, average values for 270-day lactations are between 1500 and 1700 liters; with superior herds achieving 2500 to 4000 liters, and more than 5000 liters have been reported in Brazil. The Parineiras de Ingai Farm, located in Alambari, Sao Paulo State, Brazil, is dedicated to buffalo dairy production using the Murrah breed. The area is characterized by sandy and unfertile soils. Herds are maintained on rotational grazing schemes with addition of mineral supplementation to support larger numbers of animals/hectare (6 Animal Units/hectare). Sugar cane silage is used strategically. To complement forage seasonal nutrient imbalances, forage is fertilized with manure. Forage nutritional value is monitored routinely (*Bracchiaria decumbens* sp: 12.7% protein, 34% crude fiber, 24.6% dry matter, 59% total digestible nutrients). The Santa Eliza Farm, in Dourado, Sao Paulo, Brazil, milks 600 buffalo cows, obtaining between 2000 and 3000 liters/day, which are processed by a milk plant with the Dourado trade mark, owned by the same group [23].

Due to the fact that National Research Council (U.S.A.) values are considered inadequate for buffalo, guideline values obtained from Federico II University of Naples (Italy) are now followed in Brazil. Reproduction is managed by natural mating and the average gestation length is 312.7 days. Calving interval is 392 +/- 53 days. The average number of mounts/conception (natural mating) is 1.6 and calvings are distributed throughout the year. Average milk production/buffalo cow is 3250 liters and the economic output is 6000 liters/hectare. Top producing cows produce 5142 liters/lactation (24 liters/day) [24]. In 2010, individual productions of 5613 liters (397 days) and 5647 liters (413 days) were recorded [4].

In Venezuela (2007), Castanha Grande produced an average of 2620 liters for 295-day lactation, with 8,88% butirose fat and 388-day calving interval. Animal production levels were distributed as following [25], and production levels are shown in Table **2**.

Table 2. Production level and percent of buffalo cows in a farm in Venezuela.

Production Level (KG/Lactation)	% Buffalo Cows
1600 to 2000	14.9
2001 to 3000	52.7
3001 to 4000	28.4
Over 4000	4.0

In Argentina, La Salamandra Farm, near Lujan, in Buenos Aires Province, produces 8 liters daily in two milking sessions, with 7.63% butirose fat and 4.52% protein and 2500 liters per lactation. The argentine average daily output is 5 to 6 liters, with average lactations lasting 240 days [26].

2. DAIRY BREEDS

In India, the most common breeds are Murrah, Jafarabadi and Surti. In Pakistan, the main breeds are Nili-Ravi and Kundi. In Italy and in the rest of the Mediterranean countries, the main breed is the Mediterranean, of indian origin [27].

In Italy, COFA (Cooperativa di Fecondazione Artificiale, property of Arturo Casali, Cremona, Lombardia), and CIPAB (Salerno, Campania) as well as other semen collection and commercialization companies were created for the Mediterranean breed genetic improvement to supply an increasing buffalo demand. After over 60 years of genetic selection, these companies are now producing and exporting semen from superior purebred buffalo bulls worldwide. Mediterranean is the breed that has presence in more countries in the world (in Europe, America, Asia, Africa and Oceania).

Currently in Italy, registered buffalo cows from 300 farms (controlled monthly) produce an average 2469 kg in 270-day lactation with 8.4% fat and 4.7% protein. Up until the year 2000, the genetic Herd Book was under supervision of AIA (Italian Breeders Association). This task was later transferred by the Ministry of Agriculture to ANASB (Italian Association of Buffalo Breeders) and the breed was officially named Italian Mediterranean Breed. Elite herds from this breed yield an average 3000 liters/lactation, with top producing buffalo cows reaching the 5800-liter mark [28]. In the north of Italy, 25-30 controlled farms milk an average of 170 Mediterranean buffalo cows. In 1997, the highest producing farms obtained yields higher than 5000 liters in 270-day lactations, with peak daily yields of 30 liters in two milking sessions. Although productions of 6000 liters can be obtained, this yield involved a reduction of the buffalo cow production life from 18-22 to only 12 years.

In India, the Murrah, Nili-Ravi, Surti and Jafarabadi breeds are well represented. All of them are riverine buffalo type. Although these are considered among the best dairy breeds, they are also used for meat production and draft. Indian-type Murrah, the most prevalent breed worldwide (in population), is present in Asia, Bulgaria and South America. With adequate nutrition, this breed is capable of higher yields, both in volume and fat content than the others breeds in India. Actually, it is the most numerous breed in that country. Butirose fat content ranges between 6.5 to 10.5%, with an average of 7.5; lactation yield (average 300 days) ranges from 1500 to more than 5000 liters, with production peaking by the 4$^{th>}$ lactation, and subsequently declining [29].

The Surti breed or Surati is present in the state of Gujarat, India. The Dhamrod Farm, in the Surat district, milks 177 buffalo cows with an average yield of 1577 liters for 305-day lactations, with peaks of 2883 liters. Average individual yield is 5 liters, with peaks of 16.5 liters, in two milking sessions. Average butirose fat content is 8% with a 6.5 to 11% range, which is standard for this breed.

The Mehsana breed was originated 70 years ago from the cross of Surti and Murrah. It is present in the north of Gujurat, India. Estimate yield per 300-day lactations is 1700 liters, with top herds achieving over 2800 liters and individual yields of 16 to 20 liters. Butirose fat content is 7%, and can reach 8% with nutritional supplementation. In addition, there is an artificial insemination center dedicated to this breed, with buffalo bulls whose dams produced 2800 to 4000 liters.

The Jafarabadi breed was originated in Gujarat, India. The yield in this breed ranges from 1800 to 2700 liters for 300-day lactations, with high fat content. University of Junagadh owns a 42-cow herd with reported individual yields over 5000 liters for 305-day lactations. It has been reported that one of the dams used as founder for this herd, produced yields over 7000 liters [30].

In suburban areas of Pakistan, the Nili-Ravi breed has been reported to produce 2000 liters (1700-2700 range) for 305-day lactations. For example, Kuddo, a buffalo cow owned by a local farm, produced 5820 liters for an adjusted 305-day lactation in its 3rd lactation. For the 4th lactation, yield was 5694 liters, with 6.6% butirose fat [30]. The Kundi breed is very important also in that country, with similar productions.

3. NUTRITION, REPRODUCTION AND SELECTION

Nutrition

The forage-based feeding management of the dairy buffalo cow must take into consideration the digestive characteristics of the species. Microbial rumen fermentation allows for the utilization of indigestible ingredients such as cellulose and the transformation of non-protein nitrogen (such as urea). It is therefore extremely important to conduct forage laboratory analysis in order to determine exact composition and then to accurately formulate rations according to category requirements [31].

Roughage feedstuffs are characterized by their high fiber content, generally over 18% (grasses, sugarcane, silages, *etc.*). Concentrates (fiber content under 18%) can in turn be classified as energetic (less than 20% of dry matter; corn, wheat flour, citrus pulp, *etc.*) and protein concentrates (cottonseed meal, soybean meal). The term forages includes a wide range of vegetative material, at different maturation stages. Therefore, although it is a cheap and valuable ingredient, its nutritional variability represents an extra challenge when included in dairy rations. Protein content of grasses range from 12 to 16% in early vegetative stage, these protein levels drop as the plant ages moving through blooming and seeding phases, with protein contents in this stage ranging from 5 to 7%. Energy levels follow the same trend. Total digestible nutrients (TDN) can be 60% of dry matter in young plants and 45-50% in older ones. Mineral content is also reduced during the reproductive period. Volume and composition of pastures vary throughout the year. It is important to implement optimal grazing strategies in order to maximize nutrient utilization and allow vigorous regrowth of plants.

Due to characteristics of their digestive physiology, buffalo cows (when compared to other ruminants such as sheep), are capable of higher digestive utilization coefficient with 70% roughage diets, particularly in the fibrous fraction breakdown and absorption. This competitive advantage of buffaloes tends to disappear when diets have lower fiber contents. In the center and southern regions of Brazil, calvings concentrate mostly around the end of summer and beginnings of fall, coinciding with the highest natural forage offer and allowing animals to reach parturition with a good body condition and body reserves (over conditioned). Animals that calve around this period still have 30-60 days of good quality forage supply. This in turn, translates in shortened calving-conception intervals and high fertility rates. It also allows the cow to undergo the catabolic phase of lactation with adequate body stores available for mobilization in response to heightened nutritional demand due to high milk output. It must be noted that this period also coincides with a depression in dry matter intake (usually 50-60 days post-partum) [31].

Concentrate ratios generally used in dairy buffalo cow nutrition, are formulated to guarantee an adequate level of fiber to stimulate saliva production, acetic acid production with good ruminal function and ultimately good fat content in milk. This fat content varies according to the stage of lactation; when faced with dietary restriction, the animal will compensate by modifying fat content and reducing milk output. Nutritionally-restricted animals mobilize their body fat stores, this fat metabolism translate in release of NEFAs (non-esterified fatty acids) which in turn, increase milk acidity (Dornic) and elevate cryoscopy (similar to a water:milk mixture). These transient conditions are normalized as soon as nutritional requirements are again met. Dry matter intake in dairy buffalo cows is variable, ranging from 2.2 to 3.4% of body weight (14.3 to 22.1 kg dry matter/day). The lactating buffalo cow feeding is based according to the milk production volume [31].

Compared to average animals, genetically superior buffalo cows mobilize higher proportions of the body reserves accumulated during the dry period and lose more weight during the first 60 days of lactation (catabolic phase). The decrease of live weight in the catabolic phase and ingest during the anabolic phase (in the 210 following days) of the buffalo cows of lower production, will always be lower compared to more productive animals. When comparing the average composition of *Brachiaria decumbens* sp. grass with the nutritional requirements of a buffalo cow producing 1900 liters of standardized milk with 7% fat and 4.2% protein in 270-day lactations, it can be observed that the amount of total digestible nutrients (TDN) barely covers animal requirements after the 7th month of lactation and that protein content is completely inadequate. This explains, in part, the low average production levels reported in Brazil (1714 liters), and also shortened lactations and lower fat and protein contents for animals fed exclusively on grasses in that country. Consequently, it is necessary to adopt nutritional supplementation to optimize production and achieve higher reproductive efficiency. This supplementation must be introduced carefully into the diets by allowing animals ration adaptation periods and continuously monitoring body condition, weight and milk yield [31].

In Potenza, Basilicata Region, Italy, a study was conducted to analyze the effect of diets adapted to range conditions (without irrigation) on milk production of dairy buffalo cows. Sixteen multiparous milking buffalo cows were allocated into two groups according to calving, lactation stage and milk production. Diets consisted of corn silage for group one and sorghum silage for the other; diet formulation was isocaloric and isoenergetic for both groups. Monthly milk records for production and quality were analyzed for a 5-month production period. There was no significant effect of diet composition on milk production, composition and coagulation parameters. Although not statistically significant, milk yield was higher for sorghum silage (8.78 *vs.* 8.03 kg) whereas fat content and protein content were higher for corn silage diets (8.74 *vs* 8.47% and 4.98 *vs* 4.78%, respectively). Results showed that sorghum diet does not have an effect on milk yield or quality, and it can be used in dairy buffaloes [32].

In India, the NDRI (National Dairy Research Institute) in Karnal conducted an experiment for a period of 12 weeks on two multiparous Murrah buffalo cow groups with two feeding schemes where CLA content were measured. The first group was fed with fresh Alexandria clover forage ad libitum and wheat straw. The second group was fed with a concentrate mix plus wheat straw, also ad libitum. Total CLA content was 16.38 mg/g of fat for the first group and 6.78 for the second, indicating an increase in CLA content for animals fed fresh forages of 141.59% [33].

Nutrient requirements of a dairy buffalo cow are similar to dairy cattle, although the amount of cellulose consumed by the buffalo cow is much higher. Urban dairy farms in India feed their animals with straw, sorghum stubble and concentrates. In some cases, alfalfa may be used as concentrate replacement. Reduced concentrate levels (0.3 kg/liter of milk) fed in a field trial in India resulted in profitable margins. Military-owned farms in Pakistan feed 54 kg forage (sorghum, green corn, clovers, alfalfa, chopped green oats) along with 4-6 kg straw and concentrate mix. A typical concentrate mix consists of 20 parts of cottonseed, 1 part of wheatbran or corn and grass. A typical maintenance ration would be 1.8 – 2.7 kg concentrate mix and the production ration of 1 kg per each 3 kg of milk produced. A ration of 35-40 kg of Pará grass or Guinea grass plus 1-2 kg molasses, 1-2 kg hay or straw and adequate mineral supplementation should allow a buffalo cow to produce 1200-1600 liters per lactation.

In the buffalo cow, the dry period lasts about 4 months. Nutrition during the dry period should cover, in addition to maintenance, requirements for the last third of gestation. During this period, an energy level of 0.65 Mcal/kg dry matter and a protein level of 10.5% is advised [34]. Furthermore, animals should be fed fresh forages of good quality, hay and 15% dry matter should be offered, along with concentrates. The diet during this period is characterized by its low fermentation rates. After calving, animal requirements change with diets having larger proportions of non-structural carbohydrates and protein. The latest nutritional trends indicate that rations could be modified 3 weeks prior to calving, with the buffalo cows close to parturition being fed energy levels of at least 0.90 Mcal/kg dry matter, reduced proportions of structural carbohydrates in favor of non-structural carbohydrates and protein levels of 13%.

Access to mineral supplements and adequate water are good management practices that translate into sustained milk productions. The distance animals have to walk to the milking parlor is also an important factor to consider; it should not be excessive or with excessive slopes since in both cases the animal will waste energy that would otherwise be directed to milk. Buffalo cows that are pasture-fed should receive 15-20% more energy in order to maintain production.

Studies conducted in dairy herds in India (Karnal Institute) and Bulgaria (Shumen Institute), give indication that buffalo conversion rate (utilization of fiber, protein, ether extract, calcium and phosphorus) is more efficient than cattle. In October 2007, H. Koskamp introduced 47 buffaloes (weaned heifers) into Canada from the U.S. (bought to Hugh Popenoe, Florida State). These animals, along with the 47 owned by Darrel and his wife Anthea Archer, increased by 100% the population. But in 2009 Frank Aballe, from Toronto imported for milk production 700 buffaloes from the US; and again Hoskamp imported 200 more from the same country. Actually, Canadian buffalo population is more than 1000 heads. Biofuels are driving up the cost of grains, and buffaloes are expected to give new air in dairy production, due to their ability to convert roughage into milk. The buffalo cow is the future of dairy industry [34].

In Paineiras da Ingaí Farm (Sao Paulo, Brazil), daily production increased between 30 to 35% with the introduction of a 2nd milking session. Yield (volume) is distributed such as 60-65% is obtained in the morning session of milking and 35-40% in the afternoon, with total production improving with good care to nutrition. In this study, working groups of 40 buffalo cows and one buffalo bull were kept on forage/cane based-diets. Dams had access to adequate amounts of processed roughage, mainly Cameroon grass, Tobiatä grass and sugar cane. Soy milk (500 g/animal/day or 4 liters) was used strategically to correct protein contents and enhance voluntary intake and when available, brewer's grains were offered. This feeding scheme resulted in an average production increase of 50%, and when combined with the 35% increase obtained from the introduction of a 2nd milking session, a total increase of 100% of milk yield was reported [35].

Examples of Nutritional Management Strategies in Several Regions/Continents

The Castanha Grande Ranch, in Sao Luiz do Quintude, Alagoas State, northern Brazil, is dedicated to buffalo milk production, with and intensive system of high animal loading per hectare. Voisin rotational grazing is conducted over *Brachiaria humidicola* sp. (in the hills) and Tanner Grass (in the swamp lowlands). Supplementation is based on sugar cane, molasses and urea or sugarcane cake. Dehorning, which facilitates animal handling and promotes docility, is performed using rubber ties with horns falling after 25 days (or lately using a special dehorning instrument designed by Alberto Couto). Buffalo cow producing up to 8 liters are milked once daily, 8-16 liter-producers are milked twice daily and those producing over 16 liters are milked three times a day. All milkings are done in the absence of calves, in clean and sanitary environments with experienced handlers. Animals in lactation are fed concentrates, freshly chopped grasses and are allowed nearby discretional grazing. Calves are allowed 24-48 h interaction with the dam, to ensure adequate colostrum intake. They are then moved to intensive calf raising systems. Animals are dehorned and dewormed routinely starting at 10-15 days of age. At Castanha Grande, in order to stimulate milk let-down, buffalo calves are allowed periodic contact with the dam using especially-designed pens [36].

The Laguna Farm, in Paracurú, Ceará State, Brasil, produces 1200 liters/day. Their system utilizes 12 - 13000 kg of industrial Cajunut residue monthly. Mating out of season is done in order to be able to fulfill demand during peak months, with less demand in the summer months. They perform two-milking sessions/day, with a daily average of 6.5 liters. Reproductive efficiency is 87.8%; lactation length is 294 days with average production of 2254 liters/lactation. One of their best cows, Luva, born in 1989 produced 13 calves in her lifespan. It produced 3023 liters/lactation, with peaks of 17 liters/day and a daily average of 7.23 liters. It has, so far, produced over 27300 liters, and now has reached adult body weight of 785 kg (9 years, 4 months of age). This farm, along with Ingaí Farm (Sao Paulo), owns some of best Murrah genetics in Brazil. The sandy-type soils of the region require that all forages be produced with irrigation (36 wells with 16 m diameter, pivot-type systems) and fertilization with broiler litter and buffalo manure (this allows an increase from 0 to 36 ppm phosphorus). Sugar cane is also chopped and fed to buffalo cows as nutritional supplement during the 7-month dry season (total rainfall concentrates between the months of April to June). Napier Grass (Elephant Grass) and Tanner Grass are also available for rotational grazing

[36].

The Terecay Ranch, located southwest of the State of Guárico in the heart of the Venezuelan plains, is an example of semi-intensive system. Average annual rainfall is approximately 1512 mm, concentrated between May to September, average temperature is 26°C with 75% relative humidity. About one half of the land is low, swampy-type. The milking buffalo cows are kept in semi-confinement, with access to pasture for 8 h/day. Animals are also supplemented with concentrates and hay during the night. Forages consist of Tanner Grass, German Grass (*Echinochloa polystachia* sp.) and composite pastures with *Digitaria* sp. and *Centrosema* sp. Dairy buffalo cows are fed 2 kg concentrate during milking. Dry buffalo cows are kept in native pastures (savanna) with no additional supplementation. They have 200 milking animals, with a total of over 300 heads. Lactations average 245 days, from August to March, with production peaks in October, November, December and January. Average milk production is 6.9 liters/day or 1725 kg/lactation, in two daily milking sessions. Animals are placed in production according to calving date and pregnancy status. Milking parlor has 20 milking stalls, with two parallel working trenches. Oxytocin is administered strategically. In Terecay, gathering corrals are fitted with sprinklers. Newborn buffalo calves are routinely tattooed at birth and allowed to stay 7 days with the dam. They are then moved to the calf rearing areas, where they are kept with nannies and allowed to suckle until they are 6 months of age. Nanny buffalo cows are fed the same ration as milking buffalo cows [36].

The southern region of Maracaibo Lake, Venezuela is being transformed into an extraordinary dairy region with a population of about 50000 dairy buffaloes. The region is situated 150 m above sea level, with average temperatures of 26-28° C year round (min 24° C, max 36° C) and about 2000 mm rainfall throughout the year. Most rainfall occurs during winter although the summer season cannot be considered dry, with sporadic rainfall in October, November, and December. La Fortuna Ranch, has a total of 1700 ha situated in El Vigía, Mérida State, Venezuela [36]. The farm has 1000 dairy buffalo cows and 11 vaqueras or milking parlors, 5 of which are mechanized. Buffalo graze Tanner Grass and produce about 6-7 liters/day, with mineral supplementation and without the addition of any concentrates. The price for buffalo milk is about 40% higher than cattle milk. Mortality rate is around 14% for newborn vaccine calves and 1.5% for buffalo calves (higher cost with cattle). Parturitions are concentrated around the months of August to March, although the farm is moving towards an out of season mating strategic plan. El Porvenir Ranch (Ronmer Urdaneta, 2008), owned by Agropecuaria San Rafael, in the same southern lake region (in La Fría, Táchira State) consists of a mixed bubaline and vaccine dairy farm operation. The area receives about 2100 mm annual rainfall, evenly distributed throughout the year. Cows are allowed once per day to graze 1 ha/head, whereas buffalo cows are allowed twice per day to graze 2 hectares/head, mostly Tanner Grass. Lowlands are covered with Carrizo (*Himenea amplexicauli* sp.) and Chimenea (*Paspalum fasciculatum* sp.). Currently, the farm owns 1050 buffaloes (300 dry buffalo cows, 200 milking, 189 fattening steers), with very low mortality rates (4 buffalo cows and 4 buffalo calves in 2007). Currently, they milk buffalo cows with calf present. Buffalo calves are allowed to suckle until they reach 6-7 months of age. Average birth weight is 38-40 kg and 160-180 kg at weaning. Average daily milk production is 6-7 lt., with peaks of 15-16 lt. The Agua Clara Ranch, in La Plantada, Córdoba Department, northeast of Colombia, (36) has an area of 3000 ha with 3900 buffalo heads. An area of 1200 ha, consisting of highlands with available pastures of *Brachiaria humidícola* sp., is used for buffalo cows during mating, reaching a 40-60% pregnancy rate. The remaining 1800 ha are lowland, natural pastures with good protein content levels. These lowland pastures are used to keep milking buffalo cows and second mating buffalo. They currently have 1000 buffalo cows in milking, producing an average 4 liters/day. The farm is divided in pens of 30-40 ha, each with its own water supply. Animals are supplemented with minerals and weight and individual production records are routinely kept [36].

In the year 2003, the Garofalo family owned three farms in the province of Caserta, Campania Region, Italy. Average production is 2200 liters/animal and 2000 liters/lactation. The farms produced 10,000 liters/day, with an average 8.5% butirose fat, a cheese yield of 24 - 27% (extremely high) and a protein content of 4.8% - one of the highest in Italy. They own 1300 animals in milking (1200 adults + 103 replacements). In total, they own 2500 dairy animals, and in order to expand their founder herd they decided not to sell any animal in the course of the year 2006. For a buffalo bull to be selected as breeder sire, its dam must have produced at least 3500 liters with high protein content. Milking sessions typically last 5-8 min/animal, and very seldom last more than 15 min. Animals are grouped according to their individual milking time requirements, in order to make milking sessions more efficient. One of their farms, located in Santo Amaro, has 650 buffalo cows in milking producing 2500 liters during a 270-day lactation. Individual production per animal averages 2100 liters, and this is a bit low due to the fact animals tend to skip pregnancies due to de-seasonalization. Improvements to the milking parlor, such as soaking ponds prior to milking area (renewing water continually), have helped in reducing mastitis incidence from 35 to 0%. Daily ration consists of 2 kg hay, 7-8 kg energy concentrate, 28 kg corn silage, 15 kg chopped green forage (Rye Grass). In 2007 they had another farm, Sant'Agnello Farm, in Caserta, Campania Region, with 60 ha, 3 milking parlors and 2000 buffalo head, 750 of those are milking buffalo cows producing a total of 7000 liters/day. Buffalo calf pre- and post- weaning rearing is totally automatized; animals are fed according to information contained in implanted microchips. Initial diets consist of milk consumption 8 times daily; this frequency is progressively reduced over the following weeks until animals are weaned at 13 weeks of age. Mortality rate in this production system is around 3-5%. The farm produces an average of 2650 liters for 270-day lactation. Each milking parlor has herringbone design with 12 milking stations on each side (total of 24), animals are managed with 1 operator every 100 animals. Animals are managed in groups of 48 in waiting area, with 24 entering the milking parlor at a given time; they are fitted with pedometers to record individual productions, among other parameters. Manure is managed with 1.8% slopes and two daily washings, and solids are systematically separated. Artificial insemination is conducted in the months of November, December and January; open animals are subsequently exposed to buffalo bulls in the following breeding cycle. Fifty-five percent of calvings occur during the summer months (June to September) and the remaining 45% is distributed throughout the rest of the year. De-seasonalization of animals (out of season breeding) causes losses of 30% of parturitions in older animals; these losses are reduced to 20% with young buffalo heifers in good body condition. Average production per lactation is 1800-1900 liters, with peaks after the third month. On average, animals produce 7 calves in their productive lifespan (about

12 years). Individuals that produce 3500 or more are left in the system until they die of natural causes, others are culled. This farm has records of individuals producing over 4800 liters [36].

Reproduction and Selection

Fifty years ago, the age at first service of buffalo heifers was 26 to 30 months, due to inadequate nutrition during the growth period. Today, with adequate nutrition, animals can be bred at 15 months of age although in natural range conditions it is preferred to wait until they are 22 to 24 months of age in order to allow for complete body development. Because of their longevity (buffaloes can live up to 30 years or even more) animals normally do not reach full body size until 4 years of age. According to several authors, gestation period in buffalo lasts 306 to 316 days and is not influenced by nutrition or offspring gender, although nutrition has been shown to affect calving interval [27, 37].

Mating or AI in the low breeding season is mostly done with 1st breeding heifers. Buffalo sires are often withdrawn from herds, so that there will be open animals to be bred in the spring-summer season. According to Borghese, out of mating season has been a major contribution to buffalo breeders because there is a higher monetary value of summer milk. This price difference in the value of milk compensates the losses due to lower fertility (about 30%). Breeders who have milk available during summer months, not only have higher income but also a market presence year-round. In 1997, Zicarelli reported that already 70% of buffalo herds in Italy were part of the out of mating season protocol [38]. Borghese suggested that the ideal proportion of breeding would be 30% in the fall (high breeding season) and 70% in the spring. This is a difficult goal because buffalo cows naturally tend to go back to their natural breeding season after 2 to 3 years, by prolonging the calving interval. Successive studies demonstrated that the fertility losses could be reduced to 15% using only first mating heifers during the low breeding season (spring) [5].

In the early 60's, buffalo dairy production in India, Pakistan, Azerbaijan, Italy, Bulgaria, Brazil, and other countries was a low-technology, rural setting activity characterized by inadequate nutrition. Even genetically superior animals would have low production levels, ending up with low body condition and mobilizing energy stores in order to meet milk production requirements. This, in turn, resulted in shortened lactations that made buffalo dairy production anti-economical. In the same years, bubaline dairy production witnessed a technological revolution (in India called the white revolution), that combined improvements in management, animal genetic selection and nutrition. Although intrinsic differences among countries persist to date, this technological step-up has translated into increased yields and better economic results, showing the great genetic capacity of the buffalo.

In Italy, after 2001 and despite an overall milk yield increase per farm, the industrial yield in terms of cheese production decreased slightly, giving indication that sire selection was done mainly in order to increase milk production and at the same time neglecting other important parameters; this trend is now being corrected [39]. Currently, genetic improvement in the Italian Mediterranean breed is conducted by selecting individuals based on Kilograms of Mozzarella Cheese (KMC). This parameter helps in identifying superior animals, and is obtained by multiplying milk production/lactation times the estimated cheese yield. Industrial yield is obtained applying Altiero's formula: Mozzarella cheese yield = {[(3,5 x % P in milk) + (1,25 x % F in milk)] – 0,088}. P stands for protein and F stands for fat content. Using this approach, milk controls now combine volume with chemical evaluation of samples: a buffalo cow that produces 4000 liters with a 23% cheese yield is the same as one that produces 3500 with 26% cheese yield. The study is still ongoing to evaluate a possible over-estimation of this formula on cheese yield. In addition to KMC, genetic selection is also based on morphological conformation traits such as udder, leg and hoof [28].

The breed is always important in the selection process. Repeatability of individual attributes is directly related to herd homogeneity. The selection of one defined breed is always a contributing factor to reach a major speed and robustness in the genetic improvement process [35].

Aldes Farm, in Agropoli, Salerno (Campania Region), Italy, for instance, focuses on the selection of replacement heifers with large frame and high milk production yields. In order to accelerate selection results, this farm culls 80% of first-calving heifers with low production scores (under 3000 liters), which are sold as dams. Only the best 10 animals remain in the system. If any of the remaining 10 produces more than 4000 liters, they will be dams of future superior bulls for the farm. Programmed mating favors intensive inbreeding, enhancing bloodlines with correct morphology and higher production levels. To this date, they have 12 buffalo cows considered capostipite or founder dams, all of them excellent producers and head of one line-breeding. Some of them are dams of over 30 heifers, which are now in the production system, including a total of 150 dairy buffalo cows. Production decreases after the 4th lactation. Animals are routinely culled on the 7th lactation unless they become champions (award-winning individuals). Those animals that are culled are sent directly to slaughter, to avoid other producers taking advantage of their genetics. The farm is on the lookout for potential problems derived from highly inbred animals. As soon as these problems are detected, the animals are not allowed to breed anymore and immediately culled. The highest producers (4200 liters or more) are mated in the natural season, which is normal, spontaneous and natural for them, in order to increase the milk production as much as possible, and in that way expressing their genetic capacity, allowing the necessary decisions.

Selection criteria: in a judging contest hosted in 2005 by the Bellelli farm, the following desirable female morphological traits were proposed by the ANASB (Italian Buffalo Breeders Association):

- Good hock and hoof conformation.
- Good udder conformation: correct plane of the udder in relation to the hock, good anterior and posterior insertions, and quarter development.
- Adequate bone structure: correct dorsal line, good rump development (hindquarter) and overall harmonious conformation.
- Body width (amplitude) and depth (thoracic capacity).
- Milking attributes: a thin skin, femininity, good general conformation (a good design for dairy), flattened bones with acute angles.

The udder must be well developed, with the four quarters properly framed (equidistant teats). Teats must be relatively long, flexible and easy to handle. Veins should be well marked. In addition, good hindquarter development and proper udder placement (high up, near the vulva) are desirable, since it is estimated that 60% of total milk is produced by the caudal quarters of the udder [40].

In the IIIrd National Show of Italian Mediterranean Buffalo, the Judge Dr. Massimo Neri applied the selection and conformation criteria from the Italian Buffalo Breeders Association (ANASB), consisting on a scoring system. In order to rank female conformation, the following traits with their respective scores were considered:

TRAIT	% OF TOTAL SCORE
Udder	40
Body capacity	10
Dairiness (dairy characteristics)	20
Structure	10
Hooves and legs (spur)	20

In order to rank productive ability, the following traits with their respective scores were considered:

TRAIT	% OF TOTAL SCORE
Protein index (%)	35
Fat index (%)	5
kg of milk index	15
Accuracy	15
Age	15
Ranking in its class	15

It is known that the value of mozzarella cheese can be affected by somatic cell count due to changes in the milk constituents. Somatic cell count is used as a marker for milk quality because it allows for the diagnosis of sub-clinical mastitis and the selection of mastitis-resistant individuals.

The estimated heritability of milk production trait suggests that this characteristic would improve with the implementation of selection programs. The age at first calving and interval between 1st and 2nd calving traits have low heritability, and therefore would not respond well to selection [41].

In buffalo, the heritability of milk yield ranges from 0.11 to 0.38, according to several authors. Lactation period (number of days) is of even lower heritability than milk yield, whereas heritability in growth and body weight is higher.

Other values obtained for cattle can be used for orientation purposes:

TRAIT	HERITABILITY
Birth weight	0.36
Weaning weight	0.26
Mature weight	0.28

Source: GPS, FAGB, 2010 [42].

The predictive value of lactation milk yield for buffalo sire selection (progeny test) was studied by analyzing first lactation milk yield of 685 heifer buffaloes (from 65 sires). Genetic correlation of monthly production and cumulative production for 305-day lactations was found to be close to one. This indicated that milk yield by the 4th month of lactation could be used as a tool to evaluate sires through progeny testing. This allows shortening generation intervals, increasing annual progress rates and reducing the cost of progeny testing of buffalo sires [43].

Because the buffalo is a species with little selection for milk yield, there is large variability between individual productions. This helps the application of selection programs to increase heard average milk yield through the culling of the less productive individuals and the replacement with the descendants of more productive animals.

In the year 2000, ICAR (International Committee for Animal Recording) sponsored a technical meeting in Slovenia in order to establish and standardize buffalo registries (genetic improvement programs and data registering). Some of the recommendations from the meeting were as follows: i) to achieve the knowledge of milk production at the individual herd, regional and national levels; ii) to provide information to producers to aid in their breeding strategies; iii) to make information available for national policy formulation; iiii) to focus initial efforts on large herds where owners understand the benefits of production control and the utilization of the information for their exploitation planning; v) to initiate collection of available, easy-access records such as breeding records, calving and fat content; vi) to publish information periodically so that producers can compare their performances and to standardize formulae used in milk production calculations, and to centralize data collection processing and keeping [44].

4. LACTATION: SEXUAL MATURITY, GESTATION, CALVING INTERVAL, UDDER PHYSIOLOGY, DAYS IN LACTATION AND PRODUCTION BY AGE GROUP

Planned selection has resulted in improved udder development and conformation, with quarters better adapted to mechanical milking. Buffalo cow milking tends to be a slower process than cattle, and this makes the milking nozzles to climb up the nipple. To circumvent this problem it is necessary to compensate with some kind of central weighing system. Recently, some milking systems specifically designed for buffalo have been introduced in the market.

In spite of their aspect and reputation, with good management, buffalo cows are highly tame and docile. Paineiras da Ingaí Farm works with groups of 5 untied buffalo cows in the parlor, without supplementation. Milking times average 14-17 minutes and total-milking times for 60-65 cows is about 3.5 hours. Average milk production is 8-9 liters, calves are allowed to suckle from the two quarters until 30 days of age, and then reduced to one until 3 months of age [45].

Buffalo calf suckling has traditionally been used in order to stimulate milk letdown in buffalo cow. Mammary gland output is the result of a complex stimulatory process between calf and dam; nipples are extensively innervated and have numerous receptors sensitive to touch, pressure and temperature. This stimulus is transmitted to the pituitary gland causing oxytocin release, which in turn is responsible for milk letdown through contraction of mioepithelial cells around the secretory tissue of the udder [6].

Routine parlor handling, including washing and disinfection of the udder, can also stimulate milk letdown. This aspect is extremely important in buffalo, since animals tend to be submerged in unsanitary water of ponds [27]. In Salerno, Italy, animals are fed concentrates prior to milking in order to stimulate milk letdown, although 3-4% animals withhold milk due to external negative stimuli or human presence. Oxytocin injection is needed in about 5% of animals [6].

For the mechanical milking of dairy buffalo cows, traditional milking machines (for cattle) have been used. Because dairy buffalo cows are considered slow milkers, possibly due to higher sphincter closing strength, vacuum required is higher than in dairy cattle: 48-61 cm (mercury scale) *vs.* 40-50; with pulse ratios 1:2,3 – 1:4 compression. In Italy, it is estimated an average 7 minutes of milking time per buffalo cow, taking 1.2 to 2.4 minutes per liter. N. Carvalho (2007) reported the following guidelines for dairy buffalo cow: 38-41 mm Hg and 60 pulses/minute [46].

In cattle, 20-40% of secreted milk is stored in the mammary gland cistern at the time of milking and the rest is located in the alveoli; in the buffalo cow the cistern is considerably smaller and the milk is stored mainly in the alveoli (90-95%), due to considerable less genetic improvement pressure, although cistern capacity can be improved by selection due to the high heritability of the trait. Small cistern capacity and storage make complete emptying extremely important. According to a study presented by De Laval, mechanical milking can be gradually implemented in one-week period and achieve normal production levels. Being most of the milk stored in alveoli, equipment has been designed to keep a steady low flow until reaching 200 ml/min, milking pressure is then increased and then reduced towards the end of the milking cycle, in order to drain completely the udder. This milking pattern has been designed, based on the specific lactation physiology of buffalo cow [47].

Dairy buffalo cows must have good udder and legs conformation as well as good maternal ability. Nipple length and conformation show less variability in the Mediterranean breed. (6,3 a 8,5 cm length), whereas variability is higher in Murrah breed: 60% of evaluated nipples range from 6 to 10 cm length. Overall cistern storage volume is lower in bubaline than in cattle; in the Mediterranean breed cistern capacity ranges from 75 to 220 cm^3, and alveolar tissue between 3000 to 4000 cm^3 [47]. Ten to 12 hours post-milking, 95% of milk is again stored in secretory tissue (alveoli). It is extremely important to ensure good milk ejection and complete emptying of the mammary gland in buffalo cow. Inadequate or incomplete milking results in significant losses, due to autocrine inhibition of milk secretion (alveoli deactivation) [48].

C. S. Thomas studied buffalo cow behavior in farms with automated milking, concentrate supplementation during milking routine and hydraulic manure cleaning. In a 24 h period, buffaloes spend 33% of their time laying down, resting and chewing cud, 6% sleeping, 23% feeding and 38% in other activities (walking, drinking, *etc.*). Buffaloes ruminate 5-8 hours daily, mostly during night-time [49]. When two milkings per day are done, ideally, it should be done 12 hours apart although this is not feasible in practice. In this case, it is helpful to separate animals in groups, this allows the reduction in the milking frequency in highly productive groups, and the increase in those that are not as productive [50].

The parlor facilities must obey to the requested hygienic conditions for both the environment and instruments/utensils used. It must be built with waterproof flooring, without puddles, and with a slight slope, all suitable for automatic wash and liquid runoff. Also walls must be waterproof. The area must be covered by a roof, and with an abundant clean water source, far from roads and people movements. These facilities must be protected from winds and little animals (dogs, chickens, rats, *etc.*). After every milking, the parlor must be washed, in order to remove manure and urine [50].

Good milking management can lead to a production increases up to 50%, although this has to be achieved mainly through genetic improvement. It must be noted that, compared to cattle, buffaloes have had fewer years and less resources addressed to genetic improvement. This aspect makes buffalo cows highly dependent on the presence of their calves, because it responds to a natural necessity for the species survival [25].

In Castanha Grande Ranch, after calving, the dam remains with the calf for 24 hours, to promote udder development and to let calf suckling colostrum. They also train animals to be milked without the presence of the calf since the first very days following parturition. For this purpose, they use corrals to allow cow-calf contact and interaction without allowing the calf to suckle. The dams gradually forget their calves. They regularly use nannies on a rotational scheme: buffalo cows that calve become nannies of their offspring plus one or two more. When the nannies increase, those that have being doing the task for more time, return to the milking group. This system stimulates greatly mammary gland and increases milk production. Buffalo calves are allowed to stay with nannies until 30 days of age. Animals from 30 to 60 days of age are moved to artificial calf rearing for half day (with concentrated and water ad libitum), and for the remaining part of the day they return to the nannies. By two months of age, weight is about 70 kg, and they change to a rearing system with a minimum intake of 800 g of ration and as animals have started chewing cud, they receive volume (pastures) [25].

The target in animal condition at calving should be 3-3.5 in a scale 1 to 5. Milking starts 7 days post-partum. Initial milking products could still have colostrum traces and is therefore not destined to cheese manufacturing. During those first days after birth, calves consume reduced volume of milk and the residual could remain in the alveoli. The natural physiological mechanism is that that stimulus then triggers a reduction in production. It is therefore of utmost importance to ensure complete emptying of the mammary gland during milking during that period of time (either by mechanical milking or by introducing additional calves to the buffalo cow), in order to avoid further reductions in production levels.

Animals must be handled gently, without stress or presence of dogs. It is preferable to reduce walking distances under 1 km in order not to increase energy demands. Animals must be washed and then wipe dried, prior to milking in order to provide thermal comfort and hygiene. When the udder if full of milk, the buffalo cow feels pain in the gland, and after milking they experience a comfortable condition. The dairy buffalo cow must be docile. Good environment (quiet, calm) and a friendly relationship with the operator, including an interaction between them (speaking to the animals), are very important. Any change in routine or people must be done carefully and gradually. High production buffalo cows are just as susceptible to mastitis as their cattle counterparts. Because buffaloes like to lie in mud in order to regulate heat and because nipple sphincters (in the high production dams) tend to remain open for a period of time after milking, these animals are more susceptible to environmental mastitis. A good management approach is to offer concentrate after milking, to encourage animals to remain standing while sphincters return to normal, contracted state [25].

Mammary gland physiology determines that when the gland is empty, milk production metabolism is at its peak. Progressive udder filling and increase in internal pressure determine a reduction in the milk synthesis rate, until gradually reaching an end. During milking, animals should remain calm, which is evidenced by rumination activity, sleepy eyes, lowered head and ears and a generally relaxed state [25].

These ethological observations are key in buffalo milk production. Handlers must be patient and careful when interacting with animals. Buffaloes are very sensitive to abrupt movements or physical abuse, and this is reflected in overall lowered performance. Gentle touch and positive reinforcement ease the animal´s anxiety, and in order to encourage forward movement, the use of poles with visible flags attached to the end are recommended. A buffalo under stress will exhibit the following signs: eyes wide open, erect ears and pointed to the source of distress, frequent defecation and/or urination and absence of chewing. Animals under extreme stress will open their mouth and protrude their tongues [51]. When animals are reluctant to being handled, cleaned or attached to the milking equipment, sometimes they must be restrained by tying one of their legs. Animals are moved to the dry group when production drops under 3 liters, or when they are 60 days from their calving date.

In the last century, in countries in the near and far East, lactations tended to decrease after the third production cycle mainly due to inadequate nutrition, deficient herd health or lack of sanitary conditions. Nowadays, good herd management has resulted in steady production levels over seven cycles or more. High production animals (5000 liters/lactation) are maintained in production for about 12 years *versus* 18-20 years for lower production animals. These has to be taken into account when conducting and economic analysis of the production, or when considering management or selection actions. In the Animal Production Research Centre, Rome, Italy, Maimone *et al.* (1961) have applied a quite useful measure of production persistence: comparison of the first 100 days of lactation *versus* the second 100 [27]. The Ribeira Valley, Sao Paulo State, Brazil, has been evaluated the effect of season and number of calving on average milk production and lactation persistence, and 1591 lactations (once daily milking, pasture based) were included in the study. Results showed that, for pasture-based systems, animals calving out of calving season exhibit lower production levels per lactation but higher lactation persistence; and females in first calving show lower productions [37]. In Peshawar, Pakistan, researchers evaluated the inhibiting effect of pregnancy over milk production. They recorded production of 456 pregnant and 179 open buffalo cows over a 48-week period. Milk yield of pregnant animals significantly increased during the two months after calving, and then decreased steadily at the 3rd month of gestation [52].

Artificial Calf Rearing

C. Bruna (2010) obtained encouraging results in Brazil using Sprayfo (a product from Netherlands), which has also been used in cattle. These results represent a significant improvement from local products with high soy contents that resulted in high calf mortality. Manufacturer recommendation is 4 liters product/day, in two feedings [53]. A. Paske (2010) from Brazil also recommends Sprayfo in buffalo calves, allowing them to suckle colostrum until day 7, followed by weaning and feeding 2 liters of buffalo milk combined with 2 liters of product. Animals are switched to 4 liters of product plus forage by 35 days of age. Animals are then switched to forage and concentrate diets by the age of 90 days. Under this system, average weight gain at 90 days of age is 0.5 kg/day [54].

Artificial rearing of males calves can be unprofitable. In order to lower rearing costs, Bramaderos Ranch separates males a few days after they are born and feed them colostrum and silage until 90 days of age. Then they are switched to corn silage and fresh forage diet. Colostrum is fermented at room temperature (around 25° C) under dark conditions in 60-liter, vacuum-sealed plastic bags. Product can be stored under these conditions for 30 days. In order to utilize it, it is first diluted in water (2:1 water to silage ratio) and offered in feeding bunks. Animals, who like this food, are weighted weekly, and the expected weigh gain is 638 g/day. Animals are fed colostrum until 90 days of age and 87 kg weight [55].

Mastitis

Dairy buffalo cows are considered in general more resistant to disease than cattle, although health management and prevention is similar. Mastitis has low incidence in buffalo cows; it is slightly higher in animals under mechanical milking. Subclinical inflammation of the udder makes herd screening necessary [56 - 58]. Mastitis can have several origins: infectious, allergic or trauma [46]. Infection of the mammary gland originates in the external environment and progresses through the nipple canal of the infected quarter. Operator, sanitary conditions and milking equipment are considered to be the main risk factors. External or internal trauma is sometimes caused during suckling. Buffalo cow nipples are smaller than cattle. And their sphincters have muscles with more fibers than cows, acting as protective barrier against infections. Intra-mammary antibiotic treatment is necessary upon detection of infection, and success is highly dependent of total removal of pathogen from the infected quarter [58]. Mastitis not only results in lowered production levels but also affects negatively milk quality. Milk from affected animals will have lowered fat, lactose, casein, calcium and phosphorus and will have increased undesirable traits such as somatic cell, salt, fatty acids, immunoglobulins, lipases and overall bacterial count [46, 57, 59].

Research conducted in Italy indicates levels up to 200,000 somatic cell count does not influence milk buffalo coagulation, levels up to 300,000 cells/ml are considered within normal range for mechanical milking [60]. Reports from Brazil suggest variations of 8000 to 38,000 somatic cell count/ml in buffaloes milked by hand, pasture-based and exposed to calf suckling [50].

Milk somatic cell count is primarily composed of leukocytes and mammary gland epithelium. The number of these cells present in milk indicates inflammatory response of the mammary gland to trauma, inadequate milking procedures or mastitis; this count tends to increase towards the last phase of lactation.

5. MANAGEMENT OF ENVIRONMENTAL FACTORS AND HEAT STRESS

Proper management requires adequate nutrition, health, good sanitary conditions and facilities (according to the weather conditions), trained personnel, a planned reproduction and genetic selection program, business management, *etc*. If one or more of these aspects are neglected, all efforts applied to other management factors are rendered null. Severe effects due to hot weather environments can translate into heat stress in dairy buffalo cow. Increased feed intake necessary to support high production levels results in increased metabolic heat. When air temperature is higher than 32°C, voluntary intake declines as well as milk output. Anorexia is quite common in buffaloes subjected to heat stress. Rate of passage through the digestive tract decreases when abomasal passage is reduced and milk production drops abruptly, particularly in high-producing animals.

Good management of the dairy buffalo requires effective protection against direct sunlight for at least part of the day during the summer months, with either facilities that allow complete water immersion of the animals (at least 20 min) or water sprinkler systems [27]. When buffaloes are provided thermal comfort (water sprinkler systems, ponds, mud holes or shade), it results in a significant increase in voluntary feed intake [31]. Management of heat stress (reduced rectal temperatures and heart rate) will in turn result in increased milk yields. Females with access to water-cooling have been shown to have higher pregnancy rates and shorter calving intervals. When faced with low environmental temperatures the buffalo cows have to allocate energy to keep thermal balance and thus milk production is hindered.

CONCLUSION

In Asia and Mediterranean countries, buffaloes have been utilized for centuries for milk, meat and draft. However, it wasn′t until recently that the buffalo became subject of scientific research and government promotion policies. Because domestic cattle led the way in terms of genetic selection and productive management, bubaline producers were able to rely on previously developed technologies in order to advance buffalo production and performance. This in turn paved the way for a solid buffalo dairy industry, and this trend is now being followed by producers in the world.

CONFLICT OF INTEREST

The authors confirm that they have no conflict of interest to declare for this publication.

ACKNOWLEDGEMENTS

Declared none.

REFERENCES

[1] International Dairy Federation – IDF – Statistics: the world dairy situation 2002. Bull Int Dairy Fed 2002; 378: 46-7.

[2] International Dairy Federation – IDF – Milk production: the world dairy situation 2000. Bull Int Dairy Fed 2000; 355: 5-6.

[3] Zava M. The Domestic Buffalo Publisher. Buenos Aires, Argentina: National Agricultural Research Institute 2011; p. 304.

[4] Bernardes O. Communications to the Buffalo Forum bufalos@yahoogrupos.com.br, June 22th 2010 and July 07 2010. Sao Paulo, Brazil: Paineiras da Ingaí Farm 2005.

[5] Borghese A. Buffalo Production and Research. Rome: Food and Agriculture Organization – FAO 2005.

[6] Santosh Thomas C. Machine milking buffaloes. Salerno, Italy: Published: Bubalus bubalis Magazine 2005.

[7] Zava M. The Domestic Buffalo Publisher. Buenos Aires, Argentina: National Agricultural Research Institute 2011; pp. 328-9.

[8] Casali A, Casali M. Artificial Insemination Cooperative, Catalogue, Cremona. Italy: Lombardia 2013; p. 7.

[9] Zava M. The Domestic Buffalo Publisher. Buenos Aires, Argentina: National Agricultural Research Institute 2011; pp. 340-435.

[10] Moioli B. Breeding and Selection of Dairy Buffaloes. Published in "Buffalo Production and Research", Antonio Borghese, Editor, FAO, Rome, 2005; 41

[11] Ghulam Faruque Group. Buffalo Industry. Lahore: Punjab, Pakistan, February 2011.

[12] Pasha TN. Buffalo Population in Pakistan Proceedings, VIII World Buffalo Congress. Caserta, Italy. 2007.

[13] Pasha TN. Meat Potential Production in Pakistan Proceedings, VIth American Buffalo Symposium. Mérida, Venezuela. 2008.

[14] Guglielminetti AS. 5th Germany Buffalo Day. Rome: Buffalo Newsletter, FAO 2007.

[15] Yang B, Zeng XL, Qin J, Yang C. Dairy Buffalo Breeding in countryside of Proceedings VIII World Buffalo Congress. Nanning. China, Buffalo: Research Institute 2007.

[16] Chunxi Z. Buffalo Genetic Resources. Published: Buffalo Newsletter, FAO, Rome, Italy, December 2001

[17] Chiangmai A. Development of swamp buffalo breeding improvement for sustainable use in Thailand, Department of Livestock Development, Bangkok, Thailand, Published: Buffalo Newsletter. Rome: FAO 2003.

[18] Zava M. Published, July 2013. Buenos Aires, Argentina: Argentine Buffalo Breeders Association Newsletter 2013.

[19] Drilon M. Buffalo Breeding in Philippines Proceedings, VIIth World Buffalo Congress. Manila, Philippines. 2004.

[20] Cruz L. Philippine Carabao Centre (PCC). New Delhi, India: Published: Asian Buffalo Magazine 2004.

[21] Cruz L. Proceedings, II Italian Buffalo Congress. Buffalo. 2003.

[22] El Tahir S. El Tahir Buffalo Farm. Rome, Italy: Published: Buffalo Newsletter, FAO 1999.

[23] Zava M. The Domestic Buffalo Publisher. Buenos Aires, Argentina: National Agricultural Research Institute 2011; p. 326.

[24] Bernardes O. Buffalo situation in Brazil. Proceedings III Brazilian Breeders. Recife, Pernambuco, Brazil. 2005.

[25] Couto AG. Dairy buffalo cow management and production in Castanha Grande Ranch, Sao Luiz do Quintude, Alagoas, Brazil, Published Proceedings, IV American Buffalo Symposium. Mérida, Venezuela. 2008.

[26] Zava M. The Domestic Buffalo Publisher. Buenos Aires, Argentina: National Agricultural Research Institute 2011; p. 305.

[27] Cockrill William Ross. The Husbandry and Health of the Domestic Buffalo. Rome, Italy: Published: Food and Agriculture Organization of the United Nations 1974.

[28] Casali A. COFA: the only dedicated Mediterranean buffalo stud in Italy. Rome, Italy: Buffalo Newsletter, FAO 2007.

[29] Indian Dairy Corporation (IDC). The Murrah, IDC Bulletin. Baroda, Gujarat, India: R. C. Dutt Road 1977.

[30] Dhulkhed SH, Parekh S. Gujarat Artificial Insemination Center. Gujarat, India: A. I. Center Bulletin, Rajkot 1981.

[31] Bernardes O. Grazing dairy buffalo cows management, Paineiras da Ingaí Farm, Sao Paulo, Brazil. Mérida, Venezuela: VIth American Buffalo Symposium 2008.

[32] Barile VL, Pacelli C, Palocci G, *et al.* Effects of different diets on milk yield and quality of lactating buffaloes: maize *versus* sorghum silage. Note II. Animal Production Research Center, Monterotondo, Italy. Published Proceedings, IX World Buffalo Congress. Buenos Aires, Argentina. 2010.

[33] Tyagi A. Enhancement of conjugated linoleic acid content of buffalo milk and milk product through green fodder. Proceedings, IXth World Buffalo Congress. Buenos Aires, Argentina. 2010.

[34] Zava M. The domestic buffalo Publisher. Buenos Aires, Argentina: National Agricultural Research Institute 2011; p. 318.

[35] Bernardes O. Dairy exploitation in Paineiras da Ingaí Farm, Sarapuí, Sao Paulo, Brazil. Marco Zava, The Domestic Buffalo Published. Buenos Aires: National Agricultural Research Institute 2011; p. 372.

[36] Zava Marco. Italian Mediterranean buffalo milk characteristics. Mérida, Venezuela: Published: IV American Buffalo Symposium 2008.

[37] Baruselli PS, Nagazaki E, Toledo L, Carvalho N. Effects of the season and number of calving on buffaloes milk production, UPDR-APTA-Ribeira Valley, Dept. Animal Reproduction, Sao Paulo University (USP), Brazil. Published Proceedings, VIII World Buffalo Congress. Caserta, Italy. 2007.

[38] Zicarelli L. Out of season mating. Proceedings, Vth World Buffalo Congress. Caserta, Italy. 1997.

[39] Zicarelli L. Italian Mediterranean buffalo milk characteristics. IV American Buffalo Symposium. Mérida, Venezuela. 2008.

[40] Polihronov D, Aleksiev A. Buffalo Breeding in the People's Republic of Bulgaria. Sofia, Bulgaria: National Agroindustrial Union Center for Scientific, Technical and Economic Information 1979.

[41] Oliveira Seno L, Tonhati H, Cardoso VL, El Faro L, Sesana RS. [1]Aspilcueta Borquis RR. Genetic parameters for milk yield, age at first calving and interval between first and second calving in milk buffaloes. Published Proceedings, VIII World Buffalo Congress. Caserta, Italy. 2007.

[42] Argentine Bovine Genetic Forum (FAGB) Guide of Suggested Procedures (GPS). Argentina: FAGB, Buenos Aires 2010.

[43] Jain AK, Dhilon JS. Use of part lactation records for sire evaluation. Proceedings, IIIth World Buffalo Congress. Varna, Bulgaria. 1991.

[44] International Committee for Animal Recording (ICAR). Workshop on Animal Recording for Improved Breeding and Management Strategies for Buffaloes-ICAR. Bled. Slovenia. 2000.

[45] Bernardes O. Communication to the Buffalo Forum bufalos@yahoogrupos,com.br 2010 August 2nd;

[46] Tonizza de Carvalho NA. Buffaloes Artificial Insemination Course (USP, São Paulo, Brazil). Formosa Province, Argentina: Guazú Cuá Ranch 2007.

[47] Borghese A. Milking management of dairy buffalo. Proceedings, VIII World Buffalo Congress. Caserta, Italy. 2007.

[48] Santosh Thomas C. The udder physiology. Proceedings, IVth American Buffalo Symposium. Mérida, Venezuela. 2008.

[49] Santosh Thomas C. Housing and management of lactating buffalo cows. Proceedings, Vth American Buffalo Symposium. Pedro Leopoldo, Minas Gerais, Brazil. 2009.

[50] Brazilian Buffalo Breeders Association (ABCB). Dairy buffalo cow management. Sao Paulo, Brazil: ABCB 2007.

[51] Couto AG. Ethology: A Study of Buffalo Behavior Aiming at Milk Yield. Proceedings, IX World Buffalo Congress. Buenos Aires, Argentina. 2010.

[52] Qureshi M, Khan S, Ahmad N. Pregnancy depresses milk yield in dairy buffaloes. Proceedings, VIII World Buffalo Congress. Caserta, Italy. 2007.
[http://dx.doi.org/10.4081/ijas.2007.s2.1290]

[53] Bruna C. stranho@netpoint.com.br; Communications to the Buffalo Forum bufalos@yahoo grupos.com.br 2010 June 19th;

[54] Paske A. amauripaske@yahoo.com.br, Communication to the Buffalo Forum bufalos@yahoo grupos.com.br 2010 June 20th;

[55] Ranch B. belt6769@yahoo.com; Communication to the Buffalo Forum bufalos@yahoogrupos.com.br 2010. August 24th.

[56] Calace Gallo H. Buffalo Health and. In: Zava M, Ed. Buffaloes Production. Buenos Aires, Argentina: Orientación Gráfica Editora 1992.

[57] Rodríguez R. Buffalo in Venezuela. Marco Zava, The Domestic Buffalo, Published. Buenos Aires: National Agricultural Research Institute 2011.

[58] Didonet Láu H. Buffalo Health in Brazil. 1999.

[59] Bansal DK, Hamann J, Lind O, Singh ST, Dhaliwal PS. Somatic cell count and biochemical components of milk related to udder health in buffaloes. Proceedings, VIII World Buffalo Congress. Caserta, Italy. 2007. [http://dx.doi.org/10.4081/ijas.2007.s2.1035]

[60] Terramoccia S. Milk somatic cells levels in Italy. The Domestic Buffalo, Publisher. Buenos Aires: National Agricultural Research Institute 2011; p. 347.

CHAPTER 10

Buffalo Milk Characteristics and By-Products

Marco A. Zava[1,*] and **Marina Sansinena**[2,3]

[1] *Technical Department of Argentine Buffalo Breeders Association; International Consultant, Arcos 1325, 1426, Buenos Aires, Argentina*

[2] *Animal Biotechnology Laboratory, College of Agriculture, Catholic University of Argentina, Cap. Gral. Ramón Freire 183, 1426 Buenos Aires, Argentina*

[3] *National Council for Research and Technology (CONICET)*

Abstract: This chapter covers a review of chemical composition and nutrient profile of buffalo milk; several key physical properties (freezing point, surface tension, electric conductivity and thermal stability) are described. Regional manufacturing, utilization and marketing of buffalo milk by-products such as cheese, yogurt, ghee and others are also described and step-by-step flow charts are presented.

Keywords: Breeds, Buffalo, Buffalo milk by-products, Chemical composition, Dairy.

1. INTRODUCTION

Products derived from fluid bubaline milk, such as butter and ricotta, frescal and mozzarella cheese, have outstanding attributes in terms of product quality and health benefits. Other products, such as fluid milk or ghee, have been adapted by some countries in order to satisfy local market preferences and specific human nutrition demands. In all cases, fluid buffalo milk and its by-products provide excellent nutrient profiles and unique attributes for human nutritional needs; this translates into a wide range of products with high palatability, outstanding cheese yield, and unique health benefits.

* **Corresponding author Marco A. Zava:** Technical Department of Argentine Buffalo Breeders Association; International Consultant, Arcos 1325, 1426, Buenos Aires, Argentina; Tel: +54 011 4706 2513; Fax: +54 11 4373 9982; E-mail: marcozava@gmail.com

Giorgio A. Presicce (Ed.)

2. BUFFALO MILK COMPOSITION AND NUTRIENT PROFILE

Buffalo cow milk quality is considered to be excellent due to its unique nutrient profile. It is an excellent source of protein, vitamins, minerals and other constituents and it provides calories in countries where the overall supply of essential nutrients is deficient. Bubaline milk is higher in fat, protein, lactose and total solids than milk from cattle (Fig. **1**). Its fat content is 2.5 to 3 times higher and it provides 40% more calories than its cattle counterpart [1].

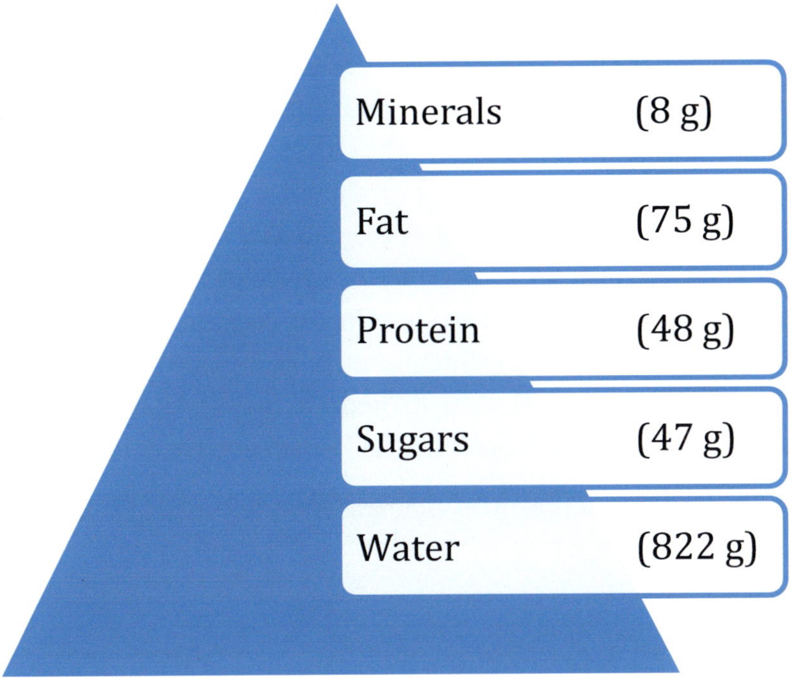

Fig. (1). Average composition of buffalo milk [3].

Studies conducted in Brazil with Murrah breed showed that buffalo milk composition includes conjugated linoleic acids (CLA), considered as anti-carcinogen compounds and shown to have beneficial effects on health problems such as obesity, arteriosclerosis and diabetes. This study also demonstrated that supplemental feeding of raw soybean oil further increases CLA content in buffalo milk [2].

The main differences between bubaline and cattle milk are:

- Higher butirose fat (107% more).
- Lower cholesterol (17 to 24% less).
- Higher protein (34% more).
- Higher lactose (19% more).
- Higher total solid content (48% more).
- Lower salts (Na, Cl, K).
- Higher overall nutrient values.

Source [4].

Buffalo cow milk is defined by its nutrient profile; this facilitates its physico-chemical and organoleptic identification. It has higher viscosity, curding strength and pH [5]. It has characteristic sensory evaluation, slightly sweet flavor and bright white color due to almost complete carotene absence in its fat fraction [3]. Buffalo cow milk differences with its cattle counterpart are present also in the colostrum. Environmental factors such as climate conditions, nutrition, breed, management and lactation period influence milk composition. Due to its high casein content, buffalo cow milk is more difficult to digest; in India it is common to add 33% water when the milk is destined for human consumption [6].

COMPOSITION	BUFFALO COW MILK	COW MILK
Water	84,5	87,5
Dry extract	16-22	11-13
Lean extract	7-12	6-10
Casein	2,8-4,2	2,6-3,0
Fat	7,0-9,6	3,3-4,3
Lactose	4,9-5,0	4,6-5,2
Total protein	4,0-4,6	3,0-3,8
Ca (mg/100 g)	180-240	120
P (mg/100 g)	120-140	65
Ca/P	1.61	1.31
Ash	0,75-0,85	0,80-0,90
Acidity (°SH/50)	4,2-5,0	3,3-3,5
Density (15°C)	1.031-1.034	1.028-1.035
pH	6,6-6,8	6,6-6,7

Fig. (2). Comparative milk composition.

The comparative milk composition of cattle and buffalo are shown in Fig. (**2**) [7], whereas changes in composition with lactation stage are shown in Fig. (**3**) [3].

Week No.	Average milk yield	Fat	Protein	Total solids	Water
	Kilograms			*(%)*	
1. (Colostrum)	-	-	-	-	-
2	9.06	7.77	5.58	19.06	80.94
4	10.85	6.74	4.41	17.26	82.74
6	10.61	6.61	3.95	16.67	83.33
8	10.31	6.30	9.82	16.23	83.77
10	9.75	6.64	9.79	16.58	83.42
11	9.54	7.11	9.88	16.94	83.06
13	9.25	7.15	9.93	17.17	82.83
15	8.97	7.22	4.01	17.22	82.78
17	7.48	7.61	4.16	17.48	82.52
19	7.95	8.01	4.20	18.07	81.93
21	7.59	8.33	4.30	18.43	81.57
23	6.92	8.68	4.48	18.84	81.16
25	6.55	8.80	4.50	18.94	81.06
27	6.51	8.90	4.48	19.02	80.98
29	6.18	9.07	4.61	19.41	80.59
31	5.65	9.10	4.66	19.63	80.37
33	5.39	9.44	4.61	19.72	80.28
35	5.13	9.70	4.86	20.42	79.58

Fig. (3). Changes in bubaline milk composition related to lactation stage.

Fat globules in buffalo cow milk are larger than in cattle counterpart. Therefore, buffalo cow milk fat has higher density and fusion values, a higher saponification and Reickert index; its butiro-refractometer index, Polenske values and Iodine values are lower (Fig. **4**) [5].

CONSTANT	BUFFALO MILK FAT	COW MILK FAT
Butiro-refractometer index	42.0	41.2
Saponification value	230.1	227.3
Reichert value	32.3	26.6
Polenske value	1.4	1.7
Kirchner value	28.5	22.1
Iodine value	29.4	33.8
Fusion point	32.0 – 43.5	28.5 – 41.0

Fig. (4). Bubaline milk fat analytic constants, compared to cattle milk.

Analyzing its nutritional value (Fig. **5**), bubaline milk shows higher resistance to damage due to oxidative conditions, and it is richer in butyric acid and long chain fatty acids such as palmitic and stearic acids. It has higher content of unsaturated fatty acids, and lower content of intermediate-length fatty acids (from C_6 to C_{12}).

Bubaline milk has higher total and colloidal calcium content, as well as iron and phosphorus. Usually, bubaline milk has more cation than anion concentration, compared to vaccine milk [5].

NUTRIENT	BUFFALO COW	COW
Fat (g)	6.9	3.3
Protein (gm)	3.7	3.2
Calcium (mg)	188	113
Iron (mg)	0.1	0
Phosphorus (mg)	117	97

Fig. (5). Nutritional values in large domestic ruminants.

Buffalo cows metabolize all nutritional carotene to vitamin A, which is then transferred to milk, making it readily accessible to the neonate [8]. A study conducted by Ezequiel Patiño, in UNNE (Corrientes University), Argentina, on 960 samples from 40 buffalo cows, described the physico-chemical description of bubaline milk for pasture-based systems (Fig. **6**) [3].

TRAIT	MEAN	SE
Density (g/ml)	1,0307	0,0039
Acidity (° Dornic)	19,65	2,96
pH	6,71	0,16
Total solids (%)	16,35	2,42
Fat (%)	7,22	1,89
Protein (%)	3,85	0,92
Lactose (%)	4,49	0,24
Ash (%)	0,83	0,08

Fig. (6). Physico-chemical composition of buffalo cow milk in pasture-based systems.

Among all the characteristics studied, titratable acidity (19,65 +/- 2,96 ° Dornic) was the trait that exhibited the most variability during lactations. Bubaline milk has a higher value of titratable acidity than cattle milk due to its higher casein content [3]; therefore, the threshold parameters used in the industry for cattle milk in Argentina (13° to 18° Dornic) are not applicable to buffalo cow. The increase in titratable acidity in the last phase of lactation coincides with a drop in milk output and with an increase in total solids due to this volume reduction and consequent protein concentration [3].

The milk used for mozzarella cheese manufacturing, must have a 2:1 fat protein ratio, a minimum fat content of 7.2% and a low value of titratable acidity. Titratable acidity values in Italian Mediterranean breed fluctuate during lactation from 12.0 to 9.0 SH° (Soux-Henkel units/ 100 ml milk) during the first 25 days after calving. Values start at 12.0 at the initiation of lactation, 10.0 by two weeks and drop to 9.0 after 25 days. Conversion used to express acidity levels in ° SH and ° Dormic (°D) can be obtained using the following formulae [3]:

- Milk acidity (°D) = (4.5 x acidity expressed in °SH)/2
- Milk acidity (°SH) = (2 x acidity expressed in °D)/4,5

LACATION PERIOD (month)	PHYSICO-CHEMICAL DETERMINATION			
	Acidity (°D)	*pH*	*Density*	*Cryoscopy(°H)*
1	20,9	6,86	1,0361	- 0,573
2	16,2	6,97	1,0344	- 0,579
3	17,1	6,94	1,0344	- 0,580
4	18,6	6,91	1,0336	- 0,575
5	18,9	6,94	1,0327	- 0,580
6	19,1	6,94	1,0337	- 0,576
7	18,6	6,90	1,0334	- 0,577
8	19,2	9,88	1,0325	- 0,574
9	19,6	6,87	1,0326	- 0,577

°D = Dornic degrees; °H = Hortvet degrees

Fig. (7). Acidity, pH, density and cryoscopic characteristics of buffalo cow milk.

Normal acidity in Italian Mediterranean breed ranges from 7.0 to 7.8 °SH (Fig. **7**) [3]. The factors affecting acidity values include a) presence of saprophyte bacteria producing lactic acid through lactose fermentation, b) conservation of milk in dirty refrigerators and slow cooling, c) transport in dirty containers and other contaminants, d) long transportation periods, e) unsanitary milking procedures, f) inadequate foodstuffs (too coarse, moldy or unbalanced mineral mixes) [9].

Colostrum is produced by the mammary gland during the early hours post-partum. It has a significant higher total solids concentration compared to milk produced during the rest of the lactation (Fig. **8**). All milk major constituents, together with the minerals (mainly calcium, phosphorus and potassium), and fat-soluble vitamins, are present in bubaline colostrum in higher concentrations compared to cattle. It also contains antibodies that protect young buffalo calf against infections [3]. In order to provide adequate immunity to the calf, it is recommended to ensure colostrum intake of at least 2 liters/calf, within 3-6 hours after birth [10].

TOTAL MILK PERCENTUAL (%)					
Days after calving	***Fat***	***Protein***	***Total solids***	***Lactose***	***Vitamin A***
Day 1	9.55	9.59	26.6	7.54	1.837
Day 7	7.61	5.55	18.9	4.41	0.280

Fig. (8). Mammary gland secretion during the first days after calving.

Buffalo cow milk has been shown to be a healthy nutrient for humans. It has 58% more calcium, 35% more protein and 20% less cholesterol than cow milk. It is also a richer source of iron, phosphorus, vitamin A and natural antioxidant tocopherol. Peroxidases are part of the mammal´s biological defense against pathogens. And peroxidase activity in buffalo cow milk is 2-4 times higher than cow milk. Bubaline milk is a perfect option for individuals that are allergic to cattle milk. Larger proportions of other bio protective compounds such as, immunoglobulins, lactoferrin, lysozyme, and lactoperoxidase make buffalo cow milk an excellent choice for a wider range of healthy diets [8].

3. CHEMICAL CONSTITUENTS AND PHYSICAL PROPERTIES OF BUFFALO MILK

3.1. Chemical Constituents

Major constituents of buffalo cow milk are those present in larger amounts: fat, protein and lactose. Minor constituents are present in relatively smaller proportions; those are minerals, vitamins, non-protein nitrogen compounds, pigments, enzymes and others. However, these minor constituents may be so important as the major. Some of them have a fundamental nutritional role, namely calcium, phosphorus and some vitamins (Fig. **9**) [1].

CONSTITUENT OR PHYSICAL PROPERTY	MEAN VALUE	RANGE
Specific gravity	1.031	1.029 – 1.033
Fat (%)	8.5	7.1 – 9.6
Total solids (%)	18.9	16.8 – 20.8
Ash (%)	0.84	0.79 – 0.90
pH	6.63	6.55 – 6.71
Total nitrogen (%)	0.710	0.571 – 0.809
Nitrogen-derivedcasein (%)	0.572	0.437 – 0.654
Non-proeicnitrogen (%)	0.031	0.009 – 0.536
Lactose (%)	4.6	4.0 – 5.1
Calcium (%)	0.203	0.179 – 0.241
Magnesium (%)	0.020	0.0126- 0.027
Potasium (%)	0.139	0.085 – 0.187
Sodium (%)	0.075	0.047 – 0.102
Phosphorus (%)	0.129	0.118 – 0.139
Chlorine (%)	0.065	0.056 - .084
Citricacid (%)	0.219	0.158 – 0.290

(%) = g / 100g milk

Fig. (9). Average values and variation of milk constituents obtained from 24 buffalo herds of Italian Mediterranean breed.

Fat globules in buffalo cow milk not only contain a spectrum of triglycerides but also small amounts of liposoluble substances such as cholesterol, vitamin A, D and α-tocopherol. The high fat content present in buffalo cow milk gives it its unique flavor and makes it a particularly valuable commodity in India and other countries where ghee, a type of clarified butter, is considered an important dairy product. This clarified butter, produced over low heat has excellent conservation properties without the need for refrigeration. In India, diluted buffalo cow milk for human consumption is preferred over cow′s milk [1].

Although similar, proteins in bubaline milk are not identical to those in cattle. Buffalo cow milk is higher in casein and serum albumins. Most bubaline casein (98.4%) is present in the form of large micelles (80 a 250 mm *vs* 70 a 110 mm in cattle). Buffalo cow milk has higher lactoferrin content. This glycoprotein plays a key role in infant protection by inhibiting bacteria such as *Escherichia coli* sp., and also plays an important role in iron absorption [8].

Some of the minor constituents such as non-protein nitrogen (NPN) of the buffalo cow milk have no major incidence in human nutrition. NPNs are compounds related to proteins without being real proteins although they are involved in some protein reactions. Some NPN compounds are present as free amino acids in small and variable quantities. Of these, tyrosine is present at a level of 46 mg/liter and does not vary significantly with lactation period. When milk is stored, this value tends to increase slowly, possibly due to enzymatic hydrolysis of protein (Ferrara *et al.*, 1964). Urea is an important compound, accounting for 40 to 50% of total NPN. Other compounds exist in small quantities: creatine, creatinine, uric acid, ammonia and those hydro soluble vitamins that have nitrogen. Urea nitrogen represents 44.8 and 41.2% of total NPN in the cow and in the buffalo cow, respectively. Creatinine nitrogen is nearly equal in cow (11.7 mg/liter) as compared to buffalo cow (9.95 mg/liter) milk. Uric acid-derived nitrogen is 5.42 mg/liter in cattle and 1.9-2.4 mg/liter in buffalo cow, and 2.5 to 2.9 mg/liter for cattle and bubaline ammonia-derived nitrogen. Some of these products are mostly considered excreted rather that secreted products. Although urea is an excreted product, it can be utilized by ruminants as a source of nitrogen by microbial conversion and further metabolized *via* saliva, food and bloodstream.

Enzymes are minor constituents of milk; two of them have commercial significance in fluid milk: peroxidase and alkaline phosphatase. Buffalo cow milk has two to four-fold higher peroxidase activity than cattle´s. The optimal pH for enzymatic activity in buffalo cow milk is 7.0 (6.5 for cattle). Only 6 at 85° C are needed for peroxidase inactivation [11]. Other minor constituents are the minerals, including macro and micro-nutrients. Calcium, very important for human consumption, is a macronutrient needed for adequate bone formation during growth of buffalo calf, and is needed for milk coagulation in the neonate´s stomach. It is also industrially important, in the first steps of cheese manufacturing. Under similar conditions, bubaline milk coagulates faster than cattle, even when diluted to double its volume [11]. Average calcium content of buffalo cow milk is 0.18-0.20%, with considerable variations out of these values towards the beginning and end of lactation, and in some animals [1].

Phosphorus, also essential to bone and teeth formation is present in bubaline milk as free phosphate, bound to other elements or in form of esterified casein or hydro soluble esterified phosphate. It may also be present as part of the phosphatide molecule, ionized or in its inorganic form. Although all of these fractions vary, average phosphorus content in bubaline milk is 0.12 – 0.13% (*versus* 0.10-0.12 in cattle) [1]. Total mineral constituents (total ash) are approximately 0.79% in bubaline milk, *versus* 0.75% in cattle. Sodium, potassium and chlorine levels are much higher in cattle than bubaline milk. Lactose content is higher in cattle´s milk.

Regarding microelements, iron and copper are needed in red blood cell formation as well as for other tissues. The levels of these elements are generally low in bubaline milk and must be provided through supplementation to ensure adequate growth of newborn calves. Other microelements are present in small quantities in milk, usually combined or associated with one or more proteins.

Values obtained for buffalo cows in the middle of lactation, expressed in parts per million, are shown in Fig. (**10**) [11]:

ELEMENT	VALUE (ppm)
Iron	1.01
Copper	0.22
Zinc	2.39
Aluminum	0.22
Manganese	0.17
Lead	0.16
Molybdenum	0.022
Silicone	0.21

Fig. (10). Microelement profile of buffalo milk.

With the exception of aluminum, silicone and lead, all of the above elements are considered essential. All of these elements are high during the first month of lactation, progressively decline towards mid lactation and tend to slightly increase by the end. Other minor constituents present in trace amounts but also considered essential nutrients are the vitamins. Most vitamins (vitamin A, Riboflavin, Vitamin C, *etc.*), with the exception of tocopherol, carotene, and probably vitamin

B_{12}, are found in lower concentration in bubaline milk compared to cattle counterpart. The content of vitamin B complex for buffalo cow milk in mid lactation has been reported [11]:

VITAMIN	CONTENT (mg/l)
Thiamine (B_1)	0.81
Riboflavin (B_2)	1.67
Biotin	2.02
B_6	0.25
Nicotinic acid	0.82
Pantothenic acid	2.02
B_{12}	4.3 (ug/l)

Fig. (11). Vitamin profile of buffalo milk.

The most apparent visual difference between buffalo cow and cattle milk is the yellowish color of the latter due to its higher carotene content. In bubaline milk, vitamin A level is higher, causing its white color. It is thought that the buffalo cow has an efficient metabolic mechanism that prevents pigments to appear in milk, whatever the carotene content of the diet may be [1]. Vitamin C (ascorbic acid) content is higher in buffalo cow milk (Fig. **12**) [11].

SPECIES	VITAMIN C VALUE (mg/l)
Buffalo	19.5 – 39.5
Domestic cow	7.1 – 7.8
Human	11.3 – 27.0

Fig. (12). Vitamin content reported for buffalo, domestic cattle and human milk.

Another minor component of bubaline milk is citric acid. This is an important constituent because it is part of non-ionic calcium, which in turn plays a role in curd formation (coagulation). It is present in significant amount, but values reported by different groups of researchers vary; some indicate that buffalo cow may have higher content than cattle, while others give indication of the opposite. Values reported for buffalo cow range between 0.180 and 0.224%. Colostrum contains quite more citric acid than the milk produced in the middle of lactation.

3.2. Physical Properties

Buffalo cow milk has a slightly sweet flavor; it is more viscous and whiter than cattle milk due to the absence of carotene in its fat globules. Just as in dairy cow, physical properties exhibit less variability around mid-lactation compared to chemical constituents.

Several studies have reported that the pH of fresh bubaline milk show great variation among individual animals. In India, on fresh milk from Murrah buffalo cows a pH values of 6.74 ± 0.08 (*vs.* Cebu cattle 6.63 ± 0.08) was reported. In Italy an average pH of 6.78 ± 0.03 for fresh milk from Italian Mediterranean buffalo cows was reported, with marked seasonal fluctuations of 6.73 in August (summer) and 6.85 in December (winter). All values were higher in buffalo cow milk. Bubaline and cattle milk tend to lose continuously carbon dioxide and to slightly increase their pH overtime. Subsequently, pH drops due to acid lactic produced by bacterial activity. A mastitis-infected animal will exhibit elevated pH values (>7.0) in the infected quarter. The pH of fresh bubaline milk does not appear to be linked to daily output, stage or number of lactation [1, 11].

Specific gravity is another physical constant of fresh bubaline milk. Average herd values are between 1.030 and 1.032, although individual animals with wider ranges may be found (*versus* 1.029 to 1.033 in cows). Low values are generally associated with higher fat percentages [1].

Freezing point of any biological fluid is found below freezing point of pure water. Freezing point depression is still utilized as an indicator of dilution of milk with water. Average freezing point for whole milk is almost the same for buffalo cow and cattle, 0.544 ºC and 0.545 ºC, respectively. Colostrum has a higher depression than milk (0.57 – 0.58 ºC). It is generally assumed that any bubaline or cattle milk with a depression of 0.530 ºC or lower should be considered altered [1, 11].

Surface tension of fresh buffalo cow milk is similar to cattle, although values may vary due to measurement techniques. On average, bubaline milk is 48.74 dynes/cm and cattle 49.36. Surface tension is inversely affected by temperature [1].

Electric conductivity is affected by hydrochloric acid content; this component tends to increase in mastitis-affected quarters. Average value for healthy samples is 6.62 milimohs for buffalo cow and 6.69 for cattle [11].

Fluorescence: When subjected to ultraviolet light, cattle's milk turns canary yellow color, whereas bubaline's turns white. When milk is heated to its boiling point, fluorescent color should not be affected. This color does change in milk that has been adulterated or diluted with water [11].

Curding time: Under similar temperature and concentration conditions, bubaline milk coagulates more rapidly than cattle; this coagulation time may be reduced by adding hydrochloric acid. Noteworthy, due to its high calcium content, buffalo cow milk stability at ambient conditions (Corrientes, Argentina) is lower than cattle, with slower coagulation times [11].

4. ELABORATION OF BUBALINE CHEESE AND OTHER BY-PRODUCTS: DESCRIPTION OF MANUFACTURING PROCESS

4.1. Manufacturing Process of White, Bubauno and Yearling Buffalo Cheese (Venezuela) [12]

- ***FIRST STAGE (same process for all three cheese types)***

Raw milk (5°C)

Heating (40°C)

Partial skimming

Polyvalent tank (36 -37 °C)

Addition of rennet (2.5 gr/100 l)

Agitation (5 minutes)

Coagulation (40-45 minutes)

Curdling

Setting period (5 minutes)

Partial removal of whey (Flor de cuajada)

- ***SECOND STAGE***

White Cheese

Addition of salt (1.2% weigh: volume)

Place in cheese molds

Pressing

Storage

Marketing

Bubauno Cheese

Heat curd (50°C 10 minutes)

Place in wicker molds

Addition of salt (rubbing)

Maturation at 18°C, skin is rubbed with vegetable oil

Marketing

Yearling Cheese

Place in molds

Pressing

Salt addition in brine (24%)

Maturation at 18°C, skin is rubbed with coffee

Marketing

4.2. Manufacturing Process for Hand-pulled Cheese (Mozzarella and Provolone) [12]

- ***FIRST STAGE (same process for all cheese types)***

Raw milk

Heating (38°C)

Coagulation starter (1%)

Addition of rennet (2.5 gr/100 l.)

Coagulation (50-60 min)

Curd cutting (size of a corn kernel)

Setting period (5 minutes)

Removal of whey

Curd kneading point

Dough kneading (in water at 85°C)

- ***Second Stage***

Mozzarella Cheese

Place in molds

Container with water (18°C)

Brine or sauce (salsetta)

Packaging

Storage and/or marketing

Provolone Cheese

Place in molds

Brine

Maturation

Storage and/or marketing

4.3. Production of Criollo (Creole) Cheese (Brazil)

The production of criollo or creole cheese (frescal for Brazil) starts with milk pasteurization. This can be accomplished by ultra-pasteurization (with the sheet equipment), 72ºC for 18, or traditional pasteurization at 65ºC for 30'. Temperature must then be lowered to 35ºC, fermentation agents must be added and after 20' rennet must be added (80% pepsin and 20% chymosin). Separation into curd and whey should be noticeable after 25-40'. Curd is then dislodged manually into pieces no bigger than 1 cm^3 (cubes). After this, 50% of whey is withdrawn and the remainder curd plus whey are placed into molds, which are then turned and salted. Product is packed in sealed plastic containers (not vacuum sealed) and kept in cold room for 24 h, after this period the product is ready to be consumed [13].

4.4. Provola Affumicata Cheese

In Italy, buffalo milk is also used to produce provola affumicata, a smoked version of mozzarella with an increasing demand in the country. It is produced by burning rice or other type of straw to produce smoke under milk containers, while covering the top with a wet cloth in order to trap humidity [13].

4.5. Mozzarella di Bufala Campana

4.5.1. Definition

The Italian Buffalo Breeders Association (ANASB: Associazione Nazionale Allevatori della Specie Bufalina) defines the Mozzarella di Bufala Campana (meaning from the entire area of Campania Region) as follows: It is a fresh stretched and kneaded cheese, produced with milk from buffalo cows raised in the region of denomination D.O.P. (Protected Denomination of Origin) and also processed in dairy plants within the same Region. The product may have several shapes and presentations that range from 10 to 800 gr. It has ivory color, a thin, smooth crust of 1mm. It is composed of thin multi-layers, slightly elastic within 8-10 h post-threading and becoming softer overtime. It should have no holes and must be produced without conservatives, inhibitors or coloring agents. It should have slight runoff of creamy whey when sliced; scent of lactic fermentation should be noticeable. According to current Italian law, preparation of mozzarella can only be done with buffalo milk.

Schematic representation of production process of "criollo" cheese (Brazil: "Queijo Minas Frescal") [13]

Filtered raw milk+ 35 % pure water

↓

Pasteurization
(73ºC/1 min or 65ºC/30 min)

↓

Cooling (35ºC) with running water

↓

Addition of
1,5% lactic fermentation agents (S. lactis y S. cremoris)
liquid or powder rennet, diluted in water (recommended quantity)

↓

Coagulation
(40 min)

↓

Separation into cubes
(1 a 2 cm)

↓

Intermittent mixing
(t = 15 min; pause every 3 – 4 minutes)

↓

"Doughy" point

↓

Removal of half of whey content

↓

Place in moulds

↓

Turn

↓

Addition of salt and removal of remainder whey till next day

↓

Finished product

Flow chart for butter production (Brazil)

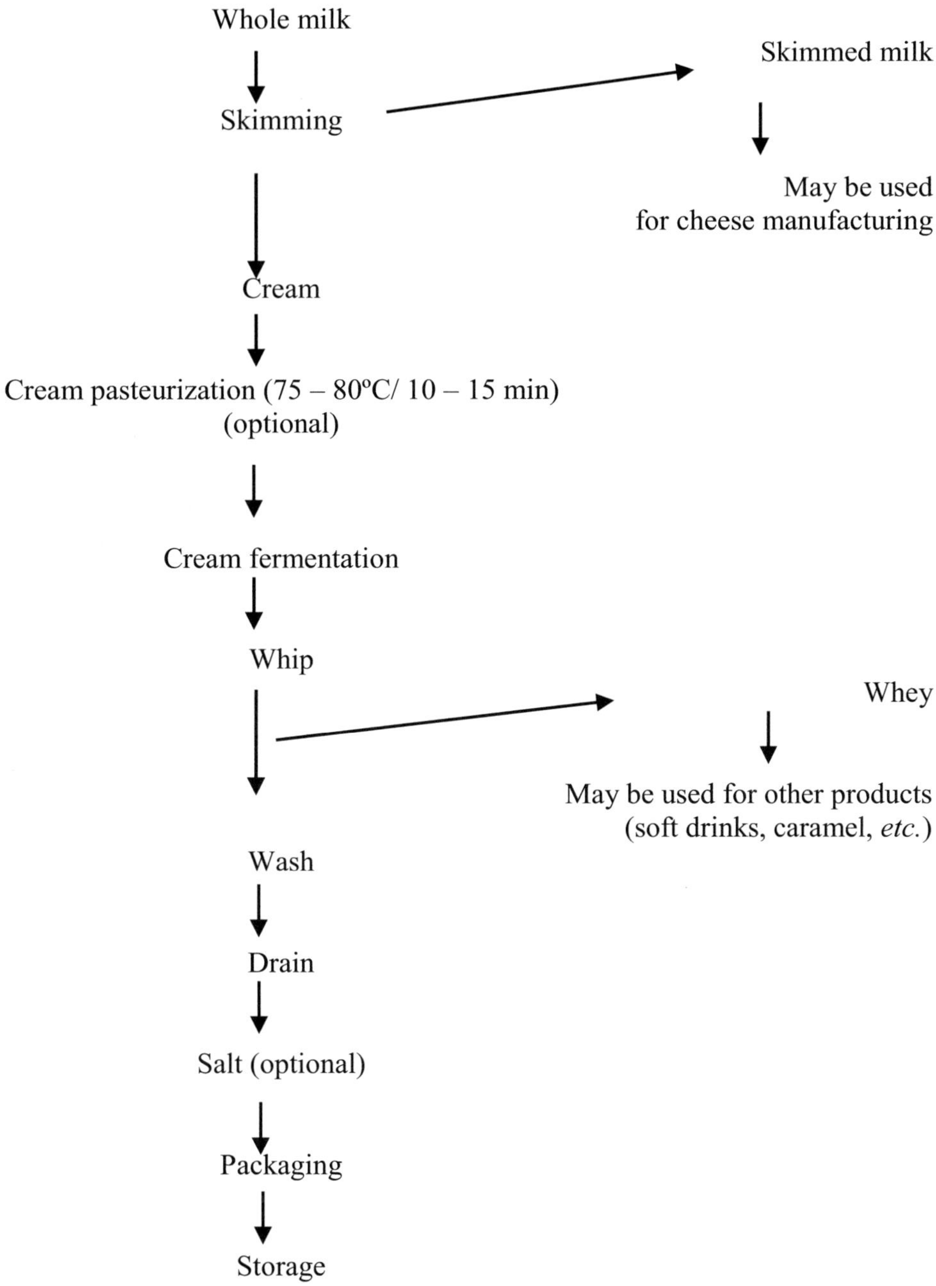

FLOW DIAGRAM – Butter Elaboration [13]

Milk quality is of upmost importance; animal health, sanitary handling, milking process and storage hygiene are key aspects of the final quality of the product. Under normal conditions, buffalo cow milk contains higher quantity and specific strains of lactobacillus, compared to cattle's. From the metabolic activity of those strains come the particular flavor and aroma, through the production of specials substances and composites, which probably have a remarkable influence in the curd acidification during the transformation. Because mozzarella manufacturing is still done using little or no mechanization (handmade), hygiene, sanitary conditions of storage and transport of the milk are essential. Microbial contamination screenings are conducted periodically year-round. Both microbiological and hygienic milk qualities are essential in mozzarella elaboration. The manufacturing of mozzarella has been termed a forward-flow process; this type of production prevents cross contamination of starting materials [7].

4.5.2. Production Examples and Aspects of Mozzarella Cheese Production

Maina della Torre Dairy Plant, owned by Prato Verde Factories, is located in Latina Province, Lazio Region, Italy. This plant only processes the milk needed to produce mozzarella within the same day. Their production inputs are: milk, enzymes and whey. After 4-5 hours, once curd and whey are separated, they cut the curd into small cubes and place them in a wooden container with water at 98° C for the handmade stretching and kneading process, where the dough will reach a temperature of 66-67°C. They produce 35-40 kg of cheese per batch. Simultaneously, they obtain the piccolo latte or small milk, a by-product from the remainder liquid. They have capacity for 5000 liters, although in winter they only process 2500 liters due to reduced demand. Mozzarella cheese yield is 1 kg of cheese of every 4 liters of milk (25% yield). Freshly made mozzarella is placed in salt-water bats (15% salt) for 2 hours; it is then transferred to a 1.5% salt-water solution, called government liquid.

La Salamandra SA, in Buenos Aires, Argentina, prepares their government liquid by adding 12 g citric acid and 320 g salt to 450 liters of water [14].

4.5.3. Liquids used in mozzarella handling and conservation [13]

Liquid from dough pulling

↓ Boil for 2 – 3 min

Rest for 24 h

↓

Remove fatty overlay

↓

"White water"

↓

Rest for 24 h

↓

"Government liquid"

↓

Pool "Government liquid"
1 % salt (others add 3-5%)

4.5.4. Mozzarella Cheese Yield

One hundred kg of buffalo milk will render from 20 (in hot days) to 25 (in cold days), sometimes even 27 kg of mozzarella cheese. In contrast, cattle's milk yield is 9-12% (100 liters of milk will yield 9-12 kg mozzarella). Ricotta cheese is produced by addition of 3% whole milk to whey. 100 kg of whey renders 1 kg of fresh ricotta. Butter is produced with the fat skimming's of whole milk; this skimming will reduce the weight of the mozzarella cheese, and therefore is not traditionally done [15].

Mozzarella (kg) = milk (kg) x [((3,5 x % protein) + (1,23 x % butirose fat) – 0,88)/100]

It must be noted that this formula was obtained from Italian elaboration standards, which accepts considerable humidity content. It is not known the extent of applicability of the formula under other conditions in other countries. Based on the formula, for each 1% increase in milk protein results in a threefold increase in cheese output. Noteworthy, it is not protein content but nitrogen level in milk that is usually routinely measured, since it is contained mainly in proteins with a ratio known to be relatively constant [15].

4.5.6. Other Aspects of the Mozzarella Cheese Production Chain

Buffalo mozzarella is considered to be of higher quality than cattle's. When the product is melted, it results in a continuous thread without clumps. In cattle's mozzarella, there is a presence of clumps and strong cheese aroma. There are continuous fluctuations in milk protein and fat content throughout the year, particularly due to the pooling of milk from buffalo cows in different stages of lactation. Milk from buffalo cows in the first stage of lactation can make up over 60% of total volume. This results in increased acidity and presents a problem for mozzarella cheese manufacturing; namely, shortened shelf-life and poor organoleptic attributes of the resulting product. Management errors such as energy and protein nutrient deficiencies, excess silage in ration during the first stage of lactation can worsen this problem because the buffalo cow will attempt to balance the nutrient imbalance by mobilizing energy stores with the consequent increase in circulating non-esterified fatty acids.

The tropical origin of the bubaline species implies poor adaptability to low ambient temperatures and wind chill; these factors can lead to an increase in milk acidity particularly in periods of transition from warm to cooler temperatures. The increase in milk acidity is a multivariate phenomenon which can be attributed to one or several factors: a) mesophyll cell count, b) chemical composition of the diet, c) poor milk handling and storage, d) poor milking hygiene leading to higher microbial counts, higher lactose fermentation and higher lactic acid production [16]. It is therefore extremely important to ensure hygiene and product quality throughout the whole cheese production chain. This is particularly true for Italy, which has stringent product quality standards for mozzarella [17]. Buffalo mozzarella consumers are a demanding clientele (particularly in Italy); cheese must arrive to markets within the day of productions, while other Italian cities have 2-3 day tolerance standards. Cheese is normally transported in brine, although vacuum-packed cheeses are now considered acceptable.

4.5.7. Process for Reception, Manufacture and Packaging for Mozzarella Cheese

As mentioned previously, mozzarella cheese production is a forward-flow process, where there is no crossing of starting materials and therefore low risk of cross-contamination [13, 18, 19].

The complete process for the manufacture of soft cheeses of threaded dough, such as mozzarella di bufala is detailed below:

1. ***Reception of Raw Milk***: milk arrives in stainless steel milk transport trucks; it has been previously cooled in the farm and shipped within a short period of time to the plant. Transport temperature should not surpass 10° C, with the exception of those farms in which the time lapse between milking and transport is under 2 hours. Milk should be kept at 0 to 4°C.
2. ***Sanitation:*** Milk is sanitized by simple filtration through fine meshes in order to separate coarse contaminant materials; it is then centrifuged at 5000 rpm to separate smaller impurities.
3. ***Pasteurization:*** Typically, pasteurization is done at 68-70° C, for a period of 15-20 seconds. In the case of Mozzarella di Bufala Campana D.O.P., treatment is conducted in a plate-type thermal exchange system, at 72° C for 15 seconds. In all cases, the thermally-treated milk must be negative to alkaline phosphatase test. Higher temperatures or longer treatment times pose risk of excessive seroprotein precipitation with casein entrapment and consequent reduction in stretching and kneading properties. The objective of pasteurization is the elimination of contaminating bacteria. However, the process also reduces the content of naturally occurring casein-utilizing microorganisms; it is then necessary to add lactic ferments or commercial yeast to counteract the depleting action of the thermal treatment. In order to maintain good spreading and kneading quality of the dough, handicraft or artisan production of mozzarella cheese does not involve pasteurization. This requires that the mesophyll cell count of the buffalo milk used for such process is under 500,000 colony forming units/ml. In addition, originating farms must be Brucellosis and Tuberculosis free. In Brazil, Oliveira recommends no pasteurization for mozzarella cheese production due to its detrimental effects on the protein matrix [13]. It must be noted that most South American farms are pasture based, as opposed to dry low/stable confined; mesophyll counts in these production systems are typically lower [20].
4. ***Fermentation Starters:*** Milk is heated in stainless steel bats at 36 a 39° C, and

lactic fermentation starters from previous batches are added (3-5 liters/100 liters of buffalo milk) (Garofalo – ANASB - 2-3 liters). The amount of added product should be enough to elevate milk´s pH to 6.3 or 11-12°SH acidity. Most natural fermentation agents contain some thermophile lactobacillus (*Lactobacillus delbrueckii Subsp. bulgaricus*), cocci (*Streptococcus* thermophiles and other mesophylls) and large yeast quantities, mostly responsible for the aroma in mozzarella. Ferments are obtained from the fermentation of sweet whey, by heating to 40 - 42° C followed by acidification to 17/18 °SH/50 and 4.3 pH and cooling 8° C.

5. ***Coagulation**:* Rennet is used as the main coagulating agent; it is added at a rate of 1:12.000 -1:15.000 parts as is, diluted in warm water. The amount of rennet added should cause milk coagulation within 15-20 minutes. Rennet is obtained from the inner mucosa of the abomasum of calves; it is rich in chymosin and pepsin. Milk coagulates and forms a curd due to a destabilization process of the calcium micelles, which occurs in response to the low pH and the enzymes present in rennet.
6. ***Curd Separation**:* Curd separation is observed when coagulated material starts detaching from the container walls, this happens when whey has reached a 7,5-8,0°SH acidity. The classic tool to dislodge curd is the herringbone mixer and sometimes the lyra-shape mixing aid. Mixing should be done slowly and in circular movements in order to gently dislodge and break the curd into pieces.
7. ***Whey Fermentation:*** After allowing curd to sediment, 2/3 of whey are separated (which can be used for ricotta cheese manufacture), the remaining whey is kept with the curd to promote fermentation.
8. ***Straining***: Once curd is set (pH close to 5) it is then removed from stainless steel bats and placed on stainless steel tables in order for remaining whey to drip (3-4 hours).
9. ***Curd Mincing**:* Curd is minced in specialized equipment with rotating blades, producing pieces of 2 x 2 cm.
10. ***Stretching and Kneading**:* It can be done in a wooden container, with a characteristic wooden stick. It can also be done automatically. In both cases, boiling water (100° C) is added to allow handling of the minced curd. Optimal stretching and kneading temperature range between 68-70° C. The dough

should never reach temperatures higher than 39° C and the process should only last 4-5 minutes. Ideal maturation of the dough is normally with pH values between 4.90 and 5.10. It is recommended to start kneading with a pH 5.2 and finish with pH 4.8 [18]. Garofalo described subtle variations to this process [19]: Stretching and kneading is the step in the manufacturing process that most greatly affects the finished product and its yield over liter of milk. Immature or overly matured curds result in loss of consistency and 2-3% reduction in overall cheese yield. Senior cheese masters are able to empirically predict the optimal point for the initiation of stretching and kneading process. Research conducted on the relation between kneading process and curd acidity demonstrated an optimal value of 4.8-4.9, which resulted in minimal weight loss in brine storage. Currently, there are several mechanical alternatives to accomplish the kneading process; all of them simulate the man-made movements of the dough. Kneading consists of submerging the curd in hot water (80-85°C) in order to acquire an elastic consistency that allow the operator to mould the dough into different shapes. The dough is kept in the kneading equipment for 15-20 minutes, approximately. In case of handmade kneading, this is done in a wooden container (45 cm height, 70 cm base diameter, 90 cm rim diameter); the dough is gently stirred with a wooden stick and a bowl, while raising it in order to incorporate water rendering a smoother, more shiny and silkier final product. Because of the limited time in small plants, it is better not to knead more than 30 kg of dough with 45 litre of water. After the necessary period of time dough is carried to the shape phase.

11. ***Cutting or Mozzatura***: This step can be done manually or mechanically, with equally satisfactory results. Cutting of mozzarella by hand is done with two operators; one of them holds large pieces of dough (3-4 kg) while another, using index and thumb fingers separates and pinches (mozza) 20-800 g pieces. Mechanization of his process results in more uniform pieces.
12. ***Cooling***: Cooling is accomplished by submerging in cold water (10-12° C) for 30 minutes. Cold shock creates a protective crust, trapping humidity within the product [13].
13. ***Salting***: Done in "salsetta": (2-5% of salt) or brine (salmoia: 10% of salt), salt concentration varies with weigh and size of pieces. Although some manufacturers combine the salting with the kneading process, mozzarella di

bufala does not render itself well to this because it requires some time exposed to brine in order to form the crust (from 5 to 15 hours). The salting process for the Mozzarella di Bufala Campana DOP [19] is done by sequential immersions in saline solutions at different concentrations (8 to 12%, acidity 9 to 11°SH/50). Salt penetrates the cheese by diffusion, speed of penetration depends on salt concentration of the brine, temperature and shape of the mozzarella piece.

14. ***Packaging and Distribution**:* Traditionally it is packaged with brine, although vacuum sealing is now available and guarantees acceptable conditions at 20°C for a maximum of 10 days. The ANASB [19] recommends using the same kneading liquids, with added salt and lactic acid. Another alternative to extend shelf life during summer months is to use salted, pasteurized water with lactic acid. Noteworthy, shelf life is primarily connected to the quality of the starting materials (raw or pasteurized milk) and the sanitary practices implemented throughout the manufacturing process [18, 19].

4.5.8. A Slightly Different Production for Mozzarella is Followed in Alagoas, Brazil [21]:

1. Add water (90% milk + 10% water).
2. Pasteurize.
3. Add 40 ml calcium chloride for each 100 liters of milk.
4. Add 3% fermented whey at 40°D (Dornic), or 2% at 60°D, or 1% at 120°D.
5. Allow fermentation for 20-30 minutes; ideally, acidity should be 21°D at the addition of rennet.
6. Temperature should be 38°C at the addition of rennet.
7. Dissolve rennet in water (2 liters).
8. Add rennet slowly, while stirring; this process should last 1-2 minutes. Let milk stand.
9. Rennet should cause the formation of curd within 30-45 minutes. If this occurs in less tan 30 minutes, the product will turn sour. If it occurs in over 45 minutes, cheese yield will be reduced.
10. Once curd is set, it is separated with a lira type tool; in sidewise and up and down motions.
11. In order to obtain a soft product, curd pieces should be 1.5 to 2 cm.

12. Curd must be allowed to set for 3 minutes, in order to allow crust formation.
13. Initial mixing: Stir slowly, increasing agitation gradually for 20 minutes.
14. Allow product to sediment to bottom of container.
15. Second mixing can be done in two ways:
    a. *By heating up the container walls:* Heat slowly, stirring gradually and increasing speed while preventing clump formation. Dough should have an ideal consistency at 38°C.
    b. *By adding hot water:* This technique is frequently termed lactose removal, because it will eliminate at least part of the lactose content. Part of the whey is removed. Water at 100°C is added with a narrow spout container. Direct contact of the dough with hot water must be avoided at all times, in order to avoid rubbery consistency. Dough is stirred slowly; speed is then increased as the temperature of the dough starts to increase. Dough should reach ideal consistency by 38°C.
16. Let dough stand with whey until it reaches kneading point (around 4-5 hours).The longer the time dough sits in whey, the longer kneading time it will require.
17. Test kneading point: dough should stretch for about a meter.
18. Kneading: Knead with water (85-90°C), the amount of water should be 1.5-2 times the weight of dough to be kneaded.
19. Salting:
    a. *Mozzarella logs for slicing:* Use 2 – 2.5% brine. Work dough, close balls and give shape. Place cheese in ice water, inside a mould for about 1 hour. Withdraw from mould and let water drain, keeping in cold room.
    b. *Mozzarella in round pieces:* Withdraw from ice water. Place in brine (20%) for 5-10 minutes, depending on the size of the ball. Place balls in brine for final storage. They should have the same acidity as the dough, to prevent brine from becoming milky.
20. Packaging: In case of mozzarella logs, packaging is vacuum sealed. In the case of mozzarella balls, they are packaged with adequate volume of brine for balls to remain fully immersed.

5. PRODUCTION AND UTILIZATION OF MILK BY-PRODUCTS IN DIFFERENT COUNTRIES

All derivatives from bubaline milk are considered functional foods: those that provide benefits for human health. The main products obtained from buffalo cow milk are fresh, frescal or criollo (creole) cheese (Argentina, Venezuela, Brazil), butter, yoghurt (Bulgaria), mozzarella, provola (Italy) and other cheeses in India, such as cheddar, karnal, brick, surati and melted.

According to their water content [11], cheese can be classified as shown in Fig. (**13**):

Another common classification of cheese is made according to the acidification type: enzymatic coagulation (curd) and acid coagulation (natural or bacterial). Many cheeses are subjected to mixed coagulations, most with higher prevalence of acid coagulation in the process [22]. Due to different characteristics of the casein micelle and fat of buffalo cow milk, the main problems associated in cheddar cheese manufacturing have been acidity, coagulation times, humidity retention and delayed proteolysis and lipolysis. Hard cheeses made with buffalo milk are more difficult to dehydrate due to the higher protein content, which in turn results in more water retention. Pasteurization is only done when the microbial count is high (this seldom occurs).

CLASSIFICATION	WATER CONTENT (%)	DENOMINATION AND COUNTRY OF ORIGIN
Soft cheeses	>45	Karish, Mish and Domiati (*Egypt*) Madhfor (*Irak*) Mozzarella (*Italy*) Alghab (*Syria*) Vladeasa (*Rumania*)
Semi-soft cheeses	40-45	Beyazpeineri (*Turkey*)
Hard cheeses	< 40	Braila (*Rumania*) Rahss (*Egypt*) White (*Bulgaria*) Akkawi (*Syria*)

Fig. (13). Cheese classification according to water content, denomination and country of origin.

Fermented dairy products have been manufactured from buffalo cow milk with good results. Yoghurt derived from bubaline milk is considered a delicacy [23], its rich and creamy texture is due to its higher calcium and casein content. Protein and vitamin E are also higher in this product, with low cholesterol. Recently, probiotics have been added to this product giving to it an unique flavor and biological properties. In Bulgaria, Rumania and Albania, buffalo milk is almost exclusively destined to yoghurt manufacture due to its high demand by local markets.

Dahi yoghurt, of superior consistency and texture, is preferably manufactured with buffalo cow milk due to its higher protein, fat and solids content and also due to the bigger size of fat globules, casein micelle and calcium in colloidal state [22]. Some typical Indian products are elaborated with buffalo cow milk, due to its quality and to the consumer preference. The most important is Khoa, a coagulated dairy product obtained by milk dehydration (water content 19-25%). Khoa prepared from buffalo cow milk has a unique quality, consistence and texture, that makes it preferred over the same product prepared from cattle´s milk. Khoa is used as a base ingredient for the preparation of widely popular sweets and candy. Paneer is another typical Indian buffalo cow dairy product. It contains an acid coagulated solid extract that is used as ingredient to cook vegetables in the north of the country. This product is obtained by acidification of milk with acid curd or lemon juice; it is then filtered and pressed without addition of salt. It must be consumed within 3 days, usually with spicy sauces and vegetables and with a special round, dry and hollow type of bread, the ciabatta. The Cottage cheese, prepared by acid coagulation in Europe and North America is a similar product [24].

India, Turkey and Iran

In India, fluid milk diluted with 33% water for human consumption is the principal destination of the production. The second product in importance is the ghee, a clarified butter with 99% fat that can be stored under ambient conditions. Buffalo cow ghee is almost translucent (as opposed to the yellowing color in cattle-derived ghee) due to absence of carotenoids. Ghee has been used since ancestral times in these countries, both as a food ingredient and as a part of the religious Hindi rituals. The product is perfectly fit to be used under tropical conditions and is the only animal fat source in the Indian predominantly vegetarian diet. The product is also steadily consumed by Muslim countries of Central Asia and Middle East. Over 40% of the milk produced in India is destined to ghee manufacture, with an annual average of 480,000,000 kg. Average human intake is 1.2 kg/head/year. Of this, 80% is destined to food preparation, 18% for bakery and 2% for religious ceremonies. Ghee contains 99-99.5% fat and no more than 0.5% humidity. Ghee is either prepared from butter or from boiled milk skin cream, following one of two methods: butter mechanical separation of skin cream hand-beaten (Desi), the latter being the method of choice for most ghee produced in India. Desi means common, or in other words, popular. In this country, buffalo milk as dry powder is also used for infant formulas. Specialists at Karnal Institute have introduced modifications in buffalo cow milk in order to make it more adequate for human consumption as fluid milk, resembling the profile of maternal milk [24]. Indian dairy cooperatives generally reduce the fat content of the product by dilution with 33% water, reaching a composition (water, fat, protein, solids) similar to cattle milk.

In Turkey, buffalo cow milk is specially sought after for its contribution to the famous Turkish breakfasts. Whipped cream is mixed with warm milk, then slowly cooled in shallow pans, re-heated and finally cut in the next morning. The result is the famous Qeymac, Keimak or Kaimak: a type of ghee, a semi-liquid clarified butter highly demanded by the population [25].

In Iran, farmers boil buffalo cow milk overnight, place it in shallow pans and collect the cream the following morning which is then sold in open markets. This ghee-type product, called Qeymac, Keimak, Kaimak in Turkish, or Sarshir in Persian, is very popular in restaurants and patisseries. Fat extracted from buffalo cow milk is partially sold to dairy product dealers, and is also used for the manufacture of salty yoghurt, a traditional product called Mast in Persia. Most of the elaboration is done by women.

Brazil, Argentina, Venezuela and Bolivia

In Brazil, in order to make better use of the advantageous properties of buffalo cow milk in the manufacture of other dairy products; a significant expansion of industrial units was undertaken in the early 90'. This expansion allowed producers to obtain a return on their product that almost doubled the return from cattle's milk. In addition, the price levels of buffalo cow milk products remained steady throughout the year. This in turn stimulated the establishment of important so-called 'cuencas' or 'hotspots' for buffalo cow milk production, particularly in the southwest of the country [26]. Noteworthy, while cattle milk demand has been dropping due to economic causes, buffalo cow milk plants have experienced an annual growth of 32.3% in processed milk between the years 2001 and 2005.

In addition to the traditional demand for mozzarella cheese, other less traditional buffalo cow products are experiencing an increase in interest and demand in Brazil, namely frescal, ricotta, provolone cheese, caramel, curd, yogurt and others. With the objective to promote buffalo cow milk, the Brazilian Buffalo Breeders Association (ABCB) has implemented a monitoring program Selo de Pureza (Purity Seal) since 2001. All products from participating farms are certified by protein electrophoresis, with guarantee of no contamination with other milk sources. As of 2007, 111 farms producing around 3.2 million liters per year were participating in the program. It is estimated that Brazil currently produces 90 million liters of bubaline milk (approximately 40,000 lactating buffalo cows), with over 150 dairy plants manufacturing some kind of bubaline dairy product. Brazilian domestic demand of buffalo cow dairy products is relatively steady throughout the year. Therefore, farmers are using reproductive biotechnologies in order to de-seasonalize calvings in order to be able to provide a more steady supply of product [26]. According to R. Amaral [27] ten years ago 80% of the producers were oriented towards meat production; today more than half of those have switched their focus towards dairy.

Santa Eliza Farm, in Dourado, Sao Paulo State, Brazil, has its own dairy plant (Dourado Buffalo Dairy Products Factory) processing 4,000 liters/day from their own and nearby milking farms. They apply standardized good manufacturing practices, taking special care of the environment; their de-seasonalization strategy allows them to maintain steady production year-round by milking 200 animals out of the breeding season. Their registered trademark, mozzarella Dourado, is one of the most prestigious products in the Brazilian market. They supply 85% of production to Sao Paulo (280 km of distance), 10% to Rio do Janeiro and the remaining production to the rest of the country. Laguna Farm [15] recently received an award by the State of Ceará. It is a family integrated production system, from farm to market, mainly supplying their products to Fortaleza, a city of 2.3 million inhabitants. Their products include frescal (regular and oregano) and criollo (creole) cheese (less humid than the frescal), ricotta and whole milk. Their production does not include mozzarella, due to its inherent lower cheese yield, compared to the other cheeses. According to their economic analysis, bubaline cheese production is more profitable than cattle's due to its lower input requirements on milk volume, forage, equipment and also because its market is about 15% higher.

A growing number of small-scale farmers are switching to bubaline milk in those regions of Brazil where dairy plants specialized in buffalo milk have settled. Even with the typical low production of poorly improved buffalo herds, their returns on investment are still higher than that obtained with cattle [26].

In Argentina, a dairy farm owned by González Fraga, in Torres, Luján, Buenos Aires Province, is the buffalo milk supplier for La Salamandra S.A. The group covers all aspects of the production chain from farm to market outlets, with a registered trademark. The industrial plant produces 22 kg mozzarella/100 liters of milk. Several niche opportunities exist today in their local market due to the significant influence of the Italian culture, especially in urban populations. This demand still remains to be satisfied. La Salamandra S.A. markets their products using top restaurants and exports 20% of their cheese production to Chile. Other dairy plants market criollo (creole) type cheeses (Formosa, Corrientes and Misiones Provinces) and flavored, semi-hardened paste cheeses (Santa Úrsula, owned by Sons of Raúl Maglietti S.R.L.) in Formosa.

Pangolares Ranch, owned by the Argentinian Alberto Duhau and brothers, is located near Maturín city, Monagas State, Venezuela, and produces Feta cheese, a Greek, salty type cheese similar to the Venezuelan criollo (creole), that yields 22-23%. They also produce white cheese (of soft consistence), Gouda cheese (semi-hard), mozzarella and ricotta. In its institutional presentation, mozzarella is packaged in a container with 2.5 liters of salt water and 16 balls of mozzarella of

160 g/each, their products are sold to the towns of Maturín, Puerto Ordaz, Puerto La Cruz, Caracas and Valencia (in Venezuela); in its home presentation is done with two balls of 160 g/each, or with 16 of 20 g [15].

El Carmen Ranch, in Santa Cruz, Bolivia, owned by Robert Haab, produces several types of cheeses such as melted cheese, ricotta and others. Their trademark, Caserti, has a strong presence in the local market [15].

Italy

Italian cheese market is complex due to market restrictions for fresh cheeses and constrains on shelf life. They key aspects of Mozzarella di Bufala Campana (MBC) are: Protected Designation of Origin (DOP) and the merge of cheese and breed, the production of mozzarella cheese from milk exclusively from buffalo cows of Italian Mediterranean breed. Another important aspect is the inclusion of mozzarella cheese in traditional Italian recipes such as pizza, caprese salad and others. Storage in salty water results in a progressive softening of the mozzarella, the degree of softening depends on the calcium content. The higher the calcium content, the firmer the cheese. Calcium content is also important in pizza preparation, because the calcium micelle aids in reducing the acidity of the tomato sauce. When baked, care should be taken not to cause browning of the cheese, through turning residual sugars (glucose and galactose) into lactic acid, using cultures of lactic acid bacterial rests [23]. Destination of Italian exports of mozzarella for the year 2005 are shown in Fig. (**14**).

COUNTRY OF DESTINATION	% OF ITALIAN EXPORTS (MOZZARELLA) (2005)	VARIATION (%) FROM PREVIOUS YEAR (2004)
France	21.4	+1
Germany	18.1	+0.7
UnitedStates	5.2	-0.8 ("Euro effect")
UnitedKingdom	12.1	-0.6
Japan	8	+2.8
Switzerland	6.8	-0.8
Spain	6.2	+2.5
Belgium	3.4	+0.7 %
Canada	2.3	+0.4

Fig. (14). country of destination of mozzarella Italian exports for 2005.

Exports to Japan have been undergoing a growing trend (2001-2005); it has grown from 2% in 2001 to 8.7% in 2005, with an increase of 2.8% respect 2004. Fifty-one percent of exports are within countries of the European Community [7].

The limitations of the Italian market are associated to the cheese industry organization and distribution problems. For this reason, many breeders (producers) and cooperatives prefer to market their products themselves in order to gain added value and improve their income. The wide diversity within typical mozzarella is a considerable marketing problem. Mozzarella produced by small plants is typically produced using unique yeasts and natural microorganisms; its shelf life is normally three to five days and may not be extended by refrigeration. On the other hand, mozzarella manufactured by larger plants is produced without yeasts and microorganisms for long-term (30 day) conservation by refrigeration. This latter product, which is destined to the large scale grocery store and export market, is not as soft and moist. Both products have the same denomination and DOP, but are quite different. Although both excellent products, the striking difference between the two may confuse the general public. Mozzarella cheese is usually presented as balls or polpettas of variable size (20-800 gr), as small bites or bocconcino and braided or treccia [22].

In Italy the price of buffalo milk is four times the price of cattle's cheese. Italian mozzarella producers started to pasteurize their milk in the early 90's. Even though pasteurization reduces milk yield significantly, it is still required by the markets due to sanitary issues and shelf life. Italian consumers have progressively learned to value the certificate of origin of their product; hence, the status of DOP (Denominazione di Origine Protetta) and DOC (Denominazione di Origine Controllata) are important accomplishments. The internal demand has also increased steadily in latest years; 63% of mozzarella is consumed in the south of Italy, with an average family intake of 1.7 kg/year in southern Italy, meanwhile the national average is of 1 kg [19].

La Garofalo Dairy Factory, in Caserta city, processing 60,000 liters/day, is the largest in Italy. The plant is completely automatized, with 20 hour-day work shifts. Forty- percent of their production goes to the export market (Germany, France, Switzerland, Belgium, Canada, USA and Russia). The price is the same for the local market and for the international trader: 8 E/kg. With the exception of the manual kneading, the rest of the manufacturing process is completely automated, including packaging. Each holding tank has a capacity of 1000 liters; pasteurization is done at 72° C for 15, and cooling at 4° C in a water-milk laminar counter flow. Riva Bianca Ranch, in Paestum, Salerno Province, processes 5000 liters/day. They consider mozzarella an excellent business: it contains 66% of water. Riva Bianca produces ricotta, mozzarella and scamorza. The last one (scamorza) has the highest shelf-life among their products; this product has an 18% yield and the production cycle lasts at least 45 days. It is a high quality cheese that allows producers the flexibility to utilize all surplus milk when the demand for mozzarella temporarily drops.

In Italy, a Technical Committee of the Scientific Consortium for the Protection of Mozzarella di Bufala Campana was established in 1999, and standardized parameters for health management, nutrition and body condition score of bubaline herds were outlined [28]. Finally, because mozzarella made form cattle's milk is 20% cheaper than its buffalo cow counterpart, it is important to be able to distinguish between the two products. 1) Color: buffalo cow mozzarella is whiter, pearlier and glossier whereas cattle's mozzarella has a yellowish color. 2) Fat content: buffalo cow mozzarella has a higher (20-30%) fat content than cattle's. 3) Texture: the surface of buffalo cow mozzarella should appear smooth, whereas cattle's is bit rougher. Its outer layer should be thin and when open, interior should be moist and creamy whey runoff should be noticeable. Fresh buffalo cow mozzarella is more elastic than cattle's. 4) Flavor: buffalo mozzarella cow is sweeter than cattle's, with a slightly acidic finish. Buffalo milk also can be differentiated from cattle's milk by protein electrophoresis. In Argentina, this test is conducted by the Industrial Technology National Institute – Dairy (INTI – LÁCTEO). In Brazil, the selo de pureza is awarded by the Breeders Association. Purity control conducted by protein electrophoresis has an accuracy of 90%. There are also molecular probes available to conduct such evaluation, with even higher accuracy [29].

CONFLICT OF INTEREST

The authors confirm that they have no conflict of interest to declare for this publication.

ACKNOWLEDGEMENTS

Declared none.

REFERENCES

[1] Cockrill WR. The Husbandry and Health of the Domestic Buffalo Published. Rome, Italy: Food and Agriculture Organization of the United Nations 1974.

[2] Lopes Oliveira R. Medicinal and nutritional qualities of the buffalo cow dairy by-products. Buffalo Bulletin, Brazilian Buffalo Breeders Association (ABCB), São Paulo, Brazil 2004.

[3] Zava M. The Domestic Buffalo Publisher. Buenos Aires, Argentina: National Agricultural Research Institute 2011; pp. 366-70.

[4] Bernardes O. Dairy Exploitation in Paineiras da Ingaí Farm. São Paulo, Brazil: Sarapui 1989.

[5] Ganguli NC. Buffalo Production Milk Processing and Marketing. Elsiever, Amsterdam: University of Melbourne, Australia. Publishing House 1992.

[6] Gimenes Fernandes A, Van Dender H, Moreno I, Do Valle JL, Borges Busani SF. Buffalo cow milk artisanal utilization Technical Manual Number 3, ITAL. Campinas, São Paulo, Brazil: São Paulo State Government, Agricultural Research Coordination Office 1989.

[7] Garofalo R. Marketing and competitivity of Mozzarella di Bufala Campana Industry IIIrd American Buffalo Symposium. Medellin, Colombia. 2006.

[8] Kumar S. Milk Buffalo Cow Composition Published in: Asian Buffalo Magazine. India: New Dehli 2007.

[9] Bastianetto E, Correa Escrivão S. Buffalo cow reproductive characteristics influence in milk production, composition and quality. Published in Buffalo Bulletin, Brazilian Buffalo Breeders Association (ABCB), São Paulo, Brazil 2005.

[10] Tonizza de Carvalho NA. Artificial Insemination Course, São Paulo University (USP). Formosa Province, Argentina: Guazú Cuá Ranch 2007.

[11] Zava M. The Domestic Buffalo Publisher. Buenos Aires, Argentina: National Agricultural Research Institute 2011; pp. 377-82.

[12] Reggeti Gómez JA. Buffalo cow milk by-products. Guárico State, Venezuela: Terecay Ranch 2009.

[13] de Oliveira JF. Artisanal processes for some milk by-products. Brazil: Agriculture Secretary of São Paulo State 2007.

[14] Erbiti L. Mozzarella elaboration proccess, La Salamandra Dairy Factory SA, Luján, Buenos Aires Province, Argentina 2008.

[15] Zava M. The Domestic Buffalo. Buenos Aires, Argentina: National Agricultural Research Institute 2011; pp. 389, 392, 399, 402-.

[16] Campanile G. Nutrition and milk production in diary buffalo. American Buffalo Symposium.

Corrientes, Argentina. 2004.

[17] Cortesi ML, Murru N. Safety and quality along the buffalo cow milk and cheese chain. Proceedings VIII World Buffalo Congress. Caserta, Italy. 2007.

[18] Citro A. Mozzarella di Bufala Camapana. Salerno, Italy: The right stretching and kneading technique for the mozzarella thermic arrangement 1999.

[19] Garofalo R. Mozzarella di Bufala Campana DOP Proceedings IIIrd American Buffalo Symposium. Medellín, Colombia. 2006.

[20] Bernardes O. Grazing dairy buffalo cow management. Proceedings, IVth Buffalo American Symposium. Mérida, Venezuela. 2008.

[21] Gusmão Couto A. Mozzarella ellaboration with buffalo cow milk. Buffalo Bulletin Number 2, Brazilian Buffalo BreedersAssociation (ABCB) 2005.

[22] Borghese A. Buffalo Production and Research. Rome: Food and Agriculture Organization of the United Nations 2005.

[23] Addeo F, Alloisio V, Chianese L. Tradition and innovation in the water buffalo dairy products. Proceedings VIIIth World Buffalo Congress. Caserta, Italy. 2007. [http://dx.doi.org/10.4081/ijas.2007.s2.51]

[24] Ganguli NC. Buffalo cow milk technology Published: World Animal Production Magazine, N° 30. Rome, Italy: Food and Agriculture Organization of the United Nations 1979.

[25] Aleksiev A. The Water Buffalo. Sophia, Bulgaria: St. Climent Ohdriski University Press 1998.

[26] Bernardes O. The importance of dairy bubaline production in the small rural property, The buffalo in Brazil IIIrd American Buffalo Symposium. Medellin, Colombia. 2006.

[27] Amaral R. Agricultural Supplement of the Estado de São Paulo Journal, São Paulo, Brazil 2007.

[28] Terramoccia S, Bartocci S, Borghese A. Nutrition requirements in buffalo cows and heifers. In: Published BA, Ed. Buffalo Production and Research. Rome: Food and Agriculture Organization of the United Nations 2005.

[29] Tonhati H. Buffalo milk purity control conducted by protein electrophoresis. Sao Paulo, Brazil: Sao Paulo State University communications 2007.

CHAPTER 11

Parasitological Scenario of Buffalo Farms in Central and Southern Italy: A Review

Antonio Bosco, Laura Rinaldi, Maria Paola Maurelli and **Giuseppe Cringoli***

Department of Veterinary Medicine and Animal Productions, University of Naples Federico II, CREMOPAR Regione Campania, Italy

Abstract: In this review, focus has been given on the diverse parasitological scenario that can be found in different buffalo farms in central and southern Italy, where the majority of buffalo heads are reared. The Geographical Information System, developed and used for the planning of sampling protocols, for data analysis and results, has been employed for the conduction of many studies performed in the course of the last twenty years. Furthermore, the copromicroscopic analyses were conducted using multivalent techniques, the FLOTAC techniques, which are characterized by high sensitivity, as well as precision, specificity, accuracy and reproducibility. Such techniques have been developed to further the capacity to quickly detect any possible parasitic infections, especially those that may pose any kind of human and veterinary public health concerns. From the results presented in this review, it is clear that we have witnessed over the last decades a significant modification of buffalo farm management and production system. Such buffalo farms have moved towards more intensive and innovative practices, such as the adoption of newly developed reproductive technologies and nutrition regimens together with increasing amounts of concentrate feeds and stored forages. The concurrent preventive use of anthelmintic treatments has greatly reduced helminth infections, which may pose a serious threat for human health such as the zoonosis caused by the larval stages of *Echinococcus granulosus*. It is worth mentioning also the witness of a parallel rise in protozoa and arthropoda infections.

* **Corresponding author Giuseppe Cringoli:** Department of Veterinary Medicine and Animal Productions, University of Naples Federico II, CREMOPAR Regione Campania, Italy; Tel: +39 081 676799; Fax: +39 081 676569; E-mail: cringoli@unina.it

Giorgio A. Presicce (Ed.)

Keywords: Buffalo, FLOTAC, Italy, Parasites.

1. INTRODUCTION

The economy of many countries across most continents is heavily influenced by the powerful zoo-economy driven by the presence of buffaloes (*Bubalus bubalis*), belonging to both the river and the swamp sub species. In some countries, and especially in Italy, the buffalo may be linked directly to some peculiar and specific product, like the mozzarella cheese. The importance of this milk-derived product is so great, that, thanks to high quality of milk produced and transformed in mozzarella cheese, the introduction of a specific designation of protected origin (DPO), has been felt mandatory, and it is used nowadays across the entire Italian territory and used abroad to identify the original product. A number of countries are paying more and more attention to buffalo milk, its quality and, equally important, to its derived products, and this is reflected in the increased funding on various areas of research activity. In addition, the buffalo species is second only to cattle in the production of milk world-wide, accounting for a 12% of the totality of milk produced all over the world [1]. In consideration of the large interest expressed for this species, its zoo-economical implications and the health issues inevitably raised, a special focus addressed into the investigation of parasitic infection is of paramount importance. In fact, in tropical and sub-tropical countries, parasitic infections are very common and are unfortunately responsible for relevant economic losses in terms of dead animals following heavy parasitic infections, consequent disposal of infected organs at slaughter, and reduced rates of weight gain [2].

In addition, some of those parasitic infections are typically zoonosis as they can have a direct clinical relevance in the human species, in some cases according to the different geographical location, such as schistosomiasis in China and the Philippines, or other infections like cystic echinococcosis, cryptosporidiosis, fasciolosis and giardiasis which are reported everywhere. Currently, in buffalo farms spread over central and southern Italy, the parasitological situation has been strongly modified in recent decades due to, as anticipated earlier, the modernization of buffalo farms together with the use of modern reproductive strategies and nutritional technologies, and the introduction of prophylactic parasitic countermeasures, especially specific anthelmintic protocols and related treatments only following a clear and accurate diagnosis [3 - 5].

Considering that most buffaloes in Italy are reared in central and southern Italy, in this review an up-to-date summary of parasitism affecting this species in that part of Italy, from protozoa to helminths and arthropoda, will be given.

In Table **1**, a list of the various parasitic species affecting the buffaloes in central and southern Italy, is made available. The data reported in Table **1** came from a study performed in the Lazio Region (central Italy) on 127 farms and from diagnostic activities performed at CREMOPAR in the Campania Region (southern Italy) from 2000 to 2013 on 1,324 farms.

Table 1. Main parasitic infections in water buffaloes in central and southern Italy [3, 6 - 11].

Parasites	**Farm Prevalence (%) (min and max)**
Protozoa	
Eimeria spp.	94.5-97.7
Helminths	
Gastrointestinal strongyles	4.7-33.1
Strongyloides spp.	3.1-4.7
Fasciola hepatica	1.1-7.1
Dicrocoelium dendriticum	0.5-2.4
Paramphistomidae	2.3-7.1
Moniezia spp.	0.5-2.4
Echinococcus granulosus (larval stages)	8.0-12.4
Arthropoda	
Lice (*Haematopinus tuberculatus*)	2.8-11.0
Mange mites (*Psoroptes* spp.)	3.0-12.6

2. PROTOZOA

Infections by intestinal protozoa are a leading cause of neonatal diarrhoea, having a negative impact on the growth performance of buffalo calves.

In particular, buffalo calves are easily hit by coccidiosis, caused by several

Eimeria species, with the result of considerable economic losses to the dairy and meat industry worldwide. In addition, such different *Eimeria* species are characterized by different pathogenicity. Almost two thousand buffaloes reared in 127 buffalo farms in the Lazio region (central Italy) were studied in the course of a cross-sectional coprological survey [9, 11]. The FLOTAC technique was used to perform copromicroscopic examinations, utilizing a solution of saturated sodium chloride (specific gravity = 1.200) [12, 13], followed by oocyst sporulation and identification of the different *Eimeria* species.

Oocysts of *Eimeria* spp. were found in 94.5% (120/127) of the farms and in 46.8% (882/1883) of the animals, and seven species of *Eimeria* have been described so far, namely *E. bareilly, E. zuernii, E. ellipsoidalis, E. subspherica, E. auburnensis, E. bovis* and *E. pellita* [4]. The following most common *Eimeria* species, such as *E. bovis*, *E. zuernii* and *E. bareilly*, which are also the most pathogenic, were found. These findings concur with findings related to similar studies carried out in the Campania region (southern Italy) on 1324 farms, and give evidence that *Eimeria* infection within buffalo farms is very common and widespread (97.7%; 1293/1324) and has to be considered the most prevalent parasitosis in water buffaloes [4].

Coccidiosis may manifest itself as clinical or subclinical infection and can affect growth performance in buffaloes as in other ruminant species. Therefore, the control of *Eimeria* infections is of fundamental importance for the health, the welfare and the productions of buffalo calves. Coccidiosis has be to fought mainly through the adoption of prophylactic and metaphylactic treatments. This is the case, as therapeutic treatments are usually ineffective due to the fact that lesions are already present in the intestinal mucosa, and therefore coccidiosis will always result in clinical disease, of which diarrhea is the most common sign [14, 15]. Controlled field trials were recently conducted to evaluate the parasitological (parasite burden reduction) and zootechnical performance (weight gain) effect of metaphylactic treatment with toltrazuril (TOL) and diclazuril (DIC) for the control of coccidiosis by *Eimeria* spp. in naturally infected water buffalo calves bred with two different management systems in a Mediterranean area (southern Italy) [16]. The study was conducted in 5 buffalo farms with a known history of coccidiosis: the farms were divided into two typologies (A and B) of management system. In farms of Typology A the buffalo calves were bred in individual boxes from birth to the seventh/eighth week of age and then transferred to the ground in multiple boxes; whereas, in the farms of Typology B the calves were bred on the ground in multiple boxes from birth. In the three buffalo farms of Typology A the calves of the groups TOL and DIC were treated only once (at the seventh/eighth week of age); whereas, in the two buffalo farms of typology B the calves of the treated groups were treated twice (once at the fifth and once at the seventh/eighth week of age). On each farm, 36 calves aged 5 weeks, were divided at random into three similar groups of 12 calves each. One group was treated with toltrazuril (TOL) at the dose of 15 mg/kg, whereas the second group was treated with diclazuril (DIC) at the dose of 1 mg/kg, and the third group remained as untreated control group (CONT). For 15 weeks calves were weekly weighed and clinically and parasitologically examined. In the five buffalo farms the average oocyst excretion decreased significantly in both treated groups (TOL and DIC) compared to the CONT groups, however the TOL groups showed intensities significantly lower than the DIC groups. The body-weight gains recorded fortnightly were significantly higher in the TOL groups (min 5.4 kg – max 8.1 kg) compared to the DIC (min 1.7 kg – max 3.1 kg) and the CONT groups which differed slightly. Therefore, subclinical coccidiosis may impair growth performance in buffalo calves reared either in individual boxes or in multiple boxes. There exists a susceptibility to metaphylactic treatment with toltrazuril and diclazuril on the reproductive cycle of *Eimeria* species in calves naturally exposed to the infection, exhibiting a growth response of treated calves. A metaphylactic treatment to be utilized in single buffalo farms, is related and has to do with specific elements of the farm involved together with the usual cost/benefit ratio. Specifically, the latter takes into consideration the balance to be achieved between the economical value of the gained body weight following treatment and the cost of the anticoccidial treatment itself, in addition to the possibility of recurrent coccidiosis outbreak.

Among intestinal protozoa, buffaloes can be affected by ubiquitous parasites such as *Giardia duodenalis* (syn. *G. intestinalis, G. lamblia*) and *Cryptosporidium parvum*, which are also responsible for infecting the human as well as other animal species. These two intestinal protozoa, which are characterized by having a direct life cycle, usually cause diarrhea and may affect the growth rate of ruminants [17]. An amplification of symptoms of concurrent infection, together with stress and nutritional deficiencies, is usually seen in buffaloes hit by these two protozoa. These are infections of considerable importance and economic concern, in consequence of the affected livestock performance caused by the most common and visible signs represented by diarrhea, and even other sub-clinical infections should be taken into serious consideration [18]. In consideration of the above, a copro-ELISAs on *G. duodenalis* and *C. parvum* in the course of a cross-sectional coprological survey, was run in 90 buffalo farms and involving 347 animals in the Lazio region [3]. *G. duodenalis* was found with a prevalence of 18.1% in animals and 30.0% in farms, whereas *C. parvum* was found with a prevalence of 14.7% in animals and 24.4% in farms. Similar values of prevalence were also found in the Campania region. Molecular techniques such as PCR and DNA sequencing, were used to characterize isolates of *G. duodenalis* and *C. parvum*, recovered from buffaloes [6]. Following the confirmed presence of both zoonotic parasites *G. duodenalis* and *C. parvum* (assemblage A) and host-specific parasite (assemblage E), it is suggested that environmental contamination with oocysts and cysts posing a threat to human health by buffalo feces, can occur if the latter are not properly disposed off. Fortunately, these two protozoa cannot affect the chain of mozzarella cheese production, considering that the process of cheese production consists of treatment of the cheese curd at a temperature of 85 to 95°C, which is sufficient to kill or inactivate the zoonotic parasites.

Another important protozoa infecting buffaloes (as an extra-intestinal coccidian) is *Neospora caninum*, which is another protozoan heavily responsible as a major cause of abortion in cattle all over the world, especially in seropositive animals when compared to seronegative ones [19]. Both dogs and coyotes are known to be the final hosts for *N. caninum* (intestinal cycle), whereas many other species among which the buffaloes, act as intermediate hosts (extra-intestinal cycle) [20, 21].

Following a serological survey on *N. caninum* by IFAT in 50 buffalo farms and involving 1377 animals in the Campania region in the south of Italy, a prevalence of infection was found in 34.6% of animals investigated and 82.0% of farms taking part in the survey [10], and only in two farms some abortions and neurological signs were recorded, together with few protozoan-like cysts observed on foetal tissue following histological examination.

3. GASTROINTESTINAL AND HEPATIC HELMINTHS

A number of several gastrointestinal and hepatic helmints such as nematoda, trematoda and cestoda can infect buffaloes: i) Nematoda: The buffalo species is commonly hit by gastrointestinal *Strongyles* and *Strongyloides* of the nematoda group, and these parasites are characterized by a direct life cycle and three different larval stages from L1 to L3 to be found in the environment; ii) Trematoda: *Fasciola hepatica, Dicrocoelium dendriticum* and *Calicophoron daubneyi* can be considered the most common flukes to be recorded among buffaloes in Italy. The liver is home for both *F. hepatica* and *D. dendriticum*, with the difference that, while the immature stages of *F. hepatica* can be found in the liver parenchyma and the adult stages in the bile ducts, *D. dendriticum* lives in bile ducts and gall bladder. Of the third most important trematoda for buffaloes, immature flukes of *C. daubneyi* are found in the upper small intestine and here are responsible of serious morbidity leading even to death of the host, whereas the adult stages can be found in the rumen and/or reticulum of the same animals. The water is the most important environmental factor for the establishment of parasitic infection due to *F. hepatica* and *C. daubneyi*. In water in fact, such parasites can find their intermediate host represented by the amphibious snails. A different environment is needed for *D. dendriticum* parasites, where they intermediate hosts are represented by land mollusks and ants, which live in biotopes characterized by dry and calcareous or alkaline soils; iii) Cestoda: of the cestoda group, the *Moniezia* genus is widely distributed, with a life cycle characterized by the presence of two different hosts, oribatid mites living in the soil as intermediate hosts, and the intestine or guts of ruminants where adult tapeworms can be found. These parasites are responsible for acute symptoms in animals like diarrhea and fleshless, which in turn may account for losses within the herd. Overall, the helminth infections above summarized are of great economic and health significance, due to the fact that the consequent digestive disorders lead to a decreased production linked to reduced weight gain, growth delay, reduced milk production, *etc.*, and all this can be reported even in case of sub-clinical parasitic infections. In the Lazio region of central Italy, almost two thousand buffaloes from 127 farms [19, 20] were investigated through a cross-sectional coprological survey, where the FLOTAC Dual technique [12, 13] was employed to perform copromicroscopic examinations characterized by a sensitivity of two eggs per gram of feces. Two floating solutions were used: i) a solution of saturated sodium chloride with a specific gravity = 1.200 needed to isolate nematode and cestoda eggs, and ii) a zinc sulphate solution with a specific gravity = 1.350 needed to detect eggs of the trematoda group.

The survey produced interesting results which are summarized in Table **1**. Among the most commonly found parasitic infections in buffaloes, gastrointestinal strongyles are the most frequent helminths recorded in buffalo farms (33.1%) and animals (5.4%). Other common parasites among buffalo farms and animals are: *F. hepatica* (7.1% and 1.3%, respectively), *C. daubneyi* (7.1% and 2.1%, respectively), *Strongyloides* species (3.1% and 0.4%, respectively), *D. dendriticum* (2.4 and 0.2%, respectively), and finally *Moniezia* species (2.4% and 0.2%, respectively). From the results obtained in the presented survey, it can be seen that helminth parasitic infection is characterized overall by low numerical values both on farms and animals. Such results recorded in the Lazio region of central Italy are similar to findings from the Caserta province in the south of Italy [22]. Collectively, results from the survey on helminth parasitic infections are quite different from the results in other geographical settings, where buffaloes are typically reared in extensive production systems and the helminth infections are generally significantly higher.

4. CYSTIC ECHINOCOCCOSIS

The genus *Echinococcus* is responsible for a cosmopolitan parasitic disease linked to both larval and adult stages of tapeworms, and within the same genus, four specific parasites can be identified, namely: *E. granulosus, E. multilocularis, E. oligarthrus* and *E. vogeli,* and the recent acquisition of a fifth species found in Tibet and named *E. shiquicus* [23, 24]. Echinococcosis can be considered one of the most important livestock parasitic infection in the entire world. In addition it is a very serious and widespread zoonosis [7] as, being the *Echinococcus* found in many host species, it can also be established in the human species. More specifically, the cystic echinococcosis (CE) is caused by the larval stages (hydatid cysts) of the parasite *E. granulosus*, and of the latter, around ten different genotypes, from G1 to G10 have been characterized by using molecular techniques [24]. Canids, among which the domestic dog, are the final hosts of the *E. granulosus* parasite life cycle, while a number of ruminants and ungulates such as cattle and buffaloes, goats and pigs, in addition to humans, are the intermediate hosts in which the hydatid cyst establishes itself [25, 26]. Some people still carry the habit of home slaughtering sheep and pigs. If such intermediate hosts have the hydatid cysts, dogs can acquire the parasitic infection by feeding on the internal organs (usually liver and lungs) [27]. In sheep, a higher frequency of CE is reported when compared to other animals [28], and this is strongly supported by surveys conducted bot in the Sardinia island and Campania regions of Italy, in which a high prevalence of CE is found: 75% of sheep sampled in Sardinia [29], and 31.2% in some areas of Campania [30].

CE in the water buffalo has been studied in the Campania region of south of Italy by performing surveys and adopting molecular approaches, with the result of evidencing a high prevalence of CE in both farms (12.4%) and animals (10.5%) [7, 31]. The rationale behind these values is worth some considerations with regard to the buffalo species. Unlike sheep, buffalo farms do not practice illegal-slaughtering and nowadays, buffaloes are sent to modern slaughterhouse facilities when needed, in addition to an efficient system of control by veterinarians and other health officers whose duty is to reinforce the chain production system and maintaining safety for both animals and humans. Therefore, canids cannot feed on buffalo internal organs following slaughter, closing the life cycle of the *Echinococcus*, and this is the case also for cattle. In a recent paper [31] Geographical Information Systems (GIS) were used in order to understand the role of sheep as a parasite reservoir. In summary, stranded dogs get infected when feeding on sheep carcasses, and then approaching and entering buffalo and dairy farms, shed their load of egg parasites infecting thus the ruminants (Table **2**). It is not surprising that many times both sheep and buffalo/dairy farms are at close distance from one another, making it easy for dogs to move from one farm to another. And in fact, the closer sheep farms are to buffalo farms, the easier the report of infection in buffalo/dairy farms and buffaloes/cattle. In addition and in support of such evidence, buffaloes/cattle and sheep in the Campania region of south of Italy, share the same *E. granulosus* genotypes such as the G1 (common sheep strain), G2 (Tasmanian sheep strain) and G3 (buffalo strain) [7, 24, 32].

Table 2. Number of sheep farms within 5 km radius buffer area around dairy and buffalo farms positive for cystic Echinococcosis in the Campania region and their distances [31].

Farm typology	Sheep farms (mean) within the buffer zone	Distances from sheep farms within each buffer zone					
		Mean	SD	25th percentile	50th percentile	75th percentile	P*
Cattle	10.7	2.2	1.8	1.0	1.9	2.7	0.001
Buffalo	6.4	4.7	2.3	2.6	5.1	6.5	

5. ARTHROPODA

The suckling lice and the mange mites in Italy are the most common arthropoda to be found in buffaloes, where they entertain their entire life cycle. Buffaloes can experience skin irritation, anaemia, anorexia, restlessness and reduced productivity when confronted with the sucking *Haematopinus tuberculatus*. Similar skin lesions, itch and irritation can be also caused by the mange mites of the *Sarcoptes, Psoroptes* and *Demodex genuses*, together with other signs such as alopecia, skin thickening and dry scab. In the Lazio region, 762 buffaloes from 127 farms were involved in a cross-sectional entomological survey [9], and standard procedures were followed for the collection and correct identification of ectoparasites [33]. In farms and animals the following ectoparasites were found: *H. tuberculatus* (lice) and *P. ovis / P. natalensis* (mange mites) on 11.0% and 12.6% of farms and 4.5% and 3.5% of animals, respectively (Table **1**). Further studies are needed in order to understand why ticks were not recorded on the tested animals. The high intensity and crowding occurring nowadays in buffalo farms is a factor favouring the diffusion of ectoparasites such as lice and mange mites, characterized by a life cycle taking place entirely on their hosts. These ectoparasites, even if they do no elicit any clinical sign, may nevertheless reduce productivity in terms of milk produced from lactating animals and weight gain in growing animals. A recent study showed the role of *H. tuberculatus* as a new host for the transmission of brucellosis [34]. The presence of DNA and RNA of *Brucella* spp. along with different developmental stages of *H. tuberculatus* was the main aim of the study, so that its possible role as vector for *Brucella* transmission could be determined. For this purpose, seropositive and seronegative buffaloes were selected and louse specimens collected from both categories of animals and divided into three different developmental stages: nits, nymphs and adults. Real Time PCR was employed in all samples to be screened in order to detect DNA and RNA of *Brucella* spp. Results show that in all developmental stages of the suckling louse *H. tuberculatus*, DNA of *Brucella* spp. was detected. The evidence of *Brucella* spp. DNA in nit samples is supportive of a hypothesis of vertical transmission of *Brucella* itself among the various stages of *H. tuberculatum* development (trans-stadial and trans-ovarial transmission). In fact, in nature an important mechanism for the diffusion of thick-borne protozoa, bacteria and viruses, is the trans-ovarial transmission [35]. There are some cases of trans-ovarial transmission in which, as in *Rickettsia* infection, this mechanism is more important and effective in maintaining and perpetuating the infection, if compared to the acquisition of the organism from natural hosts, considering that usually rickettsaemia in mammalian hosts is short lived. It is thought that *H. tuberculatus* females filled with the bacteria can transmit *Brucella* spp. to the nits, as a description of a short-lived bacteremia occurs also in the course of brucellosis. If we compare the different developmental stages of *H. tuberculatus*, the highest prevalence of bacteria presence is found in nits (around 90%) when compared to adult (66.7%) and nymphs (44.4%). Such differential rate of bacterial presence may be explained by the following: adult lice express a high rate of bacterial infection which in turn is manifested with a high rate of layed infected nits. Such high rate of infection is somewhat reduced in the course of hatching, as it has been reported in *Borrelia* infected ticks [36]. The survivability of *Brucella* spp. in the environment, and especially in some endemic areas, can be also explained by the high resistance of nits in the surrounding environment.

CONCLUSION

The parasitological scenario interesting the buffalo population in Italy has been the focus of this review. An important and representative sample of the buffalo population which has been taken into consideration in this review, reside in central and southern Italy, where the majority of the buffalo heads can be found. The shifting of buffalo farm management in the last decades, towards an intensive management system, has brought also the adoption of new and innovative practices regarding reproduction, nutrition and productive approaches. In addition, preventive measures and new health protocols have been incorporated into the new buffalo management system. Following such new guidelines, a decrease in helminth infection has been witnessed with a regular use of anthelmintic treatments, although a parallel rise of parasitic transmission from host to host has also been reported, as in the case of the protozoa *Eimeria, Giardia* and *Cryptosporidium* and the arthropoda *Haematopinus* and *Psoroptes*. Furthermore, some parasites, of which buffaloes represent intermediate hosts, have been recorded in high number, such as in the case of *Neospora* and *Echinococcus* genus. Of course the surveillance of parasitic infection in buffaloes and more generally over any livestock species must continue and is of paramount importance. Not only for the benefit of livestock species but also for us humans, as the concept worldwide known as One World – One Health in association to Animal – Human relationship. Many parasitic infections are in fact zoonosis, as seen previously in this review, some of which life threatening and pose a continuous risk of endangered health, and therefore a focus of attention in this direction can never be abandoned.

CONFLICT OF INTEREST

The authors confirm that they have no conflict of interest to declare for this publication.

ACKNOWLEDGEMENTS

Declared none.

REFERENCES

[1] CNIEL (Centre National Interprofessionnel de l'Economie Laitiere). L'economie laitiere en chiffres 2002; 183.

[2] Liu Y, Li F, Liu W, *et al.* Prevalence of helminths in water buffaloes in Hunan Province, China. Trop Anim Health Prod 2009; 41(4): 543-6. [http://dx.doi.org/10.1007/s11250-008-9219-1] [PMID: 18704740]

[3] Rinaldi L, Musella V, Condoleo R, *et al.* *Giardia* and *Cryptosporidium* in water buffaloes (*Bubalus bubalis*). Parasitol Res 2007; 100(5): 1113-8. [http://dx.doi.org/10.1007/s00436-006-0397-3] [PMID: 17211662]

[4] Cringoli G, Guarino A, Fusco G, *et al.* Diffusion of *Eimeria* spp. in buffalo breeding farms in Southern

Italy and epidemiologic role of pregnant/postpartum buffaloes. Proceedings of the 2nd Asian Buff Ass Congress 1996. 165-73.

[5] Cringoli G, Guarino A, Fusco G, Veneziano V, Rinaldi L. Diffusion dynamics of *Eimeria* spp. in infected buffalo herds. Parasitologia 1998; 40: 38.

[6] Cacciò SM, Rinaldi L, Cringoli G, Condoleo R, Pozio E. Molecular identification of *Cryptosporidium parvum* and *Giardia duodenalis* in the Italian water buffalo (*Bubalus bubalis*). Vet Parasitol 2007; 150(1-2): 146-9.
[http://dx.doi.org/10.1016/j.vetpar.2007.09.013] [PMID: 17951009]

[7] Capuano F, Rinaldi L, Maurelli MP, *et al.* Cystic echinococcosis in water buffaloes: epidemiological survey and molecular evidence of ovine (G1) and buffalo (G3) strains. Vet Parasitol 2006; 137(3-4): 262-8.
[http://dx.doi.org/10.1016/j.vetpar.2006.01.016] [PMID: 16480832]

[8] Cringoli G, Rinaldi L. Geographical Information Systems in buffalo health applications. Int J Agric Sustain 2007; 6: 217-22.

[9] Cringoli G, Musella V, Maurelli MP, *et al.* Helminths and arthropoda in buffalo farms from the Lazio region (Italy). Vet Res Commun 2009; 33 (Suppl. 1): 129-31.
[http://dx.doi.org/10.1007/s11259-009-9268-6] [PMID: 19588261]

[10] Guarino A, Fusco G, Savini G, Di Francesco G, Cringoli G. Neosporosis in water buffalo (*Bubalus bubalis*) in Southern Italy. Vet Parasitol 2000; 91(1-2): 15-21.
[http://dx.doi.org/10.1016/S0304-4017(00)00239-9] [PMID: 10889356]

[11] Rinaldi L, Musella V, Veneziano V, Condoleo RU, Cringoli G. Helmintic infections in water buffaloes on Italian farms: a spatial analysis. Geospat Health 2009; 3(2): 233-9.
[http://dx.doi.org/10.4081/gh.2009.223] [PMID: 19440965]

[12] Cringoli G. FLOTAC, a novel apparatus for a multivalent faecal egg count technique. Parasitologia 2006; 48(3): 381-4.
[PMID: 17176947]

[13] Cringoli G, Rinaldi L, Maurelli MP, Utzinger J. FLOTAC: new multivalent techniques for qualitative and quantitative copromicroscopic diagnosis of parasites in animals and humans. Nat Protoc 2010; 5(3): 503-15.
[http://dx.doi.org/10.1038/nprot.2009.235] [PMID: 20203667]

[14] Fitzgerald PR. The economic impact of coccidiosis in domestic animals. Adv Vet Sci Comp Med 1980; 24: 121-43.
[PMID: 7006338]

[15] Mundt HC, Bangoura B, Mengel H, Keidel J, Daugschies A. Control of clinical coccidiosis of calves due to *Eimeria bovis* and *Eimeria zuernii* with toltrazuril under field conditions. Parasitol Res 2005; 97 (Suppl. 1): S134-42.
[http://dx.doi.org/10.1007/s00436-005-1457-9] [PMID: 16228270]

[16] Bosco A, Rinaldi L, Morgoglione ME, *et al.* The metaphylactic efficacy of toltrazuril and diclazuril in natural infections of *Eimeria spp.* in buffalo calves: a multicenter trial in southern Italy. In: The 10th World Buffalo Congress The 7th Asian Buffalo Congress; May 6-8 2013; Phuket, Thailand. 2013; p.

276.

[17] Castro-Hermida JA, Delafosse A, Pors I, Ares-Mazás E, Chartier C. *Giardia duodenalis* and *Cryptosporidium parvum* infections in adult goats and their implications for neonatal kids. Vet Rec 2005; 157(20): 623-7.
[http://dx.doi.org/10.1136/vr.157.20.623] [PMID: 16284331]

[18] Olson ME, OHandley RM, Ralston BJ, McAllister TA, Thompson RC. Update on *Cryptosporidium* and *Giardia* infections in cattle. Trends Parasitol 2004; 20(4): 185-91.
[http://dx.doi.org/10.1016/j.pt.2004.01.015] [PMID: 15099558]

[19] Dubey JP. Review of *Neospora caninum* and neosporosis in animals. Korean J Parasitol 2003; 41(1): 1-16.
[http://dx.doi.org/10.3347/kjp.2003.41.1.1] [PMID: 12666725]

[20] McAllister MM, Dubey JP, Lindsay DS, Jolley WR, Wills RA, McGuire AM. Dogs are definitive hosts of *Neospora caninum.* Int J Parasitol 1998; 28(9): 1473-8.
[http://dx.doi.org/10.1016/S0020-7519(98)00138-6] [PMID: 9770635]

[21] Gondim LF, McAllister MM, Pitt WC, Zemlicka DE. Coyotes (*Canis latrans*) are definitive hosts of *Neospora caninum.* Int J Parasitol 2004; 34(2): 159-61.
[http://dx.doi.org/10.1016/j.ijpara.2004.01.001] [PMID: 15037103]

[22] Cringoli G, Guarino A, Fusco G, Merola A, Bani A. Endoparassiti in allevamenti bufalini della provincia di Caserta: nota 1 - zona settentrionale. Bubalus Bubalis 1995; 1: 55-64.

[23] Xiao N, Qiu J, Nakao M, *et al. Echinococcus shiquicus* n. sp., a taeniid cestode from Tibetan fox and plateau pika in China. Int J Parasitol 2005; 35(6): 693-701.
[http://dx.doi.org/10.1016/j.ijpara.2005.01.003] [PMID: 15862582]

[24] Nakao M, McManus DP, Schantz PM, Craig PS, Ito A. A molecular phylogeny of the genus *Echinococcus* inferred from complete mitochondrial genomes. Parasitology 2007; 134(Pt 5): 713-22.
[http://dx.doi.org/10.1017/S0031182006001934] [PMID: 17156584]

[25] Moro P, Schantz PM. Cystic echinococcosis in the Americas. Parasitol Int 2006; 55 (Suppl.): S181-6.
[http://dx.doi.org/10.1016/j.parint.2005.11.048] [PMID: 16376604]

[26] Craig PS, McManus DP, Lightowlers MW, *et al.* Prevention and control of cystic echinococcosis. Lancet Infect Dis 2007; 7(6): 385-94.
[http://dx.doi.org/10.1016/S1473-3099(07)70134-2] [PMID: 17521591]

[27] McManus DP, Zhang W, Li J, Bartley PB. Echinococcosis. Lancet 2003; 362(9392): 1295-304.
[http://dx.doi.org/10.1016/S0140-6736(03)14573-4] [PMID: 14575976]

[28] Daryani A, Alaei R, Arab R, Sharif M, Dehghan MH, Ziaei H. The prevalence, intensity and viability of hydatid cysts in slaughtered animals in the Ardabil province of Northwest Iran. J Helminthol 2007; 81(1): 13-7.
[http://dx.doi.org/10.1017/S0022149X0720731X] [PMID: 17381862]

[29] Scala A, Garippa G, Varcasia A, Tranquillo VM, Genchi C. Cystic echinococcosis in slaughtered sheep in Sardinia (Italy). Vet Parasitol 2006; 135(1): 33-8.
[http://dx.doi.org/10.1016/j.vetpar.2005.08.006] [PMID: 16226378]

[30] Maurelli MP, Rinaldi L, Musella V, *et al.* Geografical information system and cystic echinococcosis in southern Italy. 7th International Symposium on Geospatial Health. September 5-6, 2013; Naples.

[31] Cringoli G, Rinaldi L, Musella V, *et al.* Geo-referencing livestock farms as tool for studying cystic echinococcosis epidemiology in cattle and water buffaloes from southern Italy. Geospat Health 2007; 2(1): 105-11.
[http://dx.doi.org/10.4081/gh.2007.259] [PMID: 18686260]

[32] Rinaldi L, Maurelli MP, Capuano F, Perugini AG, Veneziano V, Cringoli S. Molecular update on cystic echinococcosis in cattle and water buffaloes of southern Italy. Zoonoses Public Health 2008; 55(2): 119-23.
[http://dx.doi.org/10.1111/j.1863-2378.2007.01101.x] [PMID: 18234031]

[33] Veneziano V, Rinaldi L, Giannetto S, Cringoli G. The first record of *Haematopinus tuberculatus* on *Bubalus bubalis* (water buffalo) in Italy. Bubalus bubalis 9: 69-75.

[34] Neglia G, Veneziano V, De Carlo E, *et al.* Detection of *Brucella abortus* DNA and RNA in different stages of development of the sucking louse *Haematopinus tuberculatus.* BMC Vet Res 2013; 9: 236.
[http://dx.doi.org/10.1186/1746-6148-9-236] [PMID: 24289112]

[35] Murray PR, Rosenthal KS, Pfaller MA. Medical Microbiology. 5th ed., United States: Elsevier Mosby 2005.

[36] Nefedova VV, Korenberg EI, Gorelova NB, Kovalevskii YV. Studies on the transovarial transmission of *Borrelia burgdorferi sensu lato* in the taiga tick *Ixodes persulcatus*. Folia Parasitol (Praha) 2004; 51(1): 67-71.
[http://dx.doi.org/10.14411/fp.2004.010] [PMID: 15139380]

CHAPTER 12

Folliculogenesis and Ovarian Physiology Applied to Reproductive Biotechnologies in Buffaloes

Pietro Sampaio Baruselli[1] and **Giorgio Antonio Presicce**[2,*]

[1] *Departamento de Reprodução Animal, FMVZ-USP, São Paulo, SP, Brazil*

[2] *ARSIAL, Regione Lazio, Via R. Lanciani, 38 - 00161 Rome, Italy*

Abstract: The review aims at illustrating the state of the art in terms of acquisition of knowledge in the reproductive physiology of the buffalo species, ranging from fetal oogenesis to prepuberal and adult follicular dynamics in river and swamp buffaloes. Such aspects are considered in parallel and compared to cattle reproductive physiology. Reproductive efficiency is presented in the light of a seasonal pattern, and affected by human intervention due to localistic differential market demands for milk and cheese production. Finally, the implementation of reproductive technologies, from the use of artificial insemination together with the development of protocols for synchronization of ovulation, to *in vivo* (MOET) and *in vitro* embryo production and Ovum Pick Up (OPU), are taken into consideration, highlighting successes and difficulties.

Keywords: Buffalo, Reproduction, Reproductive technologies.

1. INTRODUCTION

Buffalo has a great potential for milk and meat production, and in the last decade an increase of 39.1% and 15.3%, respectively, has been witnessed [1]. Despite most of the buffalo population is located in Asia (above 90%), its economical exploitation is also important in other continents (*i.e.* America and Europe). Reproductive biotechnologies have been used in this species in order to obtain a faster genetic improvement for the characters of interest. However, such newly developed strategies are not as efficiently implemented as in cattle. Some

* **Corresponding author Giorgio A. Presicce:** ARSIAL, Regione Lazio, Via R. Lanciani, 38 - 00161 Rome, Italy; Tel: +39 06 61597561; Fax: +39 06 61597561; E-mail: gpresicce@arsial.it

morphological and physiological features of buffalo reproduction could explain some of the encountered differences with the cattle counterpart and the results obtained up to now. This review focuses on the main biotechnologies applied to buffalo reproduction, emphasizing featuring aspects of reproductive physiology characterizing this species, which can affect the success of applied reproductive technologies.

2. FOLLICULOGENESIS

In the course of fetal development, germinal cells are produced following migration of primordial germ cells to the gonadal ridge. Upon colonization of the genital ridge, prophase of the first meiotic division occurs with a halt to further progression at the diplotene stage, until formation of primordial follicles [2]. Along with this progression, follicles go through a morphological modification of their anatomical structure. In the buffalo species, oogones are found within primordial follicles from 0 to 3 months of gestation, whereas preantral to antral follicles can be found between 4 to 6 months, increasing their number with the progression of gestation until its physiological end [3]. Typically, a significant decrease in the number of primordial to primary follicles is witnessed with increasing fetal age, and a concomitant increase in secondary follicles. There is a large individual variation in the number of follicles at different stages of development within different fetal ages [2].

A paucity of information is related to the number of germ cells in the buffalo species, although some authors have reported a 10-fold lower value (10,000 to 12,000) when compared to cattle [4, 5]. In addition, and typically in large ruminants, despite the thousands of available primordial follicles, the majority of them will become atretic and therefore not viable [2]. It has been reported that, in buffaloes, most follicles from ovaries collected at slaughterhouses at random stages of the reproductive cycle (92 to 95%) are estrogen inactive and atretic. The status of an atretic follicle is defined according to the molar ratio of E2 to P4 in the follicular fluid, and such atresia has been reported to be higher in small and medium rather than large follicles [5]. Le Van Ty *et al.*, also reported the existence of a lower number of antral follicles in buffalo, when compared to cattle (47.5 ± 23.8 *vs*. 233.0 ± 95.8; $P < 0.002$) [6]. Nevertheless, Presicce *et al.* [7], in prepuberal buffalo calves reported a high number of *in vivo* available antral follicles, similarly to what previously reported in cattle prepuberal calves [8]. A lower ovarian follicular pool, associated to a high level of atresia, can be accounted for the significantly lower number of antral follicles available within the follicular waves in adult buffaloes when compared to cattle. In a recent study [9], following a hormonally induced wave emergence in three different species, namely *Bubalus bubalis*, Bos indicus (Nelore) and Bos Taurus (Holstein) heifers, the mean number of antral follicles in buffaloes (13.1 ± 1.4) was similar to cattle (15.0 ± 2.8), but significantly lower than Nelore (29.7 ± 3.1).

3. ULTRASTRUCTURE OF PREANTRAL AND ANTRAL FOLLICLES

Adult buffalo ovaries have an average of less than 20 thousand preantral follicles [10]. The main modifications in the ultrastructure of preantral follicles begin with an enlargement from primordial to secondary follicles (35.0 ± 3.1 μm to 53.3 ± 12.0 μm, respectively), accomplished by an oocyte growth from 24.9 ± 3.7 μm to 29.4 ± 5.4 μm, respectively [11]. Additionally, there is an increase in the number of organelles, such as mitochondria (predominantly round-shaped), smooth and rough endoplasm reticulum, and also vesicles showing coalescence along this process. Until the primary stage, the zona pellucida cannot be seen (and after that, it is only partially developed in patches), and the oocyte and granulosa cells appear only juxtaposed. From this stage, oolemma projects into adjacent granulosa cells, which acquires a cubical form in secondary follicles [11].

With regard to antral follicles, there is a change in the organization of structures according to follicle development from 1 to 10 mm. The perivitelline space is initially formed and can be seen in 2 mm follicles and its growth is concluded in 10 mm follicles, when numerous oocyte microvilli can be found in it. The nucleus of oocyte is periferically located, and a well-developed smooth endoplasmic reticulum and Golgi apparatus can be seen in the perinuclear region. There is an increase in the proportion of pleomorphic mitochondria, instead of rounded-shape ones, reaching a peripherical location in the oolemma. Also, cortical granules (located in clusters) can be visualized in this area, increasing in number and size. Inversely, a medullar position is taken by lipid vacuoles, which increase in number and size, and coalesce as follicular growth occurs [11].

According to Mondadori *et al.* [10, 11], some of these differences such as cytoplasmic vesicles quantity, mitochondria shape and inner content, zona pellucida deposition, and granulosa cells–oocyte junctions are species-specific, and maybe responsible for some functional differences observed in *Bubalus bubalis in vitro* embryo production and follicular dynamics, when compared to *Bos taurus* or *Bos indicus* species.

4. FOLLICULAR DYNAMICS

In order to implement new reproductive technologies in the buffalo species, it is mandatory to have a thorough comprehension of follicular dynamics, so that, consequently the effectiveness of protocols used for the manipulation of the estrous cycle can be enhanced [12].

Buffaloes and cattle share a similar ovarian follicular dynamics, and although the 2-wave cycle is recorded as the most common in the buffalo species (63.3%), also 1- and 3-wave cycle can be reported [12], (Fig. **1**). Heifer and multiparous buffaloes were compared by Presicce *et al.* [13], reporting for heifers a similar number of 1- to 2-wave cycles together with some 3-wave cycles. On the contrary, adult buffaloes displayed only the 2-wave pattern. The number of waves in a cycle is typically associated to the number of days characterizing the luteal phase (10.4 ± 2.1 d *vs.* 12.7 ± 2.9 d, in 2- or 3-wave cycles, respectively) and to the estrous cycle length (22.3 ± 0.9 d *vs.* 24.5 ± 1.9 d, respectively [12].

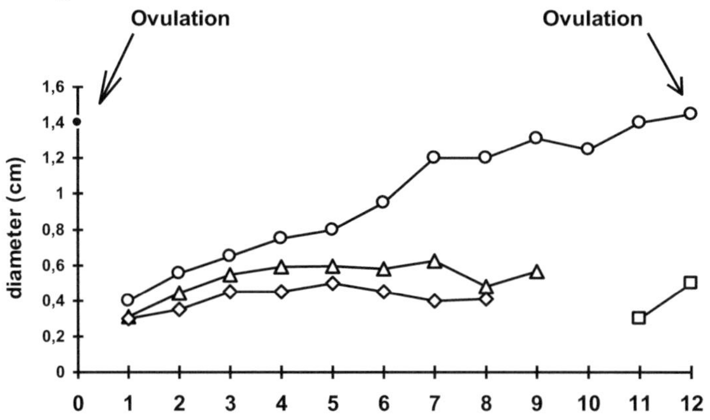

Fig. 1 contd.....

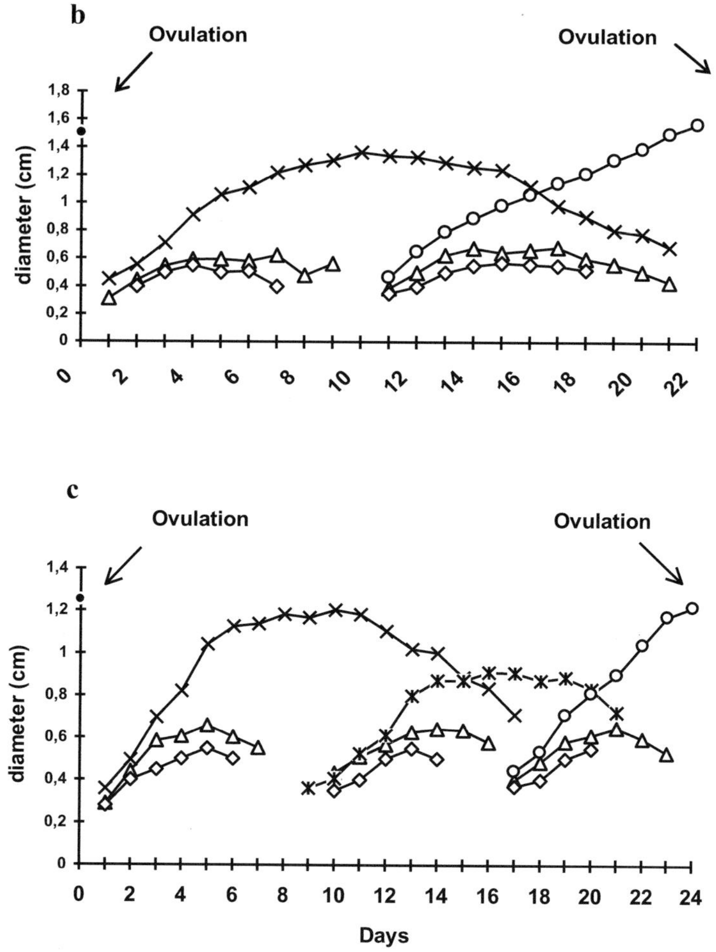

Fig. (1). Patterns of follicular wave development during buffalo cows estrous cycle. a) one wave (n=1), b) two wave (n=19), and c) three wave cycles (n=10) [12].

Some important differences in follicular dynamics can be outlined in buffaloes and compared to cattle (*Bos taurus* and *Bos indicus*), the first of which is related to the number of follicles recruited per wave, which is lower in buffalo [9]. In addition, the number of recruited follicles among buffaloes per each of the different waves shows a low variation [12], in accordance to the high repeatability of this physiological parameter [14], suggesting also that recruitment of follicles is strictly dependent on the individual, although the hereditability of such character in buffaloes has not yet been investigated. Nevertheless, such individual variability allows us to select animals before the implementation of reproductive technologies, *i.e.* superovulation treatment, due to the positive correlation reported between the number of small antral follicles and the superovulation response [15]. In line with the above represented correlation, Misra [16] reported a better response to hormonal administration in selected donors that responded to previous superovulation protocols with 4 or more ovulations.

The maximum diameter reached by the dominant follicle in each follicular wave is also an element of difference in buffaloes, considering that it varies from 11.1 to 15.5 with the number of follicular waves occurring within the animal [12, 13, 17]. These recorded diameters seem to be intermediate values between *Bos indicus* and *Bos taurus*. Different genetic groups in cattle account for the variation found in follicle diameters, being smaller in *Bos indicus* (10 to 12 mm [18 - 20]; than in *Bos taurus* (15 to 20 mm [18, 21, 22]. Furthermore, follicular diameter can also be dependent on age and reproductive status of the animals. In fact, in a study by Presicce *et al.* [13], a lower growth rate and a smaller diameter of the dominant follicle was recorded in heifers when compared to adult multiparous buffaloes. Such difference was evident for both the first follicular wave (1.3 mm *vs.* 1.7 mm/ day, and 10.5 mm *vs* 13.3 mm, respectively) and the second follicular wave (1.0 mm *vs.* 1.3 mm/ day, and 11.0 mm *vs* 13.8 mm).

In a recent trial [23], the diameter reached by dominant (DF) and subordinate follicles (SF) at follicle deviation in buffaloes, were reported following ultrasound monitoring (Fig. **2**), with follicle selection occurring 2.6 d after ovulation, similarly to *Bos taurus* [24, 25] and to *Bos indicus* [26, 27]. However, the average size of DF and SF in buffaloes at the time of deviation are larger (7.2 mm and 6.4 mm, respectively), when compared to *Bos indicus* (6.2 mm and 5.8 mm, respectively) [27] but smaller than *Bos taurus* (8.5 mm and 7.2 mm, respectively) [25].

As previously outlined, some specific features in buffalo folliculogenesis can explain the reported outcomes obtained when biotechnologies are implemented in this species, and also justify the need to modify some procedures currently and efficiently used in cattle. Swamp buffaloes, likewise their riverine counterpart, are also characterized by a reduced reproductive efficiency affected by the duration of day length, with a low breeding season from April to July characterized by reduced or absent estrus cycles, and a higher reproductive performance from November to January. Follicular dynamics in swamp buffaloes has been studied by Yindee *et al.* [28], starting postpartum until the 4th ovulation reporting a typical development of 1- and 2-wave cycles. In this sub-species and within cycles characterized by one wave of follicle development, emergence has been recorded on day 2.3±0.5 and 1.8±0.4 during the low and high breeding season, respectively ($P > 0.05$).

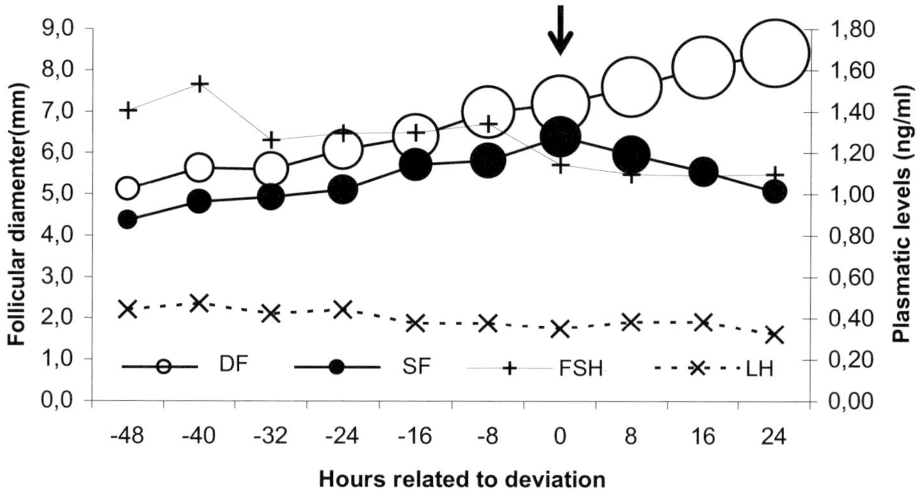

Fig. (2). Diameter (mean ± SEM) of dominant (DF) and largest subordinate (SF) follicles, and profiles of FSH and LH normalized to the day of observed deviation in 10 Murrah buffalo heifers. The arrow indicates the beginning of deviation (Gimenes *et al.* [23]).

Day of the estrous cycle when the largest size attained by the dominant follicle was reported was 13.5±1.2 and 12.6±1.5, respectively ($P > 0.05$). The largest size (mm) attained by the dominant follicle during the low breeding and high season was 14.5±2.1 and 16.4±2.7, respectively ($p>0.05$). In the course of the low breeding season, the first and second wave within cycles characterized by two waves of follicle development, emerged on day 1.2±0.3 and on day 11.4±0.8, respectively, and largest diameter of second wave dominant follicle (10.3±1.2 mm) was recorded on day 19.7±1.1. Differently, in the course of the high breeding season, the first and second wave emerged on day 0.9±0.4 and on day 10.7±0.9, respectively and the largest diameter of second wave dominant follicle (12.8±1.2 mm) was recorded on day 18.9±1.7.

5. BREEDING SEASON

The difference in reproductive performances of buffaloes with regard to the different seasons has to be taken into account, before working on any reproductive strategy within buffalo herds. In fact, buffaloes tend to display a typical differential reproductive behavior according to season, when they are found far from the equatorial line. Under such circumstances, animals perform better, from a reproductive standpoint, in the course of the year characterized by decreasing light hours [29]. Therefore, these animals are considered as short-day breeders, likewise goat and sheep. This species-specific characteristic has been previously described [30 - 32], and confirmed in a study performed with 16,487 calvings of three different breeds (Jafarabadi, n=1,771; Murrah, n=10,824 and Mediterranean, n=3,831), reared in 17 different states in Brazil, and assigned to 4 different groups according to the latitude where they were bred [33] (Fig. **3**). Results from this study give indication of a high influence of latitude on calving distribution throughout the year. In fact, the greater the latitude, the higher was the calving concentration between January and March (0° to 8°=36.4%^{a}; 8° to 16°=41.0%^{b}; 16° to 24°=62.4%^{c}; 24° to 32°=72.3%^{d}). In some countries like Italy, the highest peak of reproductive efficiency among animals and consequentially the concentration of calving and milk production, does not match the time of highest demand for milk from the market for milk processing and cheese production. Such contrast has generated the need for steering the concentration of calving, with the period of the year where milk is mostly requested by the milk industry [29]. The need to parallel milk production with market request, has generated the development and implementation of the out-of-breeding-season-mating (OBSM) technique, where bulls are included or removed from the herd according to the months of the year [29]. Similarly, in those buffalo farms where natural mating is not the only option available, AI and other reproductive technologies can be employed with reasonably good results in the period of the year (non breeding season) ordinarily considered unfavourable for a satisfactory reproductive efficiency [34].

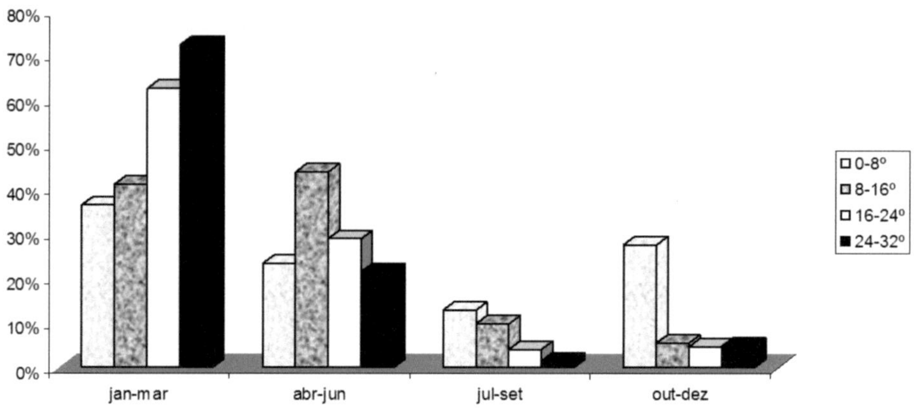

Fig. (3). Latitude and calving distribution in buffaloes during the year (n=16,487 [33]).

6. FIXED TIME ARTIFICIAL INSEMINATION (FTAI)

In cattle, artificial insemination has been the first reproductive technique successfully and widely adopted in the all world, within breeding programs. The implementation of this reproductive technique in the buffalo species has been hampered over the years by some species-specific difficulties such as the identification of estrus and the optimal time for artificial insemination. In fact, the wide acceptance in the use of artificial insemination among farmers has been impaired mostly by the failure in detecting estrus.

Therefore, the use of protocols that instead of requiring the identification of estrus, will focus on a more timely approach of artificial insemination to the event of ovulation, will contribute to expand the use and the optimization of artificial insemination itself in buffalo herds.

Synchronization of Ovulation using GnRH and Prostaglandins for FTAI

A number of trials carried out using the Ovsynch protocol in cattle have shown some efficiency in synchronizing ovulation, and have resulted in satisfactory pregnancy rates, without the need of estrus detection [35]. The same protocol has also been tested in buffaloes in various field studies [36 - 40], characterized by a hormonal treatment consisting of GnRH and prostaglandin (Fig. **4**). In such trials, an adequate response to the hormonal treatment was verified, starting with the emergence of a new follicular wave following ovulation of the dominant follicle at the time of the first GnRH. Under an optimal response to the treatment, on day 7, buffaloes will respond to PGF2α administration by CL demise (luteolysis), so that at day 9 most animal (around 80%) will respond with a synchronized ovulation within 12 hours. By employing such protocol, in cycling buffaloes a pregnancy rate (PR) of about 50% can be obtained during the breeding season. In addition, PR has been found to be influenced by body condition score (BCS of 3.5 correlated to higher pregnancy rates on a 1 to 5 scale), parity (lower PR in primiparous animals), and period of year (lower PR in the course of the off-breeding season).

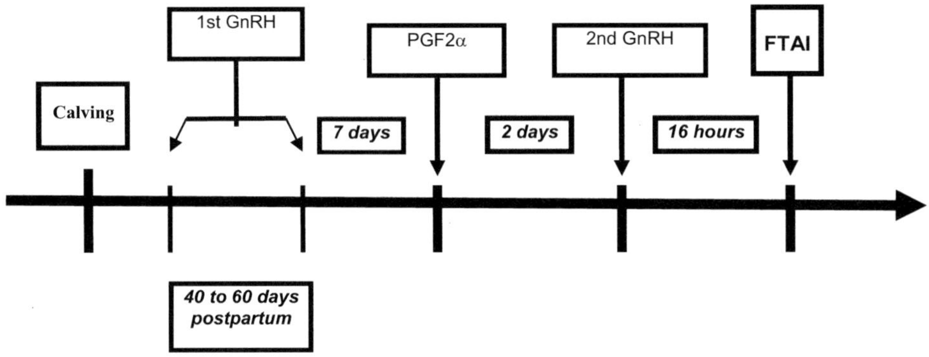

Fig. (4). FTAI protocol during the breeding season in buffalo.

Synchronization of Ovulation using Progesterone and/or Progestin Plus Estradiol

From the results available following use of the Ovsynch protocol in buffaloes, a higher efficiency can be observed from its application in breeding programs in the course of the breeding season (autumn and winter) in cycling buffaloes. A significantly lower efficiency in terms of PR, following adoption of the Ovsynch protocol can be seen in the course of the off-breeding season (spring and summer), especially in anestrous buffaloes, with rates ranging from 6.9 to 28.2% [37, 41]. These outcomes are very likely dependent on seasonal anestrus, where most buffalos will still be reported with some growth of small and medium size follicles, without ever reaching a critical size for ovulation [42]. Several studies have been carried out in order to establish an appropriate protocol for this period [39 - 41, 43 - 49].

The combined use of progesterone / progestin and estradiol at day 0 (beginning of the protocol) has been shown to be effective in inducing the emergence of a new follicular wave, interrupting both FSH and LH secretion and ushering the beginning of a new follicular wave within the ovary [50]. An increase in LH pulse frequency during and following the treatment period, consisting of progesterone administration, have been reported in studies performed in postpartum anestrous cows [51]. When compared to control animals, the treatment with progesterone of anestrous animals will result in a greater amount of follicular fluid and higher concentration of circulating estradiol, together with an increased pulsatile release of LH and increased numbers of receptors for LH in granulosa and theca cells in preovulatory follicles [52]. In addition, in the course of an anestrous period, estrus expression and follow-up physiological luteal activity are positively affected by a brief elevated progesterone level following exogenous administration [53]. According to implemented protocols, the progesterone device is removed on day 9, and to decrease blood progesterone levels and to enhance the quality of follicular growth, both PGF and eCG are administered to the animal. The above mentioned elements of follicle quality and optimal hormonal milieu, are usually compromised during the off-breeding season in non cycling buffaloes.

This is confirmed by the evidence derived from other studies, where reproductive efficiency in anestrous buffaloes was improved by the exogenous administration of eCG [54]. Additionally, in buffaloes subjected to FTAI (Figs. **5** and **6**), both CL diameter and blood progesterone level increased at diestrus (Carvalho *et al.*, 2009 unpublished data). This is in agreement with a well established concept in cattle undergoing FTAI programs, according to which the larger the CL, the higher is the secretion of progesterone, which in turn positively affects the recognition and establishment of pregnancy [55]. In Fig. (**7**), a description of the protocol mentioned above during the off-breeding season, is shown.

When adopting this protocol and following first AI, approximately 50% of pregnancies are expected in anestrous buffaloes without the need for estrus detection, around the year. A similar study by De Rensis *et al.* [40], on the use of progestin (PRID) and PMSG on non-cyclic pluriparous buffaloes in the off-breeding season, reported a higher pregnancy rate (70.5%) when compared to FTAI (Ovsynch) on cyclic nulliparous (40%) and pluriparous buffaloes (42.8%).

The strategy of breeding buffaloes during the off-breeding season is economically important, in order to meet the market demand for milk products.

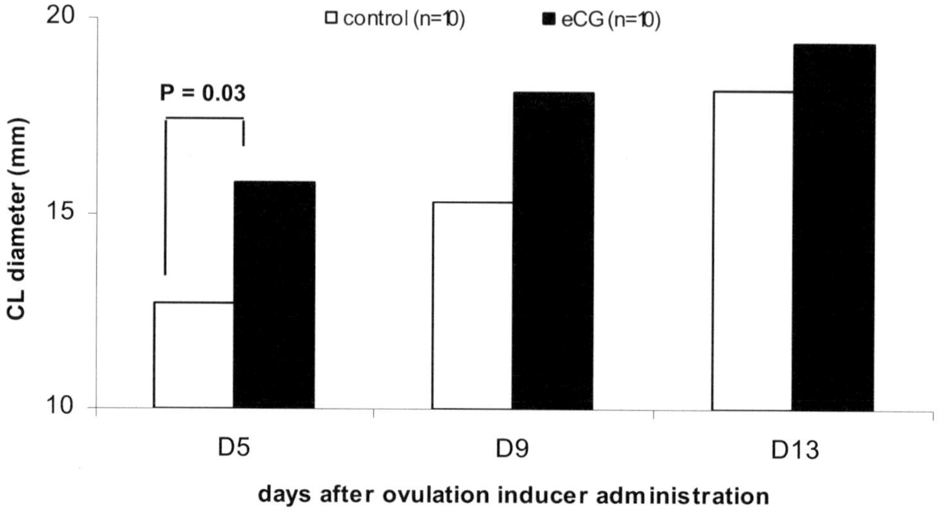

Fig. (5). CL diameter in buffaloes following synchronization protocol, characterized by eCG administration or not, at removal of progesterone device removal (Carvalho *et al.*, 2009 – unpublished data).

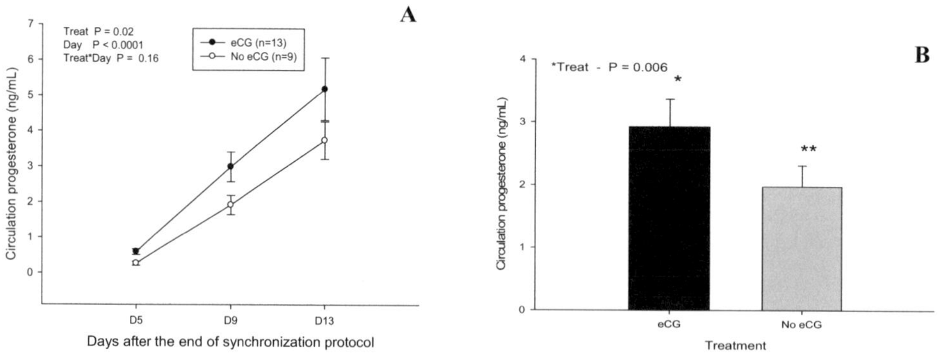

Fig. (6). eCG *vs.* no-eCG treatment in buffaloes and related serum progesterone levels (ng/ mL) **(A)**: Progesterone profile after of the synchronization protocol, and P values for treatment (Treat), day, and interaction treatment x day. **(B)**: main effect of treatment (Carvalho *et al.*, 2009 – unpublished data).

7. SUPEROVULATION (SO) AND EMBRYO TRANSFER (ET)

The adoption of multiple ovulation protocols and the recovery of embryos, allows breeders to reach and harvest the highest number of elite embryos for later transfer, enhancing thus the reproductive efficiency of their herds and consequently their genetic potential [56]. Following few decades of attempts at improving the efficiency of superovulation protocols and production of an acceptable number of good quality embryos after non surgical recovery, we are faced today with an undifferentiated level of production and expectancy. Usually, a lower rate of embryo recovery is in fact expected and reported in buffaloes, when compared to their cattle counterpart. It is true that in buffaloes, the adoption of MOET programs brings more difficulties linked to several aspects which are intrinsic to the species, such as the detection of estrus in recipients, a good donor to recipient synchronization and lastly but not less important, a functional CL at the time of embryo transfer [16]. Collectively, the above mentioned aspects contribute to a poorer embryo recovery rate in buffaloes, in comparison to cattle. Drost *et al.*, were the first to report the birth of a buffalo calf, following embryo recovery and transfer [57]. Only recently some new information on folliculogenesis in the buffalo species has been made available, and still a paucity of information exists with regard to intraovarian changes following hormonal administration. For an embryo transfer program to be successful, some elements of importance have to be taken into account in order to understand what to expect from this reproductive technology, such as an adequate response in terms of follicle development, subsequent ovulation rate and development of functional CLs. Buffalo embryos are characterized by a faster pre-implantation development, allowing thus the possibility to recover and transfer them as early as day 5 or 6 following estrus, when the CL is still young and growing [58], and difficult to detect by palpation per rectum, unless an ultrasound scanning is performed on the animal. Misra *et al.* [59], have reported so far some of the best results following MOET implementation in buffaloes. In this study 16 buffaloes, selected from their response to previous superovulation programs, were subjected to a new superovulation protocol by administering a total of 600 mg of FSH in decreasing doses in the course of five consecutive days. Each donor produced 4.37 embryos, of which 3.13 were transferable. However, this average number of produced embryos remains still lower when compared to the mean recovered embryos in cattle per each donor (10 total and 6 transferable [60]). Superovulation protocols have been extensively studied and tried on buffaloes in Brazil [12, 61 - 63]. Along with those trials, although a good response in terms of follicle development was reported with a mean number of 15 follicles > 8 mm per donor, only a moderate ovulation rate (approximately 60%), a corresponding CL development (approximately 9 CLs per donor) and a low recovery of produced embryos (34.8%), followed. Similar outcome following MOET programs in buffaloes have been reported by other authors [16, 29, 64 - 67].

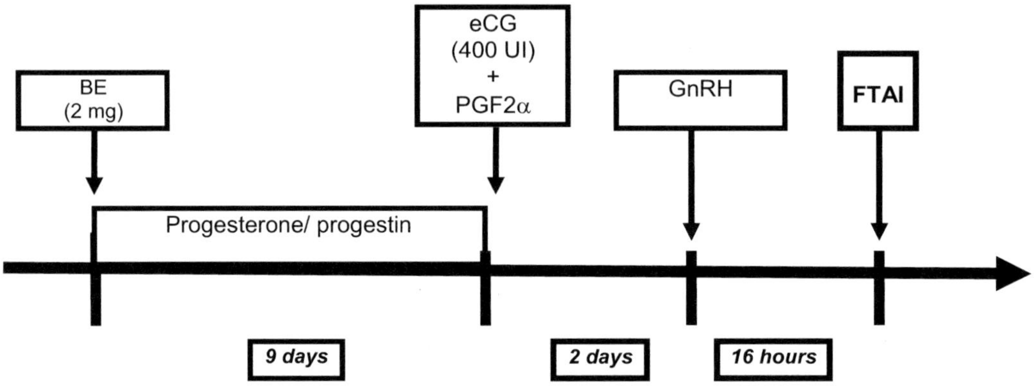

Fig. (7). FTAI protocol during the off-breeding season in buffaloes.

Collectively, it can be stated that the rate of embryo recovery in the buffalo species (around 20 to 40%) is significantly lower when confronted to cattle (63 to 80% [60, 68 - 70];). Possibly, a disturbance in the physiological mechanisms regulating oocyte entry in the oviduct following ovulation and/or its transport along the oviduct, have been hypothesized in order to explain such differential outcome between the two species [63]. The mechanism regulating oocyte transport in the oviduct are under ovarian steroids control (Hunter [71]), and such hormonal imbalances could also be the root of a disturbed uterine environment, linked also to poor embryo quality and embryo loss [60]. Such reduced efficiency in terms of embryo recovery, as suggested by Misra *et al.* [72], could possibly be linked to high estrogen levels in the course of hormonal treatment. In fact, it is possible that both oviductal and /or intrauterine environments may be modified by a prolonged exposure to continuous elevated concentrations of estrogen, and consequently affect a normal embryonic development. In addition, high 17β-estradiol levels typically recorded in the course of superstimolatory treatments, may negatively affect more buffaloes than cattle, due to a higher sensitivity of the former species [73]. Starting from this assumption, some experiments have been conducted where exogenous progesterone or deslorelin bioimplants have been employed, with the goal to lower levels of estradiol as a result of hormonal stimulation [74, 75]. However, even under such experimental circumstances, no increase in embryo recovery rate was observed. On the same line of investigation, several trials were conducted to investigate the existing anatomical and physiological relationship between ovarian steroids and the genital system in both cattle and buffaloes [3]. A detailed morphometry study in females characterized by either single or multiple ovulations, was conducted, and a comparison on oviductal ciliar movement exposed or not to estradiol in culture, was also investigated. From the above studies, it appears that neither embryo recovery nor oviductal ciliar movements are affected by estradiol, although some differences with the cattle counterpart have been evidenced, such as a higher number of an ovulatory follicles, a more rigid ovary to mesovarium connection and finally a thicker infundibulum muscle layer. All these aspects could be accountable for a lower embryo recovery rate in the buffalo species. Some studies have proved that oocyte quality in buffaloes, possibly associated to a fragile connection to granulosa cells, could be improved through a direct and/or indirect IGF-1 effect, under rbST treatment [76, 77]. The same treatment with rbST could contribute to improve embryo recovery in buffaloes following superovulation protocols, through stimulation of cumulus cell expansion [78, 79], which in turn may be responsible for enhanced oocyte adhesion to both fimbria and ciliated cells of the oviducts. In line with the above mentioned, other studies were conducted to further investigate the details of rbST effects, such as the dose employed (0, 250, or 500 mg) and its effect on hormonal treatment for superovulation [80, 81]. Controversial results have been reported as, in the first study, an increase in embryo recovery when compared to control group was reported following use of 500 mg of rbST, differently from a follow-up trial where no significant difference was observed. An increase in total number of follicles and derived CLs, together with transferable and freezable embryos was, on the contrary, reported in buffaloes when rbST was administered at a dose of 250 mg. Collectively, it can be stated that, despite the encountered intrinsic species-specific difficulties when MOET programs are applied to buffaloes and leading to reduced embryo recovery, the birth of buffalo calves following superovulation protocols have been reported, even with frozen-thawed embryos [61, 82]. This highlights the feasibility of this reproductive technology, although not yet fully commercially exploitable.

8. OVUM PICK-UP (OPU) AND *IN VITRO* EMBRYO PRODUCTION (IVEP)

The coupling of some reproductive technologies such as ovum pick-up (OPU) and *in vitro* embryo production (IVP) has already been proved feasible to a good degree of efficiency in cattle [83]. In buffaloes on the contrary, on account of several studies previously performed [84 - 89], efficiency in blastocyst production is still low, varying between 9.5% to 30.0% [88, 90 - 92]. A lower oocyte recovery from antral follicles, reduced oocyte quality, as only approximately 30% of recovered oocytes are classified as viable by Campanile *et al.* [89], and reduced embryo quality, are the main biological factors which seem to be strongly related to such inefficiency. The use of rbST in buffaloes was also tested in the course of an OPU-IVP program, aiming at improving oocyte recovery and quality [91]. OPU was performed twice a week, for a total of 10 sessions, in both control and rbST (500 mg) groups. A higher number of punctured antral follicles (12.2 ± 0.1 *vs* 8.7 ± 0.04, respectively) and retrieved oocytes (5.2 ± 0.5 *vs.* and 4.1 ± 0.5, respectively) was reported in animals treated with rbST when compared to control group.

Differently, embryo production (blastocyst rate) following *in vitro* procedures did not result in any significant difference between treatment and control animals 19.7% and 26.0%, respectively. The interval between consecutive OPU sessions (once a week or every 14 days) and rbST treatment (control or treated with 500 mg of rbST), was investigated by Ferraz *et al.* [93]. Administration of rbST increased the number of punctured follicles, although the number of blastocysts was significantly reduced on day 7 (Fig. **8A**). Number of aspirated antral follicles and total number of recovered total and viable oocytes, were reduced when OPU was performed once a week (Fig. **8B**).

Recently, the three species represented by buffaloes (*Bubalus bubalis*), Nelore (*Bos indicus*) and Holstein (*Bos taurus*) heifers, kept under similar conditions of management and nutrition, were the object of a comparison regarding the effect of synchronization of follicular wave emergence in an OPU-IVP setting [92]. The stage of the estrous cycle is a factor of paramount importance that dictates both the quantity and quality of retrieved oocytes within each OPU session, and consequently the embryo development following implementation of IVEP procedures [94 - 98]. In addition it has been established in *Bos taurus*, that oocytes recovered from follicles characterized by a slight degree of atresia, require a reduced time for maturation and give a higher rate of embryo development following IVEP [95, 98, 99]. In the same study by Gimenes *et al.* [92], the genetic make-up of the three different species under investigation did not affect their interaction nor the time of synchronization, when the animals were synchronized for follicle aspiration 1, 3 or 5 days following wave emergence.

In Table **1**, differences among the three species are summarized, and the results from that study [92] are conducive to a lower overall embryo production efficiency for both buffaloes and cattle, when compared to the Nelore genetic group.

Table 1. Effect of genetic group (Nelore/*Bos indicus*, Holstein /*Bos taurus* and Buffalo/*Bubalus bubalis*) on OPU-IVEP [92].

	Nelore (n=9)	**Holstein (n=9)**	**Buffalo (n=9)**
Mean of visualized follicles	$41.0^{a} \pm 2.1$	$22.1^{b} \pm 1.3$	$18.8^{b} \pm 0.9$
Mean of total oocytes	$37.1^{a} \pm 2.5$	$15.4^{b} \pm 1.2$	$14.8^{b} \pm 1.0$
Recovery rate (%)	89.4^{a}	73.3^{b}	82.8^{ab}
Mean of viable oocytes	$30.8^{a} \pm 2.4$	$10.7^{b} \pm 1.0$	$7.9^{b} \pm 0.7$
Mean structures on *in vitro* culture	$18.7^{a} \pm 0.8$	$8.0^{b} \pm 0.5$	$7.5^{b} \pm 0.4$
Mean of cleaved structures	$15.4^{a} \pm 0.7$	$4.6^{b} \pm 0.4$	$4.4^{b} \pm 0.3$
Cleavage rate (%)	81.8^{a}	59.1^{b}	62.3^{b}
Mean of blastocysts on D7	$5.1^{a} \pm 0.6$	$1.0^{b} \pm 0.2$	$0.6^{b} \pm 0.1$
Blastocyst rate (%)	25.8^{a}	13.6^{b}	9.1^{b}
Mean of hatched blastocysts	$2.6^{a} \pm 0.4$	$0.3^{b} \pm 0.1$	$0.3^{b} \pm 0.1$
Hatching rate (%)	50.6^{a}	23.2^{b}	31.9^{ab}

a ≠ b: superscript letters in the same row differ ($P<0.05$).

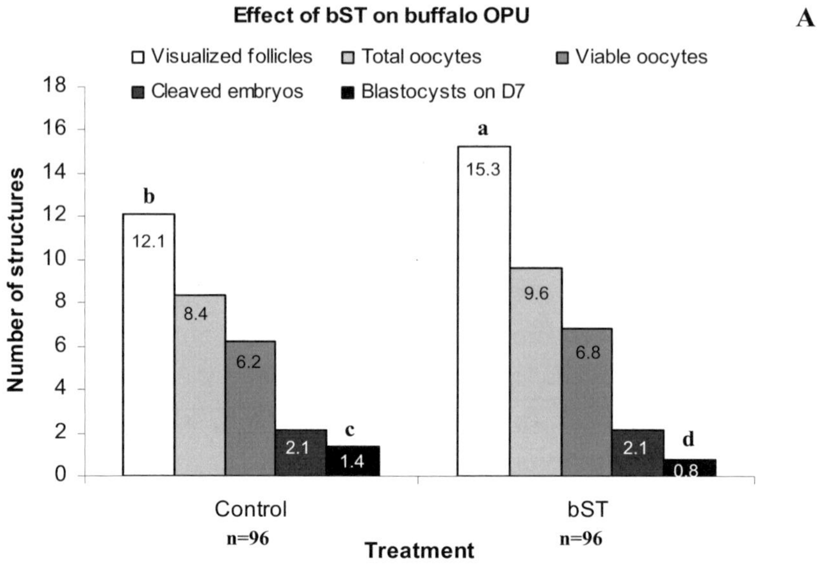

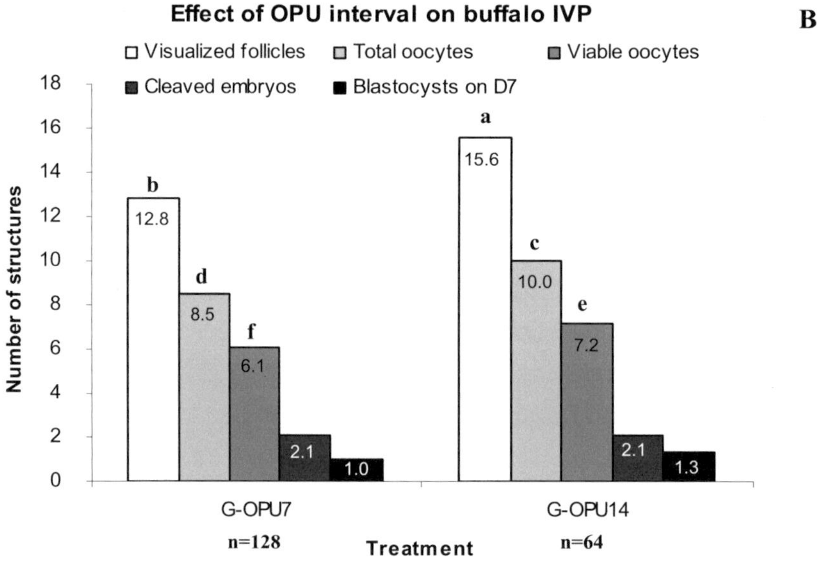

Fig. (8). **(A)** Main effects of treatment (control or 500 mg of bST; **(B)** OPU interval (G-OPU7 – OPU each 7 days or G-OPU14 – OPU each 14 days; Ferraz *et al.*, 2007). a≠b, c≠d, e≠f ($P < 0.05$).

As a result of IVEP procedure and fixed-time-embryo-transfer (FTET) in synchronized recipients by Ovsynch protocol, a pregnancy rate of 14.3% (1/7) following transfer of fresh embryos, and 8.0% (2/25) following transfer of vitrified embryos, were reported. The association of OPU-IVP resulted in the first birth of buffalo calves in the Americas from two vitrified embryos [91].

From the studies and trials reported in this review, it is evident that the coupling of both OPU and IVEP procedures is a feasible one, although further studies are still needed to develop strategies that improve embryo production in buffaloes, in an attempt to facilitate the commercial use of this biotechnology.

CONFLICT OF INTEREST

The authors confirm that they have no conflict of interest to declare for this publication.

ACKNOWLEDGEMENTS

Declared none.

REFERENCES

[1] Food and Agriculture Organization – FAO. FAOstat: FAO statistics division. disponível em: http://faostat.fao.org/site/569 Acesso em: 01/09/2009

[2] Santos SS, Biondi FC, Cordeiro MS, *et al.* Isolation, follicular density, and culture of preantral follicles of buffalo fetuses of different ages. Anim Reprod Sci 2006; 95(1-2): 1-15. [http://dx.doi.org/10.1016/j.anireprosci.2005.08.012] [PMID: 16631327]

[3] Carvalho NA. Avaliação anatomofuncional do sistema genital de fêmeas bubalinas (Bubalus bubalis), e suas implicações na múltipla ovulação e transferência de embriões Tese (Doutorado em reprodução animal) - Faculdade de Medicina Veterinária e Zootecnia. São Paulo: Universidade de São Paulo 2006.

[4] Danell B. Oestrous behaviour, ovarian morphology and cyclical variation in follicular system and endocrine pattern in water buffalo heifers 1987.

[5] Manik RS, Palta P, Singla SK, Sharma V. Folliculogenesis in buffalo (*Bubalus bubalis*): a review. Reprod Fertil Dev 2002; 14(5-6): 315-25. [http://dx.doi.org/10.1071/RD01126] [PMID: 12467356]

[6] Le Van TY, Chupin D, Driancourt DA. Ovarian follicular population in buffaloes and cows. Anim Reprod Sci 1989; 19: 171-8. [http://dx.doi.org/10.1016/0378-4320(89)90090-0]

[7] Presicce GA, Parmeggiani A, Senatore EM, *et al.* Hormonal dynamics and follicular turnover in prepuberal Mediterranean Italian buffaloes (*Bubalus bubalis*). Theriogenology 2003; 60(3): 485-93. [http://dx.doi.org/10.1016/S0093-691X(03)00034-7] [PMID: 12763162]

[8] Evans AC, Adams GP, Rawlings NC. Follicular and hormonal development in prepubertal heifers from 2 to 36 weeks of age. J Reprod Fertil 1994; 102(2): 463-70.

[http://dx.doi.org/10.1530/jrf.0.1020463] [PMID: 7861402]

[9] Gimenes LU, Fantinato Neto P, Arango JS, Ayres H, Baruselli PS. Follicular dynamics of *Bos indicus, Bos taurus* and *Bubalus bubalis* heifers treated with norgestomet ear implant associated or not to injectable progesterone. Anim Reprod 2009; 6: 256.

[10] Mondadori RG, Santin TR, Fidelis AAG, Porfirio EP, Bao SN. Buffalo (*Bubalus bubalis*) pre-antral follicle population and ultrastructural characterization of antral follicle oocyte. Reprod Dom Anim 2010; 45(1): 33-7.

[11] Mondadori RG, Luque MC, Santin TR, Báo SN. Ultrastructural and morphometric characterization of buffalo (*Bubalus bubalis*) ovarian preantral follicles. Anim Reprod Sci 2007; 97(3-4): 323-33. [http://dx.doi.org/10.1016/j.anireprosci.2006.02.010] [PMID: 16580155]

[12] Baruselli PS, Mucciolo RG, Visintin JA, *et al.* Ovarian follicular dynamics during the estrous cycle in buffalo (*Bubalus bubalis*). Theriogenology 1997; 47(8): 1531-47. [http://dx.doi.org/10.1016/S0093-691X(97)00159-3] [PMID: 16728096]

[13] Presicce GA, Senatore EM, Bella A, *et al.* Ovarian follicular dynamics and hormonal profiles in heifer and mixed-parity Mediterranean Italian buffaloes (*Bubalus bubalis*) following an estrus synchronization protocol. Theriogenology 2004; 61(7-8): 1343-55. [http://dx.doi.org/10.1016/j.theriogenology.2003.08.013] [PMID: 15036967]

[14] Boni R, Roelofsen VM, Pieterse M, Wurth Y, Kruip TH. Follicular recruitment after repeated removal of all follicles ≥ 2 mm in bovine ovary. J Reprod Fertil 1993; 12: 1993.

[15] Romero A, Albert J, Brink Z, Seidel GE Jr. Numbers of small follicles in ovaries affect superovulation response in cattle. Theriogenology 1991; 35: 265. [http://dx.doi.org/10.1016/0093-691X(91)90241-5]

[16] Misra AK. Superovulation and embryo transfer in buffalo; process, problems and future prospects in India. Buffalo J 1993; 1: 13-24.

[17] Manik RS, Madan ML, Singla SK. Ovarian follicular dynamics in water buffaloes (*Bubalus bubalis*): ultrasonically monitoring individual follicles for wave hypothesis. Theriogenology 1994; 41: 247. [http://dx.doi.org/10.1016/S0093-691X(05)80156-6]

[18] Bo GA, Martinez M, Nasser LF, Caccia M, Tribulo H, Mapletoft RJ. Follicular dynamics in bos indicus and bos taurus beef cattle under pasture conditions in Argentina. Proceedings Congresso Brasileiro de Reprodução Animal. Campo Grande. 1993.

[19] Figueiredo RA, Barros CM, Pinheiro OL, Soler JM. Ovarian follicular dynamics in Nelore breed (*Bos indicus*) cattle. Theriogenology 1997; 47(8): 1489-505. [http://dx.doi.org/10.1016/S0093-691X(97)00156-8] [PMID: 16728093]

[20] Rhodes FM, Death G, Entwhistle KW. Animal and temporal effects on ovarian follicular dynamics in Brahman heifers. Anim Reprod Sci 1995; 38: 265-77. [http://dx.doi.org/10.1016/0378-4320(94)01375-V]

[21] Ginther OJ, Kastelic JP, Knopf L. Composition and characteristics of follicular waves during the bovine estrus cycle. Anim Reprod Sci 1989; 20: 187-200. a [http://dx.doi.org/10.1016/0378-4320(89)90084-5]

[22] Kastelic JP, Knopf L, Ginther OJ. Effect of day of postaglandin F2α treatment on selection and development of the ovulatory follicle in heifers. Anim Reprod Sci 1990; 23: 169-80. [http://dx.doi.org/10.1016/0378-4320(90)90001-V]

[23] Gimenes LU, Carvalho NA, Sa Filho MF, Torres J. JRS, Ayres H, Vannucci FS, Bianconi LL, Bisinotto RS, Reichert RH, Beltran MP, Nogueira GP, Baruselli PS. Follicle selection by ultrasonography and plasmatic characteristics and ovulatory capacity in buffaloes. Ital J Anim Sci 2007; 6: 629-31. [http://dx.doi.org/10.4081/ijas.2007.s2.629]

[24] Ginther OJ, Knopf L, Kastelic JP. Temporal associations among ovarian events in cattle during oestrous cycles with two and three follicular waves. J Reprod Fertil 1989; 87(1): 223-30. b [http://dx.doi.org/10.1530/jrf.0.0870223] [PMID: 2621698]

[25] Ginther OJ, Wiltbank MC, Fricke PM, Gibbons JR, Kot K. Selection of the dominant follicle in cattle. Biol Reprod 1996; 55(6): 1187-94. [http://dx.doi.org/10.1095/biolreprod55.6.1187] [PMID: 8949873]

[26] Sartorelli ES, Carvalho LM, Bergfelt DR, Ginther OJ, Barros CM. Morphological characterization of follicle deviation in Nelore (*Bos indicus*) heifers and cows. Theriogenology 2005; 63(9): 2382-94. [http://dx.doi.org/10.1016/j.theriogenology.2004.08.017] [PMID: 15910921]

[27] Gimenes LU, Sá Filho MF, Carvalho NA, *et al.* Follicle deviation and ovulatory capacity in *Bos indicus* heifers. Theriogenology 2008; 69(7): 852-8. [http://dx.doi.org/10.1016/j.theriogenology.2008.01.001] [PMID: 18316116]

[28] Yindee M, Techakumphu M, Lohachit C, *et al.* Follicular dynamics and oestrous detection in Thai postpartum swamp buffaloes (*Bubalus bubalis*). Reprod Domest Anim 2011; 46(1): e91-6. [http://dx.doi.org/10.1111/j.1439-0531.2010.01647.x] [PMID: 20546176]

[29] Zicarelli L. Reproductive seasonality in buffalo. 1997.

[30] Abhi HL, Nagpal NP, Sharma TL, Grewal AS. A study of the breeding behaviour of *Murrah* buffaloes and their breeding efficiency through artificial insemination under farm conditions. Indian J Dairy Sci 1973; 26: 107-13.

[31] Rao BR, Patel UG, Tamhan SS. Studies on the reproductive behavior of Surti buffaloes. I. Oestrous cycle. Indian Vet J 1973; 50: 257-64.

[32] Obi-Reddy A, Tripathi VN, Raina VS. Effect of climate on the incidence of oestrus and conception rate in Murrah buffaloes. Indian J Anim Sci 1987; 57: 204-7.

[33] Baruselli PS, Bernardes O, Barufi FB, Braga D, Araujo D, Tonhati H. Calving distribution throughout the year in buffalo raised all over Brazil. In: Proc.World Buffalo Congress, 6., Maracaibo. The buffalo an alternative for animal agriculture in the third millenium; 2001; pp. 1: 234-40.

[34] Presicce GA. Reproduction in the water buffalo. Reprod Domest Anim 2007; 42 (Suppl. 2): 24-32. [http://dx.doi.org/10.1111/j.1439-0531.2007.00907.x] [PMID: 17688599]

[35] Pursley JR, Mee MO, Wiltbank MC. Synchronization of ovulation in dairy cows using PGF2α and GnRH. Theriogenology 1995; 44(7): 915-23. [http://dx.doi.org/10.1016/0093-691X(95)00279-H] [PMID: 16727787]

[36] Baruselli PS, Madureira EH, Barnabe VH, *et al.* Estudo da dinâmica folicular em búfalas submetidas à sincronização da ovulação para inseminação artificial em tempo fixo. Arq Fac Vet UFRGS 1999; 27: 210. a

[37] Baruselli PS, Madureira EH, Visintin JA, Barnabe VH, Barnabe RC, Amaral R. Inseminação artificial em tempo fixo com sincronização da ovulação em bubalinos. Rev Bras Reprod Anim 1999; 23: 360-2. b

[38] Baruselli PS, Carvalho NA, Reichert RH, Henriquez CE, Nichi M. Pre-synchronization with GnRH 7 days before Ovsynch protocol for timed insemination in buffalo. Proceedings Buffalo Symposium of Americas. Belém. 2002; pp. 414-7. a

[39] Baruselli PS, Carvalho NA, Henriquez CE, Amaral R, Nichi M, Reichert RH. Use of progesterone associated to ovsynch protocol for timed artificial insemination in buffalo (*Bubalus bubalis*). Proc. 2nd Congresso Nazionale Sull'Allevamento Del Bufalo. Roma. 2003; pp. 265-8.

[40] De Rensis F, Ronci G, Guarneri P, *et al.* Conception rate after fixed time insemination following ovsynch protocol with and without progesterone supplementation in cyclic and non-cyclic Mediterranean Italian buffaloes (*Bubalus bubalis*). Theriogenology 2005; 63(7): 1824-31. [http://dx.doi.org/10.1016/j.theriogenology.2004.07.024] [PMID: 15823341]

[41] Baruselli PS, Carvalho NA, Henriquez CE, Amaral R, Nichi M. Synchronization of ovulation for timed artificial insemination during the off breeding season in the buffalo. Proc. 1th Buffalo Symposium of Americas. Belém. 2002; pp. 418-20. b

[42] El-Wishy AB. The postpartum buffalo. II. Acyclicity and anestrus. Anim Reprod Sci 2007; 97(3-4): 216-36. [http://dx.doi.org/10.1016/j.anireprosci.2006.03.003] [PMID: 16621354]

[43] Moura AJ. Sincronização da ovulação com dispositivo intravaginal de progesterona (CIDR-B®) associado a estrógeno e prostaglandina F2α em búfalas (Bubalus bubalis) tratadas em estações reprodutivas distintas 2003 129f Tese (Doutorado). Universidade de São Paulo, São Paulo: Faculdade de Medicina Veterinária e Zootecnia 2003.

[44] Bartolomeu CC. Estudo da dinâmica folicular durante o tratamento com cidr-b e crestar visando a inseminação artificial em tempo fixo em fêmeas bubalinas (Bubalus bubalis). São Paulo 2003; p. 120. tese (doutorado) – Faculdade de Medicina Veterinária e Zootecnia, Universidade de São Paulo, 2003

[45] Porto-Filho RM. Sincronização da ovulação para a inseminação artificial em tempo fixo (IATF) durante estação reprodutiva desfavorável em fêmeas bubalinas 2004 100 f Tese (Doutorado em Medicina Veterinária). Universidade de São Paulo, São Paulo: Faculdade de Medicina Veterinária e Zootecnia 2004.

[46] Porto-Filho RM, Carvalho NA, Viel Junior JO, *et al.* eCG dosage reduction in a protocol for synchronization of ovulation for timed artificial insemination during the off breeding season in buffalo Proc. Corrientes: 2nd Buffalo Symposium of Americas 2004.

[47] Porto-Filho RM, Carvalho NA, Viel Junior JO, Reichert RH, Nichi M, Baruselli PS. Follicular responses according to hCG and eCG dosage in buffalo treated with progesterone vaginal device during the off breeding season. b

[48] Carvalho NAT, Carvalho MV, Visintin JA, *et al.* Uso de dispositivos intravaginais de progesterona

associados ao hCG ou GnRH para sincronização da ovulação em búfalas na estação reprodutiva desfavorável. Congresso Brasileiro de Reprodução Animal, 16, Goiânia, GO. Anais: resumos 2005.

[49] Carvalho NA, Nagasaku EM, Vannucci FS, Toledo LM, Baruselli PS. Conception rate according to intravaginal progesterone device and hCG or GnRH to induce ovulation in buffalo during the off breeding season. Proceedings 7th World Buffalo Congress. Caserta. 2007. b [http://dx.doi.org/10.4081/ijas.2007.s2.646]

[50] Bó GA, Baruselli PS, Martínez MF. Pattern and manipulation of follicular development in Bos indicus cattle. Anim Reprod Sci 2003; 78(3-4): 307-26. [http://dx.doi.org/10.1016/S0378-4320(03)00097-6] [PMID: 12818651]

[51] Rhodes FM, Burke CR, Clark BA, Day ML, Macmillan KL. Effect of treatment with progesterone and oestradiol benzoate on ovarian follicular turnover in postpartum anoestrous cows and cows which have resumed oestrous cycles. Anim Reprod Sci 2002; 69(3-4): 139-50. [http://dx.doi.org/10.1016/S0378-4320(01)00141-5] [PMID: 11812625]

[52] Rhodes FM, McDougall S, Burke CR, Verkerk GA, Macmillan KL. Invited review: Treatment of cows with an extended postpartum anestrous interval. J Dairy Sci 2003; 86(6): 1876-94. [http://dx.doi.org/10.3168/jds.S0022-0302(03)73775-8] [PMID: 12836922]

[53] Mcdougall S, Burke CR, Macmillan KL, Williamson NB. The effect of pretreatment with progesterone on the oestrous response to oestradiol-17*β* benzoate in the postpartum dairy cow. Proc NZ Soc Anim Prod 1992; 52: 157-60.

[54] Baruselli PS, Carvalho NA, Gimenes LU, Crepaldi GA. Fixed-time artificial insemination in buffalo. Ital J Anim Sci 2007; 6: 107-18.

[55] Baruselli PS, Reis EL, Marques MO, Nasser LF, Bó GA. The use of hormonal treatments to improve reproductive performance of anestrous beef cattle in tropical climates. Anim Reprod Sci 2004; 82-83: 479-86. [http://dx.doi.org/10.1016/j.anireprosci.2004.04.025] [PMID: 15271474]

[56] Bo GA, Adams GP, Pierson RA, Mapletoft RJ. Effect of progestogen plus estradiol-17β treatment on superovulatory response in beef cattle. Theriogenology 1996; 45(5): 897-910. [http://dx.doi.org/10.1016/0093-691X(96)00020-9] [PMID: 16727851]

[57] Drost M, Wright JM Jr, Cripe WS, Richter AR. Embryo transfer in water buffalo (*Bubalus bubalis*). Theriogenology 1983; 20(5): 579-84. [http://dx.doi.org/10.1016/0093-691X(83)90082-1] [PMID: 16725875]

[58] Knopf L, Kastelic JP, Schallenberger E, Ginther OJ. Ovarian follicular dynamics in heifers: test of two-wave hypothesis by ultrasonically monitoring individual follicles. Domest Anim Endocrinol 1989; 6(2): 111-9. [http://dx.doi.org/10.1016/0739-7240(89)90040-4] [PMID: 2659255]

[59] Misra AK, Joshi BV, Kasiraj R, Sivaiah S, Rangareddi NS. Improved superovulatory regimen for buffalo (*Bubalus bubalis*). Theriogenology 1991; 35: 245. [http://dx.doi.org/10.1016/0093-691X(91)90221-X]

[60] Boland MP, Goulding D, Roche JF. Alternative gonadotrophins for superovulation in cattle. Theriogenology 1991; 35: 5-17.

[http://dx.doi.org/10.1016/0093-691X(91)90143-2]

[61] Baruselli PS. Dinâmica folicular durante o ciclo estral e resposta superovulatória em fêmeas bubalinas (Bubalus bubalis) 96f Tese (Doutorado). Faculdade de Medicina Veterinária e Zootecnia, Universidade de São Paulo 1997.

[62] Baruselli PS, Mucciolo RG, Amaral R, *et al.* Taxa de recuperação embrionária em búfalas superovuladas 1998.

[63] Baruselli PS, Madureira EH, Visintin JA, *et al.* Failure of oocyte entry into oviduct in superovulated buffalo. Theriogenology 2000; 53: 491.

[64] Karaivanov C. Comparative studies on the superovulatory effect of PMSG and FSH in water buffalo (*Bubalus bubalis*). Theriogenology 1986; 26(1): 51-9.
[http://dx.doi.org/10.1016/0093-691X(86)90111-1] [PMID: 16726169]

[65] Alvarez RH, Nogueira JR, Araujo Filho AM. Resposta ovariana de fêmeas bubalinas (*Bubalus bubalis*) superovuladas com PMSG ou FSH-P. Boletim de Indústria Animal. Nova Odessa 1990; 47: 111-4.

[66] Madan ML. Factors limiting superovulation response in embryo transfer program in buffalo. Theriogenology 1990; 33: 280.
[http://dx.doi.org/10.1016/0093-691X(90)90704-W]

[67] Drost M. Reproductive technology in buffaloes (*Bubalus bubalis*). Bulg J Agric Sci 1996; 93-102.

[68] Adams GP. Control of ovarian follicular wave dynamics in cattle: implications for synchronization and superstimulation. Theriogenology 1994; 41: 19-24.
[http://dx.doi.org/10.1016/S0093-691X(05)80044-5]

[69] Vos PL, van der Schans A, de Wit AA, Bevers MM, Willemse AH, Dieleman SJ. Effects of neutralization of pregnant mares serum gonadotrophin (PMSG) shortly before or at the preovulatory LH surge in PMSG-superovulated heifers on follicular function and development. J Reprod Fertil 1994; 100(2): 387-93.
[http://dx.doi.org/10.1530/jrf.0.1000387] [PMID: 8021854]

[70] Shaw DW, Farin PW, Washburn SP, Britt JH. Effect of retinol palmitate on ovulation rate and embryo quality in superovulated cattle. Theriogenology 1995; 44: 51-8.
[http://dx.doi.org/10.1016/0093-691X(95)00147-Z]

[71] Hunter RH. The fallopian tubes: their role in fertility and infertility. Berlin: Springer-Verlag 1988; pp. 12-156.
[http://dx.doi.org/10.1007/978-3-642-73045-0_2]

[72] Misra AK, Kasiraj R, Rao MM, Rangareddy NS, Jaiswal RS, Pant HC. Rate of transport and development of preimplantation embryo in the superovulated buffalo (*Bubalus bubalis*). Theriogenology 1998; 50(4): 637-49.
[http://dx.doi.org/10.1016/S0093-691X(98)00168-X] [PMID: 10732154]

[73] Beg MA, Sanwal PC, Yadav MC. Ovarian response and endocrine changes in buffalo superovulated at midluteal and late luteal stage of the estrous cycle: a preliminary report. Theriogenology 1997; 47(2): 423-32.
[http://dx.doi.org/10.1016/S0093-691X(97)00001-0] [PMID: 16727995]

[74] Baruselli PS, Marques MO, Arruda RP, Carvalho NA, Oliveira CA. Plasma estradiol and progesterone concentrations in superovulated buffalo in presence of CIDR-B devices. Theriogenology 2002; 57: 761. c

[75] Carvalho NA, Baruselli PS, Zicarelli L, Madureira EH, Visintin JA, DOcchio MJ. Control of ovulation with a GnRH agonist after superstimulation of follicular growth in buffalo: fertilization and embryo recovery. Theriogenology 2002; 58(9): 1641-50. [http://dx.doi.org/10.1016/S0093-691X(02)01057-9] [PMID: 12472135]

[76] Pavlok A, Koutecka L, Krejci P, *et al.* Effect of recombinant bovine somatotropin on follicular growth and quality of oocytes in cattle. Anim Reprod Sci 1996; 41: 183-92. [http://dx.doi.org/10.1016/0378-4320(95)01464-0]

[77] Lucy MC. Regulation of ovarian follicular growth by somatotropin and insulin-like growth factors in cattle. J Dairy Sci 2000; 83(7): 1635-47. [http://dx.doi.org/10.3168/jds.S0022-0302(00)75032-6] [PMID: 10908067]

[78] Izadyar F, Hage WJ, Colenbrander B, Bevers MM. The promotory effect of growth hormone on the developmental competence of in vitro matured bovine oocytes is due to improved cytoplasmic maturation. Mol Reprod Dev 1998; 49(4): 444-53. a [http://dx.doi.org/10.1002/(SICI)1098-2795(199804)49:4<444::AID-MRD12>3.0.CO;2-U] [PMID: 9508096]

[79] Izadyar F, Zeinstra E, Bevers MM. Follicle-stimulating hormone and growth hormone act differently on nuclear maturation while both enhance developmental competence of in vitro matured bovine oocytes. Mol Reprod Dev 1998; 51(3): 339-45. b [http://dx.doi.org/10.1002/(SICI)1098-2795(199811)51:3<339::AID-MRD14>3.0.CO;2-Y] [PMID: 9771655]

[80] Baruselli PS, Carvalho NA, Cavalcante AK, Nichi M, Zicarelli L. Use of rBST associated to a protocol for multiple ovulation and embryo transfer in buffalo (*Bubalus bubalis*). Proceedings Congresso Nazionale Sull'Allevamento Del Buffalo. Roma. 2003; pp. 269-73. b

[81] Carvalho NA, Nagasaku EM, Vannucci FS, *et al.* Use of different doses of r-bST associated to a protocol for multiple ovulation and embryo transfer in buffalo (*Bubalus bubalis*). Ital J Anim Sci 2007; 6: 652-4. a [http://dx.doi.org/10.4081/ijas.2007.s2.652]

[82] Baruselli PS, Arruda RP, Sophon S, Kamonpatana M. Embryo transfer in buffaloes: a pratical approach using ultrasonography and *in vitro* culture before transplantation. Buffalo J 1994; (Suppl. 2)211-7.

[83] Kruip TA, Boni R, Wurth YA, Roelofsen MW, Pieterse MC. Potential use of ovum pick-up for embryo production and breeding in cattle. Theriogenology 1994; 42(4): 675-84. [http://dx.doi.org/10.1016/0093-691X(94)90384-U] [PMID: 16727573]

[84] Boni R, Di Palo R, Barbieri V, Zicarelli L. Ovum pick-up in deep anestrus buffaloes. Proceedings World Buffalo Congress. Caserta. 1994; pp. 480-2.

[85] Galli C, Duchi R, Crotti G, Lazzari G. Embryo production by ovum pick-up in water buffalo. Theriogenology 1998; 49: 400.

[http://dx.doi.org/10.1016/S0093-691X(98)90753-1]

[86] Ohashi OM, Souza JS, Vale WG, Silva AO. The use of assisted reproduction technology (art) in buffalo and zebu. Proceedings Follow-up Seminar on Animal Reproduction and Biotechnology for Latin America. Belém. 1998; pp. 71-9.

[87] Boni R, Roviello S, Gasparrini B, Langella M, Zicarelli L. *In vitro* production of buffalo embryos in chemically defined medium. Buffalo J 1999; 1: 115-20.

[88] Gasparrini B. *In vitro* embryo production in buffalo species: state of the art. Theriogenology 2002; 57(1): 237-56.
[http://dx.doi.org/10.1016/S0093-691X(01)00669-0] [PMID: 11775973]

[89] Campanile G, Baruselli PS, Carvalho NAT, Di Palo R, Cavalcanti RB, Vecchio D. Effect of feed restriction on ovarian activity and recovered oocyte in Murrah buffalo heifers. Bubalus bubalis 2003; 275-8.

[90] Ferraz ML, Watanabe YF, Joaquim DC, *et al.* Produção *in vitro* de embriões bubalinos – resultados preliminares. Acta Sci Vet 2005; 33 (Suppl. 1): 397.

[91] Sá Filho MF, Carvalho NA, Gimenes LU, *et al.* Effect of recombinant bovine somatotropin (bST) on follicular population and on *in vitro* buffalo embryo production. Anim Reprod Sci 2009; 113(1-4): 51-9.
[http://dx.doi.org/10.1016/j.anireprosci.2008.06.008] [PMID: 18691835]

[92] Gimenes LU, Ferraz ML, Araujo A, *et al.* OPU at different times of a synchronized follicular wave did not affect IVP in *Bos indicus, Bos taurus* and *Bubalus bubalis.* Reprod Fertil Dev 2010; 22(1): 293-4.
[http://dx.doi.org/10.1071/RDv22n1Ab273]

[93] Ferraz ML, Gimenes LU, Sa Filho MF, *et al.* Effect of OPU interval and bST treatment on embryo production in buffalo. Ital J Anim Sci 2007; 6: 766-8.
[http://dx.doi.org/10.4081/ijas.2007.s2.766]

[94] Machatková M, Jokesová E, Petelíková J, Dvorácek V. Developmental competence of bovine embryos derived from oocytes collected at various stages of the estrous cycle. Theriogenology 1996; 45(4): 801-10.
[http://dx.doi.org/10.1016/0093-691X(96)00009-X] [PMID: 16727842]

[95] Hendriksen PJ, Vos PL, Steenweg WN, Bevers MM, Dieleman SJ. Bovine follicular development and its effect on the *in vitro* competence of oocytes. Theriogenology 2000; 53(1): 11-20.
[http://dx.doi.org/10.1016/S0093-691X(99)00236-8] [PMID: 10735058]

[96] Machatkova M, Jokesova E, Horky F, Krepelova A. Utilization of the growth phase of the first follicular wave for bovine oocyte collection improves blastocyst production. Theriogenology 2000; 54(4): 543-50.
[http://dx.doi.org/10.1016/S0093-691X(00)00369-1] [PMID: 11071128]

[97] Merton JS, de Roos AP, Mullaart E, *et al.* Factors affecting oocyte quality and quantity in commercial application of embryo technologies in the cattle breeding industry. Theriogenology 2003; 59(2): 651-74.
[http://dx.doi.org/10.1016/S0093-691X(02)01246-3] [PMID: 12499010]

[98] Vassena R, Mapletoft RJ, Allodi S, Singh J, Adams GP. Morphology and developmental competence

of bovine oocytes relative to follicular status. Theriogenology 2003; 60(5): 923-32. [http://dx.doi.org/10.1016/S0093-691X(03)00101-8] [PMID: 12935869]

[99] de Wit AA, Wurth YA, Kruip TA. Effect of ovarian phase and follicle quality on morphology and developmental capacity of the bovine cumulus-oocyte complex. J Anim Sci 2000; 78(5): 1277-83. [http://dx.doi.org/10.2527/2000.7851277x] [PMID: 10834583]

CHAPTER 13

Multiple Ovulation and Embryo Transfer in the Buffalo Species

Gianluca Neglia* and **Giovanna Bifulco**

Department of Veterinary Medicine and Animal Production, Federico II University, V. Delpino 1, 80137, Naples, Italy

Abstract: Multiple Ovulation and Embryo Transfer (MOET) is one of the biotechnologies of reproduction most utilized in the world to produce a high number of *in vivo* embryos. In the buffalo species the application of this technology meets several difficulties, and the embryo recovery rate is definitely lower than that recorded in cattle. This chapter aims at discussing the state of art of MOET in buffaloes and to analyze the factors that limit and influence its efficiency.

Keywords: Buffalo, Estrous cycle, *In vivo* produced embryos, Superovulation.

1. INTRODUCTION

The Multiple Ovulation and Embryo Transfer (MOET) technique or superovulation (SO) followed by embryo transfer (ET), was designed in order to modulate the oestrous cycle and achieve a large number of ovulations in species that are usually characterized by a single ovulation (Fig. **1**) [1]. The first results on this reproductive technology in cattle have been reported more than 50 years ago [2, 3]. However, despite the new findings in oestrous cycle manipulation and follicular development in this species, some aspects related to MOET are still unknown [4, 5]. In particular, the application of this technology in the field is limited by the variability in terms of response, and represents one of the main factors limiting a widespread use of this technology in the field. In any case,

* **Corresponding author Gianluca Neglia:** Department of Veterinary Medicine and Animal Production, Federico II University, V. Delpino 1, 80137, Naples, Italy; Tel: +39 081 2536063; Fax: +39 081 292981; E-mail: neglia@unina.it

Giorgio A. Presicce (Ed.)

MOET protocols in bovine, result on average in 5 to 6 transferable embryos/donor/treatment.

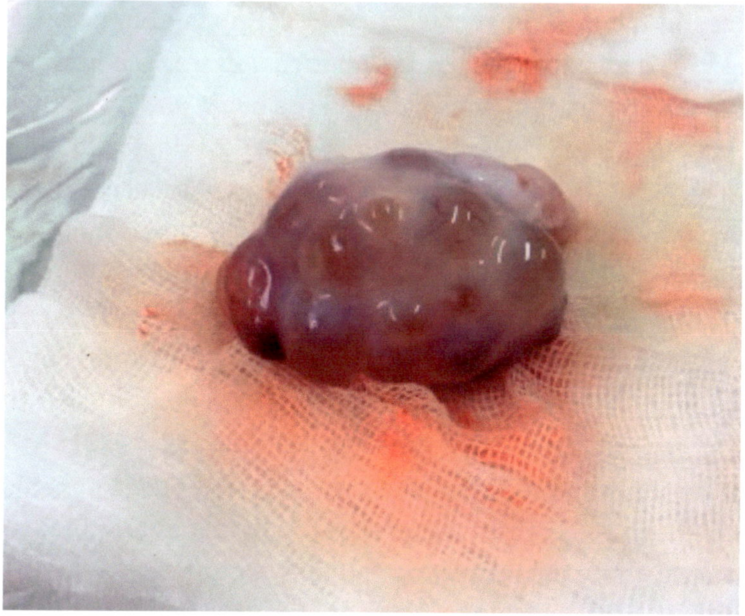

Fig. (1). Buffalo superovulated ovary.

MOET has also been applied in buffaloes. However, although the first successful embryo transfer in this species was performed in the United States of America in 1983 [6] and later in India [7], the application of MOET still results in low embryo yield when compared to cattle. In particular, following superovulatory treatment, buffaloes show good follicular response, moderate ovulatory rate and corpora lutea yield but, in contrast, low embryo recovery rate. Several attempts have been carried out in order to increase the number of recoverable embryos, but the causes for the low recovery rates are still unknown or at best speculative.

2. BASIC CONCEPTS ON SUPEROVULATION

The dynamics of follicular development occurring in waves during the oestrous cycle comes to help in achieving a better comprehension in the implementation of superovulation protocols in buffaloes. In some domestic species, like cattle and buffalo, a wave-like pattern is observed during the physiological estrous cycle [8]. Typically in cattle the estrous cycle is characterized by the development of 2 to 3 waves of follicular growth, although also cycles with 4 waves of follicle development have been observed [9].

Follicular cycles in the buffalo species are also organized in a wave-like pattern, in both natural [10] and synchronized [11] oestrus. In this species, more than 60% of animals show ordinarily two waves during the cycle and more than 30% shows three waves. The length of the cycle is typically 23-24 days, although shorter (16 days) and longer (26-30 days) cycles have been observed [11]. In buffaloes exhibiting a two-wave growth pattern, the first growth wave emerges on day 1 and the second on days 12 to 14. In those with a three-wave growth pattern, the emergence of the second and the third wave occurs on days 11 and 20, respectively [11]. During each wave, the phenomena of recruitment, selection and dominance occur [12]. During the recruitment, the growth of a cohort of 6-8 follicles is influenced by the increasing circulating levels of FSH [10]. Subsequently, the recruited follicles undergo selection and dominance processes: in the buffalo, being a monovular species, normally a single follicle develops into a dominant follicle, while the remaining follicles regress.

The phenomenon of dominance occurs when the dominant follicle reaches the diameter of approximately 7.4 mm, after 3 days of growth [13]: this phase is recognized as deviation, when the follicle acquires the receptors for LH. Interestingly, the capability of becoming a dominant follicle is retained by all growing follicles before deviation occurrence, whereas once deviation has occurred, only the largest follicle develops into a dominant follicle and the others undergo regression. It is known that during the phase of dominance, the LH plays a key role, since some studies carried out in bovine heifers demonstrated that LH receptors are expressed in granulosa cells of the future dominant follicle about 8 hours before deviation [12]. Furthermore, the intrafollicular estradiol: progesterone ratio declines, preparing the ovulation [14].

As introduced above, the aim of superovulation is to allow more ovulations within the estrous cycle of the animal. Therefore, the follicular dynamics is altered and modulated by the exogenous administration of hormones several days in advance of the anticipated normal estrus in an effort to elicit multiple ovulations in the donor animal. This is inevitably obtained by overriding the phase of dominance, allowing the growth of a large number of dominant follicles that acquire ovulatory capability.

The MOET technique allows several advantages, such as:

- increasing the number of calves from animals characterized by high genetic value;
- accelerating the genetic improvement of the herd;
- obtain newborn calves from old or wounded animals that are not able to mate or calving naturally;
- use of animals for reproductive purposes with impairment of the reproductive tract (*e.g.* salpingitis), which would otherwise be disposed of;
- increasing the farm income by the sale of embryos, that can be more easily moved across countries compared to live animals. In this regard, it is worth pointing out that Italian buffalo embryos are in particular great demand due to the intensive genetic selection in this species performed over the past years;
- reduction of semen costs.

3. HORMONAL CONTROL FOR OPTIMIZING SUPEROVULATION

The first trials carried out on superovulation in both cattle and buffaloes, foresaw conventionally the start of the treatment during midcycle. This was based on the evidence that the response to MOET treatment was greater when the hormonal treatments started 8 to 12 days after oestrus [15]. By the application of ultrasonography, it was demonstrated that this period (equivalent to 7 to 11 days after ovulation) would correspond approximately with the emergence of the second follicular wave, when a new cohort of growing follicles can be monitored on the ovary. For this reason the protocols used today involve the initiation of superstimulatory treatments after the control of follicular wave emergence by administering exogenous hormones. Different methods have been used to elude the negative consequences of the dominant follicle and reduce the atresia (see below), such as hormone administration (estradiol, progesterone, GnRH, eCG, *etc.*), or mechanical techniques, as the ablation of the dominant follicle by ovum pick-up [16].

Once the cycle has been synchronized, the superovulatory treatment can be initiated. It is common practice to carry out MOET protocols in conjunction to an intravaginal device releasing progesterone, in order to avoid an early coming into estrus of donors, and ensuring high progesterone levels that are beneficial for subsequent embryo development [5]. Several hormones have been used to manipulate the follicular development in both cattle [4, 5] and buffaloes [17, 18]. In particular, three different types of gonadotrophins are utilized:

1. pituitary extracts of porcine or other domestic animal species;
2. equine chorionic gonadotrophin (eCG);
3. human menopausal gonadotrophin (hMG).

These hormones show different characteristics that will be outlined below. Usually an administration of prostaglandin $F_{2\alpha}$ is performed one day before the end of the superovulatory treatment, to ensure corpus luteum regression and the donors are artificially or naturally inseminated about 60 and 74 hours after prostaglandin. If the buffaloes undergo artificial insemination (AI), it would be advisable to perform a GnRH injection on the day before AI, to synchronize the ovulations.

4. UTERINE FLUSHING

Six or seven days after insemination, non surgical embryo collection is carried out by performing an uterine flushing with the aid of a Foley catheter. This is inserted in the uterus by using a stiffening stylet until about 2/3 of each uterine horn. The Foley catheter is characterized by two separated channels (2-way catheter), or lumens, running down its length. One channel is open at both ends and allows the inflow and outflow of flushing medium. The other channel shows a valve on the outside end and a balloon on the opposite site (tip). By this valve, the operator can inflate the balloon with air when it lies inside the uterine horn in order to stop it from slipping out. The Foley catheter (Fig. **2**) is inserted through the genital tract till it reaches the first of the two horns, and at that point air is insufflated into the balloon. The uterine horns in buffalo are less extensible and elastic than cattle, also due to the presence of an intercornual ligament which tightly joins the two horns for a longer extension starting from their anatomical basis [19]. Therefore, the insertion of the catheter for embryo collection is not easy as in cattle and expose the basis of the horn to the risk of laceration if the balloon pressure is not suitably regulated [20]. Usually 8 to 22 cc of air are used in the buffalo species [17].

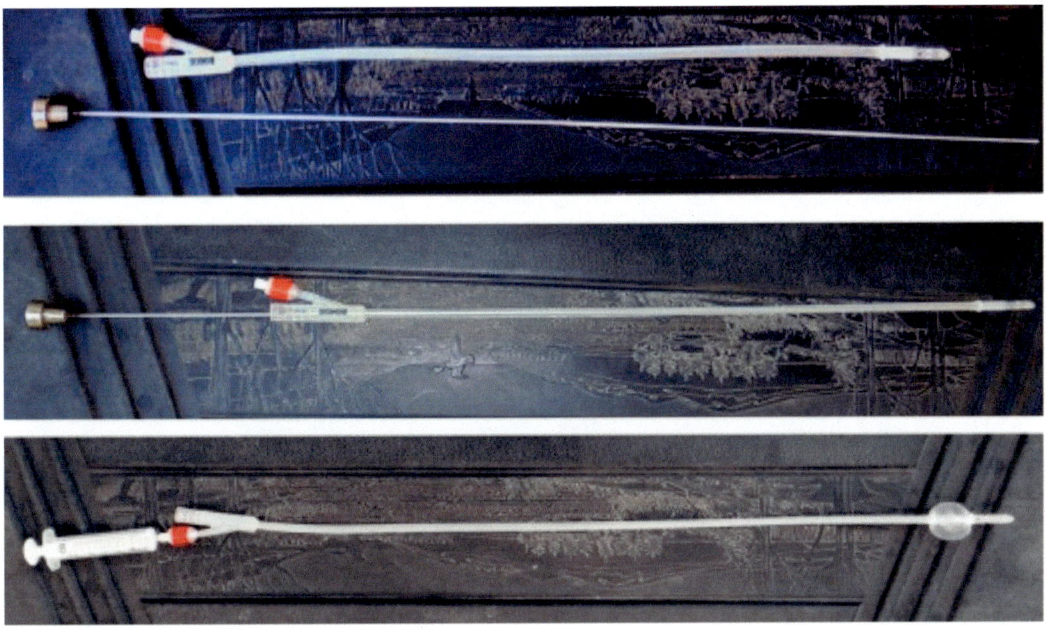

Fig. (2). Foley catheters.

The inflated balloon will seal the cranial portion of the uterine horn, in order to avoid retrograde fluid loss from the uterus, when the flushing medium is released into the uterine horn, to recover the embryos. After a small amount (100-150 ml) of flushing medium is inserted into the uterus, the fluid is recovered into a collection container. This process is repeated on each of the two uterine horns. Each uterine horn is flushed with commercially available, complete, and ready-to-use flushing media. These embryo flushing solutions also contain antibiotics and bovine serum albumin as a source of protein. Some commercial preparations of complete flush media also contain surfactants to minimize the formation of foam and bubbles in the embryo search dish. In the past, the flush media had to be prepared for each collection and consisted primarily of Dulbecco's phosphate buffered saline supplemented with antibiotics and 1% fetal/calf bovine serum (or alternatively, 0.1% bovine serum albumin). This solution is actually largely utilized in the world for its low costs. It is also important that the flushing solutions are maintained at a temperature of 30-35°C, to avoid thermal shock to the embryos (Fig. **3**).

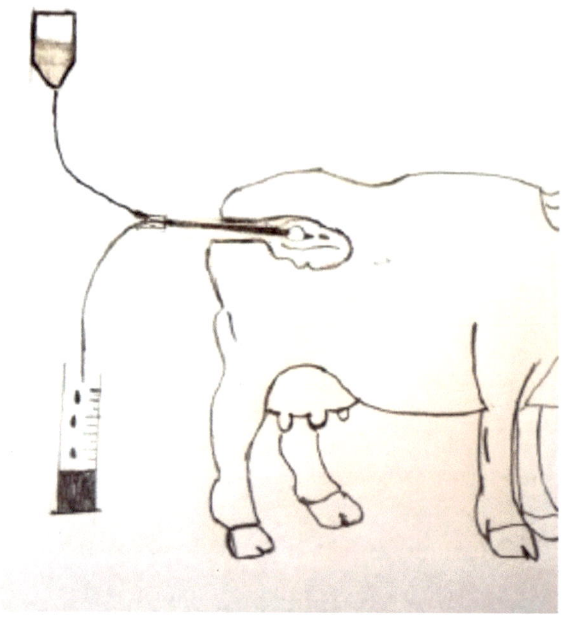

Fig. (3). Schematic representation of flushing.

Some studies performed on the development of preimplantation embryos in superovulated buffalo [21 - 24] give indication of a faster rate of development in this species when compared to cattle. These results have been confirmed in other studies on *in vitro* embryo development, showing that buffalo embryos are 12 to 24 hours more advanced than the bovine counterparts developing in parallel [25]. Oocytes and embryos in buffaloes remain in the oviduct for a period varying from 74 and 100 hours post-fertilization [26] and hence reach the uterus 4.5-5 days after fertilization. This knowledge was acquired by performing flushing on oviducts and uteri of superovulated animals at different hours post-insemination. Similarly, in Nili-Ravi buffaloes [23], at 85 hours post insemination the embryos are in the oviduct, whereas at 108 hours about 78% of the embryos descend from the oviduct into the uterus. It seems that buffalo embryos reach the uterus when they are at the developmental stage of morula [23], similarly to what described in cattle at 120 hours [27]. This would confirm the earlier development of buffalo embryos compared to cattle. Compact morulae are observed from 125 to 152 hours post-estrus and blastocysts from 141 hours. Similar data have been reported also in Nili Ravi buffaloes, in which the recovery of compact morulae occurs at about 132 hrs post estrus [28]. For this reason, it is reasonable to anticipate the flushing in buffaloes on day 6 rather than on day 7 as usually performed in cattle.

5. EMBRYO COLLECTION

Following completion of flushing, the catheter balloon is deflated and the catheter content is carefully allowed to flow into a sterile container located at the end of the outflow tubing. Usually an embryo filter is located at the end of the Foley catheter. Otherwise, the flushed medium can be decanted and subsequently filtered. The filtered medium is dispensed into a search dish with grid and visualized using a stereoscope (dissecting microscope) at 10× magnification. All embryos are moved into a clean dish containing holding media with a higher concentration of bovine fetal/calf serum (10%–20%) or bovine serum albumin (0.4%).

Embryos are then visualized at a higher magnification (40–60×) and classified according to their morphology, stage of development (unfertilized oocytes, early morula, tight morula, blastocyst, expanded blastocyst, hatched blastocyst), and quality (excellent, good, fair, poor and degenerate) [29]. The quality score is based on morphologic assessment of the physical integrity of embryos and morphologic characteristics according to the stage of embryonic development, compaction status, color of cytoplasm, areas of cellular degeneration, number of extruded blastomeres, size of perivitelline space, and the size and sphericity of the embryo.

Only embryos classified as fair, good, or excellent should be transferred. Embryos are kept in holding media after being washed at least three times. Embryo washing is performed by transferring embryos into different, clean wells containing holding media [29]. This procedure, recommended by the International Embryo Transfer Society, aids in removing cellular debris and potential pathogens adhered to the zona pellucida. Embryos are then kept in holding media at room temperature. At this point the embryos may have different fate: transfer into recipients, freezing, bisection (splitting), or determination of gender by embryo sexing [29].

It is worth pointing out that several studies demonstrated that *in vivo* produced embryos are characterized by higher resistance to cryopreservation compared to the *in vitro* counterparts, probably for the beneficial effects of some substances produced in the oviduct [30]. The possibility to cryopreserve embryos, enables a better utilization of embryos outside of the synchronization protocols required for transferring fresh embryos on a number of suitable and readily available recipients [31]. In fact, it has to be underlined that recipients need to be in the same stage of the estrous cycle of the donor, and in addition, the variability in terms of response to MOET does not allow to foresee the correct number of animals that have to be synchronized.

6. FACTORS AFFECTING MOET

Several factors are accounted for influencing the superovulatory response in buffalo. In particular we can distinguish factors that are intrinsic and extrinsic to the animal.

6.1. Intrinsic Factors

6.1.1. Age of the Donor

As in cattle, conflicting results are reported for buffaloes, regarding the influence of the age of the donor on MOET schedules. Usually buffalo heifers show high positive response to MOET in terms of ovulations and recovery rate [32], but a high incidence of oocytes rather than embryos are recovered. This is probably due to the difficulty to rely on a uniform sexual maturity among animals, due to a large variability of the population [17]. Therefore, the high oocyte recovery after hormonal administration and flushing may be explained by a failure in fertilization, caused by incompetent oocytes or not capacitated sperm cells, for inadequate uterine environment. Furthermore, it is worth noting that the reproductive tract in buffaloes has a reduced size than the bovine counterpart [19]. Therefore, if the animals do not show an adequate uterus development, it may result difficult to perform the flushing. In any case, no differences have been observed in animals of different age or parity in terms of embryo recovery [18].

6.1.2. Stage of the Estrous Cycle

The stage of the estrous cycle when MOET is initiated is one of the most important factors that can influence the response to the treatment. As specified above, the greatest embryo recovery has been observed when MOET starts 8 to 12 days after estrus, in correspondence with the emergence of the second follicular wave [33, 34], although similar results in terms of embryo recovery rate are reported when MOET treatment is initiated between days 12 and 15 after estrus [35]. However, as above reported, the day of emergence of the second wave differs between buffaloes displaying either two or three waves per cycle. This condition does not seem to be essential in order to improve MOET response in buffalo, since superovulated animals with 2 or 3 follicular waves [36] show similar number of follicles (7.50 *vs*. 7.33), ovulations (5.81 *vs*. 6.08), corpora lutea (3.94 *vs*. 4.42), recovered embryo+ova (2.69 *vs*. 2.69) and transferable embryos (1.06 *vs*. 1.17). Furthermore, because of the large variability in terms of estrus duration in buffaloes, the prediction of ovulation can be hardly foreseen [10, 37]. The response to MOET treatments is definitely greatest if hormonal treatments are administered when follicular wave emergence is recorded, rather than 1 or 2 days before or later. Therefore, the synchronization of follicular wave emergence is a key point to improve the superovulatory response [38], making it necessary to synchronise the timing of follicular wave emergence. Recently, it has been observed that the initiation of the treatment on days 7 to 8 seems to give better superovulatory response compared to 9 to 10 or 13 to 14 [39].

6.1.3. Progesterone Levels During MOET Treatment

If the stage of the estrous cycle at the initiation of MOET protocol is random, the influence of progesterone on the superovulatory response has to be taken into consideration. Although some old studies failed to highlight a significant correlation between progesterone concentration on the day of FSH administration and superovulatory response [40], a positive correlation between embryo recovery rate and progesterone circulating blood levels has been largely demonstrated in both cattle [41] and buffalo [42, 43]. In fact, it has been demonstrated *in vitro* that in the rat, progesterone is able to act on the LH β-subunits within the pituitary gland, by inducing its secretion [44] and storage. It is also known that GnRH pulsatility and the release of this hormone in the hypothalamus-pituitary circulation is diminished by P_4 levels *in vivo* [45]. As GnRH regulates the number of its receptors, it has been supposed that P4 levels may also be able to decrease pituitary responsiveness to GnRH [46]. Therefore, it is likely that high P4 levels during the first days of superovulatory treatment, may increase LH storage in pituitary gland and augment GnRH induced LH release [46]. Furthermore, high progesterone levels seem to be mandatory to improve embryo quality, by acting on oocytes developmental competence in sheep [47].

Buffaloes with more than 2 ng/ml plasma progesterone levels show better superovulatory response compared to those with less than 2 ng/ml [48]. Exogenous progesterone administered by intravaginal device can also be used to increase progesterone levels on the day of starting MOET treatment [49], resulting in higher number of corpora lutea and recovered embryos (flushing) on day 6 post-oestrus.

6.1.4. Presence or Absence of Dominant Follicle

The evaluation of the follicular population at the start of any MOET program is another factor that has to be considered. During a follicular wave, inhibin secreted by the dominant follicle causes the regression of subordinate follicles by in turn decreasing FSH level. Therefore, gonadotrophin treatment has to be initiated at the time of follicular wave emergence, optimizing the number of follicles that can be recruited overriding thus the inhibitory effect of the dominant follicle over the subordinate follicles. The presence of a dominant follicle on the day of initiation of MOET schedule, significantly influences embryo recovery rate, reducing the number of follicles that can be recruited and increasing the incidence of those that are encountering atresia. Italian Mediterranean buffaloes superovulated in the absence of a dominant follicle show higher recovery rate (3.0 *vs.* 1.87, respectively) and number of transferable embryos (2.92 *vs.* 1.74, respectively), than those superovulated in its presence [17]. Similar evidences are reported also for Egyptian buffaloes [50]. The influence of the dominant follicle is still unclear in Murrah buffaloes. Some reports highlight no differences in terms of serum progesterone concentration affecting recovery rate or transferable embryos, but only a higher number of corpora lutea on the day of flushing [51]. In other studies a similar number of corpora lutea and embryos has been observed, together with a higher number of large follicles during MOET treatment [52]. A possible hypothesis to explain these discrepant results, may be found in the functional status of the dominant follicle at the start of the superovulatory treatment. It is known that during a normal follicular wave the dominant follicle has a growth phase, followed by a static and regression phases [12]. The beginning of MOET during one of these phases results in different response, because of the different activity of the dominant follicle on the subordinates. Furthermore, in cattle the number of follicles of 3 to 8 mm in diameter is highly correlated with the absence of a dominant follicle, detected by a single ultrasound examination [53]. Nevertheless, the number of small and medium follicles prior to initiation of superovulation in buffaloes is not always different among animals that show a dominant follicle, compared to those that do not show it [52]. Therefore, it can be concluded that the morphological criteria that take into account only the size of any large follicle, are not sufficient to predict the response of buffaloes to the superovulatory treatment.

Several methods have been applied to remove the influence of the dominant follicle. Previously it has been specified that SO is usually carried out in presence of a progesterone releasing intravaginal device, with or without estradiol. The latter can also be administered before initiating treatment together with a progesterone releasing intravaginal device, causing the regression of the dominant follicle [54]. Alternatively, since in some countries the utilization of estradiol is not allowed, a single GnRH injection can be performed 36 hours before the application of a progesterone releasing intravaginal device. High progesterone levels suppress follicular growth, maintaining a high number of small follicles on the ovary when MOET treatment is initiated.

6.1.5. Genetic Factors on SO

There are two main types of domestic buffalo: the River buffalo of the Indian subcontinent with 50 pairs of chromosomes and the Swamp buffalo of the South Asian region with 48 pairs of chromosomes. Crossbreeding by mating the River and the Swamp buffalo has been practiced in many countries. This mating produces a F1 hybrid with a chromosome complement of 2n = 49. Slight differences have been observed after SO in these three genotypes. Usually, crossbred and Swamp buffaloes show a shorter ovary diameter compared to the River, although this is not a good indicator to predict the number of embryos that will be collected. In fact, both the number of corpora lutea and embryos are not different among the three genotypes (on average 6 corpora lutea and 2-2.7 embryos/donor) [55].

Genetic factors have to be considered in terms of individual differences among subjects. In fact, cows which respond poorly to the first superovulation treatment have a tendency to respond poorly to subsequent superovulations, while those which respond well to first superovulation continue to do so during subsequent treatments in both cattle [56] and buffalo [17]. Genetic constitution of a donor having more sensitivity to exogenous gonadotropins appears to be the reason for such variations. Some studies have shown that IGF-1, the main receptor of IGF, is involved in some physiological processes, including ovarian follicular development [57, 58], ovulation [59], pre-implantation embryo development [60], conception and growth. Previous reports have found a tight correlation between oocyte quality, embryo viability and IGF-1 blood levels in ruminants that had undergone hormonal treatments for superovulation.

6.2. Extrinsic Factors

6.2.1. MOET Schedules and Different Types of Gonadotrophins

As indicated above, three different types of gonadotrophins can be utilized to induce SO. Equine chorionic gonadotrophin (eCG), or pregnant mare serum gonadotrophin (PMSG), is a complex glycoprotein characterized by both FSH and LH activity [61], that has been largely used to induce SO because of its low cost and easy availability. Its main characteristic is the long half-life, which is reported to be around 40 hours in cattle. However, it persists in the bloodstream until 10 days after the end of the superovulation treatment. Although this can be considered an advantage, since one single administration is sufficient to ensure an optimal superovulatory response, facilitating animals management and handling, on the other hand the prolonged high eCG circulating levels can lead to ovarian hyperstimulation, abnormal endocrine profiles and high incidence of anovulatory follicles [26]. In fact, after eCG treatment some follicles tend to luteinize and others develop in cysts, rather than ovulate [62] by altering the estradiol:progesterone ratio. Elevated progesterone concentration in coincidence with LH surge may be responsible for asynchrony in LH peak, impaired gamete transport and both poor fertilization rate and embryo development. On the contrary high progesterone levels (more than 2.3 ng/ml) on the day of eCG administration seems to be associated with higher embryo recovery [36]. Furthermore, treatment with eCG in buffaloes for superovulation results in elevated plasma inhibin from fully developed follicles persisting for a long time and culminating in the inhibition of FSH, leading to poor ovulation of the remaining follicles [63].

A further aspect that needs to be considered is that commercial preparations of eCG are partially purified from the serum of pregnant mares [64]. Hormone concentration can be different at different times of gestation and, hence, among different batches, leading to a variability in terms of superovulatory response and embryo recovery. The treatment schedule consists in the intramuscular injection of dosages variable between 2,500 to 4,000 IU, although the 3,000 IU is the most common dose [65]. A schematic representation of eCG treatment is shown in Fig. (**4**).

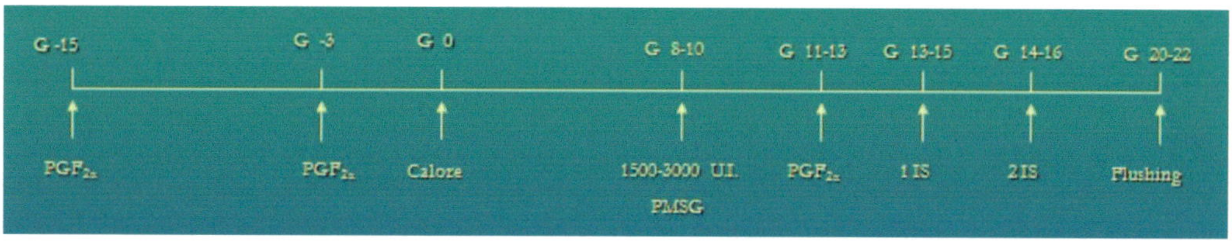

Fig. (4). Superovulation treatment by eCG.

Mean embryo recovery rate is reported between 0.7 [26] and 2 [36, 66] embryos. The ovarian response to eCG treatment has also been tested on prepubertal buffalo heifers in association with GnRH reporting a mean number of 4.5 to 5 ovulations/heifer. This allow us to believe that embryo recovery in heifers would not be so different from what reported in adult buffaloes. Furthermore, GnRH administration has no influence on the total ovulation rate, although it allows a reduction in the interval between the first and the last ovulation (about 20 hours compared to 40 in GnRH treated and control buffaloes, respectively).

To overcome the problems related with eCG prolonged half-life, some protocols have been developed. These protocols are based on the intravenous administration of monoclonal or polyclonal antibodies to eCG at the time of the first insemination, 12 to 18 hours after the onset of estrus (Fig. **5**). Treatment with Neutra-eCG results in a significant decrease in the peripheral inhibin concentration at 84 to 120 hours after prostaglandin administration and in the number of large anovulatory follicles at 168 hours, although the number of large follicles is lower than that recorded in buffaloes treated by eCG alone [68]. For this reason no differences in terms of number of corpora lutea is recorded. However, embryo recovery rate by using antibodies *versus* eCG is about 1.51/donor, with 1 transferable embryo/donor, similarly thus to what obtained with eCG alone [69].

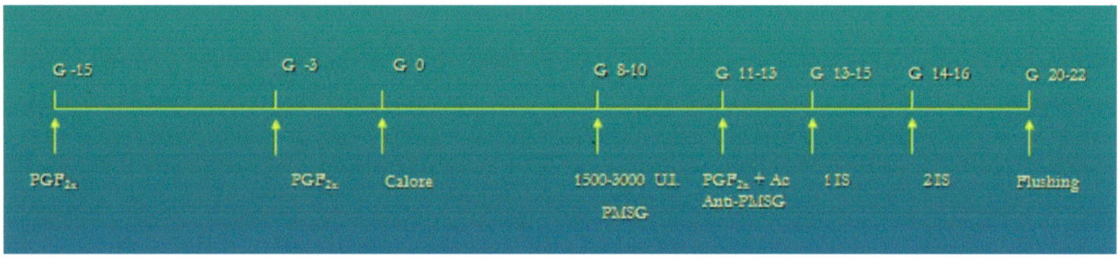

Fig. (5). Superovulation treatment by eCG and antibodies anti-eCG.

Pituitary extracts of FSH and LH are the main gonadotrophins actually utilized for MOET in buffalo. The two most commonly used commercial FSH preparations are made from porcine pituitary extracts and contain some contamination with luteinizing hormone (LH). If high amounts of LH in FSH preparations may interfere with optimal superovulatory response, it is believed though that a low level of LH contamination does not interfere and may even be needed for superovulation [70]. In any case, the maximum level of contamination of LH in pituitary extract for SO, would not exceed 15-20%. This variability may be reduced by using bovine FSH produced by recombinant DNA technology [71]. However, no trials have been performed until now in the buffalo species. As FSH is characterized by short half-life, pituitary extracts are usually administered twice daily, with schedules of 3 to 5 consecutive days

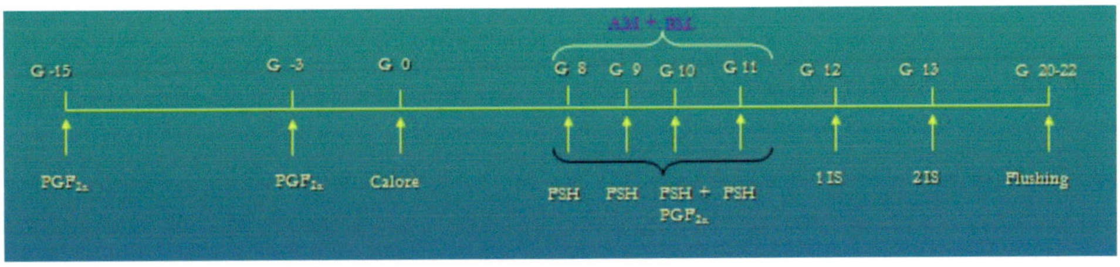

Fig. (6). Superovulation treatment by FSH or FSH+LH.

Regimens with constant, decreasing or increasing dosages have been utilized (from 800 to 1200 IU), although no differences have been observed in terms of embryo recovery [17]. It is reasonable not to administer dosages lower than 700 IU of FSH, being not able to induce a good response in buffaloes. Usually the administration of a decreasing dosage is preferred, to increase follicular recruitment and development. Furthermore, it has to be considered a further increase or decrease of about 20%, if buffaloes weighing more than 800 kg or heifers are treated, respectively. Some attempts have been made in order to reduce the number of FSH administrations, by injecting the hormone with some substances characterized by slow releasing (*eg*. PVP) subcutaneously or intramuscularly. However, single injection seems to result in lower response to MOET compared to multiple dose injection regimens [18].

Embryo recovery rate is similar to what reported for treatment by eCG, varying from 0.9 to 3.5 embryos or ova/donor [17, 49, 72, 73]. Mediterranean buffaloes treated for MOET by a commercial pituitary extract preparation [17] responded with 1.9 embryo/donor (and only 1.51 transferable embryos).

Human menopausal gonadotrophin has also been used to induce SO, with similar results to those obtained by pituitary extracts. However, commercial hMG preparations are highly expensive and are scarcely utilized in practice.

6.2.2. Influence of the Season

The season may influence the superovulatory response of buffaloes due to both the intrinsic seasonality and weather conditions. It is known that the buffalo is a short day breeder, and therefore tends to increase its reproductive activity when day light hours decrease [74]. This condition is linked to its tropical origin. In fact, buffaloes originate from north equatorial areas, where forage availability coincides with increasing dark hours. Therefore, it has been supposed that animals which calve in the most suitable period for survival of the offspring are selected [75]. Interestingly, the animals retained this behaviour even when they were transferred to places where forage is always (Italy) or less (Sud Equator areas like Sao Paulo, Br) available. In countries like Italy, the period in which day light hours are lower than dark coincides with the autumn-winter and in this period the buffalo shows its maximum reproductive efficiency [74]. Therefore, it would be reasonable to believe that also the application of reproductive biotechnologies would lead to the maximum efficiency in this period. On the contrary, embryo recovery rate after MOET in periods of decreasing daylight length may result in lower response compared to other periods of the year [76]. It is likely that in some trials, also hypofertile buffaloes may be uncorrectly considered cycling and utilized for SO, leading inevitably to low efficiency [17]. Since only cycling animals are selected for superovulation, the application of such treatments out of the breeding season allows to select high fertile animals, that are able to show high reproductive activity also when day light hours increase.

The influence of extreme weather conditions in tropical countries on the superovulatory response in buffalo is controversial. In fact, although an effect of high temperature and high humidity have been reported [77, 78], it is known that because of its tropical origin, the buffalo does not undergo heat stress like cattle. It is likely that the day light length rather than weather conditions influences the superovulatory response.

6.2.3. Days Open

The number of days open significantly affects the response to MOET [76]. The highest superovulatory response, together with the highest number of transferable embryos per donor and the highest transferable embryos/corpora lutea ratio, are obtained when animals between 61 and 220 days post-partum are superovulated [17]. Buffaloes that undergo MOET schedules within 60 days post-partum, produce mainly unfertilized oocytes, probably for the same reasons reported for heifers (inadequate uterine environment for sperm cells survival or inadequate oocyte competence). The lack of response to MOET in buffaloes at more than 220 days post-partum, may be due to uterine inflammations or deep anestrus, phenomena that these animals encounter when they are not pregnant for a long time [17].

6.2.4. Influence of Nutrition

The influence of nutrition on reproductive efficiency is actually well established [79], although some mechanisms remain to be better understood. Diets characterized by low starch content (<15.5%) and high cellulose content (>23%) allow to obtain the maximum superovulatory response in buffaloes treated by FSH [80]. This is particularly evident in buffaloes within 120 days post-partum, during the catabolic phase of lactation, when the animals encounter the negative energy balance. This interesting observation may be explained by the evidence that diets characterized by low energy density result in an increase of small follicles and high quality oocytes [81], improving blastocyst yield *in vitro*. Therefore, it is reasonable that diets with high quality forages (characterized by high nutritive value and relatively low crude fibre level), together with low concentrates content in the diet of buffaloes utilized for SO [17], would be able to meet nutritional requirements, without impairing reproductive efficiency.

Furthermore, meeting nutritional requirements is fundamental in order to ensure a proper body condition score (BCS), that was demonstrated to affect the reproductive efficiency [82]. The BCS system is a method that can be used to evaluate the body reserves of dairy animals [83].

A BCS score higher than 4 or lower than 2.5 (in a 1 to 5 scale) results in lower efficiency in Murrah buffaloes either after AI [54] or natural mating [81]. Similarly, low pregnancy rate after AI [84] has been observed in Italian Mediterranean buffaloes with a BCS score lower than 6 [85]. A lower BCS is responsible for lower LH pulsatility, impairing the efficiency of reproductive biotechnologies, such as artificial insemination and MOET.

6.2.5. r-BST Priming

In order to improve the response of the follicular population to MOET treatment, a somatotropin (r-BST) priming has been utilized in both cattle [86] and buffalo

[87]. The beneficial effect of r-BST, in fact, is due to increasing levels of Insulin-like Growth Factor I (IGF-I), which can act synergistically with FSH, *via* both increasing the number of small follicles with diameter lower than 5 mm [88] on the ovary and the number of LH receptors on the granulosa cells. Consequently, follicular growth and oocyte quality are improved. Furthermore, IGF-I favours cumulus cells expansion [89] and this can contribute to oocyte adhesion to the fimbriae after ovulation [90].

Results on r-BST influence during superovulation in buffalo are controversial. Treatment by r-BST in Swamp buffaloes has been demonstrated to slightly increase the number of corpora lutea and recovered ova and significantly the number of transferable embryos [87], leading to a mean recovery rate of about 3 transferable embryos/donor. Similarly, superovulated Mediterranean buffaloes treated by r-BST show a lower incidence of ovarian cysts and higher recovery rate, in terms of both recovered ova and transferable embryos [20].

However, the dosage utilized seems to affect the superovulatory response. Good results have been obtained by using a 250 mg dosage, administered on the day of progesterone releasing device insertion (Day 0) and starting the superovulation schedules on both day 4 [90] or day 9-11 [87]. On the contrary contrasting results are reported by the use of 500 mg, since in some studies a great improvement in terms of ovulation rate and embryo recovery is reported [91], whereas no effect has been found in other trials [90].

6.2.6. Ovum Pick-Up [OPU] Priming

OPU technology consists in the collection of oocytes by means of ultrasound guided follicular aspiration [92]. The ultrasound technology utilized during OPU allows to identify and aspirate all follicles with diameter > 2mm, resetting the estrous cycle and avoiding the phenomenon of follicular dominance (and subordinates follicle regression). It is usually performed 3 – 4 days apart, in order to allow follicular growth [25], although in buffaloes higher intervals may be necessary [93]. The reduction of atresia increases the number of cumulus oocyte complexes usable for *in vitro* embryo production (IVEP), as well as their quality [25].

OPU priming can be utilized to reset follicular population before initiating superovulation, avoiding the negative influence of the dominant follicle on the subordinates and improving oocyte quality. OPU priming in buffaloes [16] increases the number of animals that are able to respond with at least one embryo (more than 68% *vs.* 53%, in buffaloes undergone OPU priming and controls, respectively), and this is particularly evident during periods of decreasing daylight length (84 *vs.* 15%, in buffaloes undergone OPU priming and controls, respectively). In the same period, OPU primed buffaloes show a higher ova/corpora lutea ratio (47 *vs.* 12%, in buffaloes undergone OPU priming and controls, respectively) and transferable embryos (3.2 *vs.* 0.5, in buffaloes undergone OPU priming and controls, respectively). During periods of increasing daylight length no differences have been observed between buffaloes undergone OPU priming and the control counterpart. This interesting observation would be confirmed by the absence of differences between buffaloes undergone OPU priming in presence of a dominant follicle and those that do not show dominant follicles [17].

6.2.7. Influence of Interval Between PGF and Estrus

The interval between prostaglandin administration and estrus is important to foresee the superovulatory response. Usually more than 90% of animals exhibits estrus within 48 hours after $PGF_{2\alpha}$ administration [94]. Interestingly, higher recovery rate and number of viable embryos are observed in these animals compared to those that exhibit estrus later. It is likely that late estrus signs may be associated with delayed (or failure) ovulation and lack of oocyte fertilization.

6.2.8. Repeated Superovulation

Repeated SO is usually utilized to increase the number of recovered embryos from animals of high genetic value. Usually, it would be reasonable to carry out the hormonal treatment on the same animal at least 80 or 100 days apart, in cattle and buffalo respectively. The first variable that has to be considered is the type of gonadotrophin that is utilized. Swamp buffaloes, treated by eCG for four successive superovulatory treatment, undergo a high incidence of anovulatory large follicles (cysts) and reduced embryo recovery rate [95]. This is probably due to the long half-life of eCG and, consequently, the continuous ovarian stimulation. Therefore, the utilization of pituitary extracts is preferred. When buffaloes are treated repeatedly for SO by FSH for six times 77 days apart, a marked decline (about 50%) in ovulation rate, corpora lutea and embryo recovery is recorded [78]. However, it is worth pointing out that MOET treatments carried out for successive 6 sessions do not influence the reproductive efficiency of the animals, since more than 80% pregnancy rate and about 1.8 services/conception after the last treatment are reported.

6.2.9. Utilization of Exogenous LH

An improvement in MOET treatment in cattle, has been obtained by using a GnRH agonist – LH protocol [96]. It is based on the block of the preovulatory endogenous LH surge by treatment with a GnRH agonist bioimplant. The ovulation is achieved by the exogenous administration of LH after follicular superstimulation. The advantage of this protocol is that the ovulations occur over a relatively short and predictable period of time after LH administration [97]. The application of such protocol in buffaloes foresees a conventional superstimulatory protocol, followed 24 hours later by an injection of exogenous LH. It results in higher ovulation rate (about 70%) and higher embryo recovery rate (3.7 embryos on average) compared to animals treated by a conventional MOET protocol, or in those in which LH is administered 36 hours after the superstimulatory protocol [73]. A further improvement of this protocol may be obtained by an estradiol treatment, performed at the start of the superovulation protocol: in this case it is likely that higher follicular responses and ovulation rate are observed.

6.2.10. Administration of Prostaglandin on the Day of Artificial Insemination

It is known that an injection of $PGF_{2\alpha}$ or its analogues causes corpus luteum (CL) regression from day 5-6 to day 15-17 of the estrous cycle, by increasing the intraluteal production of vasoactive molecules, such as Endothelin-1 (ET-1) [98]; and Angiotensin-II (Ang-II) [99], both of which play a role during the luteolytic process. On the contrary, the role of $PGF_{2\alpha}$ administered during the estrous phase is still unclear. It has been shown that inhibitors of prostaglandin synthesis inhibit ovulation [100], and that the administration of $PGF_{2\alpha}$ on the day of AI increases corpus luteum dimensions and progesterone production at the end of a standard (Ovsynch-TAI) synchronization treatment in buffalo [101], probably *via* ET-1 and Ang-II gene expression inhibition [102 - 104]. Furthermore, the stimulation of α-receptors in the ampulla and fimbriae by prostaglandins increases the contractility of smooth muscle, thus affecting gametes transportation [105]. The influence of prostaglandin during the ovulation may be due to its action during follicular rupture. In fact, the ovulatory process involves a complex series of events that result in preovulatory follicle outbreak and cumulus oocyte complex release into the oviduct. The LH peak causes the activation of a novel form of cyclooxygenase (COX-2) enzyme, localized in the granulosa cells of the preovulatory follicle [106], increasing the intrafollicular concentrations of prostaglandin $F_{2\alpha}$ and E_2. These are responsible for the increased contraction of the myoid (smooth muscle) components of the ovary, leading to ovulation [107].

The administration of prostaglandin $F_{2\alpha}$ during the periovulatory period has been utilized also during superovulatory treatment, to verify the possibility of increasing oocyte capture by the fimbriae [108]. Although the number of follicles recruited is not influenced, a higher number of ova (3.5 *vs.* 2.3, in buffaloes treated with prostaglandin and not treated, respectively) and transferable embryos (2.7 *vs.* 1.8, in buffaloes treated with prostaglandin and not treated, respectively) are recovered in buffaloes treated with 4 doses of prostaglandins 12 hours apart, starting from the end of the superovulatory treatment. This is probably due to both: 1) improved contractions of the follicular wall, which then ruptures, expelling the ovum and accompanying follicular fluid containing high levels of $PGF_{2\alpha}$ into the tubal ampulla [109] and 2) increased contractile activity of the tubes. In fact, it is believed that elevated $PGF_{2\alpha}$ levels in the follicular fluid are necessary to enhance ovum capture by tubal fimbriae. Furthermore, the increased contractility of the oviductal smooth muscles, results in increased speed of embryonic transport and development [110, 111].

6.2.11. Immunisation Against Inhibin

Although the number of ovarian follicles recruited in a cohort wave is similar between buffalo and cattle [4, 37, 54], the number of recovered embryos in the former is very low. The developing dominant follicle produces inhibin, a substance that inhibit both pituitary FSH secretion and follicular development of subordinates. The immunoneutralisation against inhibin in cattle stimulates follicle development [112], embryo yield [113] and embryo quality [114], reducing the phenomenon of follicular atresia. The immunisation against inhibin improves superovulatory response also in water buffaloes [115], in terms of improving superovulation rates and number and percentage of transferable embryos, as well as elevating plasma E_2 concentrations during estrus and P_4 concentrations during diestrus. In particular, the utilization of primary immunisation with 2 mg inhibin fusion protein is able to increase the ovulation rate (6.5 *vs* 4.8, in treated and not treated animals, respectively), the number of recovered ova (4.5 *vs*. 2.8, in treated and not treated animals, respectively) and the number of transferable embryos (3.3 *vs*. 1.6, in treated and not treated animals, respectively). On the other hand, as described above, the utilization of antibodies anti-eCG reduces peripheral inhibin concentration and the number of anovulatory follicles [68], slightly improving the superovulatory response.

7. THE APPLICATION OF MOET IN THE BUFFALO SPECIES

As reported in the introduction of this chapter, several attempts have been performed to optimize the MOET technology in the buffalo species. However, although embryo recovery improved in the last thirty years, from less than 1 viable embryo to 2.5-3/donor, MOET in buffaloes typically results in a relatively low recovery of both embryos and unfertilized ova [17, 18, 33, 34, 43, 49, 51, 68, 72, 73, 94, 116, 117] when compared to cattle [4, 5] throughout the world. In particular, while in cattle 88% of animals produce at least 1 embryo after superstimulation, the ratio of responsive buffaloes is between 30 and 50% [17].

Several hypotheses have been formulated to explain the low embryo recovery recorded in the buffalo species after SO. It is known that oogenesis in cattle and buffalo gonads starts during the fetal life, resulting in the formation of a pool of primordial follicles, which represents the source of gametes throughout the life of the female. The number of primordial follicles represents the first great difference between cattle and buffalo. In fact, while in cattle the number of primordial follicles from the birth to about 4th year of life is 133,000 [118, 119], only 26,600 [120] or 40,000 [121, 122] primordial follicles have been recorded, in swamp and riverine buffaloes, respectively. Therefore, if buffaloes have about 20-30% of the total pool of primordial follicles compared to cattle, it would be reasonable to conclude that the response to SO treatment in terms of embryo yield in the former is about 1/5 compared to the latter. However, this hypothesis leaves some doubts, since the response of the buffalo in terms of follicles > 1cm at the end of the MOET treatment is quite satisfactory. Some studies [49, 54, 73] demonstrated that MOET programs usually result in the growth of a high number of ovulatory follicles, together with a relatively high ovulation rate (50-70%), although embryo/ova recovery rate is very low (13-35%).

Therefore, it has been supposed that follicular growth and ovulation cannot be considered the causes for low embryo recovery in buffaloes. It is more likely that the recruitment of the oocytes by the fimbriae and/or their transport within the oviduct is compromised [73]. Plasma 17-β-estradiol (estradiol) levels recorded in buffaloes are lower than those reported in cattle during normal estrous cycles [123]. On the contrary, estradiol plasma concentrations are particularly high during SO [58], resulting in an altered estradiol:progesterone ratio, that may influence oocyte recruitment by the fimbriae [24]. This would be further confirmed by the negative correlation observed between the presence of a high number of large (>8 mm) follicles on the day of embryo recovery and the number of recovered embryos [24, 54]. Furthermore, it is worth noting that the quality of the oocyte and especially the cumulus cell layers surrounding it are factors that may affect oocyte capture by the fimbriae [124]. Grade I and II oocytes (those surrounded by several granulosa cell layers) represent only about 50-60% [93] of the total oocytes retrieved in buffaloes, whereas about 80% of the same categories is retrieved in cattle.

In conclusion, the application of MOET in buffalo still needs to be improved, by increasing both the number of animals that are able to produce at least one embryo and, possibly, a higher number of recovered embryos.

CONFLICT OF INTEREST

The authors confirm that they have no conflict of interest to declare for this publication.

ACKNOWLEDGEMENTS

Declared none.

REFERENCES

[1] Bevers MM, Dieleman SJ. Superovulation of cows with PMSG: variation in plasma concentrations of progesterone, oestradiol, LH, cortisol, prolactin and PMSG and in number of preovulatory follicles. Anim Reprod Sci 1987; 15: 37-52. [http://dx.doi.org/10.1016/0378-4320(87)90004-2]

[2] Umbaugh RE. Superovulation and ovum transfer in cattle. Fertil Steril 1951; 2(3): 243-52. [http://dx.doi.org/10.1016/S0015-0282(16)30544-1] [PMID: 14831647]

[3] Gordon I. Problems and prospects in cattle egg transfer. Ir Vet J 1975; 29: 21-62.

[4] Mapletoft RJ, Bó GA. The evolution of improved and simplified superovulation protocols in cattle. Reprod Fertil Dev 2011; 24(1): 278-83. [http://dx.doi.org/10.1071/RD11919] [PMID: 22394970]

[5] Bó GA, Mapletoft RJ. Historical perspectives and recent research on superovulation in cattle. Theriogenology 2014; 81(1): 38-48. [http://dx.doi.org/10.1016/j.theriogenology.2013.09.020] [PMID: 24274408]

[6] Drost M, Wright JM Jr, Cripe WS, Richter AR. Embryo transfer in water buffalo (*Bubalus bubalis*). Theriogenology 1983; 20(5): 579-84. [http://dx.doi.org/10.1016/0093-691X(83)90082-1] [PMID: 16725875]

[7] Misra AK, Yadav MC, Motwani KT. Successful embryo transfer in a buffalo. Proceeding of II World Buffalo Congress. New Delhi, India. 1988.

[8] Evans AC, Adams GP, Rawlings NC. Endocrine and ovarian follicular changes leading up to the first ovulation in prepubertal heifers. J Reprod Fertil 1994; 100(1): 187-94. [http://dx.doi.org/10.1530/jrf.0.1000187] [PMID: 8182588]

[9] De Rensis F, Peters AR. The control of follicular dynamics by PGF2Alpha, GnRH, hCG and oestrus synchronization in cattle. Reprod Domest Anim 1999; 34: 49-59. [http://dx.doi.org/10.1111/j.1439-0531.1999.tb01383.x]

[10] Baruselli PS, Mucciolo RG, Visintin JA, *et al.* Ovarian follicular dynamics during the estrous cycle in buffalo (*Bubalus bubalis*). Theriogenology 1997; 47(8): 1531-47. [http://dx.doi.org/10.1016/S0093-691X(97)00159-3] [PMID: 16728096]

[11] Neglia G, Natale A, Esposito G, *et al.* Follicular dynamics in synchronized Italian Mediterranean buffalo cows. Italian J Anim Sci 2007; 6(1) (Suppl. 2): 61-614. [http://dx.doi.org/10.4081/ijas.2007.s2.611]

[12] Ginther OJ, Beg MA, Bergfelt DR, Donadeu FX, Kot K. Follicle selection in monovular species. Biol Reprod 2001; 65(3): 638-47. [http://dx.doi.org/10.1095/biolreprod65.3.638] [PMID: 11514323]

[13] Gimenes LU, Carvalho NA, Sá Filho MF, *et al.* Ultrasonographic and endocrine aspects of follicle

deviation, and acquisition of ovulatory capacity in buffalo (*Bubalus bubalis*) heifers. Anim Reprod Sci 2011; 123(3-4): 175-9.
[http://dx.doi.org/10.1016/j.anireprosci.2010.12.004] [PMID: 21256685]

[14] Mihm M, Baker PJ, Ireland JL, *et al.* Molecular evidence that growth of dominant follicles involves a reduction in follicle-stimulating hormone dependence and an increase in luteinizing hormone dependence in cattle. Biol Reprod 2006; 74(6): 1051-9.
[http://dx.doi.org/10.1095/biolreprod.105.045799] [PMID: 16481595]

[15] Bó GA, Adams GP, Pierson RA, Mapletoft RJ. Exogenous control of follicular wave emergence in cattle. Theriogenology 1995; 43: 31-40.
[http://dx.doi.org/10.1016/0093-691X(94)00010-R]

[16] Zicarelli L, Boni R, Campanile G, *et al.* Effect of OPU priming on superovulatory response in Italian buffalo cows. In: 5th World Buffalo Conference; Oct, 1997; Royal Palace, Caserta, Italy. 13-6.

[17] Zicarelli L. Superovulatory response in buffalo bred in Italy. Bubalus bubalis 1997; 4 (Suppl): 167-88.

[18] Misra AK, Tyagi S. *In vivo* embryo production in buffalo: present and perspectives. Ital J Anim Sci 2007; 6 (Suppl. 2): 74-91.
[http://dx.doi.org/10.4081/ijas.2007.s2.74]

[19] Vittoria A. Anatomy of the female genital tract in the buffalo. Bubalus bubalis 1997; 4 (Supp l): 15-20.

[20] Zicarelli L. Embryo transfer in Mediterranean buffaloes. Buffalo Journal 1994; 2: 87-101.

[21] Chantaraprateep P, Lohachit C, Techakumphu M, *et al.* Early embryonic development in Thai swamp buffalo (*Bubalus bubalis*). Theriogenology 1989; 31(6): 1131-9.
[http://dx.doi.org/10.1016/0093-691X(89)90081-2] [PMID: 16726630]

[22] Drost M, Elsden RP. Blastocyst development in the water buffalo. Theriogenology 1985; 23-191.

[23] Anwar M, Ullah N. Early development and location of embryos in the reproductive tract of Nili Ravi buffalo (*Bubalus bubalis*): a retrospective analysis. Theriogenology 1998; 49(6): 1187-93.
[http://dx.doi.org/10.1016/S0093-691X(98)00066-1] [PMID: 10732056]

[24] Misra AK, Kasiraj R, Rao MM, Rangareddy NS, Jaiswal RS, Pant HC. Rate of transport and development of preimplantation embryo in the superovulated buffalo (*Bubalus bubalis*). Theriogenology 1998; 50(4): 637-49.
[http://dx.doi.org/10.1016/S0093-691X(98)00168-X] [PMID: 10732154]

[25] Galli C, Crotti G, Notari C, Turini P, Duchi R, Lazzari G. Embryo production by ovum pick up from live donors. Theriogenology 2001; 55(6): 1341-57.
[http://dx.doi.org/10.1016/S0093-691X(01)00486-1] [PMID: 11327688]

[26] Karaivanov C, Vlahov K, Petrov M, *et al.* Studies on preimplantation development of buffalo embryos. Theriogenology 1987; 28(5): 747-53.
[http://dx.doi.org/10.1016/0093-691X(87)90291-3] [PMID: 16726357]

[27] Betteridge KJ, Flechon JE. The anatomy and physiology of preattachment bovine embryos. Theriogenology 1988; 29: 155-87.
[http://dx.doi.org/10.1016/0093-691X(88)90038-6]

[28] Mehmood A, Anwar M, Javed MH. Superovulation with PMSG beginning on three different days of

the cycle in Nili Ravi buffaloes. Buffalo J 1989; 5: 79-84.

[29] Stringfellow DA, Seidel SM. Manual of the International Embryo Transfer Society: a procedural guide and general information for the use of embryo transfer technology emphasizing sanitary procedures Savory. Ill. International Embryo Transfer Society 2007.

[30] Gandolfi F. The role of oviduct in farm animals reproduction. 1997; 4 (Supp l): 61-70.

[31] Neglia G. Produzione embrionale *in vivo* nella specie bufalina. Proceedings of VIII Congresso Nazionale Multisala della Società Italiana Veterinari Animali da Reddito [SIVAR]. Cremona: Italia 2006.

[32] Boni R, Roviello S, Gasparrini B, Zicarelli L. Pregnancies established after transferring embryos yielded by Ovum Pick-up and *in vitro* embryo production in Italian buffalo cows. Proceedings of V World Buffalo Congress. Caserta, Italia. 1997; pp. 787-92.

[33] Alexiev A, Vlahov K, Karaivanov Ch, *et al.* Embryo transfer in buffaloes in Bulgaria. Proceedings of the II World Buffalo Congress. Vol. 2Bulgaria. 1988; pp. : 591-5.

[34] Misra AK, Kasiraj R, Mutha Rao M, Rangareddy JN, Joshi BV. Embryo transfer in buffalo in India: progress in the last 5 years. Proceeding of IV World Buffalo Congress. 501-3.

[35] Misra AK, Joshi BV, Agrawala PL, *et al.* Multiple ovulation and embryo transfer in Indian buffalo (Bubalus buoalis). Theriogenology 1990; 33(5): 1131-41. [http://dx.doi.org/10.1016/0093-691X(90)90073-3] [PMID: 16726807]

[36] Heleil B, El Deeb Y. Superovulatory response in relation to follicular dynamics and presence of dominant follicles in Egyptian buffaloes. Adv Biol Res (Faisalabad) 2010; 4(3): 169-74.

[37] Campanile G, Baruselli PS, Neglia G, *et al.* Ovarian function in the buffalo and implications for embryo development and assisted reproduction. Anim Reprod Sci 2010; 121(1-2): 1-11. [http://dx.doi.org/10.1016/j.anireprosci.2010.03.012] [PMID: 20430540]

[38] Nasser LF, Adams GP, Bo´ GA, Mapletoft RJ. Ovarian superstimulatory response relative to follicular wave emergence in heifers. Theriogenology 1993; 40(4): 713-24. [http://dx.doi.org/10.1016/0093-691X(93)90207-L] [PMID: 16727353]

[39] Jiang H, Wei Y, Jiang Q, *et al.* Pregnancies resulted from transfer of in-vivo embryos derived from nonsurgical recovery in superovulated buffaloes. Proceeding of 5th Asian Buffalo Congress. Nanning, China. 2006; pp. 53-8.

[40] Ullah N, Wright RW Jr, Mehmood A, Baig SM. Endocrine profile in relation to ovarian response, recovery rate and quality of embryos in Nili-Ravi buffaloes treated with FSH. Buffalo J 1992; 1: 47-56.

[41] Goto K, Ohkutsu S, Nakanishi Y, *et al.* Endocrine profiles and embryo quality in superovulated Japanese Black cattle. Theriogenology 1988; 29(3): 615-29. [http://dx.doi.org/10.1016/S0093-691X(88)80009-8] [PMID: 16726384]

[42] Misra AK, Jaiswal RS, Kasiraj R, Mutha Rao M, Rangareddy NS, Pant H. C. Periovulatory steroid hormone profiles during unstimulated and superovulatory oestrous cycle in buffalo. Buffalo J 2000; 3: 371-80.

[43] Madan ML, Das SK, Palta P. Application of reproductive technology to buffaloes. Anim Reprod Sci

1996; 42: 299-306.
[http://dx.doi.org/10.1016/0378-4320(96)01534-5]

[44] Park D, Cheon M, Kim C, Kim K, Ryu K. Progesterone together with estradiol promotes luteinizing hormone beta-subunit mRNA stability in rat pituitary cells cultured *in vitro*. Eur J Endocrinol 1996; 134(2): 236-42.
[http://dx.doi.org/10.1530/eje.0.1340236] [PMID: 8630526]

[45] Karsch FJ, Cummins JT, Thomas GB, Clarke IJ. Steroid feedback inhibition of pulsatile secretion of gonadotropin-releasing hormone in the ewe. Biol Reprod 1987; 36(5): 1207-18.
[http://dx.doi.org/10.1095/biolreprod36.5.1207] [PMID: 3304436]

[46] Nett TM, Turzillo AM, Baratta M, Rispoli LA. Pituitary effects of steroid hormones on secretion of follicle-stimulating hormone and luteinizing hormone. Domest Anim Endocrinol 2002; 23(1-2): 33-42.
[http://dx.doi.org/10.1016/S0739-7240(02)00143-1] [PMID: 12142224]

[47] Gonzalez-Bulnes A, Garcia-Garcia RM, Santiago-Moreno J, Lopez-Sebastian A, Cocero MJ. Effect of follicular status on superovulatory response in ewes is influenced by presence of corpus luteum at first FSH dose. Theriogenology 2002; 58(8): 1607-14.
[http://dx.doi.org/10.1016/S0093-691X(02)01078-6] [PMID: 12374130]

[48] Madan ML, Singla SK, Singh C, Prakash BS, Jailkhani S. Embryo transfer technology in buffaloes: endocrine responses and limitations. Proceeding of II World Buffalo Congress. Vol III New Delhi. 1988; pp. : 195-211.

[49] Neglia G, Gasparrini B, Vecchio D, *et al.* Progesterone supplementation during multiple ovulation treatment in buffalo species (*Bubalus bubalis*). Trop Anim Health Prod 2010; 42(6): 1243-7.
[http://dx.doi.org/10.1007/s11250-010-9556-8] [PMID: 20411328]

[50] Heleil B, El-Kon I, El Deeb Y. Assessment of superovulatory response using hormonal profile in buffalo. Global Veterinaria 2010; 4(4): 337-42.

[51] Taneja M, Singh G, Totey SM, Ali A. Follicular dynamics in water buffalo superovulated in presence or absence of a dominant follicle. Theriogenology 1995; 44(4): 581-97.
[http://dx.doi.org/10.1016/0093-691X(95)00229-2] [PMID: 16727756]

[52] Manik RS, Singla SK, Palta P, Madan ML. Effect of presence of a dominant follicle on the superovulatory response in buffalo (*Bubalus bubalis*). Theriogenology 1998; 50(6): 841-52.
[http://dx.doi.org/10.1016/S0093-691X(98)00189-7] [PMID: 10734457]

[53] Bungartz L, Niemann H. Assessment of the presence of a dominant follicle and selection of dairy cows suitable for superovulation by a single ultrasound examination. J Reprod Fertil 1994; 101(3): 583-91.
[http://dx.doi.org/10.1530/jrf.0.1010583] [PMID: 7966012]

[54] Baruselli PS, Madureira EH, Visintin JA, Barnabe VH, Barnabe RC, Amaral R. Inseminação artificial em tempo fixo com sincronização da ovulação em bubalinos. Rev Bras Repr Anim 1999; 23: 360-2.

[55] Situmorang P. Superovulation in different buffalo genotypes. Indonesian J Animal and Veterinary Sciences 2003; 8: 40-5.

[56] Moor RM, Osborn JC, Crosby IM. Gonadotrophin-induced abnormalities in sheep oocytes after superovulation. J Reprod Fertil 1985; 74(1): 167-72.
[http://dx.doi.org/10.1530/jrf.0.0740167] [PMID: 3926997]

[57] Mazerbourg S, Bondy CA, Zhou J, Monget P. The insulin-like growth factor system: a key determinant role in the growth and selection of ovarian follicles? a comparative species study. Reprod Domest Anim 2003; 38(4): 247-58. [http://dx.doi.org/10.1046/j.1439-0531.2003.00440.x] [PMID: 12887564]

[58] Beg MA, Ginther OJ. Follicle selection in cattle and horses: role of intrafollicular factors. Reproduction 2006; 132(3): 365-77. [http://dx.doi.org/10.1530/rep.1.01233] [PMID: 16940278]

[59] Echternkamp SE, Roberts AJ, Lunstra DD, Wise T, Spicer LJ. Ovarian follicular development in cattle selected for twin ovulations and births. J Anim Sci 2004; 82(2): 459-71. [http://dx.doi.org/10.2527/2004.822459x] [PMID: 14974544]

[60] Velazquez MA, Zaraza J, Oropeza A, Webb R, Niemann H. The role of IGF1 in the *in vivo* production of bovine embryos from superovulated donors. Reproduction 2009; 137(2): 161-80. [http://dx.doi.org/10.1530/REP-08-0362] [PMID: 19029343]

[61] Murphy BD, Martinuk SD. Equine chorionic gonadotropin. Endocr Rev 1991; 12(1): 27-44. [http://dx.doi.org/10.1210/edrv-12-1-27] [PMID: 2026120]

[62] Monniaux D, Chupin D, Saumande J. Superovulatory responses of cattle. Theriogenology 1983; 19: 55-64. [http://dx.doi.org/10.1016/0093-691X(83)90124-3]

[63] Singh B, Dixit VD, Dixit VP, Singh P, George GC, Lohan IS. Changes in plasma levels of inhibin and FSH in buffaloes superovulated with eCG. Asian-Aust. J Anim Sci 2000; 13: 1205-9.

[64] Gonzales-Mencio F, Manns J, Murphy BD. FSH and LH activity of PMSG from mares at different stages of gestation. Anim Reprod Sci 1978; 1(2): 137-44. [http://dx.doi.org/10.1016/0378-4320(78)90021-0]

[65] Karaivanov C, Kacheva D, Petrov M, Vlahov K, Sapundjiev E. Superovulatory response of river bufalo (*Bubalus bubalis*). Theriogenology 1990; 33(2): 453-64. [http://dx.doi.org/10.1016/0093-691X(90)90503-L] [PMID: 16726742]

[66] Schallenberger E, Wagner HG, Papa R, Hartl P, Tenhumberg H. Endocrinological evaluation of the induction of superovulation with PMSG in water buffalo (*Bubalus bubalis*). Theriogenology 1990; 34(2): 379-92. [http://dx.doi.org/10.1016/0093-691X(90)90530-7] [PMID: 16726846]

[67] Singh C, Madan ML. The ovarian response of prepubertal buffalo (*Bubalus bubalis*) to superovulation with equine chorionic gonadotrophin with and without treatment with GnRH. Vet J 1999; 158(2): 155-8. [http://dx.doi.org/10.1053/tvjl.1998.0318] [PMID: 10489273]

[68] Palta P, Kumar M, Jailkhani S, Manik RS, Madan ML. Changes in peripheral inhibin levels and follicular development following treatment of buffalo with PMSG and Neutra-PMSG for superovulation. Theriogenology 1997; 48(2): 233-40. [http://dx.doi.org/10.1016/S0093-691X(97)84070-8] [PMID: 16728122]

[69] Palta P, Madan ML. Gonadotropic responses to GnRH in Murrah buffaloes (*Bubalus bubalis*) treated with PMSG. Buffalo J 1995; 11: 205-11.

[70] Herrler A, Elsaesser F, Parvizi N, Niemann H. Superovulation of dairy cows with purified FSH supplemented with defined amounts of LH. Theriogenology 1991; 35(3): 633-43. [http://dx.doi.org/10.1016/0093-691X(91)90459-Q] [PMID: 16726932]

[71] Looney CR, Bondioli KR, Hill KG, Massey JM. Superovulation of donor cows with bovine follicle stimulating hormone [bFSH] produced by recombinant DNA technology. Theriogenology 1990; 29: 271. [http://dx.doi.org/10.1016/0093-691X(88)90099-4]

[72] Baruselli PS, Mucciolo RG, Arruda R, Madureira RH, Amaral R, Assumpcao ME. Embryo recovery rate in superovulated buffaloes. Theriogenology 1999; 51: 401. [http://dx.doi.org/10.1016/S0093-691X(99)91960-X]

[73] Carvalho NA, Baruselli PS, Zicarelli L, Madureira EH, Visintin JA, DOcchio MJ. Control of ovulation with a GnRH agonist after superstimulation of follicular growth in buffalo: fertilization and embryo recovery. Theriogenology 2002; 58(9): 1641-50. [http://dx.doi.org/10.1016/S0093-691X(02)01057-9] [PMID: 12472135]

[74] Campanile G, Neglia G, Vecchio D, Russo M, Zicarelli L. Pregnancy in buffalo cows. In: O'Leary Marie, Arnett John, Eds. Pregnancy Protein Research. Nova Science Publishers, Inc. 2009. 978---60692-396-2. pp. 31 – 91

[75] Zicarelli L. Reproductive seasonality in buffalo. Bubalus bubalis 1974; (Supp l)29-52.

[76] Zicarelli L, Di Palo R, Palladino M, Campanile G, Esposito L. Embryo transfer in Mediterranean *Bubalus bubalis*. Proceeding of the International Symposium "Prospects of buffalo production in the Mediterranean and the Middle Est. Cairo, Egypt 1993; 9-12: 73-75

[77] Misra AK. Superovulation and embryo transfer in buffalo: Progress, problems and future prospects in India. Buffalo J 1993; 1: 13-24.

[78] Mutha Rao M, Kasiraj R, Reddy KS, Jaiswal RS, Misra AK, Ranga Reddy NS. A study on repeated superovulation and nonsurgical recovery in buffaloes. Proceeding of 4th World Buffalo Congress. Volume 3Sao Paulo, Brazil. 1994; pp. : 498-500.

[79] Campanile G, Neglia G. Influencia de la nutricion sobre las performances reproductivas de bufalos productores de leche. Proceedings of II Simposio de Bufalos de Las Americas, Facultad de Ciencias Veterinarias. Universidad Nacional del Nordeste, Argentina. 2004; pp. 78-91.

[80] Di Palo R, Campanile G, Esposito L, Barbieri V, Zicarelli L. Characteristics of diet and FSH-P superovulatory response in Italian Mediterranean buffaloes. Proceedings of IV World Buffalo Congress. Sao Paulo, Brazil. 1994; pp. 474-6.

[81] Campanile G. Di Palo, Gasparrini B, Spadetta M, Neglia G and Zicarelli L. Follicle and oocyte characteristics in buffaloes fed different diets. Proceedings of the Scientific Association of Animal Production [A.S.P.A. XIII Congress. Piacenza, Italy. 1999; pp. 241-3.

[82] Baruselli PS, Barnabe VH, Barnabe RC, Visintin JA, Molero-Filho JR, Porto R. Effect of body condition score at calving on postpartum reproductive performance in buffalo. Buffalo J 2001; 17: 53-65.

[83] Alapati A, Kapa SR, Jeepalyam S, Rangappa SM, Yemireddy KR. Development of the body condition score system in Murrah buffaloes: validation through ultrasonic assessment of body fat reserves. J Vet

Sci 2010; 11(1): 1-8.
[http://dx.doi.org/10.4142/jvs.2010.11.1.1] [PMID: 20195058]

[84] Campanile G, Neglia G, Di Palo R, *et al.* Relationship of body condition score and blood urea and ammonia to pregnancy in Italian Mediterranean buffaloes. Reprod Nutr Dev 2006; 46(1): 57-62.
[http://dx.doi.org/10.1051/rnd:2005066] [PMID: 16438915]

[85] Wagner JJ, Lusby KS, Oltjen JW, Rakestraw J, Wettemann RP, Walters LE. Carcass composition in mature Hereford cows: estimation and effect on daily metabolizable energy requirement during winter. J Anim Sci 1988; 66(3): 603-12.
[http://dx.doi.org/10.2527/jas1988.663603x] [PMID: 3378920]

[86] Gong JG, Bramley TA, Wilmut I, Webb R. Effect of recombinant bovine somatotropin on the superovulatory response to pregnant mare serum gonadotropin in heifers. Biol Reprod 1993; 48(5): 1141-9.
[http://dx.doi.org/10.1095/biolreprod48.5.1141] [PMID: 8481477]

[87] Songsasen N, Yiengvisavakul V, Buntaracha B, Pharee S, Apimeteetumrong M, Sukwongs Y. Effect of treatment with recombinant bovine somatotropin on responses to superovulatory treatment in swamp buffalo (*Bubalus bubalis*). Theriogenology 1999; 52(3): 377-84.
[http://dx.doi.org/10.1016/S0093-691X(99)00136-3] [PMID: 10734373]

[88] Gong JG, Baxter G, Bramley TA, Webb R. Enhancement of ovarian follicle development in heifers by treatment with recombinant bovine somatotrophin: a dose-response study. J Reprod Fertil 1997; 110(1): 91-7.
[http://dx.doi.org/10.1530/jrf.0.1100091] [PMID: 9227362]

[89] Izadyar F, Hage WJ, Colenbrander B, Bevers MM. The promotory effect of growth hormone on the developmental competence of in vitro matured bovine oocytes is due to improved cytoplasmic maturation. Mol Reprod Dev 1998; 49(4): 444-53.
[http://dx.doi.org/10.1002/(SICI)1098-2795(199804)49:4<444::AID-MRD12>3.0.CO;2-U] [PMID: 9508096]

[90] Carvalho NA, Nagasaku EM, Vannucci FS, *et al.* Use of different doses of rBST associated to a protocol for multiple ovulation and embryo transfer in buffalo. Ital J Anim Sci 2007; 6 (Suppl. 2): 652-4.
[http://dx.doi.org/10.4081/ijas.2007.s2.652]

[91] Baruselli PS, Carvalho NA, Cavalcante AK, Nichi M, Zicarelli L. Use of rBST associated to a protocol for multiple ovulation and embryo transfer in buffalo [*Bubalus bubalis*]. Proceedings of Proc II Congresso Nazionale sull'Allevamento del Bufalo. Monterotondo, Italy. 2003; pp. 28-30.

[92] Neglia G, Gasparrini B, Caracciolo di Brienza V, *et al.* Bovine and buffalo *in vitro* embryo production using oocytes derived from abattoir ovaries or collected by transvaginal follicle aspiration. Theriogenology 2003; 59(5-6): 1123-30.
[http://dx.doi.org/10.1016/S0093-691X(02)01170-6] [PMID: 12527061]

[93] Neglia G, Gasparrini B, Vecchio D, *et al.* Long term effect of Ovum Pick-up in buffalo species 2011.
[http://dx.doi.org/10.1016/j.anireprosci.2011.01.011]

[94] Misra AK, Pant HC. Estrus induction following PGF2α treatment in the superovulated buffalo (*Bubalus bubalis*). Theriogenology 2003; 59(5-6): 1203-7.

[http://dx.doi.org/10.1016/S0093-691X(02)01167-6] [PMID: 12527068]

[95] Cruz LC. Venturina, Jha SS, Adriano F, Duran PG, Serra P, Smith OF, Faylon PS and Lorenzon N. Successful transfer of Murrah buffalo embryos into Philippine swamp buffalo recipient. Proceedings of 3rd World Buffalo Congress. Varna, Bulgaria. 1991.

[96] DOcchio MJ, Jillella D, Lindsey BR. Factors that influence follicle recruitment, growth and ovulation during ovarian superstimulation in heifers: opportunities to increase ovulation rate and embryo recovery by delaying the exposure of follicles to LH. Theriogenology 1999; 51(1): 9-35. [http://dx.doi.org/10.1016/S0093-691X(98)00228-3] [PMID: 10729059]

[97] DOcchio MJ, Sudha G, Jillella D, *et al.* Use of a GnRH agonist to prevent the endogenous LH surge and injection of exogenous LH to induce ovulation in heifers superstimulated with FSH: a new model for superovulation. Theriogenology 1997; 47(3): 601-13. [http://dx.doi.org/10.1016/S0093-691X(97)00018-6] [PMID: 16728012]

[98] Ohtani M, Kobayashi S, Miyamoto A, Hayashi K, Fukui Y. Real-time relationships between intraluteal and plasma concentrations of endothelin, oxytocin, and progesterone during prostaglandin F2alpha-induced luteolysis in the cow. Biol Reprod 1998; 58(1): 103-8. [http://dx.doi.org/10.1095/biolreprod58.1.103] [PMID: 9472929]

[99] Hayashi K, Acosta TJ, Berisha B, Kobayashi S, Ohtani M, Miyamoto A. Real-time changes in the local angiotensin system and prostaglandin production in the regressing corpus luteum in the cow. Biol Reprod 2001; 64 (Suppl. 1): 132. [abstract 66].

[100] Ainsworth L, Tsang BK, Downey BR, Baker RD, Marcus GJ, Armstrong DT. Effects of indomethacin on ovulation and luteal function in gilts. Biol Reprod 1979; 21(2): 401-11. [http://dx.doi.org/10.1095/biolreprod21.2.401] [PMID: 486663]

[101] Neglia G, Natale A, Esposito G, *et al.* Effect of prostaglandin F2α at the time of AI on progesterone levels and pregnancy rate in synchronized Italian Mediterranean buffaloes. Theriogenology 2008; 69(8): 953-60. [http://dx.doi.org/10.1016/j.theriogenology.2008.01.008] [PMID: 18346780]

[102] Girsh E, Wang W, Mamluk R, *et al.* Regulation of endothelin-1 expression in the bovine corpus luteum: elevation by prostaglandin F 2 alpha. Endocrinology 1996; 137(12): 5191-6. [PMID: 8940334]

[103] Miyamoto A, Shirasuna K. Luteolysis in the cow: a novel concept of vasoactive molecules. Anim Reprod 2009; 6(1): 47-59.

[104] Meidan R, Milvae RA, Weiss S, Levy N, Friedman A. Intraovarian regulation of luteolysis. J Reprod Fertil Suppl 1999; 54 (Suppl.): 217-28. [PMID: 10692857]

[105] Riehl RM, Harper MJ. Changes in prostaglandin binding capacity to single oviductal smooth muscle cells after ovulation in the rabbit. Endocrinology 1981; 109(4): 1011-6. [http://dx.doi.org/10.1210/endo-109-4-1011] [PMID: 6269826]

[106] Hedin L, Gaddy-Kurten D, Kurten R, DeWitt DL, Smith WL, Richards JS. Prostaglandin endoperoxide synthase in rat ovarian follicles: content, cellular distribution, and evidence for hormonal induction preceding ovulation. Endocrinology 1987; 121(2): 722-31.

[http://dx.doi.org/10.1210/endo-121-2-722] [PMID: 3109886]

[107] Senger PL. Reproductive cyclicity—the follicular phase. Pathways to pregnancy and parturition. 2nd ed. Current Conceptions Inc. 2005; pp. 164-87.

[108] Soares JG, Carvalho NAT, Martins Junior B, *et al.* PGF2α treatment during the periovulatory period increases the number of embryos recovered from superovulated buffaloes. Buffalo Bulletin 2013; 32(2): 522-6.

[109] LeMaire WJ, Marsh JM. Interrelationship between prostaglandins, cyclic AMP and steroids in ovulation. J Reprod Fertil 1975; (Suppl. 22)53-74.

[110] Weber JA, Freeman DA, Vanderwall DK, Woods GL. Prostaglandin E2 hastens oviductal transport of equine embryos. Biol Reprod 1991; 45(4): 544-6.
[http://dx.doi.org/10.1095/biolreprod45.4.544] [PMID: 1751628]

[111] Kissler S, Wildt L, Schmiedehausen K, *et al.* Predictive value of impaired uterine transport function assessed by negative hysterosalpingoscintigraphy (HSSG). Eur J Obstet Gynecol Reprod Biol 2004; 113(2): 204-8.
[http://dx.doi.org/10.1016/j.ejogrb.2003.07.003] [PMID: 15063961]

[112] Medan MS, Akagi S, Kaneko H, Watanabe G, Tsonis CG, Taya K. Effects of re-immunization of heifers against inhibin on hormonal profiles and ovulation rate. Reproduction 2004; 128(4): 475-82.
[http://dx.doi.org/10.1530/rep.1.00232] [PMID: 15454642]

[113] Mantovani R, Enright WJ, Roche JF, Boland MP. The effect of immunization of heifers against alpha 126 inhibin conjugate on the superovulatory response to pFSH. Theriogenology 1997; 47(2): 511-9.
[http://dx.doi.org/10.1016/S0093-691X(97)00009-5] [PMID: 16728003]

[114] Li C, Zhu YL, Xue JH, Zhang SL, Ma Z, Shi ZD. Immunization against inhibin enhances both embryo quantity and quality in Holstein heifers after superovulation and insemination with sex-sorted semen. Theriogenology 2009; 71(6): 1011-7.
[http://dx.doi.org/10.1016/j.theriogenology.2008.11.003] [PMID: 19144396]

[115] Li DR, Qin GS, Wei YM, *et al.* Immunisation against inhibin enhances follicular development, oocyte maturation and superovulatory response in water buffaloes. Reprod Fertil Dev 2011; 23(6): 788-97.
[http://dx.doi.org/10.1071/RD10279] [PMID: 21791180]

[116] Beg MA, Sanwal PC, Yadav MC. Ovarian response and endocrine changes in buffalo superovulated at midluteal and late luteal stage of the estrous cycle: a preliminary report. Theriogenology 1997; 47(2): 423-32.
[http://dx.doi.org/10.1016/S0093-691X(97)00001-0] [PMID: 16727995]

[117] Qin G-S, Chen M-T, Liang X-W, *et al.* Effetcs of different hormone combinations on superovulation in River buffaloes. J Animal and Plant Sciences 2012; 22(3) (Suppl.): 257-61.

[118] Erickson BH. Development and senescence of the postnatal bovine ovary. J Anim Sci 1966; 25(3): 800-5.
[http://dx.doi.org/10.2527/jas1966.253800x] [PMID: 6007918]

[119] Driancourt MA, Gougeon A, Royere D, Thibault C. Ovarian Function. Reproduction in mammals and man C Thibault and MC levasseur, EDS RHF, Hunter. Paris: Flipses 1993; pp. 281-305.

[120] Ty LV, Nguyen BX, Son HN, Draincourt MA. Superovulation and ovarian follicular population of juvenile buffaloes and calves. Anim Reprod Sci 1994; 35: 191-9. [http://dx.doi.org/10.1016/0378-4320(94)90035-3]

[121] Samad HA, Nasseri AA. A quantitative study of primordial follicles in buffalo heifer ovaries. Comp 13th FAO/SIDA International Course Anim Reprod. Sweden: Uppsala 1979.

[122] Danell B. Oestrus behaviour, ovarian morphology and cyclical variation in the follicular system and endocrine pattern in water buffalo heifers 1987.

[123] Batra SK, Pandey RS. LH and oestradiol 17-β in blood plasma and milk during the oestrus cycle and early pregnancy in Murrah buffaloes. Anim Reprod Sci 1983; 5: 247-57. [http://dx.doi.org/10.1016/0378-4320(83)90046-5]

[124] Priedkalns J. Female reproductive system. In: Dellmann HD, Brown EM, Eds. Histologia veterinaria. Rio de Janeiro: Ciuanabera Koogen 1987; pp. 255-78.

CHAPTER 14

Applied Reproductive Technologies in the Buffalo Species

Bianca Gasparrini[*]

Department of Veterinary Medicine and Animal Production, Federico II University, Via F. Delpino 1, 80137 Naples, Italy

Abstract: In consideration of the typically low efficiency of MOET programs in buffaloes, in the past two decades there has been a mushrooming interest in the exploitation of *in vitro* embryo production procedures (IVEP), employed for a more rapid and targeted improvement and propagation of superior genetics from elite animals. Procedures that had been used in cattle successfully, were also used in the very first attempts in buffaloes, although a significant improvement in the efficiency of the entire process in the buffalo species has been achieved in the course of the intervening years through novel information on oocyte and embryo culture requirements. This review aims at describing the state of the art of IVEP in the buffalo species, the results and improvements obtained together with the difficulties and limitations still to be overcome.

Keywords: Buffalo, Cryopreservation, *In vitro* produced embryos, Sperm sexing.

1. INTRODUCTION

Buffaloes have been playing over time an important role in countries characterized by a number of disadvantages, both in terms of climate and agricultural production systems. Interest in this species has then, for these main reasons, grown up steadily in recent years. The river buffalo can be considered a dairy producer that has no match in developing countries, characterized also by

[*] **Corresponding author Bianca Gasparrini:** Department of Veterinary Medicine and Animal Production, Federico II University, *Via* F. Delpino 1, 80137 Naples, Italy; Tel: +39 081 2536284/461; Fax: +39 081 292981; E-mail: bgasparr@unina.it

Giorgio A. Presicce (Ed.)

particular environmental conditions typical of the tropics north of the equator. In those climate conditions, the buffalo is used to compensate for the lack of cattle milk in the course of the rainy season (winter to spring), enabling thus people to make use of animal proteins at competitive costs. This can happen thanks especially to the special interaction occurring between reproductive seasonality typical of this species, together with availability of forage throughout the year and external environmental conditions. A striking evidence underlining the importance of this species is given by the mushrooming increase in the total world buffalo population in the course of the last 40 years, adding up to 86% especially when compared to the cattle counterpart, with only a 34%. In Italy the Mediterranean Italian buffalo is the only livestock species that has shown a growing trend over the years; it is an important economic resource, due to the high market demand for mozzarella cheese, and its genetics is highly requested around the world due to its high milk production. The increasing demand for buffalo milk and the need to cut production costs make genetic improvement critical for successful buffalo breeding. In this scenario, programs aimed at selecting the best animals through the adoption of newly developed reproductive technologies, can be completed in shorter times than usually expected under ordinary reproductive management. In addition, developing countries require the availability of high genetic animals as quickly as possible, and in this context, reproductive biotechnologies may offer a sharp help for example in replacing the working efficiency of local swamp buffaloes with a much higher efficiency in terms of milk produced from river buffaloes. This is a possible way to enhance the availability of animal proteins for human need and consumption. In the past, one of the most applied reproductive technology in cattle, was also employed in buffaloes, in order to increase and speed up the genetic gain *via* the maternal lineage. In fact, attempts were made to induce multiple ovulations for *in vivo* embryo production in buffalo (MOET programs), although the obtained results have always been inconsistent and embryo production was always significantly reduced when compared to the cattle counterpart [1 - 3]. For this reason, and thanks to the encouraging results reported in cattle, interest has been shifting to the possibility to produce embryo following use of *in vitro* procedures (IVEP).

The first IVEP experiences were carried out on abattoir-derived oocytes mainly for research purposes and for the genetic rescue of highly valuable animals with terminal illness or characterized by reproductive inefficiency, or else for mass production of embryos. Very little impact on the genetic enhancement of animals is exerted by the use of IVEP procedures for embryo mass production, using oocytes derived from ovaries of slaughtered animals.

A boost in the spreading of IVEP procedure for the improvement of genetically important traits in production animals, has been seen thanks to the development of techniques for recovering immature oocytes from antral follicles in live animals, termed Ovum Pick Up (OPU). Indeed, the *in vivo* collection of immature oocytes by transvaginal ultrasound guided follicular aspiration, provided the lacking link between IVEP technologies and animal breeding. The genetic progress through the maternal lineage can be more efficiently and more quickly achieved through the combined use of IVEP procedure and OPU technique, thanks also to the repeatability of the procedure and its non invasive approach, leading to a higher number of embryos produced on a long term basis. In addition to the poor embryo output of MOET [1 - 3], and in comparison to MOET programs, characterized in buffaloes by a low efficiency in terms of embryos produced and recovered [1 - 3], the synergistic coupling of IVEP and OPU allows a consistent and wider production of embryos from animals that would have been otherwise discarded, such as in the case of acyclic females, reproductive failures due to salpingitis or infections of the genital tract, unresponsiveness to hormonal administration for superovulation. In addition, even pregnant animals within their first trimester can be used for embryo production through OPU.

The introduction of OPU in cattle dates back to the late 1980s, and became operational in the early 1990s. OPU was first adopted in 1994, in buffaloes found in deep anestrus characterized by hypotrophic ovaries [4, 5], and since then it has spread in many other countries other than Italy [6 - 13], like Brazil [14, 15], China ([16, 17], Argentina [18] and India [19, 20]. Therefore, in light of some of the above mentioned aspects, the coupling of IVEP and OPU techniques is the most productive and efficient approach for elite embryo production (transferable embryos) on an animal-donor basis and over long period of times. In addition, and especially in the buffalo species, this is a very competitive combined technology in terms of embryo yield when compared to MOET programs, due to the fact that these animals may be less responsive to hormonal stimulation for superovulation, less amenable to the procedure due to seasonal anestrus, and overall produce less embryos. Additionally, the procedure can be made even more efficient if, prior to its implementation, animals can be monitored and selected on the basis of their follicular dynamics and follicle count on the ovaries, bypassing thus the intrinsic variability among animals in follicular recruitment per each wave, consequent retrieval of immature oocytes and final embryo production (1 to 25 blastocysts per donor in 3.5 months) [13]. Interestingly, it was recently demonstrated that the initial number of follicles and cumulus-oocyte-complexes (COCs) might predict the blastocyst yields in a long-term period. This means that a preliminary screening, performed through a simple ultrasonic examination of the animals, allows the selection of the best oocyte donors and embryo producers [13].

Despite all the success in the exploitation of this procedure in buffaloes in recent decades, as witnessed by the ever increasing blastocyst yield [21] and production of offspring [10, 14, 16, 22], the viability of the same technology is still far from reaching a commercial consistency. An intrinsic and insuperable limitation in buffaloes, is given by the reduced amount of recruitable follicles per wave, when compared to cattle, together with a poorer viability of buffalo embryos possibly caused by inadequate culture conditions, and a higher susceptibility to cryopreservation when buffalo embryos are produced *in vitro*, due mostly to their greater lipid content [23]. All the above concurs to a poor pregnancy rates when cryopreserved IVP embryos are transferred into synchronized recipients. Embryonic mortality following natural mating is a major cause for low birth rate in buffaloes in Italy in the course of the long day length seasons (spring to summer). Such embryo loss is further increased when reproductive technologies, from AI to transfer of IVP embryos, are used in this species [24, 25]. This phenomenon is due to the concourse of several factors such as the poor quality of the retrieved oocytes [12, 26] and the poor quality of the developing CL characterized by lower and insufficient progesterone production [24, 25]. In addition, the buffalo embryo shows a marked reduced viability when its production derives from the implementation of *in vitro* procedures, and a possible major cause for such sub-optimal viability can be attributed to the use of sub-optimal culture conditions, that are known to negatively affect all the events related to post-implantation [27].

As an additional remark on the delay reported in this species with regard to the scientific improvement through the use of the above mentioned newly developed reproductive technologies, it is the lack or insufficient availability of experimental material and animals needed. This is in part related to the small number of buffaloes and to the low culling rate compared to cattle. In Italy, for instance, the estimated population of buffaloes is slightly less than 400,000 *versus* 7.2 million cattle, and the culling rate is < 15% *vs.* > 35% for cattle. This scarcity is also due to differences in breeding systems, such as small farms scattered over large territories in the majority of the countries with high buffalo population (China, India). One of the reasons for the low availability of viable buffaloes is to be found in their long reproductive lifespan (approximately 12 years in Italy, and even longer in other countries like China and South East Asia, where swamp buffaloes are typically raised). Such animals are slaughtered only when old, at the end of their career, due to compromised health or impaired reproductive efficiency. Under such conditions, the rate of viable competent oocytes is quite low when recovered from the ovaries of slaughtered animals. Other factors impacting on the velocity of scientific gain over the past years are given by: i) the relative recent appreciation of buffalo as an animal species of particular economic importance, delaying thus the application of specific studies and consequent application of advanced reproductive techniques, which have started only in the late 90s; ii) the highest availability of buffalo heads in countries characterized by competent scientists dealing though with low funding for scientific enquiries and lack of facilities. These aspects, together with the attitude to consider buffaloes as ruminants very similar to cattle, has brought scientists to adopt the same strategies and procedures to produce embryos *in vitro*, with the inevitable result of an overall low efficiency. Differently, when laboratory procedures have focused on species-specific differences, improvements have been reported over the last years with a significant increase in the rate of late stage preimplantation embryo development [21].

In this chapter the latest advancements of the last decades in procedures and technologies related to *in vitro* embryo production and OPU will be given, while a second part will be devoted to additional technologies evolving around oocyte and embryo cryopreservation, together with embryo and sperm sexing.

2. OOCYTE SOURCE AND QUALITY

A major limitation in the exploitation of the OPU / IVEP technology in buffaloes is given by their intrinsic physiological reduced follicular population when compared to cattle, which corresponds to a lower number of retrieved immature oocytes from live animals, with a reported average of 0.7 and 4.3 per animal [5, 28 - 30]. In addition, another physiological limitation is linked to the higher incidence of follicular atresia, resulting in a consequent reduced recovery of good quality oocytes, which, according to several authors is 0.4 [28, 30], 0.9 [29], 1.76 [31], and 2.4 [32]. When considering our laboratory setting and our working conditions, ovaries of slaughtered buffaloes give us a mean of 4.3 oocytes recovered of which 2.4 of good quality, per ovary [32]. Breeds may account for a reported difference in these parameters in addition to age of the animals, health conditions and nutritional status [33], known to affect follicular dynamics and its hormonal inner working [34].

Several factors affect oocyte recovery, such as the ovarian status [35], the postpartum period [6 - 8], season [20, 36], *etc*. There is a significant difference between cattle and buffaloes with regard to the average number of good quality oocytes obtained per ovary (approximately 10 per ovary in cattle) [37], which is similar to the average number recovered per donor animal when OPU is applied to the two species (approximately 4.5 in buffaloes *vs.* 10 in cattle) [38].

What has been anticipated so far in this review, finds its reason in some physiological features typical of the buffalo species, like: i) the approximately 10-fold lower number of primordial follicles when compared to cattle (10,000 to 19,000 [39, 40] *vs.* 150,000 [41], respectively), ii) corresponding lower number of available antral follicles throughout the estrous cycle [42], iii) higher incidence compared to cattle of follicular atresia [43, 44] as observed in slaughterhouse ovaries and, iiii) not surprisingly smaller size of ovaries in comparison to the cattle counterparts [45]. Such intrinsic species-specific features represent somehow a sort of obstacle to the diffusion of the OPU technology in conjunction to the IVEP procedures in buffaloes. Of course these are limitations that cannot be bypassed, other than maybe, selecting the future oocyte donors on the basis of their follicular population to start with, by ultrasound monitoring of their ovaries [13]. With the same goal of overcoming the physiological limitations, earlier attempts have shown that in deep anestrus buffaloes a slight improvement in the number of punctured follicles, recovered oocytes and oocyte quality by priming OPU donors with FSH-P [4], can be achieved. It has also been reported that rBST pretreatment of buffalo donors [14, 15] has a significant effect in promoting follicular growth (12.2 *vs.* 8.7 total follicles punctured; 9.1 *vs.* 6.5 small follicles) with the consequent increase in the number of recovered oocytes per session (5.2 *vs.*. 4.1; p=0.07). Despite the increase in those parameters, and similarly to what already reported in cattle [46, 47], the rate of late stage development embryos was not increased in buffaloes on an OPU session basis. This result was confirmed also when buffaloes were treated with rbST and subjected to once a week OPU session [48]. All of this amply demonstrates the need for additional studies and trials in the same topic, although it is worth mentioning that one of the strong asset of the OPU technology, is just the possibility to avoid hormonal stimulation to the donors and all the consequences linked to this practice.

Finally, for completeness of the topic, Baruselli *et al.* [48], have recently reported that, by increasing the interval between OPU session to once a week or even every two weeks, the total number of recovered oocytes can be significantly increased (one week interval: 8.5 and 6.1 total and viable oocytes, respectively; two week interval: 10 and 7.2 total and viable oocytes, respectively).

The same authors demonstrated that the aspiration at 1, 3 and 5 days after the follicular emergency in heifers gave the same results [48] but also in this case the average number of follicles, total oocytes recovered and viable oocytes was much higher than in any other report. It is likely that such differences may be attributed to many concurring factors, other than the length of interval between OPU sessions, such as the genetic potential of the animals part of the trial, together with breed and the surrounding environment. It has to be underlined though that, other than the higher number of available antral follicles and related recovered oocytes, a longer interval between OPU sessions is accountable for a reduced rate of late stage embryo development. This is due to a much higher heterogeneity of follicle population within ovaries, as dominance over other follicles of the same wave occurs, and consequent follicular atresia leading to reduced quality of the recovered oocytes. Furthermore, in the buffalo species the quality of the recovered oocyte can be considered a major factor affecting the overall efficiency of the OPU/IVEP procedure.

The morphology of the oocytes is used to build a classification of quality that is employed worldwide. Such classification in turn, to some extent, can be predictive of oocyte viability and its future developmental potential. Therefore, according to this classification, a decrease in the efficiency of embryo production can be foreseen when, from the highest grades of oocyte quality (grade A and B which are suitable for IVEP), it goes down to grades C and D [9] (Fig. **1**).

Ideally, only the best grade oocytes should be used in order to reliably count on the highest possible embryo production. In reality, due to the very limited number of retrieved oocytes, they are almost all used, in order to optimize the efforts practiced in the field. Embryo production can also be optimized by selecting the most competently available oocytes following their recovery from slaughterhouse ovaries, by using the non invasive brilliant cresyl blue (BCB) staining [49].

The rate of good quality oocytes (grades A and B) in buffaloes is usually lower when compared to cattle and anyway not exceeding 50% of the total number of retrieved oocytes. In fact, in a retrospective analysis of data generated in our lab following 3 years of laboratory activity, over a total of 116 replicates consisting of oocytes recovered from slaughterhouse ovaries, 46.3% belonged to grade A and B, while of the remaining oocytes, grade C represented 6.4% of the total number of oocytes and collectively 47.3% of them were judged unsuitable for *in vitro* processing [26].

In another trial an even lower proportion of good quality oocytes (33.7% of Grade A+B), together with a higher incidence (37.9%) of Grade C was reported [50]. When BCB staining was used for oocyte selection, the percentage of good quality oocytes was slightly higher (57%), on equal blastocyst yields.

A number of variables are responsible for determining the final quality of the retrieved oocytes, like the pressure needed to aspirate the oocytes by mechanical vacuum, the time needed to move oocytes from the OPU site to the lab and their processing, environmental temperature and temperature of the collection vials during transport of the oocytes, season of the year, *etc*. The source of the oocytes is another variable of importance, as we have seen in our experience, that OPU-derived oocytes appear to show a worse overall quality (*i.e.* reduced number of granulosa cells surrounding the oocyte) when compared to oocytes from slaughterhouse ovaries.

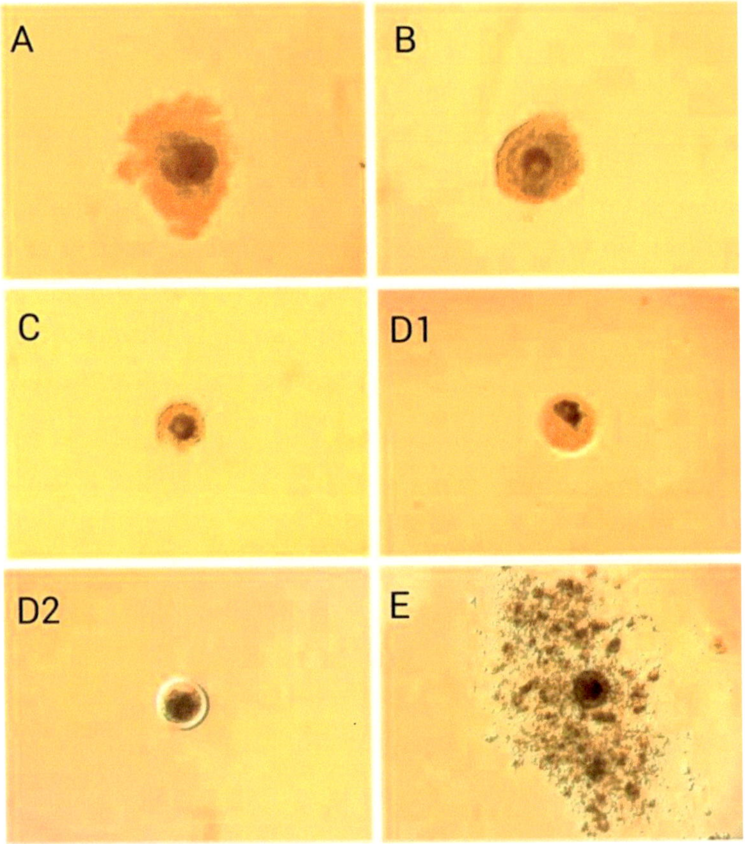

Fig. (1). (A) Oocytes with more than three layers of cumulus cells and homogenous cytoplasm; **(B)** Oocytes with at least 2 layers of cumulus cells and homogenous cytoplasm; **(C)** Oocytes partially denuded, but still showing homogenous cytoplasm; **(D1)** Degenerated oocytes (oocytes with irregular shrunken cytoplasm); **(D2)/E** Naked (totally denuded oocytes), and abnormally expanded oocytes with particularly clustered cumulus cells.

In cattle too, a higher prevalence of good quality oocytes was reported when retrieved from slaughterhouse ovaries, compared to OPU derived oocytes [51]. It seems then that this difference in oocyte source is not species-specific and not due to OPU techniques or media employed to stock oocytes. It has been speculated that a post-mortem effect may be accountable for a better quality of retrieved COCs, as they are less tightly anchored to the inner follicle wall and finally recovered with a better preserved morphology. This explanation may be found even more applicable to the buffalo species, as in these animals a reduced adhesion of cumulus cells to the follicle wall has been described [52]. This aspect allows us to speculate, additionally, that under mechanical retrieval of oocytes from antral follicles in buffaloes, and according to other variables such as the length of the needle and suction line attached to the vacuum pump, a greater loss of granulosa cells may occur, leading to an underestimation of their quality score. This latter aspect may give an explanation of a higher developmental potential of OPU derived oocytes in buffaloes as opposed to cattle [51], as indicated by both increased blastocyst yields [9, 19] and improved blastocyst cryotolerance compared to abattoir-derived buffalo oocytes [19].

Embryo yield is higher when oocytes are recovered by OPU performed at an interval of twice a week. This can be explained by the mechanical interfering with wave follicular dynamics, and the resetting of the beginning of a new follicular wave when OPU is performed. When the new OPU session is repeated, usually 3 days later, follicular dominance has not occurred yet the effect of follicular atresia over the remaining follicular population, and therefore a homogeneity of follicular population is witnessed, accounting for a higher oocyte developmental potential and consequent embryo yield. Differently, when using ovaries of slaughtered animals, a heterogeneous follicular population is encountered and consequently, a more heterogeneous oocyte quality is recorded, accounting for a lower developmental potential and reduced embryo yield. The oocyte competence is in fact dependent on the morpho-functional state of the ovaries, and this is so true that an improved embryo yield is witnessed when oocytes are recovered from ovaries characterized by absence of a dominant follicle and having either a functional CL or a corpus hemorragicum [53]. The lower embryo yield in buffaloes from abattoir ovaries-derived oocytes, has also to contend with the fact that animals are brought to the slaughterhouse usually at the end of their productive career or due to some reproductive failures. A further element of consideration in the arena of embryo yield in ruminants, is the higher embryo production in cattle when using oocytes from slaughterhouse ovaries when compared to OPU derived oocytes. This difference may be related to the early atresia occurring during post-mortem, which has been shown to positively affect developmental competence [54], differently from what has been reported in buffaloes, highlighting thus the need for further in-depth studies aimed at elucidating the timing of atresia in buffaloes and its consequential effect on the oocyte. Differently, a shorter exposure to environmental stressing factors may account for a higher developmental competence of OPU derived oocytes, when compared to oocytes derived from slaughterhouse ovaries. In the latter case in fact, usually the time needed from ovaries to reach any laboratory from slaughtering of the animal, excision from the peritoneal cavity and their transport, may be so prolonged that autolytic processes occur, leading to cell damage affecting very likely the oocytes residing still in the excised ovaries. Therefore, another element to be considered within the overall efficiency process in *in vitro* embryo production, is the time interval needed from excision of the ovaries at the slaughterhouse and the beginning of oocyte processing in the lab following follicle aspiration. In our experience and within our experimental setting, the time needed for receiving the ovaries in the lab from the slaughterhouse is from 3 to 6 hours. We ran a retrospective analysis of data generated in the last four years of work with slaughterhouse ovaries and *in vitro* embryo production, and although the quality of retrieved oocytes, as judged by a higher incidence of grade A and B COCs, was superior when the time needed for the ovaries to reach the lab was not higher than 3 hours, the final rate of late stage embryo development was not significantly different when confronted to 4.5 to 6 hours [55]. In addition, to reduce the risk of lowering the efficiency of the IVEP session, whenever OPU is carried distantly from the lab, an improvement in embryo yield can be achieved when they are immediately placed, following follicle puncture and retrieval, in hepes-buffered *in vitro* maturation medium in a portable incubator. This allows oocytes to start the maturation process very close in time with their removal from the antral milieu, and optimize thus their developmental potential [56].

Another factor to be considered that is part of the many variables affecting *in vitro* embryo production, is the holding temperature for oocytes recovered either by

OPU or for ovaries to be taken to the lab after their excision from the slaughtered animal. Usually, oocytes from OPU sessions are held in tubes within warm boxes or mechanical devices maintaining the wanted temperature. Differently, excised ovaries are usually held in physiological saline at 30 to 35°C until they reach the lab, although it has been recently reported that lowering such temperature during transportation to the lab from 25 to 29.5°C, positively influences the final outcome in terms of cleavage and blastocyst development after IVF [55].

Again, buffaloes are animals affected in their reproductive performances by season and exposure to either short or long period of light, and therefore also applied reproductive technologies such as MOET and AI can be consequently affected by the season, when such practices are being implemented [24, 25]. At our latitudes, season significantly affects oocyte competence, without influencing the follicular population and oocyte yield. In fact, both a retrospective study on abattoir ovaries and an OPU trial demonstrated that both the number of retrieved COCs and their quality were not affected by performing OPU during the season characterized by long days, but oocyte developmental competence was influenced when oocytes were collected in the course of the short-day season, as judged by a higher rate of cleavage and blastocyst development [12, 26].

From these results it is then suggested to focus on OPU and IVEP session during the short-day seasons of the year at our latitudes, in order to capitalize on resources and favor the benefit/costs ratio.

This is in line with the well known seasonality of buffaloes at our latitudes, where they exhibit the highest reproductive efficiency during the season of the year characterized by short days (autumn/winter).

On the other hand, Indian [20] authors reported a seasonal effect on IVEP efficiency from OPU-derived oocytes that was, though, mainly due to decreased follicular population. In fact, blastocyst rate was not affected, although the number of follicles, COCs and blastocysts per animal per session decreased during the unfavorable season. It was previously reported [57] that hot ambient temperature (> 40°C) on day of slaughter negatively affects both cleavage and blastocyst development following IVF, confirming previous observations in buffalo [58]. It is likely that reproductive efficiency at different latitudes may be affected by other variables, other than photoperiod and climate, like feed availability. In addition, it has to be emphasized that in our country nutrition plans in buffaloes are well established and followed, and that these animals are kept under continuous nutrition regimen throughout the year.

3. *IN VITRO* MATURATION (IVM)

A correct maturation of the oocytes at the time they encounter the sperm is unquestionably a critical prerequisite for effective fertilization. The maturation process, that encompasses both the nuclear and cytoplasmic compartments, is fundamental for the oocyte to attain the developmental competence. Buffalo oocytes are matured *in vitro* in complex media, such as the worldwide used Tissue Culture Medium 199 and Ham's F- 10, supplemented with different sources of serum [31, 59 - 61], hormones and other additives. Different sources of serum have been utilized as supplements of IVM medium [31, 59 - 61]. Although *in vitro* maturation occurs even in the absence of hormones [30], increased maturation and fertilization rates are recorded when oocytes are matured in the presence of gonadotrophins and 17β -estradiol [28, 60]. It is known that hormones receptors are sited on the somatic cells, and that signals transduction to the oocyte occurs through gap junctions or extracellular mechanisms. It follows that the presence of cumulus cells is fundamental for the oocyte to acquire the developmental competence during IVM, as indicated by the decreased cleavage and post-IVF embryo development of denuded *vs.* cumulus-enclosed oocytes [62, 63]. This is very important in buffalo due to the high percentage of totally or partially denuded oocytes generally recruited in this species. A possible approach to save poor quality oocytes is to carry out IVM on a cumulus cells monolayer [64]. It has also been reported that expensive hormones and serum additives can be replaced with buffalo follicular fluid, a waste product of oocyte collection, with similar maturation, fertilization, and blastocyst rates [65]. It is known that ovarian-derived growth factors, such as IGF-l, IGF-2 and insulin improve oocyte maturation, fertilization and blastocyst development [66]. Furthermore, the inclusion of EGF in the IVM medium has beneficial effects on cumulus expansion, nuclear maturation, and cleavage rate of cumulus-enclosed buffalo oocytes, without influencing the post-fertilization embryonic development [67]. In another study blastocyst yields increased when IVM was enriched with EGF either alone or in combination with fibroblast growth factor (FGF) and vasoactive intestinal peptide (VIP), and the cleaved embryos were cultured in a complex co-culture system [68].

A significant improvement of IVM in buffalo has been achieved by enriching the medium with thiol compounds, known to act as antioxidants factors by stimulating glutathione (GSH) synthesis. This is likely due to the fact that buffalo oocytes and embryos, characterized by high lipid content [23], are highly sensitive to oxidative damages. It is well known that GSH plays a pivotal role in the protection of mammalian cells from oxidative stress, that is a major element affecting *in vitro* mammalian embryo development. Indeed, the oocyte GSH reservoir created during IVM is the only source of antioxidant power for the embryos until genomic activation [69, 70]. In an earlier trial the addition of cysteamine during IVM improved blastocyst rates in buffalo [32], by increasing intracytoplasmic GSH content [71], without nevertheless influencing cleavage rate. However, when the IVM medium was supplemented with both cystine and cysteamine [21] the GSH reservoir of the oocytes further increased, leading to improved penetration (81%), cleavage rate (78%) and blastocyst yield (30%). A beneficial effect of other antioxidants, such as taurine and melatonin, during IVM was also demonstrated [72].

Another approach [73] to improve maturation of buffalo oocytes is given by the inclusion in the IVM medium of mitogenic lectin, shown to enhance cumulus expansion and cleavage rate following IVF and upregulate the expression of genes involved in important physiological activities, like gap junction and cell communication protein (Cx43), cumulus-expansion enabling factor and cell cycle protein (GDF-9), basic growth factor (FGF-4) and cell membrane protein (fibronectin).

IVM and its temporal acquisition, has a fundamental role, among other variables, exerting an effect on *in vitro* development of mammalian embryos. In fact, an inadequate maturation time may lead to abnormal chromatin configuration [74], oocyte aging [75] and reduced development [76]. In addition, early development following penetration of partially matured oocytes [77], is usually reduced and therefore as a consequence it can be stated that the highest rate of early embryo development follows from the *in vitro* fertilization (IVF) of oocytes that have fully completed meiosis, which typically occurs at different times according to the species, such as 18-24 hours in cattle [78, 79] and 36-48 hours in pig [80]. In buffaloes, a different maturation time has been reported by several authors, although the highest rate of completed meiosis has been reported between 16 and 24 hours [79, 81, 82], and consequently most authors tend to fertilize *in vitro* buffalo oocytes at the end of 24 hours of IVM. Very likely it is the quality of the oocytes that accounts for the variability reported in the timing of IVM. The quality itself can be affected by many variables such as environmental conditions and the season, being the buffalo a seasonal species. Based on these well known elements of knowledge, our lab has been involved in a number of studies on the kinetics of oocyte maturation and IVM timing and their effect on embryo development. We have ascertained that MII stage is reached around 18-19 hours of IVM and that a full cytoplasmic and nuclear maturation is usually completed between 20 to 24 hours. In addition, we have proven that the developmental competence of oocytes, fertilization ability and early stage embryos potential are affected by the duration in time of *in vitro* maturation, being progressively decreased as the time of IVM is increased from 18 to 30 hours [82]. From the above it can be stated that the best time for IVF falls at 18 hours of IVM and definitely not later than 24 h. This is also substantiated by the poor appearance of oocytes that had been kept in maturation medium over 24 hours, resulting in reduced rate of fertilization following IVF. The possibility of dealing with an intrinsic species-specific characteristic, related to the attainment of oocyte developmental competence at an earlier time, was taken into consideration by evaluating the increased incidence of degenerated oocytes following increasing times for IVM [79]. A confirmation of the importance of timing in IVM for oocyte developmental competence and further developmental ability, is given by the evidence of deterioration of parthenogenetic embryos in correspondence to increased *in vitro* maturation time [79]. All the above proves to be of paramount importance when we are dealing with oocytes recovered from several animals in the course of OPU sessions. In fact, when a good number of animals are part of the OPU session, inevitably recovered oocytes from each individual donor animal are put into maturation medium at different times, adding up to a difference of few hours from the first batch of oocytes to the last one. Therefore, in order to catch with the optimal time for IVM, usually the following day IVF is performed so that the range in maturation time between the last batch of oocytes recovered and the first one is 19 to 20 and 23 to 24 hours, respectively.

4. *IN VITRO* FERTILIZATION (IVF)

The low cleavage rates widely reported in the buffalo species in the past [9, 38, 83, 84] suggested that fertilization was the most critical step of the IVEP technology. In our former studies, although maturation rates were similar in buffalo and cattle (87% *vs.* 94%), cleavage rates significantly decreased in buffalo (65% *vs.* 84%) [9]. The overall poorer IVEP efficiency in buffalo compared to cattle (26 *vs.* 34%, respectively) was mainly due to the low proportion of oocytes cleaving; indeed, the proportion of cleaved embryos developing into blastocysts was similar in the two species (about 40%). The *in vitro* fertilization efficiency depends on several factors, such as the appropriate environment for gametes survival, the sperm viability and fertilizing ability, the optimal insemination time, the length of sperm-oocyte co-incubation, the presence of cumulus cells and the attainment of oocyte developmental competence during the delicate process of cytoplasmic maturation. In fact, although fertilization failure may be due to inadequacies of the IVF system, the appropriate maturation of the egg is compulsory.

The most common IVF media used are Tyrode's modified medium (TALP) and Brackett Oliphant (BO) medium, enriched with heparin as capacitating agent and sperm motility inducing factors, such as combined hypotaurine-penicillamine or caffeine. The results of a comparison trial indicated the superiority of TALP medium, supplemented with heparin, hypotaurine and penicillamine, in terms of both cleavage and blastocysts yields [84]. When frozen-thawed sperm are employed it is important to preliminarily select the motile spermatozoa either by the swim-up method or by Percoll density gradient. Although the proportion of motile sperm is higher with Percoll separation, swim-up separated sperm display a higher motility, membrane integrity and cleavage rate [85]. However, a greater bull effect is observed on cleavage rate and cleavage index with swim-up separated sperm. In our laboratory both separation methods have been widely utilized over the years, with comparable embryo yields. However, we also observed a strong bull effect with swim-up, with several bulls failing to separate well, providing low concentrated sperm and hence requiring more straws/IVF. It results that the choice of the method may also depend on the bull chosen for the IVF program. In former times the quality of cryopreserved semen was thought to be a major factor impairing IVF, because of the proven cryopreservation-induced sperm damages [86], together with the dramatic decrease of cleavage rate reported with frozen *vs.* fresh semen [28]. Currently, the quality of cryopreserved semen has greatly improved, as shown by similar fertility parameters, recorded for fresh compared to frozen semen [87], suggesting that other factors negatively influence fertilization. However, despite the improved quality of frozen sperm, an important limiting factor persists, *i.e.* the so-called bull effect, consisting in the high individual variability recorded among buffalo bulls in the *in vitro* fertilizing ability [60]. As a consequence, as only few bulls have good fertilizing capability *in vitro* (around 10%), a preliminary screening of sperm of several bulls is necessary to identify a suitable semen for IVF programs. Although several fertility tests have been developed, the most accurate assessment still goes through IVF trials, with different bulls tested on the same batch of eggs, and because of the poor number of oocytes recovered, such tests are very time-consuming. Interestingly, the easy and quick Trypan-blue/Giemsa staining technique [88] can be used to predict the fertilizing capability *in vitro* of buffalo bulls, as indicated by the correlation existent between the percentages of acrosome-intact viable sperm cells at thawing and the blastocyst rates [89].

It is well known that sperm attain the fertilizing ability through the process of capacitation, that *in vivo* occurs within the female genital tract. Although several agents may induce sperm capacitation *in vitro*, heparin is still the most widely used capacitating agent in most domestic species. In order to evaluate whether *in vitro* capacitation is improved by agents different than heparin, buffalo sperm cells have been incubated under different conditions and capacitation has been indirectly assessed by estimating the capacity of sperm to acrosome react following incubation with lysophosphatidilcholine, a fusogenic lipid, known to induce acrosome reaction in capacitated sperm without affecting motility.

Doing such a test, it was demonstrated that progesterone, sodium nitroprusside, a well known generator of nitric oxide *in vitro* and melatonin, trigger *in vitro* sperm capacitation and may be used as alternative capacitating agents for buffalo IVF [90 - 92]. As buffalo is a short-day breeder, it would be worth investigating the influence of melatonin also in relation to the season of semen collection.

The most promising results, however, came from a study in which sperm were incubated with biological fluids, such as follicular fluid (FF) recovered from a pool of dominant follicles and buffalo estrus serum (BES) [93]. Indeed, the proportion of capacitated sperm significantly increased for sperm treated with both FF and BES compared to heparin (94.5, 84.3, *vs.* 50.1%, respectively). This beneficial effect may be accounted for by the presence in the oviduct at the time of fertilization of factors deriving from BES and FF, that play a key role during *in vivo* capacitation. A possible strategy to improve IVF efficiency is to mimic the oviduct environment. This was achieved by incubating buffalo sperm on a 6-day bovine oviduct epithelial cells monolayer, as indicated by improved sperm capacitation [94] and oocyte penetration rate after heterologous IVF [95]. A more practical approach to mimic the oviduct environment is the enrichment of IVF medium with oviduct-derived factors, known to play a pivotal role during fertilization. A potential candidate is osteopontin (OPN), an acidic single-chain phosphorylated glycoprotein, identified in both the oviductal fluid and epithelium in cattle, known to increase IVEP efficiency and promote sperm capacitation [96]. Osteopontin is also a marker of male fertility in cattle, as its expression in semen is correlated with bull fertility [97]. Osteopontin was also identified in buffalo semen, at higher concentration in seminal plasma than in spermatozoa [98], suggesting that ampullae and seminal vesicles are the major sources, like in cattle [97]. Following standard cryopreservation, the concentration of OPN in buffalo semen decreases by around 50% [98]. It was subsequently reported that OPN enhances the *in vitro* capacitation efficiency and that its incorporation in the IVF medium significantly improves synchronous pronuclei formation, cleavage rate and blastocyst yields [99].

Proteolytic enzymes are also known to exert a fundamental role during the subsequent events of fertilization. An increased proportion of acrosome-reacted sperm and enhanced motility were observed when plasmin, the active enzyme of the plasminogen activation system, was added to heparin-capacitated buffalo sperm [100]. However, the effect of plasmin supplementation during IVF on IVEP efficiency in buffalo has still not been evaluated.

Like in cattle [101], the presence of cumulus cells at the time of IVF is critical in buffalo as shown by the decreased cleavage and blastocyst yields recorded with denuded compared to cumulus-enclosed oocytes [63]. However, the fertilizing ability and embryo development of denuded oocytes can be restored by co-culture with bovine intact COCs in a 1:1 ratio [102]. This strategy can be utilized for manipulations requiring cumulus removal, such as oocyte cryopreservation.

The length of sperm-oocyte co-incubation is another factor that may influence embryo development. As high sperm concentrations in small volumes are used *in vitro*, long co-incubation times should be avoided, to limit the production of hydrolytic enzymes [103] and free radicals [104] that damage the eggs. In a former study, the optimal gametes co-incubation time for optimizing the blastocyst output in buffalo was 16 hours [82]. Shortening the gamete co-incubation length to 8 hours reduced cleavage rate, as previously reported in cattle [105, 106]. However, oocytes that cleaved developed into viable embryos at the same rate as in the 16 hours group. In contrast, prolonging co-incubation time to 20 hours negatively affected blastocyst production, despite similar cleavage rates. Furthermore, at this time a higher incidence of polyspermy was observed, confirming previous findings [107]. It is worth underlining, however, that in this study semen from a single bull previously tested for IVF was used. Afterwards, marked differences in the kinetics of sperm penetration among buffalo bulls were recorded [108]. It was also observed that kinetics of penetration is correlated to the blastocyst yield [109], suggesting that this parameter is a reliable marker to predict the *in vitro* fertility of buffalo bulls. It follows the importance of evaluating the sperm kinetics before enrollment of bulls in IVF programs. It is worth pointing out that among 6 buffaloes tested the bull with the fastest penetration rate (64% penetration at 3 hours pi with the peak 72-77% –between 6 and 9 hours pi) gave a marked increase in polyspermy at longer insemination intervals. Therefore, it is strongly suggested to choose the most appropriate sperm-oocyte co-incubation length for each bull.

Finally, the poor cleavage rate may also result from the failure in the acquisition of oocyte developmental competence, that is attained during maturation. Parthenogenetic activation is a valid tool to evaluate oocyte competence. Therefore, to better comprehend the reasons behind the lower IVF efficiency in buffalo, in a former trial oocytes were either *in vitro* fertilized or chemically activated with both ethanol and ionomycin, followed by 4 h-exposure to 6-DMAP [83]. The improved cleavage (71% *vs.* 56%, respectively) and blastocyst rate (33 *vs.* 23%, respectively) recorded with ethanol-induced activation *vs.* IVF, suggest that oocyte developmental competence was acquired during IVM. However, ionomycin gave intermediate cleavage and blastocyst rates (59 and 26%, respectively). Subsequently, activation with different methods was reported to increase cleavage and blastocyst rates compared to IVF, indicating a paternal rather than a maternal origin [50]. However, the marked difference observed by these authors may have been related to the poor sperm quality, suggested by very low cleavage (< 37%) and blastocyst rates (< 16%) recorded following IVF.

However, it is worth emphasizing that, after several ineffective attempts carried out over the years, the fertilization efficiency has finally improved (around 80% of cleavage rate), by supplementing the IVM medium with cystine and cysteamine. The beneficial effect of thiols was demonstrated to be due to increased intracytoplasmic GSH concentration [21]. This suggests that an inappropriate maturation of the female gamete was the main cause of the low cleavage rate so far recorded of this species. It is well known, in fact, that the GSH reservoir is fundamental for attainment of oocyte developmental competence [110] and that the GSH concentration at the end of IVM is a recognized marker of cytoplasmic maturation [111].

5. *IN VITRO* CULTURE (IVC)

The *in vitro* culture system in buffalo has been developed like in other ruminant species. In the very early attempts, embryos were cultured in the oviduct of an intermediate host (*in vivo*), generally the sheep [112], until the blastocyst stage. However, although embryo quality and cryotolerance is improved when development occurs in the oviduct, this system is not suitable for large scale *in vitro* embryo production. The first approach to culture buffalo embryos entirely *in vitro* was co-culture with cumulus and oviductal cells [28, 30, 59] or with established cell lines such as BRL [113]. Subsequently, the co-culture systems were replaced by serum and cells–free defined media, to better understand the specific needs of buffalo embryos, fundamental to develop an optimal species-specific culture system. In 1999 buffalo embryos were successfully cultured in Synthetic Oviduct Fluid (SOF) medium [113], a well known defined medium created by Tervit in 1972 [114]. Lately, similar blastocysts yields were obtained by culturing buffalo embryos in SOF and in Potassium Simplex Optimized Medium (KSOM), another defined cell-free medium [115]. The high increase in blastocysts rates recorded over the years (35-40%) is mainly related to the improvement of the IVM and in part of the IVF systems rather than to optimization of the IVC system. Indeed, more than 40 years passed and currently the most appropriate medium for embryo culture in buffalo is still the original SOF [114]. It is likely that the low percentage of pregnancy to term after transfer of frozen buffalo embryos is due to poor viability of IVP embryos, originating from suboptimal culture conditions. At present, in spite of many attempts to optimize the embryo culture system in several species, the oviduct is still inimitable for embryo development. It follows that the analysis of oviduct fluid (ODF) composition at different estrous cycle phases is critical to satisfy the needs of buffalo embryos *in vitro* [116]. Species-specific differences in ODF composition may justify adjustments of the media used for buffalo IVEP. As an example, the protein concentration and the total amount of proteins secreted in 24 hours were 5 and 3.5 times lower respectively in buffalo ODF than in cattle [117]. Remarkably, the protein concentration in buffalo ODF was also 4.4 times lower than the BSA concentration (8 mg/ml BSA) commonly used in both IVF and IVC media. This suggests to evaluate the effect of reducing protein concentration in media destined to buffalo IVEP. It has been previously reported that one of the major factors affecting viability of IVP embryos, likely to be associated to the large offspring syndrome, is the ammonium derived from protein metabolism [27, 118, 119]. It has been suggested to change medium more often during IVC in order to limit the increase of free radicals, ammonium and other catabolites that are toxic to the embryos. This approach, successful in other species, did not improve embryo development in buffalo, with a tendency to higher yields when medium is changed less frequently, suggesting not to disturb the embryos during IVC [120]. This is likely due to the fact that buffalo embryos are very sensitive to fluctuations of temperature and/or pH that may take place during a culture change.

Although toxic effects of glucose have been reported, most of the embryo culture media contain this sugar as energy source [121 - 123]. In cattle blastulation is facilitated when embryo are cultured without glucose up to the morula stage [124] and blastocyst production is impaired when embryos are cultured in the presence of high concentration of glucose (5-6 mmol) [122, 124, 125]. In buffalo, relatively high concentrations of glucose (1.5 mM, *i.e.* the standard concentration in SOF medium) are required, particularly during the early embryonic development, *i.e.* up to Day 4 [126]. In fact, the absence of glucose throughout culture or limitedly to early culture dramatically decreased blastocyst rates. In contrast, when glucose was absent during late culture, blastocyst yields were similar to the control (SOF). After this earlier trial, we modified the experimental design to evaluate the influence of reducing glucose concentrations during IVC on buffalo embryos, because a certain amount of glucose is fundamental for ribose and NADH production through the pentose-phosphate pathway. Decreasing the sugar concentration by 1/3, *i.e.* to 0.5 mM was uninfluential, whereas further decreasing it to 0.15 mM(1/10), *i.e.* the concentration utilized in most dynamic media for bovine embryos, throughout culture and only during early culture, negatively affected development. In contrast, embryo development was not affected by decreased glucose concentration during late culture. These results highlight important differences in energy requirements of buffalo embryos during IVC compared to those of other ruminants, known to exhibit a substantial increase in glucose consumption during late culture, *i.e.* just around compaction [125, 127, 128]. According to a more recent study, an even much higher concentration of glucose (5.6 mM) is constantly required throughout the IVM and IVC steps to maximize blastocyst rates in buffalo [129, 130]. Interestingly, this concentration is deleterious for bovine embryos, with a selective embryo-toxicity towards females [131]. Furthermore, the expression of metabolism-related genes indicates that the major pathway of glucose metabolism during early embryonic stages is glycolysis, which shifts towards oxidative phosphorylation during post-embryonic genome activation (EGA) stages in buffalo embryo [130]. In contrast, in bovine and sheep embryos a change to an enhanced contribution of glycolysis to ATP production is observed during compaction and blastulation [125, 132, 133], leading to increased glucose consumption. These relevant differences may provide useful hints to formulate a more suitable *in vitro* culture system for buffalo embryos.

It was proven that oxidative stress-induced DNA damage occurs in buffalo oocytes and embryos during IVC, that increases with time as development goes on [134]. It was also reported that enriching culture medium with cysteamine in part overcomes the injure [134], as indicated by decreased DNA damage in 8-16 cell embryos. This embryonic stage is particularly critical, corresponding to the developmental block [135]. It was also reported that the beneficial effect on embryo development of both lowering O_2 concentration and adding cysteamine is due to reduced apoptosis, as suggested by the higher expression of anti-apoptotic genes and lower expression of pro-apoptotic genes in the embryos [136]. The enrichment of the buffalo culture medium with either taurine or melatonin has been shown to improve blastocyst yield [72]. A beneficial effect of vitamins A, E and C on blastocyst production has also been recorded in the presence of high O_2 concentration [137, 138].

It is known that embryonic genome activation (EGA) takes place at species-specific developmental stages. It was recently reported that the major EGA in buffalo embryos occurs between the 4 and 8-cell stages, with a minor activation between the 2 and 4-cell stages [139]. This is considerably different from the EGA event in cattle and explains why the blastocyst development in this species occurs earlier than in cattle, both in superovulated animals [140 - 142] and under *in vitro* conditions [38, 143]. Buffalo embryos *in vitro* develop faster than bovine counterparts, reaching the blastocyst stage about 12-24 hours earlier [38, 143]. In our setting, the majority of the embryos develop into blastocysts on Day 7 (Day 0 = IVF), although advanced stage embryos, including hatched blastocysts can be seen since Day 6 (Fig. **2**). A small percentage of embryos reach the blastocyst stage on Day 8 but the delayed development indicates poorer quality, reflected in lower cryotolerance [143]. It was demonstrated that early cleaving embryos give higher blastocyst yields, develop faster and have higher cell number [144]. In contrast, slower-developing buffalo embryos have decreased total cell number and abnormal expression of development-related genes such as HSP-70.1 and GLUT-1 [145]. This confirms that blastocyst production may be enhanced, extending the incubation time, but at the cost of embryo viability. Hatching is also a good marker of embryo viability. It is possible to increase hatching rate of Day 7 late morulae/early blastocysts by supplementing the IVC medium with FBS, BSA and insulin the [146].

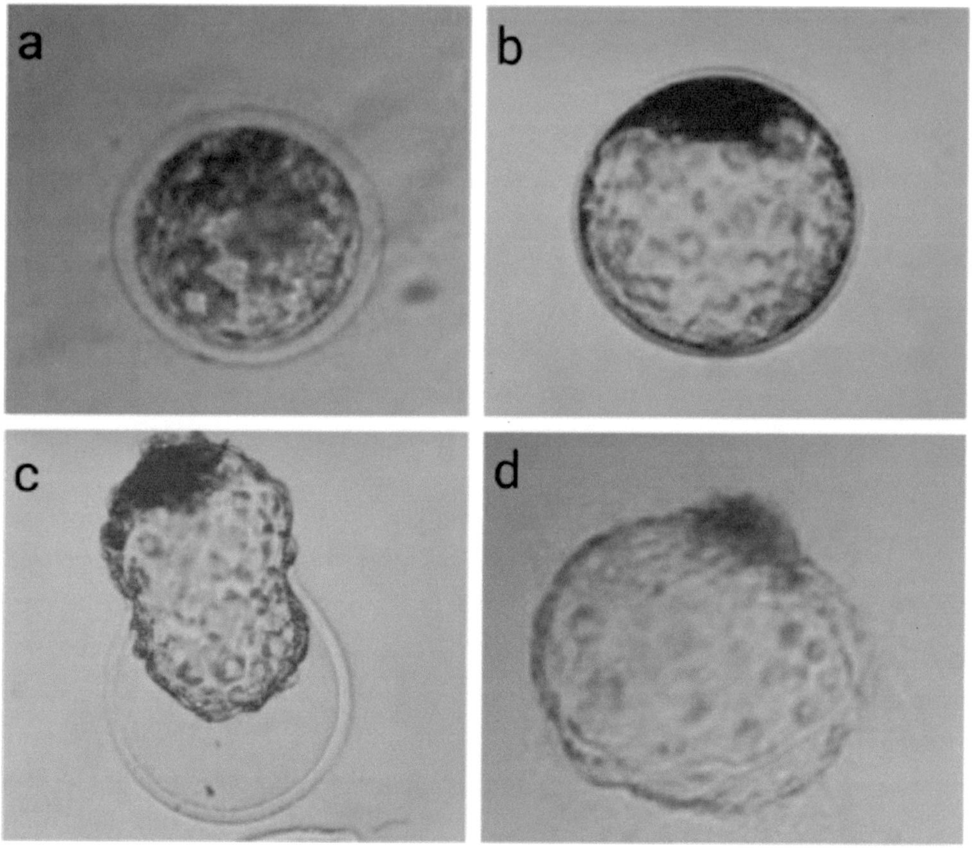

Fig. (2). Buffalo early blastocyst **(a)**, blastocyst **(b)**, hatched blastocyst **(c)** and expanded blastocyst **(d)**.

It is known that blastocyst quality more than blastocyst production has an impact on pregnancy outcome. A recent study reported that the inclusion of leukaemia inhibitory factor to the IVC medium improves blastocyst development and quality [147]. An improvement of embryo quality, indicated by faster development and increased cryotolerance, was obtained by high concentration of hyaluronic acid during late culture [148]. Finally, we recently observed that the addition of L-carnitine during IVC also improves the cryotolerance of IVP buffalo embryos, likely facilitating the proper consumption of endogenous lipid reserves [149].

6. EMBRYO CRYOPRESERVATION AND PREGNANCY TO TERM

Embryo cryopreservation is the best tool to overcome the major factor limiting the commercial use of embryo transfer (ET), that is the low number of available recipients. This is particularly true in buffalo, due to both the poorer response to hormonal stimulation and hence to synchronization programs and to the seasonality, that suggests to restrict the period of ET in the breeding season. As previously mentioned, the cryotolerance of IVP embryos is reduced compared to the *in vivo* embryos, due to the poorer viability, determined by suboptimal culture conditions. In addition, the high intracytoplasmic lipid concentration makes buffalo IVP embryos even more sensitive to cryopreservation [23]. It is known that *in vivo* culture in the sheep oviduct increases cryotolerance of buffalo embryos [112]. However, although *in vivo* culture of *in vitro* matured and fertilized oocytes allows the production of high quality embryos, this system has several constraints, such as the need to possess adequate facilities, higher costs, as well as ethical issues. Buffalo IVP embryos have been effectively cryopreserved by vitrification, as indicated by their survival after post-warming *in vitro* culture [143] and by the production of offspring following ET [10, 14, 22] (Fig. **3**). However, even if pregnancies to term have been recorded, it is still necessary to optimize the efficiency for the diffusion of OPU-IVEP technologies in the field. Among other factors, the culture conditions are known to significantly affect the efficiency; in fact, improved survival rates following cryopreservation are observed for embryos cultured in serum-free defined media compared to co-culture systems [68], like in other species. This is likely due to the increased intracytoplasmic lipid concentration of embryos cultured in the presence of cells and serum, reflected in their darker color. The source of oocytes also influences the cryopreservation efficiency, with OPU-derived oocytes giving more cryotolerant blastocysts than abattoir-derived oocytes [19].

In an earlier study, buffalo IVP blastocysts were cryopreserved by vitrification in French straws, with a method formerly employed in the sheep [150]. Briefly, blastocysts were first incubated for 5 min into 1.4 M glycerol, then into 1.4 M glycerol and 3.6 EG for further 5 min before being transferred for 25 sec into the final vitrification solution (3.4 M glycerol and 4.6 EG) and loaded into the straws. For warming, the embryos were expelled from the straws into a 0.5 M sucrose solution and then exposed for 5 min to 0.25 sucrose. After warming, embryos were cultured and viability was evaluated at 24 and 48 hours on the basis of blastocoele re-expansion, resumption of morphology, and hatching. Survival rates after 24 and 48 hours post-warming culture were respectively 64% and 52% [143]. However, increased survival rates were recorded for faster developing embryos (Day 6), confirming that delayed embryos, *i.e.* those developing later to the blastocyst stage, are less viable. Lately, eight IVP vitrified embryos derived from OPU-derived oocytes were transferred into recipients [10], giving three pregnancies (pregnancy rate of 37.5%), one of which was interrupted at 180 days, while the other two reached full term (25% development to term).

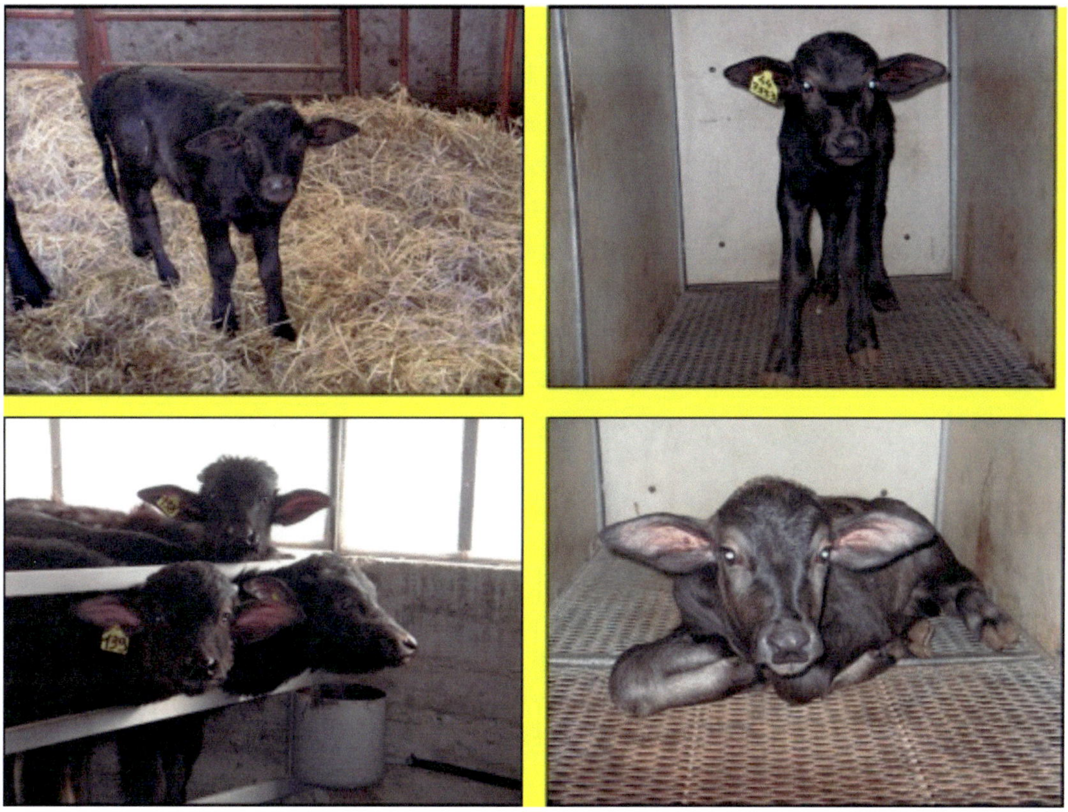

Fig. (3). Buffalo calves born following OPU/IVEP/vitrification procedures.

Hufana-Duran *et al.* [22] reported pregnancy to term following ET of IVP embryos that were vitrified in EFS40 vitrification solution (40% EG; 18% ficoll and 0.3 M sucrose) using pointed-shape open straws. The hatching rate after 72 h post-warming culture on a cumulus cell monolayer was 83% with no differences among developmental stages. To assess the *in vivo* developmental competence 95 embryos were transferred into 55 recipients (1-3 embryos per cow) after natural and synchronized estrus. Pregnancy and calving rates were on average 16.4% and 10.9%. No differences were observed in relation to the number of embryos transferred per animal but this was likely due to the limited number of transfers per group. In fact, it is worth noting that out of the 2 recipients that received 3 embryos one gave birth to a viable calf, hence with 50% pregnancy to term. In this work, five out of six calves were born when ET was carried out after natural estrus whereas only one calf was born from a synchronized recipient (16 *vs.* 4% pregnancy to term). It was hypothesized that the lower pregnancy rate in synchronized animals may be related to higher incidence of a short luteal phase, caused by earlier corpus luteum regression [150, 152], as well as to an improper timing of ET. The latter may be the result of the difficulty to detect estrus in synchronized buffaloes, because estrus signs are even weaker. It is known that embryo-recipient synchrony is a critical factor for embryo survival after ET. Kasiraj *et al.* [153] reported that an asynchrony of 12 h is the maximum that *in vivo* buffalo embryos cryopreserved by slow freezing can tolerate. It is worth pointing out that embryos developed in a co-culture system, and this in part may account for the lower development to term despite the higher hatching rates. Similar pregnancy to term (2/25; 8%) was reported after ET of buffalo IVP embryos cultured in a medium supplemented with serum and vitrified with the same method we previously utilized [14]. However, it is worth noting that pregnancy to term was also low after transfer of fresh embryos (1/7; 14.3%).

In another study the effects of different vitrification solutions (40% EG; 25% glycerol + 25% EG, and 25% EG + 25% DMSO) and exposure times (2, 4 and 6 min in the equilibration solution) on embryo survival were evaluated [154]. The higher expansion (72%) and hatching rates (46%) after 72 h culture were observed for blastocysts vitrified in 25% EG + 25% DMSO with an exposure time of 4 min. Furthermore, an effect of the stage of embryonic development was observed, as shown by the lower hatching rate of morulae (maximum hatching rate of 22%). In a more recent trial that compared different cryoprotectants and cryopreservation methods, using vitrification in pointed-shape open straws, the most favorable solution for cryopreservation of buffalo IVP embryos was 20% EG, 20% DMSO and 0.5 M sucrose [155].

It is known that cryoprotectants (CPs) damage the cytoskeleton, that is fundamental for appropriate cytokinesis and karyokinesis. The disruption of the cytoskeletal components interferes with the mitotic cell cycles, junctional complexes and solute transport systems. Therefore, it is very important to preserve the cyto-architecture integrity of the embryos during cryopreservation. In swine an improved development was recorded when embryos were treated with cytochalasin-B before cryopreservation [156]. In contrast, cytoskeleton stabilization with cytochalasin-B did not affect the post-culture development of buffalo embryos that were cryopreserved by a two-step vitrification method in 25% EG and 25% DMSO and 0.3 M sucrose [157]. However, the expansion and hatching rates of cytochalasin-B-treated vitrified-warmed morulae were similar to those recorded for their non-vitrified counterparts.

Finally, minimum volume vitrification methods, such as Open Pulled Straw [158] and Cryotop [159, 160] significantly increased the survival of buffalo IVP embryos. Similar embryo survival rates (70% *vs.* 62% respectively) were recorded after 24 h post-warming culture of buffalo embryos vitrified in OPS with the vitrification/warming solutions formerly used for buffalo embryos in French straws [143], and with those utilized for OPS vitrification of cattle embryos [161]. Subsequently, very promising results were obtained when IVP buffalo embryos were cryopreserved by Cryotop (Fig. **4**) vitrification [159]. The embryos were equilibrated for 3 min in 7.5% GE and DMSO and then transferred into the final vitrification solution (16.5% EG, 16.5% DMSO and 0.5 M). After 25 sec the embryos were picked up in a minimum volume (less than 0.1 μl), put on the top of a Cryotop and immediately plunged into liquid nitrogen. Warming was carried out in decreasing sucrose solutions (0.25 M for 1 min and 0.15 M for 5 min). Also in this trial the developmental stage affected freezability of IVP embryos, with enhanced survival for advanced embryos [158, 159, 162], such as expanded and hatched blastocysts (around 75%), known to be higher quality embryos as they develop faster *in vitro*. Interestingly, OPU-derived blastocysts vitrified by this method gave higher pregnancy rate at 25 days than in all former studies: pregnancy rate was 50%, to increase up to 75% after ET of fast developing embryos [162]. In addition, pregnancies established by fast embryos were maintained high (62.5%) also at 45 days. Nevertheless, calving rate was only 5.3%, to increase to 12.5% in case of faster developing embryos.

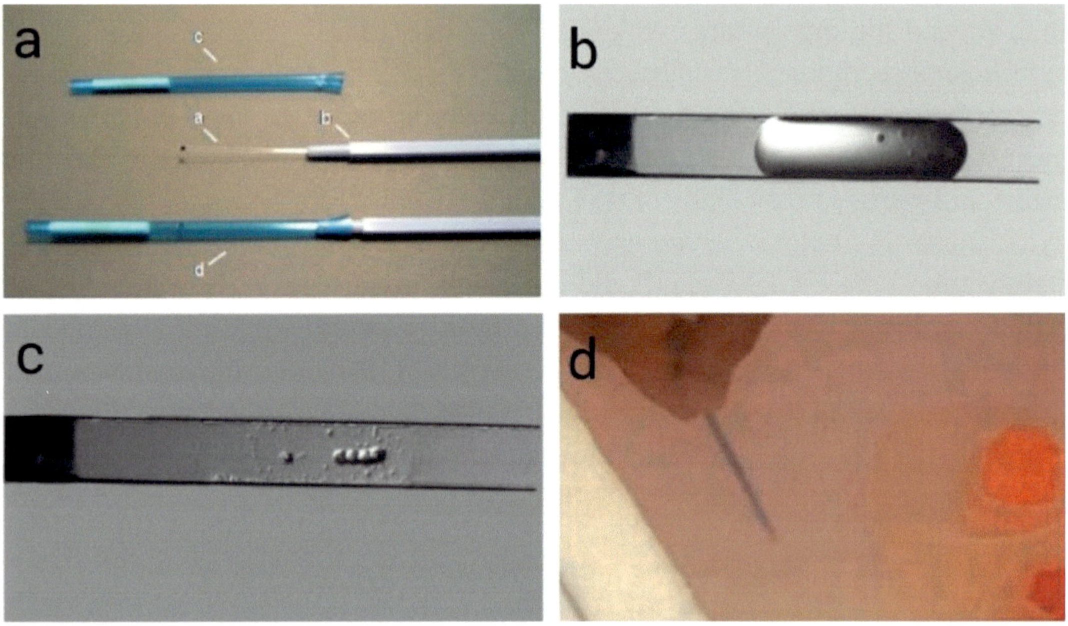

Fig. (4). Cryotop vitrification.

Finally, unprecedented results came from an OPU trial carried out in Brazil, where 70 embryos vitrified by CTV were transferred into recipients by fixed time embryo transfer (FTET), using eCG in estradiol/progestin-based protocol [163]. With regard to the embryo-recipient synchrony, day 5 and 6-embryos were transferred into recipients on day 6 and 7 after ovulation, respectively. Pregnancy rates were 37.1% on day 30 and 31.4% on day 60, with 15.4% late embryonic mortality. Development to term was higher than ever reported in literature, with 12 female and 10 male healthy calves born. These results completely changed the scenario, opening opportunities for the application in the field of OPU-IVEP. It is known that the final pregnancy outcome is in part due to the embryo vitality, affected by culture conditions, and in part to the recipient status and to the appropriate embryo-recipient synchrony. Therefore, encouraged by the excellent results, we planned an OPU trial and subsequent ET, to start with a better status of both donors and recipients, and we used FTET, with eCG in GnRH based protocol (as oestradiol is not allowed in our country) [164]. We transferred 46 blastocysts (25 fresh and 21 vitrified). The ET of fresh blastocysts resulted in 32% and 24% pregnancy rates on day 25 and 45, respectively. However, faster developing embryos, *i.e.* expanded and hatched, gave higher pregnancy rates than slower developing embryos, *i.e.* early blastocysts and blastocysts (40 *vs.* 26.7% on day 25 and 30 *vs.* 20% on day 45, respectively). Pregnancy rates after ET of vitrified embryos were 23.8% on day 25 and 19.0% to term. However, the difference related to the chronology of development was greater for vitrified embryos: in fact, faster embryos gave 45.5% pregnancy rate on day 25 and 36.4% to term, whereas no pregnancy was obtained from slower embryos. In contrast with the other trial (involving higher numbers), in this study the sex ratio was skewed towards males (66%). The overall improvement of pregnancy rate and the higher efficiency of faster embryos suggest that both the embryo viability and the recipient management play an important role.

In conclusion, there are no clear proofs indicating the supremacy of a particular cryopreservation method for buffalo embryos. In this regard, it is worth reminding that it is not possible to compare results because different laboratories employ different tools, and combinations of CPs/exposure times *etc*. In addition, the use of different culture systems, proven to influence embryo viability further complicates the scenario. The choice of a specific tool also depends on the future destination of the cryopreserved embryos. In fact, methods based on direct contact of embryos with LN_2 are not permitted for embryo movement across countries, due to potential sanitary risks. Nevertheless, if the superiority of these methods is proven also in terms of births after ET, strategies may be developed to eliminate these risks, such as the use of sterile filtered LN_2 and a safe sealing system before storage. Furthermore, it is well known that the major factor influencing the cryopreservation efficiency is undoubtedly the embryo quality. In buffalo, a severe selection of superior quality embryos for cryopreservation, currently practiced in cattle, would further limit the number of embryos, affecting the benefit cost ratio. Therefore, as embryo quality depends in part on the oocyte quality but mainly on the culture environment, the optimization of culture system is still required.

7. OOCYTE CRYOPRESERVATION

Cryopreservation of mammalian oocytes represents a fundamental technology, because of its potential implications for a faster development of biomedical research. In fact, the possibility of cryopreserving oocytes may increase the availability of female gametes for a wide range of reproductive biotechnologies, including IVEP, nuclear transfer and gene banking for the preservation of endangered species. Although embryo cryopreservation has been successful in several species, the high sensitivity of oocytes to cooling injuries still makes oocyte cryopreservation an open challenge in most mammals. Nevertheless, live offspring have been obtained after ET of embryos produced from cryopreserved mouse [165], rabbit [166], cattle [167, 168], equine [169], and human oocytes [170]. The interest in oocyte cryopreservation in buffalo has increased over the years because this technology, by enhancing the availability of gametes, may in part overcome the major limitation of IVEP in this species, *i.e.* the poor number of oocytes that can be recruited [52]. The possibility to store large number of competent oocytes may allow to plan IVF trials at the most convenient time and, hence to reduce strongly the lab costs: indeed, the cost for processing 10 *vs.* 100-200 oocytes is basically the same. Nevertheless, oocyte cryopreservation in buffalo is an open challenge as buffalo oocytes are highly sensitive to chilling injuries, due to their high intracytoplasmic lipid concentration [23]. Although the superiority of vitrification for oocyte cryopreservation has been clearly demonstrated in several species [171, 172], slow freezing of immature [173] and *in vitro*-matured buffalo oocytes [174] has been only recently reported. It was first demonstrated that slow freezing is not effective for immature buffalo oocytes, as indicated by impaired maturation and development to morulae [175]. Then it was proven that vitrification is more efficient than slow freezing for cryopreserving *in vitro*-matured buffalo oocytes [176]. The former studies on oocyte cryopreservation in buffalo were performed on immature oocytes that were vitrified in traditional French straws, using a variety of CPs at different concentrations and different exposure times, resulting in poor maturation rates despite the high post-warming survival [175, 176]. Among the cell damages described, oocytes cracking of the zona pellucida was the abnormality observed most frequently [175], followed by leakage of cellular contents, change of shape and splitting into two halves. Subsequently, the influence of different CPs at different concentrations on survival, *in vitro* maturation [177] as well as on cleavage and blastocyst production [178] of vitrified-thawed immature buffalo oocytes was evaluated. For all CPs used, higher maturation and cleavage rates were recorded at higher concentrations: 7M of DMSO, EG, PROH and glycerol. Furthermore, blastocysts were produced for the first time from immature vitrified oocytes although the efficiency was low and not affected by treatments [178]. Then it was demonstrated that it is preferable to combine two permeable CPs and that the best combination is EG and DMS in a 2-step vitrification (equilibration in half the concentration of the final vitrification solution) both in French straws and OPS [179]. More recently, it was demonstrated the superiority of CTV compared to SSV for immature buffalo oocytes in terms of post-warming survival rates and that a pre-treatment with cytochalasin B does not improve the efficiency that remained very low in terms of maturation, cleavage and blastocyst rates [180]. All these studies, however, confirmed the extremely high sensitivity of buffalo immature oocytes to cryopreservation.

In order to evaluate the effect of meiotic stage, buffalo immature oocytes were vitrified at different maturation times (0, 6, 12, 18 and 24 h) in 40% propanediol and 0.25 mol/L trehalose, and then matured for an additional time to reach 24 h of IVM [181]. Improved post-thaw survival and maturation rate were observed at higher interval of maturation. It has been suggested that the low permeability [182] and low stability [183] of plasma membrane may be responsible for higher susceptibility to osmotic damage [184 - 186] and, hence poor cryotolerance of immature oocytes. The poorer maturation rate of oocytes that did not accomplish maturation may be related to several factors, such as loss of association between oocyte and cumulus cells [187, 188], loss of cell structure integrity, increasing the ooplasm porosity [189], higher vulnerability of the cytoskeleton and cytoplasmic damages [190, 191].

Recently, studies on buffalo oocyte cryopreservation have intensified, shifting to *in vitro* matured oocytes and, parallel to the advancements in vitrification technology achieved in other species, to the use of innovative methods. It is well documented that fast cooling and warming rates decrease the CPs toxicity and allow to bypass the exposure of oocytes to temperatures toward which they are particularly sensitive [184, 192]. Therefore, several methods have been proposed to enhance cooling and warming rates, based on the use of minimal volumes and direct contact with LN_2 [193]. Electron microscopy grids [194], glass capillaries [195], open-pulled straws [196], cryoloops [197] and cryotop [198] have, as common denominator, the use of small volumes. Another recently developed method is the solid surface vitrification (SSV), that combines the advantages of the containerless microdrop-vitrification and of a precooled metal surface that increases heat exchange [199]. Minimum volumes vitrification methods such SSV and Cryoloop vitrification (CLV) have been used to effectively cryopreserve *in vitro*-matured buffalo oocytes, as shown by their capacity to cleave and develop into blastocysts following IVF [63]. For SSV, oocytes were vitrified in 35% EG, 5% PVP and 0.4% trehalose and warmed in a 0.3 M trehalose. For CLV, vitrification solution consisted of 16.5% EG and 16.5% DMSO and warming was carried out in decreasing sucrose concentrations. Survival rates of denuded and cumulus enclosed oocytes were high with both methods. However, CLV significantly improved cleavage rate compared to SSV with denuded oocytes (45% *vs.* 26%, respectively), but similar values were recorded with cumulus-enclosed oocytes (14% *vs.* 15%, respectively). Although blastocyst production from *in vitro* matured vitrified-warmed buffalo oocytes was described for the first time, the efficiency was very low.

Blastocyst development was also achieved following parthenogenetic activation of *in vitro*-matured Swamp buffalo oocytes vitrified by SSV and in-straw vitrification (ISV). Both methods caused ultrastructural damages to microvilli, mitochondria, oolemma and cortical granules, resulting in decreased competence. However, the SSV damaged mitochondria to a lesser extent, and increased blastocyst rate [200]. It was then demonstrated that OPS is a more efficient cryodevice than French mini straws and that EG +DMSO is better than propylene glycol + DMSO to cryopreserve matured buffalo oocytes, as suggested by reduced morphological changes and DNA damage and improved developmental competence [201]. Nevertheless, cleavage rates were still low and blastocyst rates very poor.

Cryotop vitrification (CTV) is certainly one of the most efficient ultrarapid vitrification techniques, as suggested by the excellent survival and developmental rates reported for human and bovine MII phase oocytes [198]. Lately, this method was effectively employed to cryopreserve horse [202], ovine [203] and pig oocytes [204]. It was demonstrated that *in vitro* matured Swamp buffalo oocytes vitrified by CTV are able to cleave and reach the blastocyst stage after activation and nuclear transfer [205]. Thereafter, the capacity of *in vitro* matured River buffalo oocytes vitrified by CTV to cleave and to develop into blastocysts after IVF was proven [206]. In particular, higher efficiency was obtained by using a two-step equilibration in 20% DMSO, 20% EG, and 0.5 M sucrose during vitrification and a multistep decreasing sucrose concentrations starting from 1.25 M for warming. However, in spite of high survival (93%) and cleavage rates (55%), the percentage of blastocysts (8%) still need to be enhanced.

Another study reported that in a 2-step vitrification in microdrops, with 1 min in the first solution (10% DMSO and EG) an improved efficiency after activation and ICSI was obtained when oocytes were placed in the final vitrification solution (20% DMSO and EG +0.5 M sucrose) for 30 s compared to 45 or 60 s [207]. Furthermore, it was reported that microdrops and CTV in a mixture of EG and Me_2SO are equally effective on survival and embryo development [208], although the embryo development was very poor.

Another important aspect to consider is the critical role played by cumulus cells during both oocyte maturation and fertilization. In fact, the presence of cumulus investments may interfere with the diffusion of CPs within the oocyte, resulting in insufficient cell protection [209]. Accordingly, buffalo oocytes should be freed of cumulus cells before cryopreservation to increase the efficiency [63]. However, it is well known that the removal of cumulus cells affects fertilization and embryo development [62]. In our previous experience, non vitrified denuded oocytes gave cleavage and blastocyst rates as low as those obtained from vitrified-warmed oocytes [63]. Impaired fertilization of denuded oocytes is due to the lack of cumulus cells, known to attract and select sperm [210, 211], promote sperm capacitation, acrosome reaction and penetration [211, 212] and prevent earlier hardening of the zona pellucida [213]. Indeed, zona pellucida hardening occurs following cryopreservation, decreasing fertilization rate [214, 215]. This problem may be in part overcome by partial removal of cumulus cells prior vitrification in other species but the scarce adhesion of somatic cells to the buffalo egg [52] makes this procedure hard to perform.

Based on these observations, we evaluated whether providing cumulus cells support during IVF of vitrified-warmed denuded oocytes would improve the efficiency. The most efficient somatic support that totally restored the fertilizing ability of buffalo denuded vitrified oocytes was demonstrated to be the co-culture with bovine intact COCs (1:1 ratio) during IVF. In fact, this method significantly improved cleavage rate up to values similar to those of fresh oocytes (61 *vs.* 68%), without though improving blastocyst development [102]. The beneficial effect of this co-culture approach on the fertilizing capability of denuded oocytes is likely due to the fact that within the COCs physiological interaction between the oocytes and cumulus cells is maintained. On the other hand, post-fertilization embryo development is impaired because of many cryopreservation-induced damages, such as spindle disruption, chromatin fragmentation, spontaneous activation [216] alterations of microvilli, mitochondria, oolemma and cortical granules [200]. It results that although the replacement of cumulus cells during IVF of vitrified denuded oocytes is efficient to restore their capability to be fertilized *in vitro*, other strategies still need to be developed to improve the developmental competence of buffalo oocytes undergoing vitrification.

8. SEX PREDETERMINATION: EMBRYO AND SPERM SEXING

The predetermination of the sex of offspring has immense potentials in the livestock industry. In the past, manipulation of the sex ratio went through selective abortion of the fetus of the undesired gender. With the improvement of the IVEP system and the possibility to sex pre-implantation stage embryos, the manipulation of the sex ratio has become a reality. For the buffalo species, sexing embryos has been, likewise cattle, a landmark for the embryo transfer industry as well as for the enhancement of the genetic merit. A number of techniques developed in order to select embryos according to their gender, such as blastomere cytogenetic analysis [217 - 219], male-specific antigens [220, 221], X-linked enzyme activities [222] and hybridisation by specific Y-linked probes [223], have been found to be of no practical value or not reliable in a commercial setting. With the advent and development of the polymerase chain reaction (PCR) [224], a new scenario has opened within the embryo sexing technology, allowing the possibility to amplify Y-chromosome-specific DNA sequences and therefore differentiating male from female cells. The efficiency and potential of this new technique has been shown in several species [225], such as in human [226], bovine [227 - 231], equine [232], ovine [227, 233] and porcine embryos [234].

A novel methodology for buffalo embryo sexing was developed by Appa Rao *et al.* [235], by amplification of the Y-chromosome-specific sequence. DNA amplification is an ideal and sensitive technique based on repetitive sequences found on the Y chromosome, for the development of sexing protocols [228, 236, 237]. A particular repetitive sequence found on the Y chromosome (BRY) is evolutively conserved in a number of species such as sheep, goat and deer [238, 239]. In buffaloes a sequence (BuRY.I), homologue of the BRY.1 sequence, has been reported by Appa Rao and Totey [240], and consequently a PCR procedure for embryo sexing in buffaloes has been developed using specific BuRY.I primers. In doing so, a nested and multiplex PCR was developed as an efficient and sensitive procedure to sex buffalo embryos, by using a single blastomere. In a subsequent study [241] primers derived from bovine Y-chromosome-specific sequences (BRY4.a and BRY.1) were used on 359 IVP buffalo embryos along with the available PCR assay. A comparison on two different methods for DNA extraction was performed: i) a standard procedure (ST) where an ordinary extraction was used by mean of phenolchloroform, isoamyl alcohol and a final precipitation in absolute ethanol; and a ii) direct procedure (DT), where a commercial kit (Qiaquik-qiagen mini blood) was used. Sufficient amounts of target DNA was recovered using both procedures at all stages of embryo development, although the commercial kits required much less time needed for its execution when compared to the standard procedure: 5 h *vs.* 24 h, respectively.

Hirayama *et al.* reported a loop mediated isothermal amplification (LAMP) in order to sex buffalo embryos [242], which is a novel approach enabling the amplification of a specific target sequence under isothermal conditions. These authors have established an efficient protocol for sexing buffalo embryos with the LAMP approach, by identifying Y chromosome-specific sequences in this species. It only takes 1 hour for the procedure of DNA extraction and embryo sexing to be performed, with LAMP reaction requiring approximately 45 min. It can conclusively be stated that the protocol established, with unneeded procedure for thermal cycling and electrophoresis, is feasible and reliable and can therefore be conducted in buffalo embryos.

The SRY gene can be considered the dominant functional region of the Y-chromosome. Therefore, to be able to correctly conduct sex determination, it is logical to consider that male specific SRY (Sry) fragments have to be amplified. Within this framework, embryo sexing was reported by Utsumi and Iritani, by employing PCR and a male-specific (SRY) primer [243]. Finally, it was recently demonstrated that the so-called multiplex-nested PCR procedure is also highly reliable for sexing swamp buffalo embryos, by adjusting MG^{2+} and dNTPs concentrations, primers ratio and number of cycles [244]. Therefore, efficient methods for embryo sexing in buffalo are available but data are still lacking on pregnancy rates after ET of sexed embryos.

To be able to determine gender prior to conception, is the most efficient mean to reach the desired result in terms of wanted offspring. In this line, at present, the only correct and reliable method to a very large extent for sex preselection, is based on the possibility to separate X- and Y-chromosome-bearing sperm cells by flow cytometry. Preselected sperm cells can be then used in the realm of modern reproductive technologies, ranging from AI to IVF, followed by ET. Sperm sexing combined with IVF or ICSI, can be accounted for a more efficient and higher number of produced embryos of the desired gender when compared to traditional and older technology for embryo sexing. The latter nowadays is only marginally performed, due to its limited usefulness if we consider the number of discarded embryos of unwanted gender, which makes the procedure in its whole highly inefficient. In 2003 [245], X- and Y-bearing spermatozoa were detected in water buffalo spermatozoa by fluorescence *in situ* hybridization, using an X- and Y-specific probe set derived from yak chromosomes, and a cattle Y- chromosome repeat sequence (BC1.2).

In a following study it was shown that X- and Y- painting probes can be used for sexing procedures and analysis of spermatozoa belonging to different species of the Bovidae family including buffalo [246]. In 2005 [247] pregnancies following

AI with sexed semen were reported for the first time in buffaloes synchronized by Ovsynch. In particular, low doses of sexed frozen spermatozoa, previously sorted by flow cytometry, were deposited near the utero-tubal junction, reaching conception rates not significantly different from those reported ordinarily with the use of a full dose of unsorted semen following conventional AI (42.8 *vs.* 43.3%, respectively).

Following fetal sexing and final confirmation at birth, eight of the nine fetuses corresponded to the predicted sex. Further investigations on the validity and reliability of the procedure of sexing sperm cells and follow-up production of buffalo calves of the wanted gender, were carried out [248]. In an additional trial, sorted buffalo X-sperm cells was used for AI in buffaloes following spontaneous estrus, resulting in a 69.7% conception rate and 82.8% sexing accuracy. Individual bulls were found to be a determining factor for conception rate, although similar results were obtained when considered both sorted and unsorted semen as well as heifers *vs.* pluriparous buffalo cows. Similar pregnancy rates with sexed and conventional semen were also recorded after AI in Mediterranean buffalo heifers synchronized by Presynch; in this trial pregnancy rates were higher when sexed semen was deposited into the body of the uterus rather than the horn [249]. Recently, similar pregnancies after AI with sexed and conventional semen were also reported in pluriparous Mediterranean buffaloes during different seasons [250].

Finally, sexed sperm were used for IVF of OPU-derived buffalo oocytes to produce sex-preselected embryos [17]. No differences in cleavage (50.5 *vs.*. 50.9%) and blastocyst (15.3 *vs.*. 19.1%) development were recorded between frozen-thawed sexed and unsexed semen. More importantly, pregnancies were established after ET of sex preselected embryos at the same rate of the unsexed embryos (26.5 *vs.* 26.9%, respectively with fresh embryos; 11.6 *vs.* 15.4%, respectively with frozen-thawed embryos).

The results here reported indicate the feasibility of the application of the sexing technology to accelerate the genetic improvement in buffalo both *via* maternal and paternal lineage. However, data are still limited and more extensive studies should be carried out to allow optimization of the procedure before it is commercially applied.

CONCLUSION

An incredible improvement in the efficiency of a number of embryo related and reproductive technologies, such as IVEP in the buffalo species has been achieved. The recent results in terms of pregnancy rates after ET of cryopreserved IVP buffalo embryos are unprecedented in science and open alternative reproductive strategies and new possibilities for the commercial use of OPU and IVEP in buffalo. Nevertheless there is still a need to continue to improve and optimize culture conditions in order to increase the viability and cryotolerance of IVP embryos, so that this newly developed reproductive technologies will become more attractive and diffuse in the buffalo breeding industry.

The major current limitation is the low number of oocytes recovered that depends on the scarce follicular reservoir of the species. It follows that the human intervention is strongly limited to overcome the innate limitation of the species to yield competent oocytes, although some expedients may increase the recovery rate to a certain extent. In future perspective, the optimization of the oocyte cryopreservation efficiency may lead to increased oocyte availability for IVEP, allowing to better plan IVF trials and save resources. Furthermore, the use of sexed semen for IVF may further optimize the competitiveness of this technology.

CONFLICT OF INTEREST

The author confirm that the author has no conflict of interest to declare for this publication.

ACKNOWLEDGEMENTS

Declared none.

REFERENCES

[1] Misra AK. Application of biotechnologies to buffalo breeding in India. Third Course on Biotechnology of Reproduction in buffaloes. Italy: Caserta 1997; pp. 141-66.

[2] Zicarelli L. Superovulatory response in buffaloes bred in Italy. Third Course on Biotechnology of Reproduction in buffaloes. Italy: Caserta 1997; pp. 167-88.

[3] Perera BM. Reproduction in domestic buffalo. Reprod Domest Anim 2008; 43(2) (Suppl. 2): 200-6. [http://dx.doi.org/10.1111/j.1439-0531.2008.01162.x] [PMID: 18638124]

[4] Boni R, Di Palo R, Barbieri V, Zicarelli L. Ovum pick-up in deep anestrus buffaloes. Proc IV World Buffalo Congress. 480-2.

[5] Boni R. *In vitro* production in bovine and buffalo species. Buffalo J 1994; 2: 147-60.

[6] Boni R, Roviello S, Campanile G, Di Palo R, Zicarelli L. Single ovum pick-up performed from the sixth to the eleventh estrous cycle day in buffalo cows. Proc Symp on Reprod Animal Breeding: Advances and Strategies. 357-8.

[7] Boni R, Roviello S, Zicarelli L. Repeated ovum pick-up in Italian Mediterranean buffalo cows. Theriogenology 1996; 46(5): 899-909. [http://dx.doi.org/10.1016/S0093-691X(96)00248-8] [PMID: 16727954]

[8] Boni R, Roviello S, Gasparrini B, Zicarelli L. Pregnancies established after transferring embryos yielded by ovum pick-up and *in vitro* embryo production in Italian buffalo cows. Proc V World Buffalo Congress. Caserta, Italy. 1997; pp. 787-92.

[9] Neglia G, Gasparrini B, Caracciolo di Brienza V, *et al.* Bovine and buffalo *in vitro* embryo production using oocytes derived from abattoir ovaries or collected by transvaginal follicle aspiration. Theriogenology 2003; 59(5-6): 1123-30. [http://dx.doi.org/10.1016/S0093-691X(02)01170-6] [PMID: 12527061]

[10] Neglia G, Gasparrini B, Caracciolo di Brienza V, Di Palo R, Zicarelli L. First pregnancies to term after transfer of buffalo vitrified embryos entirely produced *in vitro.* Vet Res Commun 2004; 28: 233-326. [http://dx.doi.org/10.1023/B:VERC.0000045414.65331.6a] [PMID: 15372965]

[11] Neglia G, Gasparrini B, Vecchio D, *et al.* Long term effect of Ovum Pick-up in buffalo species. Anim Reprod Sci 2011; 123(3-4): 180-6. [http://dx.doi.org/10.1016/j.anireprosci.2011.01.011] [PMID: 21306842]

[12] Di Francesco S, Novoa MV, Vecchio D, *et al.* Ovum pick-up and *in vitro* embryo production (OPU-IVEP) in Mediterranean Italian buffalo performed in different seasons. Theriogenology 2012; 77(1): 148-54. [http://dx.doi.org/10.1016/j.theriogenology.2011.07.028] [PMID: 21872310]

[13] Gasparrini B, Neglia G, Di Palo R, *et al.* Influence of oocyte donor on *in vitro* embryo production in buffalo. Anim Reprod Sci 2014; 144(3-4): 95-101. [http://dx.doi.org/10.1016/j.anireprosci.2013.11.010] [PMID: 24374181]

[14] Sá Filho MF, Carvalho NA, Gimenes LU, *et al.* Birth of the first buffalo calves after transfer of vitrified embryos produced *in vitro* in America. Proceedings of 3° Congresso Nazionale sull'Allevamento del Bufalo and 1° Buffalo Symposium of Europe and the Americas; Capaccio-Paestum (SA), Italy, October 2005

[15] Sá Filho MF, Carvalho NA, Gimenes LU, *et al.* Effect of recombinant bovine somatotropin (bST) on follicular population and on *in vitro* buffalo embryo production. Anim Reprod Sci 2009; 113(1-4): 51-9. [http://dx.doi.org/10.1016/j.anireprosci.2008.06.008] [PMID: 18691835]

[16] Huang Y, Zhuang X, Gasparrini B, Presicce GA. Oocyte recovery by ovum pick-up and embryo production in Murrah and Nili-Ravi buffaloes (*Bubalus bubalis*) imported in China. Reprod Fertil Dev 2005; 17(1,2): 273.

[17] Liang XW, Lu YQ, Chen MT, *et al. In vitro* embryo production in buffalo (*Bubalus bubalis*) using sexed sperm and oocytes from ovum pick up. Theriogenology 2008; 69(7): 822-6. [http://dx.doi.org/10.1016/j.theriogenology.2007.11.021] [PMID: 18336893]

[18] Pellerano G, Gasparrini B, Crudeli G, *et al.* Ovum pick-up and *in vitro* embryo production technology in field conditions in the North East of Argentina. Proc of the 8th World Buffalo Congress, Caserta, October 19-22. Ital J Anim Sci 2007; 6(2): 743-6. [http://dx.doi.org/10.4081/ijas.2007.s2.743]

[19] Manjunatha BM, Gupta PS, Ravindra JP, Devaraj M, Nandi S. *In vitro* embryo development and blastocyst hatching rates following vitrification of river buffalo embryos produced from oocytes recovered from slaughterhouse ovaries or live animals by ovum pick-up. Anim Reprod Sci 2008; 104(2-4): 419-26. [http://dx.doi.org/10.1016/j.anireprosci.2007.06.030] [PMID: 17689038]

[20] Manjunatha BM, Ravindra JP, Gupta PS, Devaraj M, Nandi S. Effect of breeding season on *in vivo* oocyte recovery and embryo production in non-descriptive Indian river buffaloes (*Bubalus bubalis*). Anim Reprod Sci 2009; 111(2-4): 376-83. [http://dx.doi.org/10.1016/j.anireprosci.2008.03.003] [PMID: 18440168]

[21] Gasparrini B, Boccia L, Marchandise J, *et al.* Enrichment of *in vitro* maturation medium for buffalo (*Bubalus bubalis*) oocytes with thiol compounds: effects of cystine on glutathione synthesis and embryo development. Theriogenology 2006; 65(2): 275-87. [http://dx.doi.org/10.1016/j.theriogenology.2005.05.036] [PMID: 15979699]

[22] Hufana-Duran D, Pedro PB, Venturina HV, *et al.* Post-warming hatching and birth of live calves following transfer of *in vitro*-derived vitrified water buffalo (*Bubalus bubalis*) embryos. Theriogenology 2004; 61(7-8): 1429-39. [http://dx.doi.org/10.1016/j.theriogenology.2003.08.011] [PMID: 15036974]

[23] Boni R, Santella L, Dale B, Roviello S, Di Palo R, Barbieri V. An ultrastructural study of maturation in buffalo oocytes. Acta Med Vet (Napoli) 1992; 38: 153-61.

[24] Campanile G, Neglia G, Gasparrini B, *et al.* Embryonic mortality in buffaloes synchronized and mated by AI during the seasonal decline in reproductive function. Theriogenology 2005; 63(8): 2334-40. [http://dx.doi.org/10.1016/j.theriogenology.2004.10.012] [PMID: 15826694]

[25] Campanile G, Baruselli PS, Neglia G, *et al.* Ovarian function in the buffalo and implications for embryo development and assisted reproduction. Anim Reprod Sci 2010; 121(1-2): 1-11. [http://dx.doi.org/10.1016/j.anireprosci.2010.03.012] [PMID: 20430540]

[26] Di Francesco S, Boccia L, Campanile G, *et al.* The effect of season on oocyte quality and developmental competence in Italian Mediterranean buffaloes (*Bubalus bubalis*). Anim Reprod Sci 2011; 123(1-2): 48-53. [http://dx.doi.org/10.1016/j.anireprosci.2010.11.009] [PMID: 21168984]

[27] McEvoy TG, Robinson JJ, Carolan C, Staines ME, Broadbent PJ, Sinclair KD. Ovine fetal

development following embryo culture in synthetic oviduct fluid with added ammonium. Theriogenology 1999; 51: 247.
[http://dx.doi.org/10.1016/S0093-691X(99)91806-X]

[28] Totey SM, Singh G, Taneja M, Pawshe CH, Talwar GP. *In vitro* maturation, fertilization and development of follicular oocytes from buffalo (*Bubalus bubalis*). J Reprod Fertil 1992; 95: 597-607.

[29] Das GK, Jain GC, Solari VS, Tripathi VN. Efficacy of various collection methods for oocytes retrieval in buffalo. Theriogenology 1996; 46: 1403-11.
[http://dx.doi.org/10.1016/S0093-691X(96)00319-6]

[30] Madan ML, Singla SK, Chauhan MS, Manik RS. *In vitro* production and transfer of embryos in buffaloes. Theriogenology 1994; 41: 139-43.
[http://dx.doi.org/10.1016/S0093-691X(05)80059-7]

[31] Samad HA, Khan IQ, Rehman NU, Ahmed N. The recovery, *in vitro* maturation and fertilization of Nilli-Ravi buffalo follicular oocytes. J Anim Sci 1998; 11: 491-7.

[32] Gasparrini B, Neglia G, Palo RD, Campanile G, Zicarelli L. Effect of cysteamine during *in vitro* maturation on buffalo embryo development. Theriogenology 2000; 54(9): 1537-42.
[http://dx.doi.org/10.1016/S0093-691X(00)00473-8] [PMID: 11191875]

[33] Goswami SL, Manik RS, Balakrishnan CR. Status of buffalo and goat ovaries collected from slaughterhouse. Proc of the Symposium on embryo transfer technology held at IVRI Izatnagar. 1992, April 16–17;

[34] Smith JF. Protein, energy and ovulation rate. In: Land RB, Robinson DW, Eds. Genetics of Reproduction in Sheep London. Butterworth 1984; pp. 349-59.

[35] Nandi S, Chauhan MS, Palta P. Effect of a corpus luteum on the recovery and developmental potential of buffalo oocytes. Vet Rec 2000; 147(20): 580-1.
[http://dx.doi.org/10.1136/vr.147.20.580] [PMID: 11104045]

[36] Misra AK. Embryo transfer technology in buffaloes. Process and developments. National Seminar on Recent Advances in Conservation of Biodiversity and Augmentation of Reproduction and Production in Farm Animals, Sardarkrushinagar, India, March 6–7, 2005. 37. Gordon I. Aspiration techniques: Old and new. In Laboratory Production of Cattle Embryos. Wallingford, UK 1994: CAB International, 71-72

[37] Gordon I. Aspiration techniques: Old and new. Laboratory Production of Cattle Embryos. Wallingford, UK: CAB International 1994; pp. 71-2.

[38] Galli C, Crotti G, Notari C, Turini P, Duchi R, Lazzari G. Embryo production by ovum pick up from live donors. Theriogenology 2001; 55(6): 1341-57.
[http://dx.doi.org/10.1016/S0093-691X(01)00486-1] [PMID: 11327688]

[39] Samad HA, Nasseri AA. A quantitative study of primordial follicles in buffalo heifer ovaries. Compendium 13 FAO/SIDA Int Course. Anim Reprod 1979.

[40] Danell B. Oestrus behaviour, ovarian morphology and cyclic variations in follicular system and endocrine pattern in water buffalo heifers. PhD thesis, Uppsala, Sweden, Sveriges Lantbruksuniversiter 1987.

[41] Erickson BH. Development and senescence of the postnatal bovine ovary. J Anim Sci 1966; 25(3): 800-5.
[http://dx.doi.org/10.2527/jas1966.253800x] [PMID: 6007918]

[42] Kumar A, Solanki VS, Jindal SK, Tripathi VN, Jain GC. Oocyte retrieval and histological studies of follicular population in buffalo ovaries. Anim Reprod Sci 1997; 47(3): 189-95.
[http://dx.doi.org/10.1016/S0378-4320(96)01588-6] [PMID: 9329860]

[43] Ocampo MB, de Asis AT, Ocampo LC, Kanagawa H. Histological observation of follicular atresia in Swamp buffalo. Buffalo Bull 1994; 13: 51-5.

[44] Palta P, Banzai N, Prakash BS, Manik RS, Madan ML. Endocrinological observation of atresia in individual buffalo ovarian follicles. Indian J Anim Sci 1998; 68: 444-7.

[45] Vittoria A. Anatomy of the female genital tract in the buffalo. Third Course on Biotechnology of Reproduction in Buffaloes. Italy: Caserta 1997; pp. 15-20.

[46] Bols PE, Ysebaert MT, Lein A, Coryn M, Van Soom A, de Kruif A. Effects of long-term treatment with bovine somatotropin on follicular dynamics and subsequent oocyte and blastocyst yield in an OPU-IVF program. Theriogenology 1998; 49(5): 983-95.
[http://dx.doi.org/10.1016/S0093-691X(98)00047-8] [PMID: 10732106]

[47] Tripp MW, Ju JC, Hoagland TA, Riesen JW, Yang X, Zinn SA. Influence of somatotropin and nutrition on bovine oocyte retrieval and in vitro development. Theriogenology 2000; 53(8): 1581-90.
[http://dx.doi.org/10.1016/S0093-691X(00)00299-5] [PMID: 10883845]

[48] Baruselli PS, Gimenes LU, Carvalho NA, Sa Filho MF, Ferraz ML. Control of ovarian function for assisted reproductive technologies in buffalo.

[49] Manjunatha BM, Gupta PS, Devaraj M, Ravindra JP, Nandi S. Selection of developmentally competent buffalo oocytes by brilliant cresyl blue staining before IVM. Theriogenology 2007; 68(9): 1299-304. a
[http://dx.doi.org/10.1016/j.theriogenology.2007.08.031] [PMID: 17920672]

[50] Mishra V, Misra AK, Sharma R. A comparative study of parthenogenic activation and in vitro fertilization of bubaline oocytes. Anim Reprod Sci 2008; 103(3-4): 249-59.
[http://dx.doi.org/10.1016/j.anireprosci.2006.12.019] [PMID: 17321079]

[51] Merton JS, de Roos AP, Mullaart E, *et al.* Factors affecting oocyte quality and quantity in commercial application of embryo technologies in the cattle breeding industry. Theriogenology 2003; 59(2): 651-74.
[http://dx.doi.org/10.1016/S0093-691X(02)01246-3] [PMID: 12499010]

[52] Gasparrini B. *In vitro* embryo production in buffalo species: state of the art. Theriogenology 2002; 57(1): 237-56.
[http://dx.doi.org/10.1016/S0093-691X(01)00669-0] [PMID: 11775973]

[53] Manjunatha BM, Gupta PS, Ravindra JP, Devaraj M, Ramesh HS, Nandi S. *In vitro* developmental competence of buffalo oocytes collected at various stages of the estrous cycle. Theriogenology 2007; 68(6): 882-8. b
[http://dx.doi.org/10.1016/j.theriogenology.2007.07.001] [PMID: 17706758]

[54] Blondin P, Coenen K, Guilbault LA, Sirard MA. *In vitro* production of bovine embryos: developmental competence is acquired before maturation. Theriogenology 1997; 47(5): 1061-75. [http://dx.doi.org/10.1016/S0093-691X(97)00063-0] [PMID: 16728056]

[55] Di Francesco S, Boccia L, Di Palo R, *et al.* Influence of temperature and time during ovary transportation on *in vitro* embryo production efficiency in the buffalo species (*Bubalus bubalis*). Proc of the 8th World Buffalo Congress, Caserta, October 19-22, 2007. Ital J Anim Sci 2007; 6(2): 755-8. [http://dx.doi.org/10.4081/ijas.2007.s2.755]

[56] Gasparrini B. Advances on *in vitro* embryo production in water buffalo. Proc of the 5th Asian Buffalo Congress on "Social economic contribution of buffalo to rural areas", April 18-22, Nanning, China 2006; 1:15-21

[57] Mishra V, Misra AK, Sharma R. Effect of ambient temperature on *in vitro* fertilization of Bubaline oocyte. Anim Reprod Sci 2007; 100(3-4): 379-84. [http://dx.doi.org/10.1016/j.anireprosci.2006.10.020] [PMID: 17125942]

[58] Nandi S, Chauhan MS, Palta P. Effect of environmental temperature on quality and developmental competence *in vitro* of buffalo oocytes. Vet Rec 2001; 148(9): 278-9. [http://dx.doi.org/10.1136/vr.148.9.278] [PMID: 11292091]

[59] Chuangsoongneon U, Kamonpatana M. Oocyte maturation, *in vitro* fertilization and culture system for developing preimplantation Swamp buffalo embryos using frozen-thawed semen. Buffalo J 1991; 7: 189-98.

[60] Totey SM, Pawshe CH, Singh GP. *In vitro* maturation and fertilization of buffalo oocytes (*Bubalus bubalis*): Effects of media, hormones and sera. Theriogenology 1993; 39(5): 1153-71. [http://dx.doi.org/10.1016/0093-691X(93)90014-V] [PMID: 16727284]

[61] Chauhan MS, Singla SK, Palta P, Manik RS, Madan ML. *In vitro* maturation and fertilization, and subsequent development of buffalo (*Bubalus bubalis*) embryos: effects of oocyte quality and type of serum. Reprod Fertil Dev 1998; 10(2): 173-7. a [http://dx.doi.org/10.1071/R97080] [PMID: 9801269]

[62] Nandi S, Chauhan MS, Palta P. Influence of cumulus cells and sperm concentration on cleavage rate and subsequent embryonic development of buffalo (*Bubalus bubalis*) oocytes matured and fertilized *in vitro*. Theriogenology 1998; 50(8): 1251-62. [http://dx.doi.org/10.1016/S0093-691X(98)00224-6] [PMID: 10734439]

[63] Gasparrini B, Attanasio L, De Rosa A, Monaco E, Di Palo R, Campanile G. Cryopreservation of *in vitro* matured buffalo (*Bubalus bubalis*) oocytes by minimum volumes vitrification methods. Anim Reprod Sci 2007; 98(3-4): 335-42. [http://dx.doi.org/10.1016/j.anireprosci.2006.04.046] [PMID: 16698202]

[64] Pawshe CH, Totey SM. Effects of cumulus cells monolayer on *in vitro* maturation of denuded oocytes of buffalo (*Bubalus bubalis*). Theriogenology 1993; 39: 281. [http://dx.doi.org/10.1016/0093-691X(93)90136-S]

[65] Chauhan MS, Palta P, Das SK, Katiyar PK, Madan ML. Replacement of serum and hormone additives with follicular fluid in the IVM medium: effects on maturation, fertilization and subsequent development of buffalo oocytes *in vitro*. Theriogenology 1997; 48(3): 461-9.

[http://dx.doi.org/10.1016/S0093-691X(97)00255-0] [PMID: 16728142]

[66] Pawshe CH, Rao KB, Totey SM. Effect of insulin-like growth factor I and its interaction with gonadotropins on *in vitro* maturation and embryonic development, cell proliferation, and biosynthetic activity of cumulus-oocyte complexes and granulosa cells in buffalo. Mol Reprod Dev 1998; 49(3): 277-85.
[http://dx.doi.org/10.1002/(SICI)1098-2795(199803)49:3<277::AID-MRD8>3.0.CO;2-L] [PMID: 9491380]

[67] Chauhan MS, Singla SK, Palta P, Manik RS, Madan ML. Effect of epidermal growth factor on the cumulus expansion, meiotic maturation and development of buffalo oocytes *in vitro.* Vet Rec 1999; 144(10): 266-7.
[http://dx.doi.org/10.1136/vr.144.10.266] [PMID: 10209821]

[68] Nandi S, Ravindranatha BM, Gupta PS, Raghu HM, Sarma PV. Developmental competence and post-thaw survivability of buffalo embryos produced *in vitro*: effect of growth factors in oocyte maturation medium and of embryo culture system. Theriogenology 2003; 60(9): 1621-31.
[http://dx.doi.org/10.1016/S0093-691X(03)00148-1] [PMID: 14580645]

[69] Gardiner CS, Reed DJ. Status of glutathione during oxidant-induced oxidative stress in the preimplantation mouse embryo. Biol Reprod 1994; 51(6): 1307-14.
[http://dx.doi.org/10.1095/biolreprod51.6.1307] [PMID: 7888510]

[70] Telford NA, Watson AJ, Schultz GA. Transition from maternal to embryonic control in early mammalian development: a comparison of several species. Mol Reprod Dev 1990; 26(1): 90-100.
[http://dx.doi.org/10.1002/mrd.1080260113] [PMID: 2189447]

[71] Gasparrini B, Sayoud H, Neglia G, Matos DG, Donnay I, Zicarelli L. Glutathione synthesis during *in vitro* maturation of buffalo (*Bubalus bubalis*) oocytes: effects of cysteamine on embryo development. Theriogenology 2003; 60(5): 943-52.
[http://dx.doi.org/10.1016/S0093-691X(03)00098-0] [PMID: 12935871]

[72] Manjunatha BM, Devaraj M, Gupta PS, Ravindra JP, Nandi S. Effect of taurine and melatonin in the culture medium on buffalo *in vitro* embryo development. Reprod Domest Anim 2009; 44(1): 12-6.
[http://dx.doi.org/10.1111/j.1439-0531.2007.00982.x] [PMID: 18507802]

[73] Pandey A, Gupta N, Gupta SC. Improvement of *in vitro* oocyte maturation with lectin supplementation and expression analysis of Cx43, GDF-9, FGF-4 and Fibronectin mRNA transcripts in Buffalo (*Bubalus bubalis*). J Assist Reprod Genet 2009; 26(6): 365-71.
[http://dx.doi.org/10.1007/s10815-009-9314-x] [PMID: 19629675]

[74] Dominko T, First NL. Timing of meiotic progression in bovine oocytes and its effect on early embryo development. Mol Reprod Dev 1997; 47(4): 456-67.
[http://dx.doi.org/10.1002/(SICI)1098-2795(199708)47:4<456::AID-MRD13>3.0.CO;2-U] [PMID: 9211431]

[75] Hunter RH, Greve T. Could artificial insemination of cattle be more fruitful? Penalties associated with aging eggs. Reprod Domest Anim 1997; 32: 137-42.
[http://dx.doi.org/10.1111/j.1439-0531.1997.tb01271.x]

[76] Marston JH, Chang MC. The fertilizable life of ova and their morphology following delayed insemination in mature and immature mice. J Exp Zool 1964; 155: 237-51.

[http://dx.doi.org/10.1002/jez.1401550211] [PMID: 14131458]

[77] Chian RC, Niwa K, Nakahara H. Effect of sperm penetration *in vitro* on completion of first meiosis by bovine oocytes arrested at various stages in culture. J Reprod Fertil 1992; 96(1): 73-8. [http://dx.doi.org/10.1530/jrf.0.0960073] [PMID: 1432976]

[78] Sirard MA, Florman HM, Leibfried-Rutledge ML, Barnes FL, Sims ML, First NL. Timing of nuclear progression and protein synthesis necessary for meiotic maturation of bovine oocytes. Biol Reprod 1989; 40(6): 1257-63. [http://dx.doi.org/10.1095/biolreprod40.6.1257] [PMID: 2775818]

[79] Neglia G, Marino M, Di Palo R, *et al.* A comparison of *in vitro* maturation in buffalo (*Bubalus bubalis*) and bovine oocytes using confocal microscopy. Theriogenology 2001; 55: 488.

[80] Prather RS, Day BN. Practical considerations for the *in vitro* production of pig embryos. Theriogenology 1998; 49(1): 23-32. [http://dx.doi.org/10.1016/S0093-691X(97)00399-3] [PMID: 10732118]

[81] Yadav BR, Katiyar PK, Chauhan MS, Madan ML. Chromosome configuration during *in vitro* maturation of goat, sheep and buffalo oocytes. Theriogenology 1997; 47(4): 943-51. [http://dx.doi.org/10.1016/S0093-691X(97)00050-2] [PMID: 16728044]

[82] Gasparrini B, De Rosa A, Attanasio L, *et al.* Influence of the duration of *in vitro* maturation and gamete co-incubation on the efficiency of *in vitro* embryo development in Italian Mediterranean buffalo (*Bubalus bubalis*). Anim Reprod Sci 2008; 105(3-4): 354-64. [http://dx.doi.org/10.1016/j.anireprosci.2007.03.022] [PMID: 17481834]

[83] Gasparrini B, Boccia L, Rosa AD, Palo RD, Campanile G, Zicarelli L. Chemical activation of buffalo (*Bubalus bubalis*) oocytes by different methods: effects of aging on post-parthenogenetic development. Theriogenology 2004; 62(9): 1627-37. a [http://dx.doi.org/10.1016/j.theriogenology.2004.03.005] [PMID: 15511550]

[84] Gasparrini B, Boccia L, De Rosa A, Vecchio D, Di Palo R, Zicarelli L. *In vitro* fertilization of buffalo (*Bubalus bubalis*) oocytes: effects of media and sperm motility inducing agents. Reprod Fertil Dev 2004; 16: 255. b [http://dx.doi.org/10.1071/RDv16n1Ab270]

[85] Mehmood A, Anwar M, Naqvi SM. Motility, acrosome integrity, membrane integrity and oocyte cleavage rate of sperm separated by swim-up or Percoll gradient method from frozen-thawed buffalo semen. Anim Reprod Sci 2009; 111(2-4): 141-8. [http://dx.doi.org/10.1016/j.anireprosci.2008.02.011] [PMID: 18378413]

[86] Muer SK, Roy SB, Mohan G, Dhoble RL. Cryogenic changes in seminal protein of cattle and buffalo. Theriogenology 1988; 30(5): 1005-10. [http://dx.doi.org/10.1016/S0093-691X(88)80063-3] [PMID: 16726543]

[87] Wilding M, Gasparrini B, Neglia G, Dale B, Zicarelli L. Mitochondrial activity and fertilization potential of fresh and cryopreserved buffalo sperm. Theriogenology 2003; 59: 466.

[88] Kovács A, Foote RH. Viability and acrosome staining of bull, boar and rabbit spermatozoa. Biotech Histochem 1992; 67(3): 119-24. [http://dx.doi.org/10.3109/10520299209110020] [PMID: 1377502]

[89] Boccia L, Di Palo R, De Rosa A, Attanasio L, Mariotti E, Gasparrini B. Evaluation of buffalo semen by Trypan blue/Giemsa staining and related fertility *in vitro*. 8th World Buffalo Congress, Caserta, Italy October 19-22, 2007. Ital J Anim Sci 2007; 6(2): 739-42. [http://dx.doi.org/10.4081/ijas.2007.s2.739]

[90] Boccia L, Attanasio L, De Rosa A, Pellerano G, Di Palo R, Gasparrini B. Effect of sodium nitroprusside on buffalo sperm capacitation *in vitro*. Reprod Fertil Dev 2007; 19: 276. [http://dx.doi.org/10.1071/RDv19n1Ab322]

[91] Boccia L, Attanasio L, Monaco E, De Rosa A, Di Palo R, Gasparrini B. Effect of progesterone on capacitation of buffalo (*Bubalus bubalis*) spermatozoa *in vitro*. Reprod Domest Anim 2006; 41(4): 311.

[92] Di Francesco S, Mariotti E, Tsantarliotou M, *et al.* Melatonin promotes *in vitro* sperm capacitation in buffalo (*Bubalus bubalis*). 36th Annual Conference of the International Embryo Transfer Society, 9-12 January, Cordoba, Argentina. Reprod Fertil Dev 2010; 22(1): 311-2. [http://dx.doi.org/10.1071/RDv22n1Ab311]

[93] Boccia L, De Rosa A, Attanasio L, Di Palo R, Zicarelli L, Gasparrini B. Capacitation of buffalo spermatozoa *in vitro*. Reprod Fertil Dev 2005; 17(1,2): 270.

[94] Siniscalchi C, Mariotti E, Boccia L, *et al.* Co-culture with oviduct epithelial cells promotes capacitation of buffalo (*Bubalus bubalis*) sperm. Proc of 36th Annual Conference of the International Embryo Transfer Society, 9-12 January, Cordoba, Argentina. J Reprod Fert Dev 2010; 22(1): 316. [http://dx.doi.org/10.1071/RDv22n1Ab321]

[95] Mariotti E, Di Francesco S, De Blasi M, *et al.* Fertilizing capacity of buffalo (*Bubalus bubalis*) sperm co-cultured with oviduct epithelial cells. Proc of 36th Annual Conference of the International Embryo Transfer Society, 9-12 January 2010, Cordoba, Argentina. J Reprod Fert Dev 2010; 22(1): 299a. [http://dx.doi.org/10.1071/RDv22n1Ab284]

[96] Monaco E, Gasparrini B, Boccia L, *et al.* Effect of osteopontin (OPN) on *in vitro* embryo development in cattle. Theriogenology 2009; 71(3): 450-7. [http://dx.doi.org/10.1016/j.theriogenology.2008.08.012] [PMID: 18835636]

[97] Cancel AM, Chapman DA, Killian GJ. Osteopontin localization in the Holstein bull reproductive tract. Biol Reprod 1999; 60(2): 454-60. [http://dx.doi.org/10.1095/biolreprod60.2.454] [PMID: 9916014]

[98] Pero ME, Killian GJ, Lombardi P, Zicarelli L, Avallone L, Gasparrini B. Identification of osteopontin in water buffalo semen. Proc of the 33th Annual Conference of the Internation Embryo Transfer Society, Kyoto, Japan, 6-10 January. Reprod Fertil Dev 2007; 1: 279. [http://dx.doi.org/10.1071/RDv19n1Ab327]

[99] Boccia L, Di Francesco S, Neglia G, *et al.* Osteopontin improves sperm capacitation and *in vitro* fertilization efficiency in buffalo (*Bubalus bubalis*). Theriogenology 2013; 80(3): 212-7. [http://dx.doi.org/10.1016/j.theriogenology.2013.04.017] [PMID: 23726297]

[100] Venditto I, Mariotti E, Boccia L, *et al.* Effect of plasmin on acrosome reaction of buffalo (*Bubalus bubalis*) spermatozoa *in vitro*. Proc of 36th Annual Conference of the International Embryo Transfer Society, 9-12 January, Cordoba, Argentina. J Reprod Fert Dev 2010; 22(1): 317.

[http://dx.doi.org/10.1071/RDv22n1Ab322]

[101] Zhang L, Jiang S, Wozniak PJ, Yang X, Godke RA. Cumulus cell function during bovine oocyte maturation, fertilization, and embryo development *in vitro*. Mol Reprod Dev 1995; 40(3): 338-44. [http://dx.doi.org/10.1002/mrd.1080400310] [PMID: 7772344]

[102] Attanasio L, De Rosa A, De Blasi M, *et al.* The influence of cumulus cells during *in vitro* fertilization of buffalo (*Bubalus bubalis*) denuded oocytes that have undergone vitrification. Theriogenology 2010; 74(8): 1504-8. [http://dx.doi.org/10.1016/j.theriogenology.2010.05.014] [PMID: 20615538]

[103] Rehman N, Collins AR, Suh TK, Wright RW Jr. Effect of sperm exposure time on *in vitro* fertilization and embryo development of bovine oocytes matured *in vitro*. Theriogenology 1994; 41(7): 1447-52. [http://dx.doi.org/10.1016/0093-691X(94)90195-O] [PMID: 16727498]

[104] Aitken RJ. A free radical theory of male infertility. Reprod Fertil Dev 1994; 6(1): 19-23. [http://dx.doi.org/10.1071/RD9940019] [PMID: 8066217]

[105] Ward F, Enright B, Rizos D, Boland M, Lonergan P. Optimization of *in vitro* bovine embryo production: effect of duration of maturation, length of gamete co-incubation, sperm concentration and sire. Theriogenology 2002; 57(8): 2105-17. [http://dx.doi.org/10.1016/S0093-691X(02)00696-9] [PMID: 12066869]

[106] Kochhar HS, Kochhar KP, Basrur PK, King WA. Influence of the duration of gamete interaction on cleavage, growth rate and sex distribution of *in vitro* produced bovine embryos. Anim Reprod Sci 2003; 77(1-2): 33-49. [http://dx.doi.org/10.1016/S0378-4320(03)00006-X] [PMID: 12654526]

[107] Sumantri C, Boediono A, Ooe M, Murakami M, Saha S, Suzuki T. The effect of sperm-oocyte incubation time on *in vitro* embryo development using sperm from a tetraparental chimeric bull. Anim Reprod Sci 1997; 48(2-4): 187-95. [http://dx.doi.org/10.1016/S0378-4320(97)00052-3] [PMID: 9452872]

[108] Di Fenza M, De Rosa A, Boccia L, *et al.* Kinetics of sperm penetration in buffalo (Bubalus bubalis) species: effect of bull. Annual Conference of European Society of Domestic Animal Reproduction (ESDAR); Reprod Dom Anim 2008; 43(5):56

[109] Rubessa M, Di Fenza M, Mariotti E, *et al.* Kinetics of sperm penetration is correlated with *in vitro* fertility of buffalo (*Bubalus bubalis*) bulls. Reprod Fertil Dev 2009; 21(1): 206-7. [http://dx.doi.org/10.1071/RDv21n1Ab217]

[110] Eppig JJ. Coordination of nuclear and cytoplasmic oocyte maturation in eutherian mammals. Reprod Fertil Dev 1996; 8(4): 485-9. [http://dx.doi.org/10.1071/RD9960485] [PMID: 8870074]

[111] de Matos DG, Furnus CC, Moses DF. Glutathione synthesis during *in vitro* maturation of bovine oocytes: role of cumulus cells. Biol Reprod 1997; 57(6): 1420-5. [http://dx.doi.org/10.1095/biolreprod57.6.1420] [PMID: 9408249]

[112] Galli C, Duchi R, Crotti G, Lazzari G. Embryo production by Ovum Pick-up in Water Buffalo. Theriogenology 1998; 50: 259.

[113] Boni R, Roviello S, Gasparrini B, Langella M, Zicarelli L. *In vitro* production of buffalo embryos in

chemically defined medium. Buffalo J 1999; 1: 115-20. a

[114] Caracciolo di Brienza V, Neglia G, Masola N, Gasparrini B, Di Palo R, Campanile G. *In vitro* embryo production in chemically defined media. Atti 1° Congresso Nazionale sull'Allevamento del Bufalo, 3-5 ottobre 2001, Eboli (SA), Italy: 341-344

[115] Tervit HR, Whittingham DG, Rowson LE. Successful culture *in vitro* of sheep and cattle ova. J Reprod Fertil 1972; 30(3): 493-7.
[http://dx.doi.org/10.1530/jrf.0.0300493] [PMID: 4672493]

[116] Vecchio D, Neglia G, Di Palo R, *et al.* Ion, protein, phospholipid and energy substrate content of oviduct fluid during the oestrous cycle of buffalo (*Bubalus bubalis*). Reprod Domest Anim 2010; 45(5): e32-9.
[PMID: 19761531]

[117] Killian GJ, Chapman DA, Kavanaugh JF, Deaver DR, Wiggin HB. Changes in phospholipids, cholesterol and protein content of oviduct fluid of cows during the oestrous cycle. J Reprod Fertil 1989; 86(2): 419-26.
[http://dx.doi.org/10.1530/jrf.0.0860419] [PMID: 2760872]

[118] McEvoy TG, Robinson JJ, Aitken RP, Findlay PA, Robertson IS. Dietary excesses of urea influence the viability and metabolism of preimplantation sheep embryos and may affect fetal growth among survivors. Anim Reprod Sci 1997; 47(1-2): 71-90.
[http://dx.doi.org/10.1016/S0378-4320(96)01627-2] [PMID: 9233507]

[119] Farin PW, Piedrahita JA, Farin CE. Errors in development of fetuses and placentas from *in vitro*-produced bovine embryos. Theriogenology 2006; 65(1): 178-91.
[http://dx.doi.org/10.1016/j.theriogenology.2005.09.022] [PMID: 16266745]

[120] Boccia L, Monaco E, Attanasio L, De Rosa A, Gasparrini B. Influenza del cambio di coltura (doppio *vs.* singolo) sullo sviluppo di embrioni bufalini *in vitro*. XII Giornate scientifiche", Università degli Studi di Napoli Federico II, Polo delle Scienze e delle Tecnologie per la Vita, Facoltà di Medicina e Chirurgia, 15-16 Giugno 2006b Napoli:171b

[121] Schini SA, Bavister BD. Two-cell block to development of cultured hamster embryos is caused by phosphate and glucose. Biol Reprod 1988; 39(5): 1183-92.
[http://dx.doi.org/10.1095/biolreprod39.5.1183] [PMID: 3219389]

[122] Takahashi Y, First NL. *In vitro* development of bovine one-cell embryos: Influence of glucose, lactate, pyruvate, amino acids and vitamins. Theriogenology 1992; 37(5): 963-78.
[http://dx.doi.org/10.1016/0093-691X(92)90096-A] [PMID: 16727096]

[123] Rubessa M, Boccia L, Campanile G, *et al.* Effect of energy source during culture on *in vitro* embryo development, resistance to cryopreservation and sex ratio. Theriogenology 2011; 76(7): 1347-55.
[http://dx.doi.org/10.1016/j.theriogenology.2011.06.004] [PMID: 21820719]

[124] Kim JH, Niwa K, Lim JM, Okuda K. Effects of phosphate, energy substrates and amino acids on development of *in vitro*-matured, *in vitro*-fertilized bovine oocytes in a chemically defined medium. Biol Reprod 1993; 48: 1320-5.
[http://dx.doi.org/10.1095/biolreprod48.6.1320] [PMID: 8318585]

[125] Thompson JG, Partridge RJ, Houghton FD, Cox CI, Leese HJ. Oxygen uptake and carbohydrate

metabolism by *in vitro* derived bovine embryos. J Reprod Fertil 1996; 106(2): 299-306. [http://dx.doi.org/10.1530/jrf.0.1060299] [PMID: 8699414]

[126] Monaco E, De Rosa A, Attanasio L, Boccia L, Zicarelli L, Gasparrini B. *In vitro* culture of buffalo (*Bubalus bubalis*) embryos in the presence or absence of glucose. Reprod Domest Anim 2006; 41(4): 332.

[127] Thompson JG, Simpson AC, Pugh PA, Wright RW Jr, Tervit HR. Glucose utilization by sheep embryos derived *in vivo* and *in vitro*. Reprod Fertil Dev 1991; 3(5): 571-6. [http://dx.doi.org/10.1071/RD9910571] [PMID: 1788397]

[128] Thompson JG, Simpson AC, Pugh PA, Tervit HR. Requirement for glucose during *in vitro* culture of sheep preimplantation embryos. Mol Reprod Dev 1992; 31(4): 253-7. [http://dx.doi.org/10.1002/mrd.1080310405] [PMID: 1571159]

[129] Kumar P, Verma A, Roy B, *et al.* Effect of varying glucose concentrations during *in vitro* maturation and embryo culture on efficiency of *in vitro* embryo production in buffalo. Reprod Domest Anim 2012; 47(2): 269-73. [http://dx.doi.org/10.1111/j.1439-0531.2011.01849.x] [PMID: 21762215]

[130] Kumar P, Rajput S, Verma A, De S, Datta TK. Expression pattern of glucose metabolism genes in relation to development rate of buffalo (*Bubalus bubalis*) oocytes and *in vitro*-produced embryos. Theriogenology 2013; 80(8): 914-22. [http://dx.doi.org/10.1016/j.theriogenology.2013.07.018] [PMID: 23992643]

[131] Gutiérrez-Adán A, Granados J, Pintado B, De La Fuente J. Influence of glucose on the sex ratio of bovine IVM/IVF embryos cultured *in vitro*. Reprod Fertil Dev 2001; 13(5-6): 361-5. [http://dx.doi.org/10.1071/RD00039] [PMID: 11833931]

[132] Gardner DK, Lane M, Batt P. Uptake and metabolism of pyruvate and glucose by individual sheep preattachment embryos developed *in vivo*. Mol Reprod Dev 1993; 36(3): 313-9. [http://dx.doi.org/10.1002/mrd.1080360305] [PMID: 8286112]

[133] Thompson JG. *In vitro* culture and embryo metabolism of cattle and sheep embryos - a decade of achievement. Anim Reprod Sci 2000; 60-61: 263-75. [http://dx.doi.org/10.1016/S0378-4320(00)00096-8] [PMID: 10844200]

[134] Mukherjee A, Kumar D, Singh KP, *et al.* Assessment of DNA damage during in vitro development of buffalo (*Bubalus bubalis*) embryos: effect of cysteamine. Reprod Domest Anim 2010; 45(6): 1118-21. [http://dx.doi.org/10.1111/j.1439-0531.2009.01484.x] [PMID: 19515031]

[135] Eyestone WH, First NL. Characterization of developmental arrest in early bovine embryos cultured *in vitro*. Theriogenology 1991; 35(3): 613-24. [http://dx.doi.org/10.1016/0093-691X(91)90457-O] [PMID: 16726930]

[136] Elamaran G, Singh KP, Singh MK, *et al.* Oxygen concentration and cysteamine supplementation during in vitro production of buffalo (*Bubalus bubalis*) embryos affect mRNA expression of BCL-2, BCL-XL, MCL-1, BAX and BID. Reprod Domest Anim 2012; 47(6): 1027-36. [http://dx.doi.org/10.1111/j.1439-0531.2012.02009.x] [PMID: 22452597]

[137] Thiyagarajan B, Valivittan K. Ameliorating effect of vitamin E on *in vitro* development of preimplantation buffalo embryos. J Assist Reprod Genet 2009; 26(4): 217-25.

[http://dx.doi.org/10.1007/s10815-009-9302-1] [PMID: 19252977]

[138] Thiyagarajan B, Valivittan K. Effect of all-trans retinol on *in vitro* development of preimplantation buffalo embryos. Animal 2009; 3(3): 385-92. [http://dx.doi.org/10.1017/S1751731108003455] [PMID: 22444309]

[139] Verma A, Kumar P, Rajput S, Roy B, De S, Datta TK. Embryonic genome activation events in buffalo (*Bubalus bubalis*) preimplantation embryos. Mol Reprod Dev 2012; 79(5): 321-8. [http://dx.doi.org/10.1002/mrd.22027] [PMID: 22461405]

[140] Drost M, Elsden RP. Blastocyst development in water buffalo (*Bubalus bubalis*). Theriogenology 1985; 23: 191. [http://dx.doi.org/10.1016/0093-691X(85)90097-4]

[141] Misra AK, Kasiraj R, Rao MM, Rangareddy NS, Jaiswal RS, Pant HC. Rate of transport and development of preimplantation embryo in the superovulated buffalo (*Bubalus bubalis*). Theriogenology 1998; 50(4): 637-49. [http://dx.doi.org/10.1016/S0093-691X(98)00168-X] [PMID: 10732154]

[142] Heleil B, Deeb EI. Superovulatory response in relation to follicular dynamics and presence of dominant follicles in Egyptian buffaloes. Adv Biol Res (Faisalabad) 2010; 4: 169-74.

[143] Gasparrini B, Neglia G, Caracciolo di Brienza V, Campanile G, Di Palo R, Zicarelli L. Preliminary analysis of vitrified *in vitro* produced embryos. Theriogenology 2001; 55: 307.

[144] Totey SM, Daliri M, Appa Rao KB, Pawshe CH, Taneja M, Chillar RS. Differential cleavage and developmental rates and their correlation with cell numbers and sex ratios in buffalo embryos generated *in vitro*. Theriogenology 1996; 45(2): 521-33. [http://dx.doi.org/10.1016/0093-691X(95)00388-O] [PMID: 16727815]

[145] Rajhans R, Kumar GS, Dubey PK, Sharma GT. Effect of timing of development on total cell number and expression profile of HSP-70.1 and GLUT-1 in buffalo (*Bubalus bubalis*) oocytes and preimplantation embryos produced *in vitro*. Cell Biol Int 2010; 34(5): 463-8. [http://dx.doi.org/10.1042/CBI20090295] [PMID: 20100172]

[146] Chauhan MS, Palta P, Das SK, Tomer OS. Effect of culture conditions on the hatching ability of *in vitro* produced buffalo (*Bubalus bubalis*) embryos. Vet Rec 1998; 142(7): 169-71. b [http://dx.doi.org/10.1136/vr.142.7.169] [PMID: 9519431]

[147] Eswari S, Sai Kumar G, Sharma GT. Expression of mRNA encoding leukaemia inhibitory factor (LIF) and its receptor (LIFRβ) in buffalo preimplantation embryos produced *in vitro*: markers of successful embryo implantation. Zygote 2013; 21(2): 203-13. [http://dx.doi.org/10.1017/S0967199412000172] [PMID: 22892066]

[148] Boccia L, Rubessa M, De Blasi M, *et al.* Hyaluronic acid improve cryotolerance of buffalo (*Bubalus bubalis*) *in vitro* derived embryos. 38th Annual Conference of the International Embryo Transfer Society, 7-10 January 2012, Phoenix, Arizona. Reprod Fertil Dev 2012; 24(I): 138. [http://dx.doi.org/10.1071/RDv24n1Ab52]

[149] Gasparrini B, Longobardi V, Zullo G, *et al.* Effect of L-carnitine on buffalo *in vitro* embryo development. Proceedings of 20th ASPA Congress. Bologna, Italy. 2013.

[150] Naitana S, Loi P, Ledda S, *et al.* Effect of biopsy and vitrification on *in vitro* survival of ovine

embryos at different stages of development. Theriogenology 1996; 46(5): 813-24. [http://dx.doi.org/10.1016/S0093-691X(96)00239-7] [PMID: 16727945]

[151] Behrman HR, Grinwich DL, Hichens M. Studies on the mechanism of PGF2alpha and gonadotropin interactions on LH receptor function in corpora lutea during luteolysis. Adv Prostaglandin Thromboxane Res 1976; 2: 655-66. [PMID: 185887]

[152] Beal WE, Milvae RA, Hansel H. Estrus cycle length and plasma progesterone concentration following administration of PGF2alpha early in the bovine estrous cylcle. J Reprod Fertil 1980; 59: 383-96. [http://dx.doi.org/10.1530/jrf.0.0590393] [PMID: 7431294]

[153] Kasiraj R, Misra AK, Mutha Rao M, Jaiswal RS, Rangareddi NS. Successful culmination of pregnancy and live birth following the transfer of frozen-thawed buffalo embryos. Theriogenology 1993; 39(5): 1187-92. [http://dx.doi.org/10.1016/0093-691X(93)90016-X] [PMID: 16727286]

[154] Manjunatha BM, Gupta PS, Ravindra JP, Devaraj M, Nandi S. Effect of vitrification medium composition and exposure time on post-thaw development of buffalo embryos produced *in vitro*. Vet J 2009; 179(2): 287-91. c [http://dx.doi.org/10.1016/j.tvjl.2007.08.031] [PMID: 17933564]

[155] Yang CY, Pang CY, Yang BZ, Li RC, Lu YQ, Liang XW. Optimization of cryopreservation of buffalo (*Bubalus bubalis*) blastocysts produced by *in vitro* fertilization and somatic cell nuclear transfer. Theriogenology 2012; 78(7): 1437-45. [http://dx.doi.org/10.1016/j.theriogenology.2012.05.032] [PMID: 22925650]

[156] Dobrinsky JR, Pursel VG, Long CR, Johnson LA. Birth of piglets after transfer of embryos cryopreserved by cytoskeletal stabilization and vitrification. Biol Reprod 2000; 62(3): 564-70. [http://dx.doi.org/10.1095/biolreprod62.3.564] [PMID: 10684796]

[157] Manjunatha BM, Ravindra JP, Gupta PS, Devaraj M, Nandi S. Effect of breeding season on *in vivo* oocyte recovery and embryo production in non-descriptive Indian river buffaloes (*Bubalus bubalis*). Anim Reprod Sci 2009; 111(2-4): 376-83. [http://dx.doi.org/10.1016/j.anireprosci.2008.03.003] [PMID: 18440168]

[158] De Rosa A, Di Palo R, Attanasio L, Monaco E, Campanile G, Gasparrini B. Open pulled straw vitrification for *in vitro* produced buffalo (*Bubalus bubalis*) embryos. Reprod Fertil Dev 2006; 39(1,2): 153.

[159] De Rosa A, Attanasio L, Boccia L, Pellerano G, Campanile G, Gasparrini B. Cryotop vitrification for *in vitro* produced buffalo (*Bubalus bubalis*) embryos. Reprod Fertil Dev 2007; 19: 174. [http://dx.doi.org/10.1071/RDv19n1Ab114]

[160] Laowtammathron C, Lorthongpanich C, Ketudat-Cairns M, Hochi S, Parnpai R. Factors affecting cryosurvival of nuclear-transferred bovine and swamp buffalo blastocysts: effects of hatching stage, linoleic acid-albumin in IVC medium and Ficoll supplementation to vitrification solution. Theriogenology 2005; 64(5): 1185-96. [http://dx.doi.org/10.1016/j.theriogenology.2005.02.001] [PMID: 16125561]

[161] Vajta G, Holm P, Kuwayama M, *et al.* Open Pulled Straw (OPS) vitrification: a new way to reduce cryoinjuries of bovine ova and embryos. Mol Reprod Dev 1998; 51(1): 53-8.

[http://dx.doi.org/10.1002/(SICI)1098-2795(199809)51:1<53::AID-MRD6>3.0.CO;2-V] [PMID: 9712317]

[162] Boccia L, De Rosa A, Attanasio L, *et al.* Developmental speed affects the cryotolerance of *in vitro* produced buffalo (*Bubalus bubalis*) embryos. Ital J Anim Sci 2013; 12(4): 492-6. [http://dx.doi.org/10.4081/ijas.2013.e80]

[163] Saliba W, Gimenes L, Drumond R, *et al.* Efficiency of OPU-IVEP-ET of fresh and vitrified embryos in buffaloes. Proc of 10th World Buffalo Congress and the 7th Asian Buffalo Congress 2013, Phuket, Thailand. Buffalo Bull 2013; 32(2): 385-8.

[164] Gasparrini B. *In vitro* embryo production in buffalo: Yesterday, today and tomorrow. Buffalo Bull 2013; 32(1): 188-95.

[165] Whittingham DJ. Fertilization *in vitro* and development to term of unfertilized mouse oocytes previously stored at -196°C. J Rreprod Fertil 1977; 49(1,2): 89-94.

[166] al-Hasani S, Kirsch J, Diedrich K, Blanke S, van der Ven H, Krebs D. Successful embryo transfer of cryopreserved and *in-vitro* fertilized rabbit oocytes. Hum Reprod 1989; 4(1): 77-9. [PMID: 2708506]

[167] Hamano S, Koikeda A, Kuwayama M, Nagai T. Full-term development of *in vitro*-matured, vitrified and fertilized bovine oocytes. Theriogenology 1992; 38(6): 1085-90. [http://dx.doi.org/10.1016/0093-691X(92)90122-8] [PMID: 16727206]

[168] Vieira AD, Mezzalira A, Barbieri DP, Lehmkuhl RC, Rubin MI, Vajta G. Calves born after open pulled straw vitrification of immature bovine oocytes. Cryobiology 2002; 45(1): 91-4. [http://dx.doi.org/10.1016/S0011-2240(02)00109-8] [PMID: 12445553]

[169] Maclellan LJ, Carnevale EM, Coutinho da Silva MA, Scoggin CF, Bruemmer JE, Squires EL. Pregnancies from vitrified equine oocytes collected from super-stimulated and non-stimulated mares. Theriogenology 2002; 58(5): 911-9. [http://dx.doi.org/10.1016/S0093-691X(02)00920-2] [PMID: 12212891]

[170] Katayama KP, Stehlik J, Kuwayama M, Kato O, Stehlik E. High survival rate of vitrified human oocytes results in clinical pregnancy. Fertil Steril 2003; 80(1): 223-4. [http://dx.doi.org/10.1016/S0015-0282(03)00551-X] [PMID: 12849831]

[171] Vajta G, Kuwayama M. Improving cryopreservation systems. Theriogenology 2006; 65(1): 236-44. [http://dx.doi.org/10.1016/j.theriogenology.2005.09.026] [PMID: 16289262]

[172] Vajta G, Nagy ZP. Are programmable freezers still needed in the embryo laboratory? Review on vitrification. Reprod Biomed Online 2006; 12(6): 779-96. [http://dx.doi.org/10.1016/S1472-6483(10)61091-7] [PMID: 16792858]

[173] Gautam SK, Verma V, Singh B, *et al.* Effect of slow freezing on morphology and developmental competence of buffalo (*Bubalus bubalis*) immature oocytes. Anim Reprod Sci 2008; 105(3-4): 311-8. a
[http://dx.doi.org/10.1016/j.anireprosci.2007.03.014] [PMID: 17449204]

[174] Gautam SK, Verma V, Palta P, Chauhan MS, Manik RS. Effect of type of cryoprotectant on morphology and developmental competence of *in vitro*-matured buffalo (*Bubalus bubalis*) oocytes subjected to slow freezing or vitrification. Reprod Fertil Dev 2008; 20(4): 490-6. b

[http://dx.doi.org/10.1071/RD07203] [PMID: 18462611]

[175] Dhali A, Manik RS, Das SK, Singla SK, Palta P. Vitrification of buffalo (*Bubalus bubalis*) oocytes. Theriogenology 2000; 53(6): 1295-303. a
[http://dx.doi.org/10.1016/S0093-691X(00)00273-9] [PMID: 10832754]

[176] Dhali A, Manik RS, Das SK, Singla SK, Palta P. Post-vitrification survival and *in vitro* maturation rate of buffalo (*Bubalus bubalis*) oocytes: effect of ethylene glycol concentration and exposure time. Anim Reprod Sci 2000; 63(3-4): 159-65. b
[http://dx.doi.org/10.1016/S0378-4320(00)00170-6] [PMID: 10989226]

[177] Wani NA, Misra AK, Maurya SN. Maturation rates of vitrified-thawed immature buffalo (*Bubalus bubalis*) oocytes: effect of different types of cryoprotectants. Anim Reprod Sci 2004; 84(3-4): 327-35. a
[http://dx.doi.org/10.1016/j.anireprosci.2004.02.007] [PMID: 15302375]

[178] Wani NA, Maurya SN, Misra AK, Saxena VB, Lakhchaura BD. Effect of cryoprotectants and their concentration on *in vitro* development of vitrified-warmed immature oocytes in buffalo (*Bubalus bubalis*). Theriogenology 2004; 61(5): 831-42. b
[http://dx.doi.org/10.1016/j.theriogenology.2003.06.002] [PMID: 14757469]

[179] Mahmoud KG, Scholkamy TH, Ahmed YF, Seidel GE Jr, Nawito MF. Effect of different combinations of cryoprotectants on in vitro maturation of immature buffalo (*Bubalus bubalis*) oocytes vitrified by straw and open-pulled straw methods. Reprod Domest Anim 2010; 45(4): 565-71.
[PMID: 19090828]

[180] Liang Y, Rakwongrit D, Phermthai T, Somfai T, Nagai T, Parnpai R. Cryopreservation of immature buffalo oocytes: effects of cytochalasin B pretreatment on the efficiency of cryotop and solid surface vitrification methods. Anim Sci J 2012; 83(9): 630-8.
[http://dx.doi.org/10.1111/j.1740-0929.2012.01013.x] [PMID: 22943529]

[181] Sharma GT, Loganathasamy K. Effect of meiotic stages during *in vitro* maturation on the survival of vitrified-warmed buffalo oocytes. Vet Res Commun 2007; 31(7): 881-93.
[http://dx.doi.org/10.1007/s11259-007-0059-7] [PMID: 17285244]

[182] Hochi S, Ito K, Hirabayashi M, Ueda M, Kimura K, Hanada A. Effect of nuclear stages during IVM on the survival of vitrified-warmed bovine oocytes. Theriogenology 1998; 49(4): 787-96.
[http://dx.doi.org/10.1016/S0093-691X(98)00028-4] [PMID: 10732087]

[183] Hong SW, Chung HM, Lim JM, *et al.* Improved human oocyte development after vitrification: a comparison of thawing methods. Fertil Steril 1999; 72(1): 142-6.
[http://dx.doi.org/10.1016/S0015-0282(99)00199-5] [PMID: 10428163]

[184] Arav A, Shehu D, Mattioli M. Osmotic and cytotoxic study of vitrification of immature bovine oocytes. J Reprod Fertil 1993; 99(2): 353-8.
[http://dx.doi.org/10.1530/jrf.0.0990353] [PMID: 8107016]

[185] Arav A, Rubinsky B, Seren E, Roche JF, Boland MP. The role of thermal hysteresis proteins during cryopreservation of oocytes and embryos. Theriogenology 1994; 41: 107-12.
[http://dx.doi.org/10.1016/S0093-691X(05)80055-X]

[186] Le Gal F, Massip A. Cryopreservation of cattle oocytes: effects of meiotic stage, cycloheximide

treatment, and vitrification procedure. Cryobiology 1999; 38(4): 290-300.
[http://dx.doi.org/10.1006/cryo.1999.2172] [PMID: 10413572]

[187] Cooper A, Paynter SJ, Fuller BJ, Shaw RW. Differential effects of cryopreservation on nuclear or cytoplasmic maturation *in vitro* in immature mouse oocytes from stimulated ovaries. Hum Reprod 1998; 13(4): 971-8.
[http://dx.doi.org/10.1093/humrep/13.4.971] [PMID: 9619556]

[188] Ruppert-Lingham CJ, Paynter SJ, Godfrey J, Fuller BJ, Shaw RW. Developmental potential of murine germinal vesicle stage cumulus-oocyte complexes following exposure to dimethylsulphoxide or cryopreservation: loss of membrane integrity of cumulus cells after thawing. Hum Reprod 2003; 18(2): 392-8.
[http://dx.doi.org/10.1093/humrep/deg071] [PMID: 12571179]

[189] Fuku E, Xia L, Downey BR. Ultrastructural changes in bovine oocytes cryopreserved by vitrification. Cryobiology 1995; 32(2): 139-56.
[http://dx.doi.org/10.1006/cryo.1995.1013] [PMID: 7743816]

[190] Frydman N, Selva J, Bergere M, Auroux M, Maro B. Cryopreserved immature mouse oocytes: a chromosomal and spindle study. J Assist Reprod Genet 1997; 14(10): 617-23.
[http://dx.doi.org/10.1023/A:1022593004528] [PMID: 9447465]

[191] Isachenko EF, Nayudu PL. Vitrification of mouse germinal vesicle oocytes: effect of treatment temperature and egg yolk on chromatin and spindle normality and cumulus integrity. Hum Reprod 1999; 14(2): 400-8.
[http://dx.doi.org/10.1093/humrep/14.2.400] [PMID: 10099987]

[192] Parks JE, Ruffing NA. Factors affecting low temperatures survival of mammalian oocytes. Theriogenology 1992; 37: 59-73.
[http://dx.doi.org/10.1016/0093-691X(92)90247-O]

[193] Riha J, Landa V, Kneissl J, Matus J, Jindra J, Kloucek Z. Vitrification of cattle embryos by direct dropping into liquid nitrogen and embryo survival after nonsurgical transfer. Zivoc Vic 1991; 36: 113-20.

[194] Martino A, Pollard JW, Leibo SP. Effect of chilling bovine oocytes on their developmental competence. Mol Reprod Dev 1996; 45(4): 503-12.
[http://dx.doi.org/10.1002/(SICI)1098-2795(199612)45:4<503:AID-MRD13>3.0.CO;2-X] [PMID: 8956289]

[195] Hochi S, Fujimoto T, Braun J, Oguri N. Pregnancies following transfer of equine embryos cryopreserved by vitrification. Theriogenology 1994; 42(3): 483-8.
[http://dx.doi.org/10.1016/0093-691X(94)90686-D] [PMID: 16727555]

[196] Vajta G, Booth PJ, Holm P, Greve T, Callesen H. Successful vitrification of early stage bovine *in vitro* produced embryos with the open pulled straw (OPS) method. Cryo Lett 1997; 18: 191-5.

[197] Lane M, Bavister BD, Lyons EA, Forest KT. Containerless vitrification of mammalian oocytes and embryos. Nat Biotechnol 1999; 17(12): 1234-6.
[http://dx.doi.org/10.1038/70795] [PMID: 10585728]

[198] Kuwayama M, Vajta G, Kato O, Leibo SP. Highly efficient vitrification method for cryopreservation

of human oocytes. Reprod Biomed Online 2005; 11(3): 300-8.
[http://dx.doi.org/10.1016/S1472-6483(10)60837-1] [PMID: 16176668]

[199] Dinnyés A, Dai Y, Jiang S, Yang X. High developmental rates of vitrified bovine oocytes following parthenogenetic activation, in vitro fertilization, and somatic cell nuclear transfer. Biol Reprod 2000; 63(2): 513-8.
[http://dx.doi.org/10.1095/biolreprod63.2.513] [PMID: 10906058]

[200] Boonkusol D, Faisaikarm T, Dinnyes A, Kitiyanant Y. Effects of vitrification procedures on subsequent development and ultrastructure of *in vitro*-matured swamp buffalo (*Bubalus bubalis*) oocytes. Reprod Fertil Dev 2007; 19(2): 383-91.
[http://dx.doi.org/10.1071/RD06097] [PMID: 17257525]

[201] Sharma GT, Dubey PK, Chandra V. Morphological changes, DNA damage and developmental competence of *in vitro* matured, vitrified-thawed buffalo (*Bubalus bubalis*) oocytes: A comparative study of two cryoprotectants and two cryodevices. Cryobiology 2010; 60(3): 315-21.
[http://dx.doi.org/10.1016/j.cryobiol.2010.02.006] [PMID: 20178778]

[202] Bogliolo L, Ariu F, Rosati I, *et al.* Vitrification of immature and *in vitro* matured horse oocytes. Reprod Fertil Dev 2006; 18(1,2): 149-50.

[203] Succu S, Bebbere D, Bogliolo L, *et al.* Vitrification of *in vitro* matured ovine oocytes affects *in vitro* pre-implantation development and mRNA abundance. Mol Reprod Dev 2008; 75(3): 538-46.
[http://dx.doi.org/10.1002/mrd.20784] [PMID: 17886274]

[204] Fujihira T, Nagai H, Fukui Y. Relationship between equilibration times and the presence of cumulus cells, and effect of taxol treatment for vitrification of *in vitro* matured porcine oocytes. Cryobiology 2005; 51(3): 339-43.
[http://dx.doi.org/10.1016/j.cryobiol.2005.08.002] [PMID: 16183050]

[205] Muenthaisong S, Laowtammathron C, Ketudat-Cairns M, Parnpai R, Hochi S. Quality analysis of buffalo blastocysts derived from oocytes vitrified before or after enucleation and reconstructed with somatic cell nuclei. Theriogenology 2007; 67(4): 893-900.
[http://dx.doi.org/10.1016/j.theriogenology.2006.11.005] [PMID: 17161454]

[206] Attanasio L, Boccia L, Vajta G, *et al.* Cryotop vitrification of buffalo (*Bubalus bubalis*) *in vitro* matured oocytes: effects of cryoprotectant concentrations and warming procedures. Reprod Domest Anim 2010; 45(6): 997-1002.
[http://dx.doi.org/10.1111/j.1439-0531.2009.01475.x] [PMID: 19473307]

[207] Liang YY, Phermthai T, Nagai T, Somfai T, Parnpai R. *In vitro* development of vitrified buffalo oocytes following parthenogenetic activation and intracytoplasmic sperm injection. Theriogenology 2011; 75(9): 1652-60.
[http://dx.doi.org/10.1016/j.theriogenology.2010.12.028] [PMID: 21356549]

[208] Liang YY, Srirattana K, Phermthai T, Somfai T, Nagai T, Parnpai R. Effects of vitrification cryoprotectant treatment and cooling method on the viability and development of buffalo oocytes after intracytoplasmic sperm injection. Cryobiology 2012; 65(2): 151-6.
[http://dx.doi.org/10.1016/j.cryobiol.2012.04.006] [PMID: 22568927]

[209] Hyttel P, Vajta G, Callesen H. Vitrification of bovine oocytes with the open pulled straw method: ultrastructural consequences. Mol Reprod Dev 2000; 56(1): 80-8.

[http://dx.doi.org/10.1002/(SICI)1098-2795(200005)56:1<80::AID-MRD10>3.0.CO;2-U] [PMID: 10737970]

[210] Chian RC, Park CK, Sirard MA. Cumulus cells act as a sperm trap during *in vitro* fertilization of bovine oocytes. Theriogenology 1996; 45: 258. [http://dx.doi.org/10.1016/0093-691X(96)84731-5]

[211] Cox JF, Hormazabal J, Santa Maria A. Effect of the cumulus cells on *in vitro* fertilization of bovine matured oocytes. Theriogenology 1993; 40: 1259-67. [http://dx.doi.org/10.1016/0093-691X(93)90296-H]

[212] Fukui Y. Effect of follicle cells on the acrosome reaction, fertilization, and developmental competence of bovine oocytes matured in vitro. Mol Reprod Dev 1990; 26(1): 40-6. [http://dx.doi.org/10.1002/mrd.1080260107] [PMID: 2346644]

[213] Katska L, Kauffold P, Smorag Z, Duschinski U, Torner H, Kanitz W. Influence of hardening of the zona pellucida on *in vitro* fertilization of bovine oocytes. Theriogenology 1989; 32(5): 767-77. [http://dx.doi.org/10.1016/0093-691X(89)90465-2] [PMID: 16726723]

[214] Carroll J, Depypere H, Matthews CD. Freeze-thaw-induced changes of the zona pellucida explains decreased rates of fertilization in frozen-thawed mouse oocytes. J Reprod Fertil 1990; 90(2): 547-53. [http://dx.doi.org/10.1530/jrf.0.0900547] [PMID: 2250252]

[215] Matson PL, Graefling J, Junk SM, Yovich JL, Edirisinghe WR. Cryopreservation of oocytes and embryos: use of a mouse model to investigate effects upon zona hardness and formulate treatment strategies in an in-vitro fertilization programme. Hum Reprod 1997; 12(7): 1550-3. [http://dx.doi.org/10.1093/humrep/12.7.1550] [PMID: 9262294]

[216] De Blasi M, Mariotti E, Rubessa M, *et al.* Exposure to ethylene glycol (EG) and dimethyl sulfoxide (DMSO) causes activation and spindle anomalies in buffalo (*Bubalus bubalis*) oocytes. Reprod Fertil Dev 2009; 21: 131. [http://dx.doi.org/10.1071/RDv21n1Ab62]

[217] Betteridge KJ, Hare WC, Singh EL. Approaches to sex selection in farm animals. In: Brackett BG, Seidel GE, Seidel SM, Eds. New Technologies in Animal Breeding. New York: Academic Press 1981; pp. 109-25. [http://dx.doi.org/10.1016/B978-0-12-123450-8.50011-3]

[218] King WA. Sexing embryos by cytological methods. Theriogenology 1984; 21: 7-17. [http://dx.doi.org/10.1016/0093-691X(84)90302-9]

[219] Hare WC, Mitchell D, Betteridge KJ, Eaglesome MD, Randall GC. Sexing two-week old bovine embryos by chromosomal analysis prior to surgical transfer: preliminary methods and results. Theriogenology 1976; 5: 243-53. [http://dx.doi.org/10.1016/0093-691X(76)90236-3]

[220] Wachtel SS. H-Y antigen in the study of sex determination and control of sex ratio. Theriogenology 1984; 21: 18-27. [http://dx.doi.org/10.1016/0093-691X(84)90303-0]

[221] White KL, Anderson GB, Bondurant RH. Expression of a male-specific factor on various stages of preimplantation bovine embryos. Biol Reprod 1987; 37(4): 867-73.

[http://dx.doi.org/10.1095/biolreprod37.4.867] [PMID: 3318944]

[222] Williams TJ. A technique for sexing mouse embryos by a visual colorimetric assay of the X-linked enzyme, glucose 6-phosphate dehydrogenase. Theriogenology 1986; 25(5): 733-9. [http://dx.doi.org/10.1016/0093-691X(86)90131-7] [PMID: 16726164]

[223] Bondioli KR, Ellis SB, Prior JH, Williams MW, Harpold MM. The use of male specific chromosomal DNA fragments to determine the sex of bovine preimplantation embryos. Theriogenology 1989; 31: 95-104. [http://dx.doi.org/10.1016/0093-691X(89)90567-0]

[224] Saiki RK, Gelfand DH, Stoffel S, *et al.* Primer-directed enzymatic amplification of DNA with a thermostable DNA polymerase. Science 1988; 239(4839): 487-91. [http://dx.doi.org/10.1126/science.2448875] [PMID: 2448875]

[225] Bondioli K. Embryo sexing: a review of current techniques and their potential for commercial application in livestock production. J Anim Sci 1992; 70(2): 19-29. [http://dx.doi.org/10.2527/1992.70suppl_219x]

[226] Handyside AH, Pattinson JK, Penketh RJ, Delhanty JD, Winston RM, Tuddenham EG. Biopsy of human preimplantation embryos and sexing by DNA amplification. Lancet 1989; 1(8634): 347-9. [http://dx.doi.org/10.1016/S0140-6736(89)91723-6] [PMID: 2464730]

[227] Herr CM, Matthaei KI, Bradley MP, Reed KC. Rapid accurate sexing of livestock embryos. Proc of the 4th World Congress on Genetics Applied to Livestock Production.

[228] Peura T, Hyttinen JM, Turunen M, Jänne J. Areliable sex determination assay for bovine preimplantation embryos using the polymerase chain reaction. Theriogenology 1991; 35(3): 547-55. [http://dx.doi.org/10.1016/0093-691X(91)90451-I] [PMID: 16726924]

[229] Macháty Z, Páldi A, Csáki T, *et al.* Biopsy and sex determination by PCR of IVF bovine embryos. J Reprod Fertil 1993; 98(2): 467-70. [http://dx.doi.org/10.1530/jrf.0.0980467] [PMID: 8410812]

[230] Thibier M, Nibart M. The sexing of bovine embryos in the field. Theriogenology 1995; 43: 71-80. [http://dx.doi.org/10.1016/0093-691X(94)00008-I]

[231] Collins ME, Stevens DA, Jenner LJ, Brownlie J. A rapid method for mRNA detection in single-cell biopsies from preimplantation-stage bovine embryos. Theriogenology 1995; 43(7): 1227-38. [http://dx.doi.org/10.1016/0093-691X(95)00094-O] [PMID: 16727708]

[232] Peippo J, Huhtinen M, Kotilainen T. Sex diagnosis of equine preimplantation embryos using the polymerase chain reaction. Theriogenology 1995; 44(5): 619-27. [http://dx.doi.org/10.1016/0093-691X(95)00242-Z] [PMID: 16727760]

[233] Bredbacka P, Peippo J. Sex diagnosis of ovine and bovine embryos by enzymatic amplification and digestion of DNA from the ZFY/ZFX locus. Agric Sci Finl 1992; 2: 233-8.

[234] Fajfar-Whetstone CJ, Lane Rayburn A III, Schook LB, Wheeler MB. Sex determination of porcine preimplantation embryos *via* Y-chromosome specific DNA sequences. Anim Biotechnol 1993; 4: 183-93. [http://dx.doi.org/10.1080/10495399309525795]

[235] Rao KB, Pawshe CH, Totey SM. Sex determination of in vitro developed buffalo (*Bubalus bubalis*) embryos by DNA amplification. Mol Reprod Dev 1993; 36(3): 291-6.
[http://dx.doi.org/10.1002/mrd.1080360302] [PMID: 8286109]

[236] Kageyama S, Yoshida I, Kawakura K, Chikuni K. A novel repeated sequence located on the bovine Y chromosome: its application to rapid and precise embryo sexing by PCR. J Vet Med Sci 2004; 66(5): 509-14.
[http://dx.doi.org/10.1292/jvms.66.509] [PMID: 15187360]

[237] Bradbury MW, Isola LM, Gordon JW. Enzymatic amplification of a Y chromosome repeat in a single blastomere allows identification of the sex of preimplantation mouse embryos. Proc Natl Acad Sci USA 1990; 87(11): 4053-7.
[http://dx.doi.org/10.1073/pnas.87.11.4053] [PMID: 2349218]

[238] Matthews ME, Reed KC. Sequences from a family of bovine Y-chromosomal repeats. Genomics 1992; 13(4): 1267-73.
[http://dx.doi.org/10.1016/0888-7543(92)90045-T] [PMID: 1505958]

[239] Matthews ME, Reed KC. A DNA sequence that is present in both sexes of Artiodactyla is repeated on the Y chromosome of cattle, sheep, and goats. Cytogenet Cell Genet 1991; 56(1): 40-4.
[http://dx.doi.org/10.1159/000133043] [PMID: 2004555]

[240] Appa Rao KB, Totey SM. Cloning and sequencing of buffalo male-specific repetitive DNA: sexing of in-vitro developed buffalo embryos using multiplex and nested polymerase chain reaction. Theriogenology 1999; 51(4): 785-97.
[http://dx.doi.org/10.1016/S0093-691X(99)00027-8] [PMID: 10729003]

[241] Manna L, Neglia G, Marino M, Gasparrini B, Di Palo R, Zicarelli L. Sex determination of buffalo embryos (*Bubalus bubalis*) by polymerase chain reaction. Zygote 2003; 11(1): 17-22.
[http://dx.doi.org/10.1017/S0967199403001035] [PMID: 12625525]

[242] Hirayama H, Kageyama S, Takahashi Y, *et al.* Rapid sexing of water buffalo (*Bubalus bubalis*) embryos using loop-mediated isothermal amplification. Theriogenology 2006; 66(5): 1249-56.
[http://dx.doi.org/10.1016/j.theriogenology.2006.03.036] [PMID: 16672158]

[243] Utsumi K, Iritani A. Embryo sexing by male specific antibody and by PCR using male specific (SRY) primer. Mol Reprod Dev 1993; 36(2): 238-41.
[http://dx.doi.org/10.1002/mrd.1080360219] [PMID: 8257576]

[244] Fu Q, Zhang M, Qin WS, *et al.* Cloning the swamp buffalo SRY gene for embryo sexing with multiplex-nested PCR. Theriogenology 2007; 68(9): 1211-8.
[http://dx.doi.org/10.1016/j.theriogenology.2007.07.007] [PMID: 17928043]

[245] Révay T, Kovács A, Presicce GA, Rens W, Gustavsson I. Detection of water buffalo sex chromosomes in spermatozoa by fluorescence *in situ* hybridization. Reprod Domest Anim 2003; 38(5): 377-9.
[http://dx.doi.org/10.1046/j.1439-0531.2003.00442.x] [PMID: 12950688]

[246] Di Berardino D, Vozdova M, Kubickova S, *et al.* Sexing river buffalo (*Bubalus bubalis* L.), sheep (*Ovis aries* L.), goat (*Capra hircus* L.), and cattle spermatozoa by double color FISH using bovine (*Bos taurus* L.) X- and Y-painting probes. Mol Reprod Dev 2004; 67(1): 108-15.
[http://dx.doi.org/10.1002/mrd.20016] [PMID: 14648881]

[247] Presicce GA, Verberckmoes S, Senatore EM, Klinc P, Rath D. First established pregnancies in Mediterranean Italian buffaloes (*Bubalus bubalis*) following deposition of sexed spermatozoa near the utero tubal junction. Reprod Domest Anim 2005; 40(1): 73-5. [http://dx.doi.org/10.1111/j.1439-0531.2004.00560.x] [PMID: 15655005]

[248] Lu Y, Zhang M, Lu S, *et al.* Sex-preselected buffalo (*Bubalus bubalis*) calves derived from artificial insemination with sexed sperm. Anim Reprod Sci 2010; 119(3-4): 169-71. [http://dx.doi.org/10.1016/j.anireprosci.2010.01.001] [PMID: 20137870]

[249] Campanile G, Gasparrini B, Vecchio D, *et al.* Pregnancy rates following AI with sexed semen in Mediterranean Italian buffalo heifers (*Bubalus bubalis*). Theriogenology 2011; 76(3): 500-6. [http://dx.doi.org/10.1016/j.theriogenology.2011.02.029] [PMID: 21497388]

[250] Campanile G, Vecchio D, Neglia G, *et al.* Effect of season, late embryonic mortality and progesterone production on pregnancy rates in pluriparous buffaloes (*Bubalus bubalis*) after artificial insemination with sexed semen. Theriogenology 2013; 79(4): 653-9. [http://dx.doi.org/10.1016/j.theriogenology.2012.11.020] [PMID: 23265928]

CHAPTER 15

Buffalo Cloning and Transgenesis

Gautam Kumar Deb[1,4], Rangsun Parnpai[3] and Il Keun Kong[1,2,*]

[1] *Division of Applied Life Science (BK21plus Program), Graduate School of Gyeongsang National University, Jinju, Gyeongsangnam-do, Republic of Korea*

[2] *Institute of Agriculture and Life Sciences, Jinju 660-701, Gyeongnam, Republic of Korea*

[3] *Embryo Technology and Stem Cell Research Center, School of Biotechnology, Suranaree University of Technology, Nakhon Ratchasima 30000, Thailand*

[4] *Bangladesh Livestock Research Institute, Savar, Dhaka–1341, Bangladesh*

Abstract: Somatic cell nuclear transfer (SCNT) is a relatively new technique applied to the buffalo species. The current oocyte maturation, enucleation and nuclear transfer, and *in vitro* embryo culture systems for buffalo reconstructed embryos, are comparable with bovine SCNT. However, there are very few reports on delivery of normal live cloned buffalo calves. The inducible pluripotent stem cells (iPS), which made a major breakthrough in the remodeling of somatic cell nucleus by inducing different transcription factors, have not been applied in the buffalo cloning. Moreover, the application of SCNT in transgenesis of buffalo is limited to the development of transgenic blastocysts. In this chapter, we described recent advances and novel approaches in SCNT and transgenic buffalo productions in connection with the concurrent advances in other relevant mammalian species.

Keywords: Buffalo, Cloning, Induced pluripotent stem cells, Somatic cell nuclear transfer, Transgenesis.

1. INTRODUCTION

Buffaloes (*Bubalus bubalis*) are characterized by a series of physiological fea-

* **Corresponding author Il Keun Kong:** Division of Applied Life Science (BK21plus Program), Graduate School of Gyeongsang National University, Institute of Agriculture and Life Sciences, Jinju 660-701, Gyeongnam, Republic of Korea; Tel: +82 055 772 1942 and +82 010 3785 3567; Fax: +82 055 772 1949; E-mail: ikong@gnu.kr.ac

Giorgio A. Presicce (Ed.)

tures such as late onset of puberty, silent estrus, seasonal anestrus, long post partum anestrus and long calving interval [1]. Moreover, the ovaries of buffaloes present lower numbers of follicles, leading to few oocytes available for *in vitro* embryo manipulation. Consequently, progress in the application of assisted reproductive technologies has been slow in this species [2]. The first cloned buffalo calves were born in 2007 [3], approximately 16 years after the first buffalo calf born from *in vitro* fertilization [4]; however, there is no report of a live transgenic buffalo clone to date.

When any organism is genetically identical to another, it is considered to be a biological clone. Cloning is a complex process leading the to the production of an identical genetic organism through the procedure of somatic cell nuclear transfer (SCNT), as defined by the American Medical Association. Often though, the term cloning is also used, in a broader definition, to include the production of tissues and organs from cells or tissue cultures adopting stem cells. The first cloning experiment in farm animals was conducted in the late 1980s to produce monozygotic twins by cutting an embryo into two halves and each half then transferred in an empty zona pellucida in sheep [5] and cows [6]. A tremendous advance in farm animal cloning was reached with the birth of Dolly the sheep in 1996, by using the SCNT procedure [7]. Dolly was produced by transferring an adult somatic cell nucleus into an enucleated oocyte. Since then, clones have been born in different farm animal species using various somatic cell nuclei derived from fetuses to adult animals. The birth of Polly was considered the second landmark in biology and farm animal cloning, as this animals was a genetically modified clone, which opened a new horizon in farm animal cloning [8]. Transgenic farm animals, which are a group of animals which have been genetically modified, are characterized by having inserted in their genome, one or more genes derived from another organism, and following the birth of Polly, more farm animals have been cloned by SCNT such as goat [9], pig [10 - 12] and cattle [13 - 15].

Recently, the reprogramming of somatic cells in animals has been achieved through the forced induction of several transcription factors. The reprogrammed cells present the properties of embryonic stem cells and are known as induced pluripotent stem cells (iPS) [16]. IPS cells are able to produce live mouse chimeras [17 - 19]. Why such excitement in a successful cloning? In breeding programs, in order to quicken the disseminations of genes from superior genetic animals to less valuable genetic animals within commercial populations for generating transgenic animals, cloning is instrumental due to its intrinsic features of increasing the accuracy of selection and the genetic progress. Unfortunately, the main limitation of this novel strategy, is the low success rate of the overall process and consequently the high cost per single transgenic animal produced to be ready for reproduction [20]. In this chapter, the authors describe the current state of cloning and transgenesis in the buffalo species.

2. SOMATIC CELL NUCLEAR TRANSFER

By SCNT is meant a laboratory procedure performed in order to de-differentiate a somatic cell, like a fibroblast or any other adult somatic cell, so that a nuclear reprogramming can occur when subsequently, the same somatic cell is inserted into an enucleated recipient oocyte [21]. By employing such technical procedure, a number of genetically identical animals can be obtained. Nuclear transfer is a powerful tool for studying genomic imprinting, nuclear-cytoplasmic interaction, totipotency, and the contribution of paternal and maternal genomes to developing embryos. However, it is an inefficient method for cloning farm animals, achieving 0 to 4% live births [22]. Parameters affecting the success rate include the age of donor cells, cell cycle stage, ploidy and developmental stage of recipient cells [23], and activation schedule following fusion [22]. The SCNT procedure includes several steps as described below (Fig. **1**).

2.1. Oocyte Recovery

Three methods are widely used for retrieving immature oocytes from abattoir ovaries in buffalos (Table **1**): 1) slicing, 2) follicle puncture, and 3) follicle aspiration. The follicular aspiration method is commonly used for the retrieval of COCs for SCNT and transgenic operations in buffalos. The mean recovery of good quality oocytes per abattoir ovary is between 0.4 to 2.4 [24 - 28], which is lower than cattle (8–12 good quality oocytes/abattoir-derived ovary). Ultrasound-guided ovum pick (OPU) from live animals slightly increases the number of oocytes retrieved [29 - 31]. The buffalo ovary is smaller in size [32] and contains fewer follicles than cattle, resulting in fewer follicles recruited in each cycle [33]. The low number of good quality oocytes available per ovary is further decreased in the presence of corpus luteum [29]. The cumulus cell attachment and cytoplasmic structure of immature oocytes correlate with its developmental competence. According to Chauhan *et al.* [34], the developmental competence of oocytes declines from Grade 1 to Grade 3. Grade 1 and 2 oocytes are generally used for *in vitro* maturation (Table **2**).

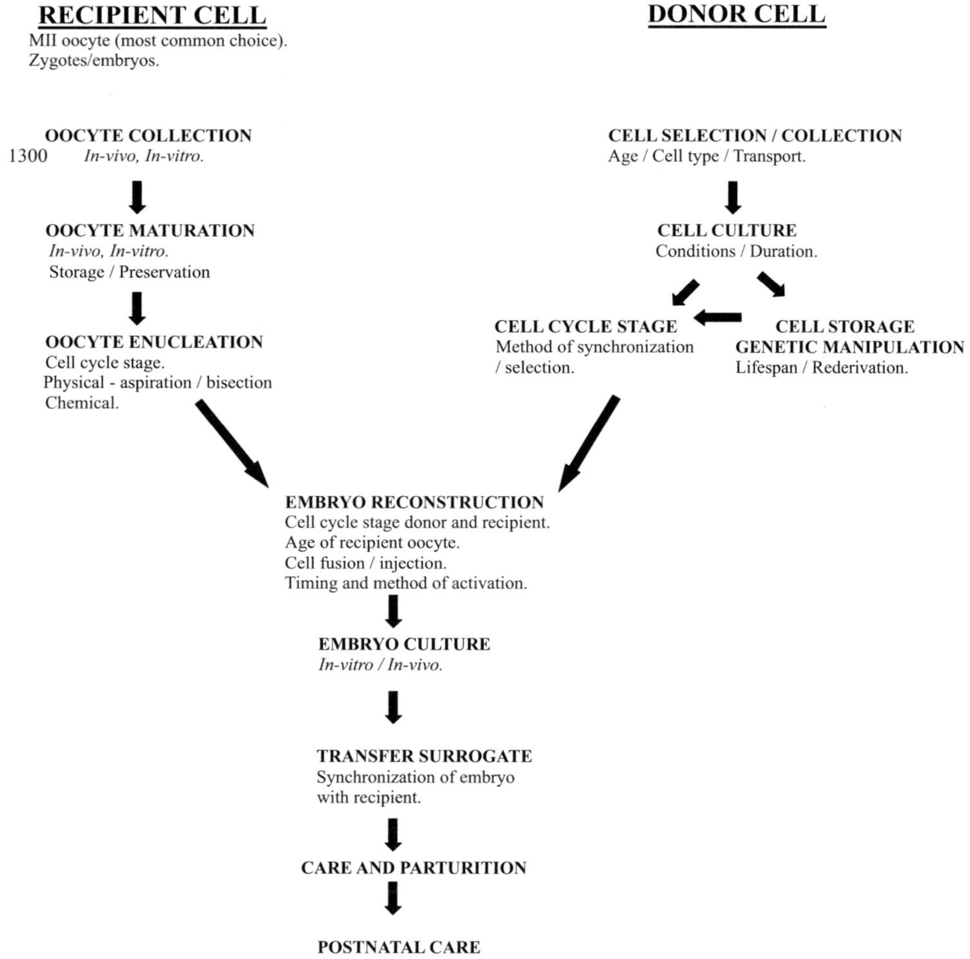

Fig. (1). Somatic Cell Nuclear Transfer (SCNT) and the steps needed for multiple identical offspring production. Cited from Campbell *et al.* [45], Theriogenology 2007, 68S: S214–S231.

Table 1. Methods of oocyte retrieval from slaughterhouse buffalo ovaries.

Parameter	Slicing	Follicle puncture	Follicle aspiration
Definition	Ovaries are sliced into small pieces using a surgical blade in a Petridish containing normal saline solution. The sliced stromal tissues are discarded and the oocytes are selected under a stereomicroscope	Follicles are punctured with an 18 or 20 gauge needle. Oocytes with follicular fluids are allowed to escape into the normal saline solution of Petri dish by applying gentle pressure on the adjacent stroma of punctured follicle	Follicular fluids are aspirated through a sterile 18 to 20 gauge needle attached to a syringe or vacuum pump. Finally, the oocyte is collected from the aspirated content under a stereomicroscope
Follicle source	Follicles in the ovarian surface as well as in the deeper cortical stroma	Follicles in the ovarian surface	Follicles in the ovarian surface
Time required for oocyte collection (min)	High (2.8 ± 0.09)	Low (1.5 ± 0.06)	Low (1.6 ± 0.07)
Efficiency	Higher number of oocyte/ ovary (6.25/ovary)	Low number of oocytes/ ovary (3.10/ovary)	Low number of oocytes/ ovary (2.35/ovary)
Oocyte morphology	Higher chance of poor quality oocytes	Lower chance of poor quality oocytes	Lower chance of poor quality oocytes
Follicle size	Slice all follicles, irrespective of size	Puncture follicles of the desired size	Aspirate follicles of the desired size

Summarized from Kumar *et al.* [29] and Das *et al.* [26].

Table 2. Classification of immature buffalo oocytes.

	Grade 1	Grade 2	Grade 3
Cumulus cell	Compact cumulus cell attachment More than five layers of cumulus cells	Compact cumulus cell attachment Less than five layers of cumulus cells	Oocyte without a cumulus cell or with an expanded cumulus cell, or that is partially denuded
Cytoplasm	Homogenous cytoplasm	Homogenous cytoplasm	Uneven cytoplasm
	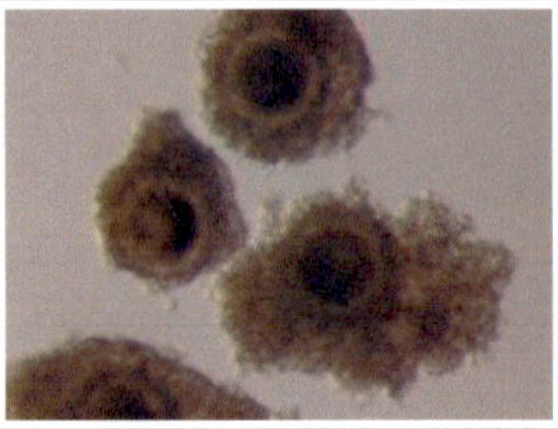	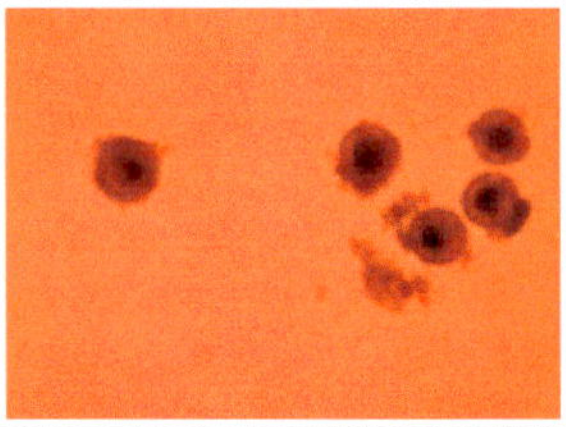	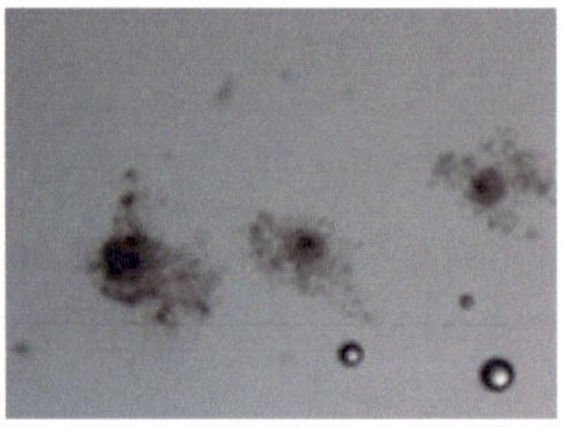

(Table 2) contd.....

	Grade 1	Grade 2	Grade 3
Photo courtesy of Dr. Bianca Gasparrini			

Summarized from Chauhan *et al.* [34]

2.2. Effect of Donor Cell Types on Efficiency of Embryo Development

Different cell types are used as nuclear donors to generate farm animal clones by SCNT. The cell cycle phase of the donor cells at the time of nuclear transfer affects the efficiency of SCNT. Donor cells in G0/G1 provide greater cloning efficiency than cells in other phases [35]. Variation in cloning efficiency was also observed between different sub-populations of the same cell line [36] and between different clonal lines of transgenic fibroblasts originating from the same fetus [37]. Moreover, the genetic origin of the donor cells affects the success of SCNT in mouse and sheep [38]. The donor cells used for SCNT in different species can be divided into three groups according to their origin:

2.2.1. Embryo-Derived Donor Cells

The first cloned mammal offspring was derived by transferring embryonic blastomeres to recipient oocytes [39]. Nuclei from 8- to 16-cell stage sheep embryos produced live lambs following transfer into recipient sheep. Nuclei of embryonic blastomeres are more efficient than somatic cell nuclei and achieve higher embryo production rates, higher pregnancy rates and lower incidences of death and developmental abnormalities. However, the low number of clones has limited its use in farm animal cloning. No buffalo calf was born from transfer of embryonic nuclei to date.

2.2.2. Somatic Cells

A variety of differentiated somatic cell types have been successfully reprogrammed into recipient enucleated oocytes (Table **3**). Thanks to their rapid growth in culture, fibroblast have been chosen and used extensively in the course of SCNT. In cattle, skin fibroblasts >12 passages tend to lose their chromosomal structure, resulting in the developmental failure of the clone offspring [40], and usually decapitated and eviscerated fetuses at around 40 to 60 days of gestation, are the source of these cells to be used in SCNT. In 1999, Parnpai *et al.* [41] first reported of producing cloned swamp buffalo blastocysts from fetal fibroblasts which had been used up to passage 8.

Table 3. ***In vitro*** **culture of buffalo reconstructed embryos.**

Reference	*In vitro* culture condition	Donor cells	% blastocyst	Comment
1	Twenty couplets per 100 µL mSOFaa medium for 2 days Ten 8-cell embryo/ 100-µL droplet of mSOFaa, cell free system or co-cultured with cattle or buffalo oviductal epithelial cells for additional 5 days	Buffalo FF	Cell free: 20 Cattle OEC: 30.9 Buffalo OEC: 30.9	% blastocyst from cultured 8-cell stage
2	Twenty couplets per 100 µL mSOFaa medium for 2 days. Ten 8-cell embryo/ 100-µL droplet of mSOFaa + cattle oviductal epithelial cells for additional 5 days	Buffalo FF	21.8	CC nuclei reprogrammed more efficiently
		EF	26.8	
		GC	24.5	
		CC	27.9a	
3	a. Hepes-modified TCM199 + 10% FBS	Buffalo ovarian granulose cells	22.3a	Compared to IVC media 100 µL droplet for 7 days
	b. Hepes-modified TCM199 + 0.1% PVA		13.0	
	c. CR1aa + 0.3% BSA		19.2a	
4	30 µL mSOFaa medium for 2 days Ten 8-cell embryo droplets of TCM199 + 3% ECS + GC monolayer 50% medium was replaced with fresh medium every 24 h until Day 8	Buffalo FF/Buffalo GC	Conf: 8.7/9.8	Donor cells were subjected to confluent (Conf), serum starvation (SS) and aphidicolin + serum starvation (ASS)
			SS: 10.6/10.3	
			ASS: 21.3/22.2	
5	Embryos were cultured in 100 µl droplets of mSOF for 2 days 8-cell embryos were transferred into 100 µl droplets of mSOF with bovine oviductal epithelial cells for 5 days.	Buffalo ear skin	35.0	Evaluated epigenetic characteristics of SCNT and IVF embryos

(Table 3) contd.....

Reference	*In vitro* culture condition	Donor cells	% blastocyst	Comment
6	Embryos were cocultured with BRL cells in 50 μL droplets of TCM199 + 10% FCS for 2 days 8-cell embryos were transferred in 50 μL droplets of TCM199 + 10% FCS + buffalo oviductal epithelial cells for 5 days	Buffalo FF	BO: 39.0	Evaluated SCNT efficiency of buffalo FF on buffalo oocyte (BO) and cow oocyte (CO)
			CO: 33.0	
7	10–15 re-constructed embryos/400 μL K-RVCL-50 + 1.0% fatty acid free BSA in a 4 well dish covered with mineral oil for 7 days	Fetal skin (60 days)	24.0	Different donor cells were compared according to SCNT efficiency. Cumulus cell was more efficient
		Newborn skin	33.0	
		Adult skin	21.0	
		Cumulus cells	49.6	
8	20 embryos/ 100 μL droplets of mSOFaa + 0.3% fatty acid-free BSA for 2 days. 8-cell embryos were cocultured with bovine oviductal epithelial cells (BOEC) for 5 days. Half of the medium was changed with fresh medium every day	Adult ear skin	23.0	Evaluated vitrification effect of oocyte on SCNT efficiency. Fresh control development rate was presented in this table
9	30 μL droplets of TCM199 + 10% FBS+ buffalo granulose cell monolayer 50% medium was changed every two days until day 8 of embryonic development	EG-like cells	13.3a	EG-like cells showed a similar efficiency to that of the nuclear donors, at least until 8 passages
		EGFP EG-like cells	11.0a	
		Buffalo FF	7.1a	
		EGFP Buffalo FF	0b	
10	30 μL droplets of TCM199 + 10% FBS+ buffalo granulose cell monolayer 50% medium was changed every two days until day 8 of embryonic development.	Freshly-thawed ear fibroblasts	9.5	
		Serum-starved ear fibroblast	16.2a	
		Cumulus cells	17.9a	
		G1 ear fibroblasts	16.2a	
11	a. TCM199 + 10% FBS + buffalo oviductal epithelial cells	Media was changed every 2 days	a38%	Cumulus cell nuclei were used in cloning
	b. TCM199 + 10% FBS + buffalo cumulus cells		[a]35%	
	c. TCM199 + 10% FBS + Vero cell		a35%	
	d. Ligated buffalo oviduct culture		a35%	
	e. TCM199 + 10% FBS		17%	

(Table 3) contd.....

Reference	*In vitro* culture condition	Donor cells	% blastocyst	Comment
12	a. TCM199 + 20% FBS + 10 ng/mL EGF + 100 μM cysteamine + 50–100 cylinder of buffalo oviductal epithelial cells	Media was changed every 2 days	0%	Nuclei of FF were used in cloning
	b. SOFaa + 4 mg/mL FAF BSA + 10 ng/mL EGF+ 100 μM cysteamine		0%	
	c. G1/G2 + 0.5% FAF BSA		3%	

1: Parnpai *et al.* [41]; 2: Srirattana *et al.* [93]; 3: Pandey *et al.* [94]; 4: Shi *et al.* [3]; 5: Suteevun *et al.* [95]; 6: Kitiyanant *et al.* [96]; 7: Shah *et al.* [61]; 8: Muenthaisong *et al.* [97]; 9: Huang *et al.* [87]; 10: Yang *et al.* [98]; 11: Wadhwa *et al.* [83]; 12: Simon *et al.* [52]. FF: Follicular fluid; EF:; GC: granulose cell CC: cumulus cell; OEC: oviductal epithelial cells.

2.2.3. Stem Cells

Nuclear reprogramming in SCNT has been playing a pivotal role, since it was observed that more differentiated (adult) somatic cells are more difficulty reprogrammed than less differentiated cells. The finding that less differentiated cells can be more easily reprogrammed than more differentiated cells supports the critical role of nuclear reprogramming in SCNT [42, 43]. SCNT embryos and their development are easily affected by the state of differentiation and the type of donor cell, and this is due to the nature of the donor cell itself and its epigenetic state at the time of embryo reconstruction [44]. All the above are supportive of the idea that the oocyte milieu following SCNT can more easily reprogram less differentiated cells, such as stem cells.

2.3. Preparation of Recipient Oocytes

Metaphase II (MII) oocytes are generally used as recipient cytoplasts for SCNT. Fertilized zygotes and 2-cell embryos are also able to reprogram differentiated somatic cells [45]; however, the efficiency of reprogramming is very low compared to MII oocytes. In buffalo, MII oocytes are commonly used for cloning and transgenic animal production. Buffalo oocytes with more than three to five compact cumulus layers and an even cytoplasm recovered from 2 to 8 mm follicles are mostly cultured in groups (5 to 20 oocytes) for 21–24 h in 50 to 100 μL droplets of commercially available complex medium such as tissue culture medium 199 (TCM 199), Ham's F-10 medium, G_1/G_2, or minimum essential medium (MEM). These media were originally designed for cell culture and are not capable of supporting high levels of oocyte maturation. Therefore, these basic media are often supplemented with sera (fetal calf serum, fetal bovine serum, estrus buffalo serum, estrus cow serum, human serum, steer serum or super ovulated buffalo serum), a hormone such as FSH alone or in combination with LH, or a combination of FSH, LH or estradiol. Feeder cells and in some cases follicular fluids can also supplement basic medium. TCM199 with supplements is commonly used for IVM of buffalo oocytes in cloned and transgenic animal production protocols (Table **4**). Immature buffalo oocytes need to be cultured *in vitro* for 18 to 24 h for proper maturation [46]. After IVM, the cumulus cells are removed either mechanically by repeated pipetting in 0.2% hyaluronidase using a fine-tip pipette or by vortexing in a 1.5 mL microcentrifuge tube containing 500 µL of medium supplemented with hyaluronidase (0.5 mg/mL). The oocytes are then sequentially washed five times in TCM199 medium. For enucleation, matured oocytes with first polar bodies are placed into culture medium containing 5 µg of cytochalasin B/mL for 5–15 min.

Table 4. ***In vitro* maturation media used for *in vitro* maturation of buffalo oocyte for cloning and transgenesis.**

Composition	Formulation											
	1	2	3	4	5	6	7	8	9	10	11	12
Base medium	TCM199	TCM199	TCM199	TCM 199	TCM 199	TCM199	TCM199	TCM199	TCM 199	TCM199	TCM199	$NaHCO_3$ buffered TCM199
Hepes	-	-	-	5 mM	-	-	-	-	5 mM	-	-	-
$NaHCO_3$	25 mM	25 mM	-	26.2 mM	25 mM	-	-	25 mM	26.2 mM	-	-	-
Sera	10% FBS	10% FBS	10% FBS	5% ECS	10% FBS	10% FBS	10% FBS	10% FBS	5% ECS	10% FBS	10% FCS	10% FBS
FSH	0.02 AU/mL	0.02 AU/mL	500 IU/mL	0.1 lg/mL	0.02 AU/mL	5 mg/mL	5 mg/mL	0.02 AU/mL	0.1 µg/mL	5 ug/mL	1 µg/mL	1 µg/mL
LH	50 iu/mL hCG	50 iu/mL hCG	500 IU/mL	-	50 iu/mL hCG	5 mg/mL		50 iu/mL hCG	-	10 ug/mL	5 µg/mL	0.02 IU/mL
Estradiol 17β	1 µg/mL	1 µg/mL	1000 IU/mL	-	1 µg/mL	1 mg/mL	1 mg/mL	1 µg/mL	-	1 µg/mL	0.5 µg/mL	1 µg/mL
Sodium pyruvate	0.2 mM	0.2 mM	-	-	0.2 mM	0.2 mM	0.8 mM	0.2 mM	-	0.2mM	27.5 µg/mL	
Follicular fluid (FF)	-	-	-	2% bovine FF	-	-	5% Buffalo FF	-	2% bovine FF	-	-	
Cysteine	-	-	-	-	-	-	-	-	-	50 mM	-	100 µM

(Table 4) contd.....

Composition	Formulation											
	1	2	3	4	5	6	7	8	9	10	11	12
Growth factor	-	-	-	-	-	-	-	-	-	25 ng/mL EGF	10 ng/mL EGF	10 ng/mL EGF
Antibiotic	50 µg/mL penicillin G+100 µg/mL streptomycin sulphate	-	-	-	-	-	50 mg/mL gentamicin	-	60 µg/mL penicillin G+100 µg/mL streptomycin sulphate	-	-	-
Others	-	-	-	-	-	-	-	-	-	-	10% post maturation medium	-
Follicle size	2-8 mm	2–8 mm	2–8 mm		2–6 mm	2–8 mm		2–6 mm	-	-		
Culture period	19 h	22 h	24 h	20–22 h	22 h	24 h	21 h	21 h	22 h	22-24 h	18-22 h	
Reference	1	2	3	4	5	6	7	8	9	10	11	12

Post maturation medium: supernatant medium previously collected from the cultures of mature oocytes; BFF: buffalo follicular fluid.

1: Parnpai *et al.* [41]; 2: Srirattana *et al.* [93]; 3: Pandey *et al.* [94]; 4: Shi *et al.* [3]; 5: Suteevun *et al.* [95]; 6: Kitiyanant *et al.* [96]; 7: Shah *et al.* [61]; 8: Muenthaisong *et al.* [97]; 9: Huang *et al.* [87]; 10: Yang *et al.* [98]; 11: Wadhwa *et al.* [83]; 12: Simon *et al.* [52].

2.4. Enucleation of Oocytes

Enucleation of oocytes can be conducted using either zona-intact or zona-free oocytes. The use of zona-intact oocytes is known as traditional cloning and that of zona-free oocytes is known as handmade cloning (HMC).

2.4.1. Zona-Intact Oocytes

The metaphase II spindle of an *in vitro*-matured oocyte is removed by maintaining the oocyte in the appropriate position by applying to it a minimal vacuum force through the polished end of holding pipette. Then, the chromatin within the oocyte is aspirated by mean of a sharp enucleation pipette going through the zona pellucida. Different techniques have been developed to optimize the enucleation process in different species including: 1) enucleation of oocyte at MII, 2) enucleation of activated oocyte at telophase of the second meiotic division, 3) enucleation at anaphase/telophase of the first meiotic division, and 4) chemical enucleation using etoposide, a combination of etoposide and cycloheximide or ethanol and demecolcine. Recently, techniques have been developed to visualize the MII spindle during enucleation (Fig. **2**).

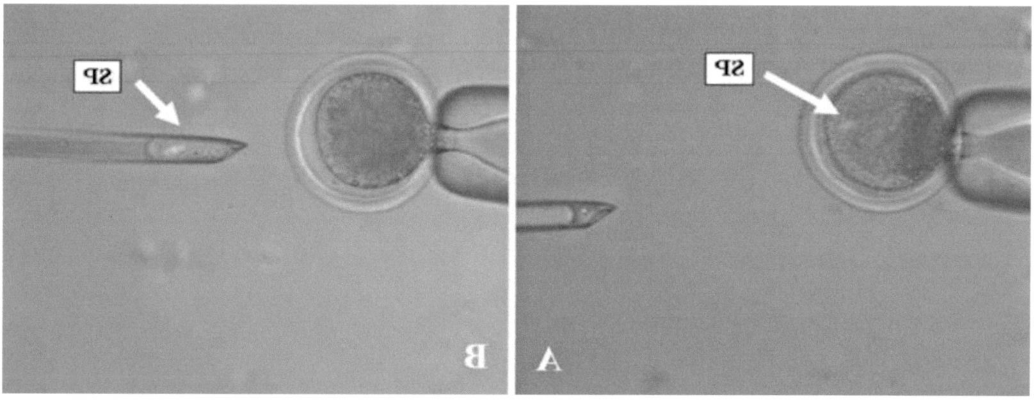

Fig. (2). Enucleation of buffalo oocytes under the Spindle View System. **(A)** Spindle (SP) of a buffalo oocyte prior to enucleation. Original magnification 3200. **(B)** Spindle inside the 25 μm beveled glass pipette diameter, following enucleation. Original magnification 3200. Cited from Shi *et al.* [3], Biology of Reproduction 2007, 77, 285–291.

For example, the exposure of oocytes to 3% sucrose allows the visualization of the meiotic spindle with a light microscope. A POL-scope and XY clone laser system can also be used (detail reviewed in Campbell *et al.* [45]). Most published studies of buffalo cloning and transgenesis report the enucleation of oocytes at the MII stage using a glass pipette. The oocytes are placed in 30–50 μL droplets of enucleation medium containing 5 to 7.5 μg cytochalasin B (CB) per milliliter of medium for 5–15 min before micromanipulation. An inverted miscroscope set up on a micromanipulator is used to remove both first polar body and metaphase II plate thanks to a sharp beveled pipette with an inner diameter of 20 to 25 μm. Alternatively, enucleation can be performed by squeezing out a small volume (~10%) of cytoplasm where the first polar body is visualized, following a small dissection of the zona pellucida and a glass needle used to exert a slight pressure above the opening that has been created (Fig. **3**). The successful enucleation of each oocyte is confirmed by staining by fluorescence the squeezed out cytoplasm with Hoechst 33342 [41, 47].

2.4.2. Zona-Free Oocytes

Two methods are used to enucleate zona-free oocytes:

2.4.2.1. Enucleation by Bisecting

To our knowledge, three different enucleation methods have been reported for manually bisecting denuded oocytes:

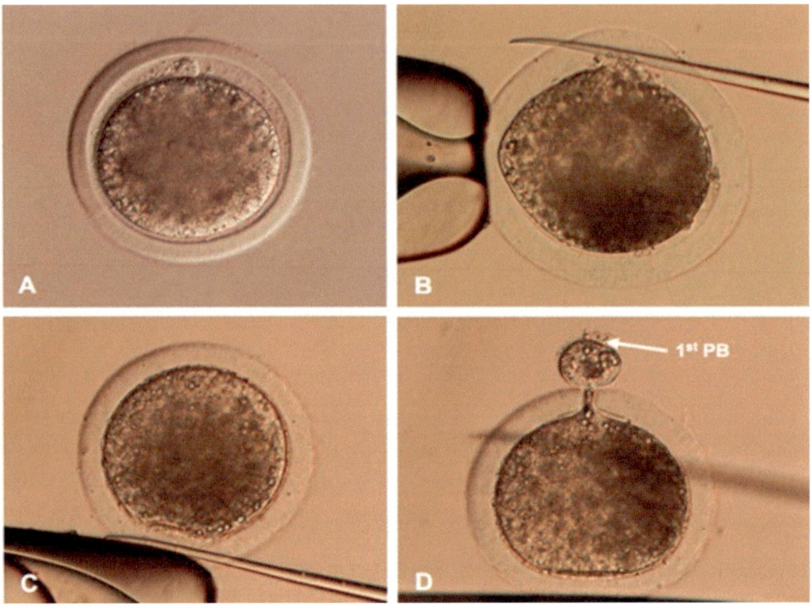

Fig. (3). Enucleation of buffalo oocytes by squeeze out technique **(A)** Matured swamp buffalo oocytes **(B-C)** dissection of the zona pellucida by using a glass needle, close to first polar body **(D)** squeezing out of cytoplasm (~10% of volume) following mechanical opening of the zona pellucida in correspondence to the first polar body. Courtesy of Parnpai, R (unpublished data).

2.4.2.1.1. Blind Bisection

In this process, the *in vitro*-matured oocytes are denuded and oocytes with first polar bodies are selected for bisection prior to zona removal and enucleation. The selected oocytes are bi-sectioned manually and the chromosome complements are removed under UV light. Finally, a single somatic cell and two cytoplasts are fused to develop a cloned embryo. Inevitably, some errors in the selection process of the enucleated cytoplasm have to be contemplated when this approach is used. In fact, it is mandatory to quickly identify the nucleated halves through UV exposure by reducing as much as possible the time needed, in addition to the possible misidentification of the human eye of the cytoplast to be disposed of.

2.4.2.1.2. Combined Blind Bisection and Hoechst 33342 Staining

This is a modification of the blind bisectioning method. In this process, enucleation is conducted after visualizing genetic material by staining with Hoechst 33342 under UV light. Following enucleation, a single somatic cell and two cytoplasts are fused to develop a cloned embryo. Enucleation following Hoechst staining has improved the accuracy of the technique.

2.4.2.1.3. Protrusion Cone-Guided Bisection

In this method, denuded matured oocytes are directly subjected to pronase digestion without polar body selection. An oocyte with a polar body exhibits a prominent surface protrusion when the zona is digested. The cumulative effect of pronase and subsequent incubation in culture medium facilitates protrusion on the surface of the oocyte. Oocytes exhibiting a surface protrusion cone are then selected for manual bisection. In this method, the oocytes are not subjected to Hoechst 33342 and UV light. The labeling and enucleation of oocytes with Hoechst 33342 have no adverse effect on SCNT success rate, but a loss of membrane integrity can be caused by direct exposure to UV light, together with a decreased methionine incorporation and altered protein synthesis in bovine oocytes [48].

2.4.2.2. Enucleation with Simple Blunt Micropipette

In this method (Fig. **4**), the metaphase II plate is directly aspirated from the zona removed oocyte under a UV light system with very little cytoplasm. This method is similar to classical method of enucleating zona-enclosed oocytes. However, it is less complicated and much faster than enucleating a zona-enclosed oocyte [49].

2.5. Donor Cell Transfer

The cultured donor cells are usually serum-starved (in DMEM + 0.5% FCS for 24-72 h) to arrest them at G0/G1 stage. Following serum starvation, the cells are digested with an enzymatic solution (0.25% trypsin and 0.05% EDTA) for 5 to 7 min. A micropipette is used to insert a fibroblast cell into the perivitelline space of the enucleated oocyte, through the opening made in the zona pellucida in the course of enucleation (Fig. **5**).

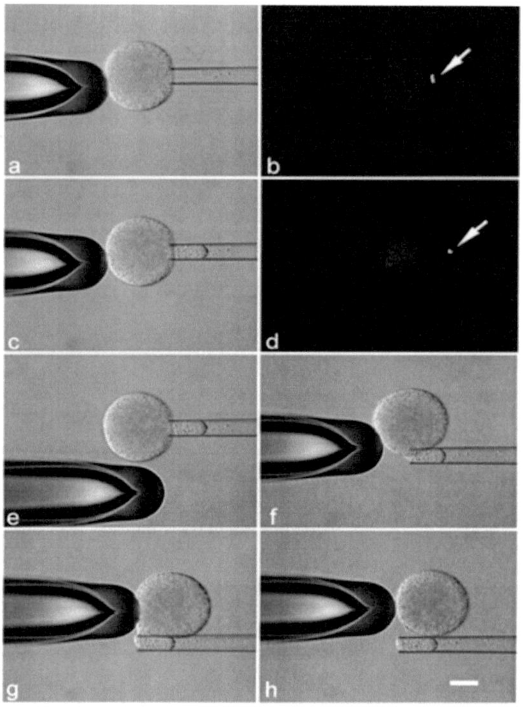

Fig. (4). Zona-free enucleation. Removal of the metaphase plate by adoption of a blunt enucleation pipette and a separation needle **(a-c-e-h)**. **(a)** Both the enucleation pipette and the metaphase plate are adjusted in order to be on the same focal plane. **(c)** The metaphase plate is aspirated inside the glass pipette together with a small amount of cytoplasm. **(e,g)** In one single and smooth movement, the separation needle is pushed upward **(f)** and rightward **(g)** to completely detach the karyoplast **(h)**. Removal of the metaphase plate (arrows) is confirmed by Hoechst 33342 staining **(b,d)**. Bar 5 40 *m*m. Cited from Oback *et al.* [56], Cloning and Stem Cells 2003, 5: 3-12.

2.6. Fusion

In buffalo, the fusion of donor nucleus and recipient cytoplasm is generally achieved with an alternative pulse followed by one or two DC electric pulses or a DC pulse alone. Zimmermann fusion medium or 0.28–0.3 M mannitol supplemented with $CaCl_2$, $MgSO_4$ with or without Hepes, and BSA are mostly used for the fusion of reconstructed oocytes. Parnpai *et al.* [41] reported of using a pair of fusion electrode instead of fusion chamber led to achieve the high fusion rate (Table **5**).

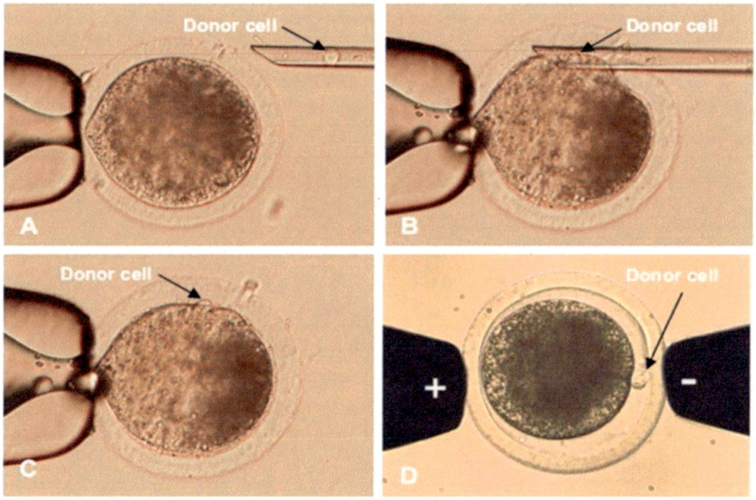

Fig. (5). Injecting donor cell into enucleatated swamp buffalo oocyte and fusion **(A-C)**. A single donor cell is inserted into the perivitelline space of enucleated oocyte through the opening in the zona pellucida created at enucleation **(D)**. The coupled donor cell-enucleated oocyte is placed and fused between the fusion electrode in a Zimmermann medium, by using a 2 direct current pulses of 26 V for 17 μsec. Courtesy of Parnpai, R (unpublish data).

Table 5. Protocol for fusion of reconstructed buffalo couplets.

Reference	Fusion protocol	Fusion medium
1	Two DC pulses of 30 V for 15 μsec	Zimmermann fusion medium (Zimmermann & Vienken, 1982)
2	Two DC pulses of 26 V for 17 μsec	Zimmermann fusion medium (Zimmermann & Vienken, 1982)
3	2 DC pulses of 1.8–2 KV/cm^2 for 15 μsec each, 15 sec apart	0.3 M mannitol + 0.05 mM $CaCl_2$ + 0.1 mM $MgSO_4$
4	An AC pulse of 2 V for 1 sec + 3 DC pulses of 1 kV/cm for 15 μsec	0.28 M mannitol + 0.1 mM $CaCl_2$ + 0.1 mM $MgSO_4$ + 5 mM Hepes + 0.1% BSA
5	Two DC pulses of 26 V for 17 μsec	Zimmermann fusion medium (Zimmermann & Vienken, 1982)
6	Two DC pulses of 2.1 kV/cm for 20 μsec (1 sec apart)	0.3 M mannitol + 0.05 mM $CaCl_2$ + 0.1 mM $MgSO_4$, 7 H_2O + 0.5 mM Hepes + 0.05% fatty acid free BSA 2 h cocultured with buffalo rat liver cells in TCM199 + 10% FCS
7	An AC pulse of 4 V followed by a single DC pulse of 3.36 kV/cm for 4 μsec	0.3 M D-mannitol + 0.05 mM $CaCl_2$ + 0.1 mM $MgCl_2$ + 1 mg/mL polyvinyl alcohol Cultured in Hepes-modified TCM199 + 20% FBS for 4 h

(Table 5) contd.....

Reference	Fusion protocol	Fusion medium
8	Two DC pulses of 26 V for 17 μsec donor-cytoplast couplets were checked for successful fusion after 1 h of electric pulse	Zimmermann fusion medium
9	An AC pulse of 2 V for 1 sec + 3 DC pulses of 1 kV/cm for 15 μsec	0.28 M mannitol + 0.1 mM $CaCl_2$ + 0.1 mM $MgSO_4$ + 5 mM Hepes + 0.1% BSA
10	5 min equilibration in fusion medium Two DC pulses of 1 kV/cm for 10 μsec Fusion check after 1 h	250 mM sorbitol + 0.1 mM calcium acetate + 0.5 mM magnesium acetate + 0.5 mM Hepes + 0.1% BBSA
11	One AC pulse of 3.3 V, 600 kHz for 15 sec One DC pulse of 0.6 kV/cm for 30 μsec followed by second DC pulse of 1.2 kV/cm for 30 μsec, 1 h after first pulse	0.3 M mannose, 0.1 mM $MgSO_4$, and 1% (v/v) serum
12	Two DC pulses of 1.4–1.6 kV/cm for 35 μsec	0.3 M mannitol + 0.05 mM $CaCl_2$, 2 H_2O + 0.1 mM Mg Cl_2 + 0.5 mM Hepes + 4 mg/mL fatty acid free BSA

CD: cytochalasin D; CLH: cycloheximide; CB: cytochalasin B; 6-DMAP: 6-dimethylaminopurine; $mSOF_{aacis}$: modified synthetic oviductal fluid containing essential and nonessential amino acids, myoinositol, sodium citrate, and 5% (v/v) cattle serum; mSOFaa: modified oviduct synthetic fluid with amino acids medium;K-RVCL-50: Research Vitro Cleave medium (Cook® Australia, Queensland, Australia).

1: Parnpai *et al.* [41]; 2: Srirattana *et al.* [93]; 3: Pandey *et al.* [94]; 4: Shi *et al.* [3]; 5: Suteevun *et al.* [95]; 6: Kitiyanant *et al.* [96]; 7: Shah *et al.* [61]; 8: Muenthaisong *et al.* [97]; 9: Huang *et al.* [87]; 10: Yang *et al.* [98]; 11: Wadhwa *et al.* [83]; 12: Simon *et al.* [52].

2.7. Activation

Several artificial activation protocols have been developed in different laboratory and farm animals to activate reconstructed oocytes with the aim of maximizing developmental competence [45]. Activation protocols can be grouped into three categories: 1) chemical treatment, 2) electrical stimulation, and 3) sperm-mediated activation [45, 50, 51]. Ionomycin in combination with 6-dimethylaminopurine (6-DMAP) is routinely used in buffalo with few exceptions. Ethanol followed by a combination of cytochalasin B or D and cycloheximide is also successfully used in buffalo.

The different activation protocols for buffalo reconstructed embryos are summarized in Table **6**. A recent study found that embryo developmental competence was increased upon delayed activation after 3-4 h of fusion compared to immediate activation following fusion [52].

Table 6. Protocol for activation of buffalo reconstructed oocytes.

Ref.	Acceleration of intra cellular Ca^{++}			Inhibition of MFP protein			Comment
	Treatment	Period	Medium	Treatment	Period	Medium	
1	7% ethanol	5 min	Hepes-modified TCM199	1.25 μg/mL CD + 10 μg/mL CYH	5 h	mSOFaa	
2	7% ethanol	5 min	Hepes-modified TCM199	1.25 μg/mL CD + 10 μg/mL CYH	5 h	mSOFaa	
3	5 μM ionomycin	10 min	TCM199 + 10% FBS	2.5 mM 6-DMAP + 10 ug/ml CYH + 7.5 μg/mL CB	3.30 h	TCM199 + 10% FBS	
4	5 μM ionomycin	5 min	TCM199 + 3% ECS+60 ug/mL penicillin G + 100 ug/mL streptomycin sulphate	2 mM 6-DMAP	3 h	TCM199 + 3% ECS + 60 ug/mL penicillin G + 100 μg/mL streptomycin sulphate	Activation was done 3 h after fusion
5	7% ethanol	5 min	Hepes-modified TCM199	1.25 μg/mL CD + 10 μg/mL CYC	5 h	mSOFaa + 3 mg/mL BSA	
6	5 μM ionomycin	5 min		2 mM 6-DMAP	5 h		
7	5 μM calcimycin A23187	5 min	Hepes-modified TCM199 + 20% FBS	2 mM 6-DMAP	4 h	Hepes-modified TCM199 + 20% FBS	
8	7% ethanol	5 min	Emcare holding medium	1.25 μg/mL CD + 10 μg/mL CYC	5 h	mSOFaa + 10% FBS	
9	5μM ionomycin	5 min	TCM199 + 3% ECS+60 ug/mL penicillin G + 100 ug/mL streptomycin sulphate	2 mM 6-DMAP	3 h	TCM199 + 3% ECS+60 ug/mL penicillin G + 100 ug/mL streptomycin sulphate	Activation was done 3 h after fusion
10	5 μM ionomycin	5 min	TCM199 + 10% FBS	2 mM 6-DMAP	3–4 h	TCM199 + 10% FBS	

(Table 6) contd.....

Ref.	Acceleration of intra cellular Ca^{++}			Inhibition of MFP protein			Comment
	Treatment	Period	Medium	Treatment	Period	Medium	
11	10 µM calcium ionophore A23187	1.5–5 min	Hepes-modified TCM199 + 30 mg/mL Penicillin G + 50 mg/mL streptomycin + 40 mg/mL gentamycin	2 mM 6-DMAP + 5 µg/mLCB	4 h	Hepes-modified TCM199 + 30 mg/mL Penicillin G + 50 mg/mL streptomycin + 40 mg/mL gentamycin	Activation was done 2 h after fusion
12	5 µM ionomycin	4 min	SOFaa + 1 mg/mL fatty acid free (FAF) BSA or TCM199 + 2% FBS or G1+ 1 mg/mL FAF BSA	2 mM 6-DMAP	4 h	SOFaa + 30 mg/mL FAF BSA or G1+ 30 mg/mL FAF BSA	

1: Parnpai *et al.* [41]; 2: Srirattana *et al.* [93]; 3: Pandey *et al.* [94]; 4: Shi *et al.* [3]; 5: Suteevun *et al.* [95]; 6: Kitiyanant *et al.* [96]; 7: Shah *et al.* [61]; 8: Muenthaisong *et al.* [97]; 9: Huang *et al.* [87]; 10: Yang *et al.* [98]; 11: Wadhwa *et al.* [83]; 12: Simon *et al.* [52].

2.8. *In Vitro* Culture

A number of base culture media can support the development of reconstructed buffalo embryos *in vitro*. Base media commonly used for buffalo embryo culture include TCM199, mSOF, CR1aa, KRVCL50 and G1/G2 (Table **6**). These culture media generally require supplementation to support high embryo development. Serum (FCS, ECS), which is a complex undefined mixture of hormones, growth factors, vitamins and numerous other identified or non-identified factors [45], and BSA are routinely added to the IVC medium. Co-culture of reconstructed embryos with buffalo oviductal epithelial cells improves the *in vitro* culture system. Parnpai *et al.* [41] showed that reconstructed swamp buffalo embryos cultured in mSOF alone (cell free system) gave lower blastocyst rates than those co-cultured with bovine or buffalo oviductal epithelial cells. Furthermore, Simon *et al.* [45] showed that G1/G2, a commercially available sequential medium, increased the cleavage of cloned embryos compared to TCM-199 with oviduct epithelial cell co-culture and synthetic oviduct fluid. A representative photograph of cloned hatched buffalo blastocyst is given in Fig. (**6**), followed by born cloned buffalo calves (Fig. **7**).

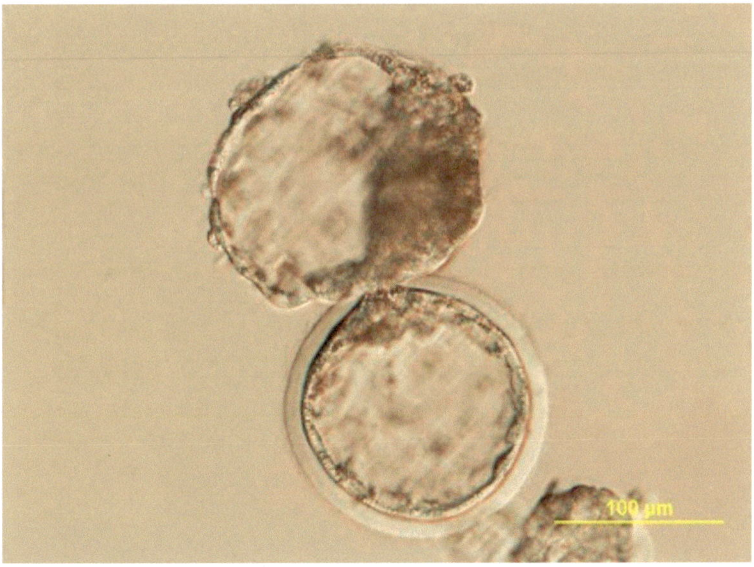

Fig. (6). Cloned swamp buffalo blastocyst. Photos from Parnpai, R (published data).

2.9. Hand-Made Cloning

The hand made cloning (HMC) technique is a simplified nuclear transfer process that does not require micromanipulators. The HMC technique fuses an enucleated matured oocyte, with a zona removed manually, and a single donor nucleus to develop a cloned embryo. The method was developed following the successful activation/*in vitro* fertilization of zona-free oocytes and *in vitro* culture of zona-removed embryos in different species (for review [53]). Tatham *et al.* [54] first produced cloned embryos by fusing zona-free enucleated oocytes and embryonic cell nuclei. They first positioned the metaphase II spindle for enucleation by centrifugation. Subsequently, a Percoll density gradient-centrifugation of oocytes deprived of the zona pellucida was performed. This produced the result of stretching the oocytes so that a cytoplast and metaphase II spindles were formed. Finally, the enucleated cytoplasts were aggregated with blastomere to produced cloned embryos. However, this method was unreliable and no calves were born after the transfer of cloned embryos.

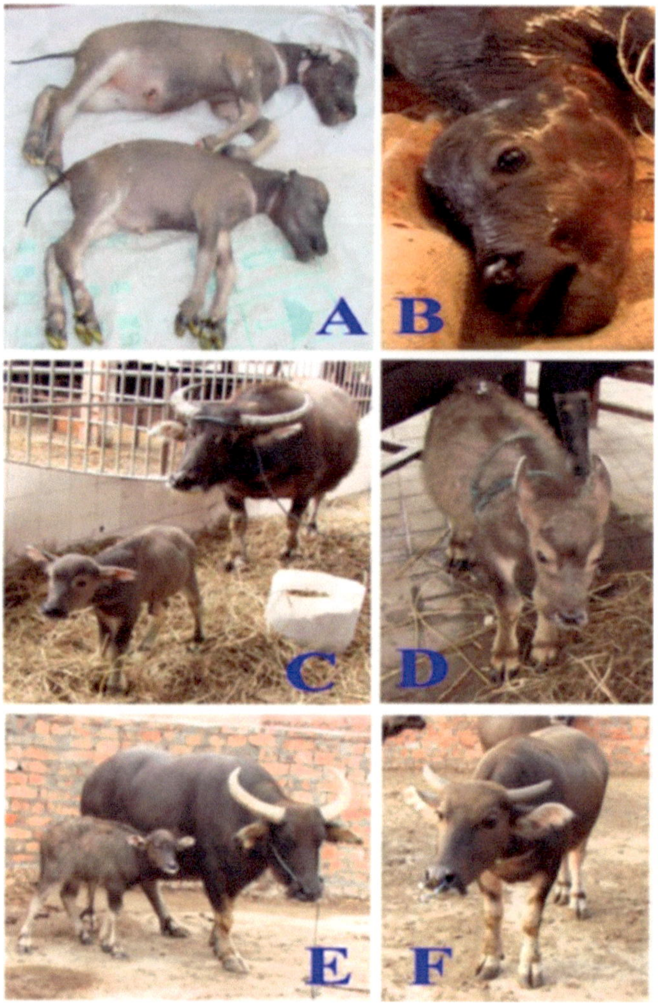

Fig. (7). Cloned buffalo calves derived from fetal fibroblasts and granulosa cells. **(A)** Premature twin cloned buffalo calves derived from fibroblasts of a fetus aborted on Day 300 of gestation. **(B)** Cloned buffalo calf (CB1) derived from fetal fibroblasts, delivered by cesarean section on Day 343 of gestation. **(C)** Cloned buffalo calf (CB2) derived from granulosa cells, delivered on Day 349 of gestation. **(D)** Cloned calf CB2 showing rough hairs on Day 14 after birth. **(E)** Cloned buffalo calf (CB3) derived from fetal fibroblasts, delivered on Day 338 of gestation. **(F)** Cloned calf CB3, still alive. Cited from Shi *et al.* [3], Biology of Reproduction 2007, 77: 285–291.

An efficient and reliable reconstruction process was established by Peura *et al.* [55], consisting in the fusion of two enucleated oocytes to one blastomere. Phytohaemagglutinin is used to glue the polar body to the oolemma, and thereafter a metal blade is employed to manually cut in half the zona-freed oocytes, in order to have the part linked to the polar body with approximately 25% of the total volume of the oocyte. This fragment is meant to be discarded, so that the remaining cytoplast presumptively free from the chromatin is used for fusion with an embryonic blastomere. More recently, Oback *et al.* [56] produced a live calf from HMC embryos where the enucleation of zona-free oocytes was performed with a simple blunt micropipette without bisectioning. The process of bovine HMC with chemically-assisted enucleation are shown in Fig. (**8**) and photographs of HMC buffalo embryos are given in Fig. (**9**).

2.10. Benefits and Drawbacks of Handmade Cloning

HMC is a more efficient and economical technique than the traditional micromanipulator-based approach. Live cloned offspring was delivered by this technique in cattle [57], pig [58], horse [49], sheep [59] and goat [60]. Recently, Shah *et al.* reported the successful pregnancy establishment of cloned buffalo embryos constructed by HMC in recipient uterus [61]. Vajta *et al.* [53] summarized the potential advantages and limitations of HMC.

2.10.1. Advantages

1. Equipment: less expensive than micromanipulation-based cloning.
2. Procedure: simple, rapid, easy to learn and perform.
3. Efficiency: reduced time and workforce required, and lower investment needed when confronted to traditional cloning. Rates of transferable embryos per oocyte are roughly similar, but in order to reconstruct one embryo, two oocytes are required.
4. Embryo cryopreservation: both in cattle and pigs healthy offspring has been produced.
5. Pregnancy and calving and/or farrowing rates: based on evidence and available data, such rates are similar to those produced using traditional cloning procedure (micromanipulation).
6. Special benefits: automation of the process is likely to be achieved in the future, in connection to the microchannel–microfluidics technology.

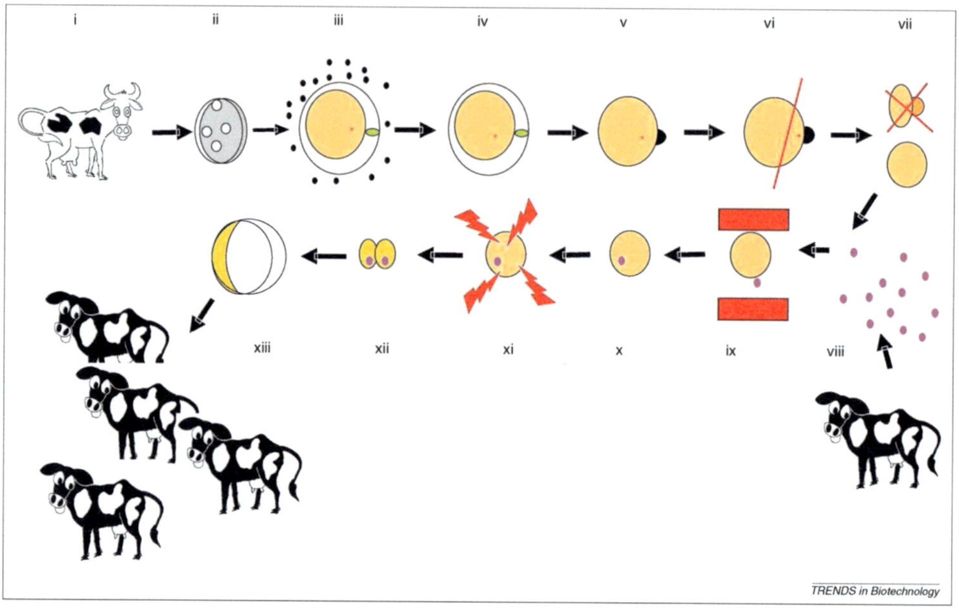

Fig. (8). The process of bovine HMC with chemically-assisted enucleation. Ovaries are collected from slaughtered animals **(i)** and transported to the laboratory, and oocytes are aspirated from the visible 2–7 mm diameter follicles **(ii)**. After 22 h of maturation, cumulus cells are removed by vortexing **(iii)**, denuded oocytes are incubated for a further 1 to 2 h in demecolcine **(iv)**, and the zonae pellucidae are digested by pronase **(v)**. Through the joint effect of demecolcine and pronase, an extrusion cone occurs on the surface, which serves as an orientation point for enucleation by hand with a disposable blade **(vi)**. Karyoplasts containing the chromatin are discarded, whereas cytoplasts are used as recipients **(vii)**. Somatic cells, derived from another cattle, calf or fetus, are cultured on monolayers **(viii)**. After trypsinization, these cells are individually attached to cytoplasts that have been briefly submerged into phytohemagglutinin to make their surface sticky, and then the pairs of cells are transferred to between the electrodes of a fusion chamber **(ix)**. After electrofusion, reconstructed embryos **(x)** are subjected to chemical activation **(xi)** and then cultured *in vitro* (xii) for one week. Emerging blastocysts **(xiii)** are transferred into recipients to produce animals (almost) identical to the somatic cell donor. (Cow cartoons drawn by Poul Maddox-Hyttel). Cited from Vajta [53], Trends in Biotechnology 2007, 25, 250–253.

2.10.2. Limitations

1. Possibility of attachment to each other of zona-free oocytes, cytoplasts and reconstructed embryos, and consequent loss of time or, occasionally, of products in the course of the mechanical separation process.
2. The lack of zona pellucida in the HMC embryos may allow disease transmission.
3. Some concerns may be generated by the resulting heteroplasmy, following use of three different sources of mitochondria, although up to date, no drawbacks or

misadvantages with regard to the above mentioned heteroplasmy, have been reported.

4. The need for two oocytes to produce a single cloned embryo may limit the use of this technique in species where a limited number of oocytes are available for manipulation.

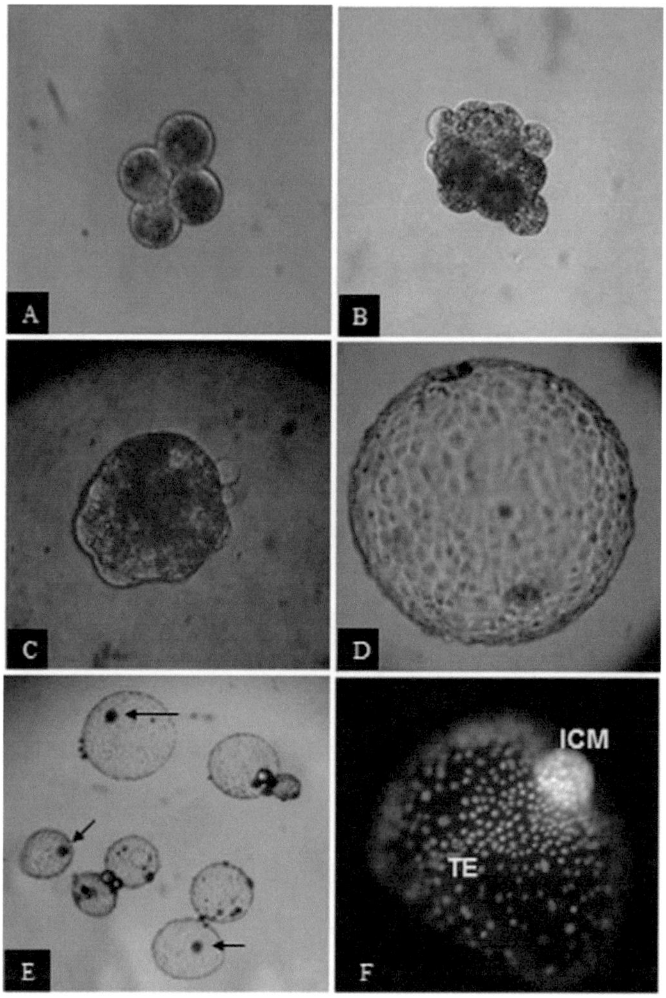

Fig. (9). HMC buffalo embryos at different stages of development: (**A**) four-cell, (**B**) 16-cell, (**C**) compact morula, (**D**) day 7 blastocyst, (**E**) group of blastocysts showing prominent ICM (arrow), and (**F**) single blastocyst after differential staining. ICM: inner cell mass and TE: trophectoderm cited from Shah *et al.* [99], Cloning and Stem Cells 2008, 10: 435-442.

3. INDUCED PLURIPOTENT STEM CELLS

The induced pluripotent stem cell (iPS) is a relatively new process of reprogramming adult somatic cells into pluripotent stem cells. IPS are the result of genetic reprogramming of adult cells into an embryonic stem cell-like state, characterized by the expression of genes and resulting factors needed to maintain the properties that define any embryonic stem cells. Yamanaka and his team [16] first reported the reprogramming of mouse embryonic and adult fibroblasts into iPS in 2006. They induced the expression of four key genes (OCT3/4, SOX2, KLF4 and c-MYC) using a retroviral system. The following year, they also reprogrammed adult human dermal fibroblasts into iPS using the same four factors [62]. IPS cells are functionally equivalent to embryonic stem cells in terms of their morphology, expression of pluripotent marker genes, telomerase activity and ability to form teratomas [16, 62]. Moreover, iPS cells are able to develop chimeras in mice through tetraploid complementation [17 - 19]. The work of Yamanaka and his team was confirmed by Thomson and colleagues at the University of Wisconsin [63], who expressed OCT4, SOX2, NANOG and LIN28 using a lentiviral system. The risks of retroviral and lentiviral transfection systems, which may trigger the expression of cancer-causing genes or oncogenes, limit the use of iPS cells in humans [62, 64]. To avoid such risks, adult cells can be reprogrammed using adenovirus [64] or plasmid [65]. Adenovirus does not recombine any of its own genes with those of the host. The efficiency of reprogramming is low when reprogramming is accomplished *via* plasmid. Page *et al.* [66] successfully reprogrammed adult human fibroblasts into stem cells without any genetic alteration of the adult cell. They showed that pluripotency can be induced by treating repeatedly the cells with some proteins that have been channeled into them *via* poly-arginine anchors. Protein-induced iPS in mouse was also reported by the Sheng Ding group. To date, there are no reports of adult buffalo cell reprogramming into iPS. Once established, buffalo somatic cell-derived iPS could be used as donor cells to clone buffalo or transgenic buffalo.

4. TRANSGENESIS

Transgenesis is the alteration of animal characteristics through the direct manipulation of the genetic makeup of an individual. A transgenic animal is characterized by containing within its genome some DNA of another different organism, introduced by means of laboratory manipulations [67]. The exogenous gene introduced into the genome of the transgenic animal is known as the transgene. The transgene is transmitted to offspring. The universality of the genetic code allows the transgene to function in the transgenic animal, meaning that the same protein will be specified by that specific DNA sequence in any organism. A number of taken laboratory actions can ease the process of transgenesis, such as liposomes, plasmid vectors, viral vectors, pronuclear injection, protoplast fusion and ballistic DNA injection. The first transgenic mouse was produced in the early 1980s. Thereafter, extensive studies were carried out on mice transgenesis. Three basic methods of inserting transgenes are widely used in the production of transgenic animals, including pronuclear microinjection [68], retrovirus-mediated gene transfer [69] and embryonic stem cell-mediated gene transfer [70]. However, these methods are less efficient for farm animals. Since the production of Polly, the transgenic sheep [8], the SCNT technique is commonly used for the production of transgenic farm animals. Two main procedures are involved in the production of transgenic animals by SCNT: i) introducing DNA into somatic cells and then selecting the ones that have properly incorporated the transgene, or ii) using transgenic donor cells within the cloning process to produce transgenic embryos. In this process, cultured cells are genetically modified *in vitro* by liposomes or electroporation. Thereafter, a modified cell is inserted into an enucleated oocyte and fused to the recipient cytoplasm. Transfection *in vitro* of somatic cells (often fibroblast cells) can be achieved by using different procedures such as use of liposomes or electroporation. Thereafter the same presumed transfected cells are screened for gene targeting and then transferred into enucleated oocytes. Fusion of the couplets is then accomplished by use of electric pulses, following activation and subsequent progression of *in vitro* or *in vivo* development. Finally, developed preimplantation embryos are then transferred into recipients until birth of offspring that will carry the mutations from the gene-targeted somatic cells [71]. Nuclear transfer technology has been used to create transgenic animals in a number of different species including sheep [8], goats [9], cows [13, 72], pigs [73] and mice [74].

4.1. Methods for Production of Transgenic Animals

4.1.1. Pronuclear Microinjection

In this method, multiple copies of the gene construct (a single gene or a combination of genes) are directly microinjected into the male pronucleus of a fertilized egg. The reconstructed eggs are cultured *in vitro* up to the blastocyst stage and then transferred into the uterus of recipient animals for development of the embryos. This process allows random insertion of transgenes into the host genome. This method has been successfully applied in mouse, rats, rabbit, sheep, pigs, cattle, birds and fish. However, transgene expression patterns and uncertain gene transmission through the germ line preclude widespread application of this technology [75].

4.1.2. Retrovirus-Mediated Gene Transfer

In this method, the transgene is inserted into the host genome using a carrier or vector. The most widely used vectors are viruses or plasmids. Retroviruses are commonly used in transgenic animal production for transferring target genes into the host genome. This method produces chimera, which requires outbreeding to obtain pure transgenic animals. Retrovirus mediated gene transfer were done in mice and human fibroblast cells [76].

4.1.3. Embryonic Stem Cell-Mediated Gene Transfer

In this method, a stem cell line is established from the inner cell mass (ICM) of blastocysts. Embryonic stem cells are transfected with the desired gene constructs by homologous recombination and then inserted into blastocyst stage embryos. The blastocysts develop into live transgenic animals once transferred into the recipient uterus. The offspring are chimera and require outbreeding to obtain a pure transgenic line. For example, transgenic mice carrying neomycin phosphotransferase gene were generated from embryonic stem cell derived from blastocyst injected with genetically modified cell for the target gene [70]. The main feature of this method is that genetically modified cells can be screened before reintroducing the embryonic stem cells into the animals.

4.2. Advantages of Scnt in Transgenic Animal Production

Bosch *et al.* [77] summarized the potential advantages of SCNT over other methods of transgenic animal production.

1. SCNT allows the production of transgenic animals with the desired sex. The sex of the animal depends on the source of the donor material (*i.e.*, male or female tissue). The efficiency and effectiveness of transgenesis will increase dramatically if we can produce animals with a desired sex. For example, the production of a specific human protein in cow milk requires the production of transgenic cows rather than bulls.
2. Many transgenic cells that can be later frozen and stored for long periods of time, are produced starting from few donor cells. As a result, many cloned transgenic animals can be produced when SCNT is employed in conjunction to the use of transgenic donor cells.
3. SCNT allows 100% accuracy in the production of transgenic animals. Molecular technology and its various approaches such as PCR, Southern blot analysis, Western blot analysis and Fluorescent *in situ* Hybridization (FISH), can be used to test both transgene structure and expression, prior to NT procedure and embryo transfer.
4. Variations among animals in levels of transgene expression are decreased when SCNT is employed. In addition, whenever a clonal population of transgenic cells is used, the same transgene insertion site for each clone is guaranteed.
5. Transgenes can be inserted into animals with specific genetic background, like a good dairy milk producer characterized by a level above average of protein content, could be used and considered the genetic background on which the transgene is inserted.
6. SCNT allows both random and targeted insertion of DNA by homologous recombination. Targeted insertion of DNA enables the modulation of specific gene expression as well as the creation of gene knockouts.

4.3. Risk of Transgenic Animal Production

Van Reenen *et al.* [78] reviewed the risk factors related to the welfare of transgenic animals.

1. Possibility to loose host gene function (insertional mutation) whenever a transgene is integrated within an endogenous gene.
2. Inappropriate transgene expression.
3. Actions of foreign biologically active proteins, derived from inserted transgene, to the host organism.
4. Larger incidence of altered and abnormal aspects related to parturition (difficulty), embryo and fetal development (losses and abortions), birth of debilitated offspring or carrying anatomical defects (Large Offspring Syndrome), when newly developed reproductive technologies are applied and employed with the aim of producing transgenic farm animals.

4.4. Application of Transgenesis

4.4.1. Medicine

4.4.1.1. Gene Therapy

Success of transgenic animal production has enabled researchers to correct genetic diseases of human and animals. A defective gene can be replaced by inserting a normal functional copy of the same gene into the genome carrying the defective gene. For example, the A. I. Virtanen Institute in Finland produced transgenic cattle having the gene coding for the erythropoietin that promote the growth of red cells in humans [79].

4.4.1.2. Xenotransplantation

Transgenic technology can be used to develop animals carrying human organs, for example heart, liver or kidney. Transgenic pigs are considered to be a good source of transplant organs. However, the problem of donor rejection caused by a protein needs to be solved.

4.4.1.3. Pharmaceuticals

Animals can be used as bioreactors to produce proteins. Genes for desired proteins are introduced *via* transgenesis to target cells. For example, transgenic cows and goats produce the recombinant human protein AT III, which prevents blood clotting, in their milk.

4.4.2. Agricultural

4.4.2.1. Breeding

The gene for a desired character can be transferred into the genome of an animal to achieve higher productivity. Transgenesis can allow the rapid improvement of farm animals compared to conventional selective breeding, which has been practiced for hundreds of years. The scope of transgenesis in animal breeding includes the following: faster growth rate, high milk yield, improved food-conversion rates; increased muscle mass; improved wool quality; and improved nutritional quality or appeal (reviewed by [80]).

4.4.2.2. Disease Resistance

The development of farm animals capable of resisting disease outbreaks or preventing disease spread will increase return rates in animal farming. Every year, large numbers of farm animals die in disease outbreak or are sacrificed to control outbreak; for example, in 2010, thousands of cattle and pigs were killed in the Republic of Korea to prevent foot and mouth disease. Therefore, transgenesis may be used to produce animals resistant to common diseases, such as mastitis [81]. However, the challenge is that most agriculturally relevant traits are complex and controlled by more than one gene [82].

4.4.2.3. Quality

Human beings are becoming more concerned about the quality of foods of animal origin. For example, the demand for low fat milk, lean meat, cholesterol free milk, and eggs with high quality protein is increasing. Transgenesis can allow the satisfaction of consumer demands by genetically modifying farm animals.

4.4.3. Industrial

Transgenesis may be used for the production of industrial products for human wellbeing. For example, Nexia Biotechnologies of Canada developed a high-strength based fiber material made of the recombinant spider silk-like protein

MaSpI or MaSpII, which was extracted from the milk of transgenic goats (biosteel). The technique may provide light weight, strong and versatile materials for a variety of medical and industrial applications, including bullet proof vests and in suture silk for stitching wounds.

4.5. Transgenesis in Buffalo

The first transgenic cloned buffalo embryos were produced in 2009 by the transfer of buffalo oviductal epithelial cell (BOEC) nuclei transfected with enhanced green fluorescent protein (EGFP) into enucleated oocytes [83]. The EGFP transgene was inserted into the BOEC genome through electroporation. Embryonic germ cells were derived from primordial germ cells isolated from fetuses [84]. Embryonic stem (ES) cell lines derived from the inner cell mass (ICM) of blastocysts were reported in buffalo [85 - 88]. Both of these cell lines are pluripotent in nature, maintain an undifferentiated state in culture, can differentiate into various types of cells [89, 90], and contribute to different tissues of healthy chimeric animals born after blastocyst injection or morula aggregation [91, 92]. Recently, Huang *et al.* [87] showed that transgenic cloned buffalo chimera could be produced by transferring embryonic germ (EG)-like cells expressing the green fluorescent protein gene into *in vitro*-derived buffalo blastocysts. In this study, the embryonic germ-like cell was transfected with plasmid (pCE-EGFP-IRES-NeodNdB) using Lipofectamine™2000. They injected ten to fifteen EGFP-positives, EG-like cells into the perivitelline space of embryos at the 8- to 16-cell stage. The reconstructed embryos were then cultured *in vitro* until the blastocyst stage. However, they did not transfer these embryos into any recipient animals. These developments suggest that transgenesis may be achievable in buffalo.

CONCLUSION

The number of usable immature oocytes available per ovary is limiting the application of reproductive biotechnology tools in the buffalo species. Different oocyte aspiration methods, *in vitro* oocyte maturation protocols, enucleation and nuclear transfer protocols and *in vitro* embryo culture system were adapted for production of buffalo cloned offspring. The SCNT are also being used for transgenic buffalo production. However, the success remained up to transgenic blastocyst development. Further development in the cloning and transgenesis in buffalo species is important for exploiting beneficial use of SCNT in the fields of medicine, agriculture and industry.

CONFLICT OF INTEREST

The authors confirm that they have no conflict of interest to declare for this publication.

ACKNOWLEDGEMENTS

Declared none.

REFERENCES

[1] Drost M. Bubaline *versus* bovine reproduction. Theriogenology 2007; 68(3): 447-9. [http://dx.doi.org/10.1016/j.theriogenology.2007.04.012] [PMID: 17482253]

[2] Drost M. Advanced reproductive technology in the water buffalo. Theriogenology 2007; 68(3): 450-3. [http://dx.doi.org/10.1016/j.theriogenology.2007.04.013] [PMID: 17481722]

[3] Shi D, Lu F, Wei Y, *et al.* Buffalos (*Bubalus bubalis*) cloned by nuclear transfer of somatic cells. Biol Reprod 2007; 77(2): 285-91. [http://dx.doi.org/10.1095/biolreprod.107.060210] [PMID: 17475931]

[4] Madan ML, Singla SK, Jailkhani S, Ambrose JD. *In vitro* fertilization and birth of first ever IVF buffalo calf. Proc Third World Buffalo Congress. Varna, Bulgaria. 1991; pp. 11-7.

[5] Willadsen SM. A method for culture of micromanipulated sheep embryos and its use to produce monozygotic twins. Nature 1979; 277(5694): 298-300. [http://dx.doi.org/10.1038/277298a0] [PMID: 570249]

[6] Ozil JP, Heyman Y, Renard JP. Production of monozygotic twins by micromanipulation and cervical transfer in the cow. Vet Rec 1982; 110(6): 126-7. [http://dx.doi.org/10.1136/vr.110.6.126] [PMID: 6892266]

[7] Wilmut I, Schnieke AE, McWhir J, Kind AJ, Campbell KH. Viable offspring derived from fetal and adult mammalian cells. Nature 1997; 385(6619): 810-3. [http://dx.doi.org/10.1038/385810a0] [PMID: 9039911]

[8] Schnieke AE, Kind AJ, Ritchie WA, *et al.* Human factor IX transgenic sheep produced by transfer of nuclei from transfected fetal fibroblasts. Science 1997; 278(5346): 2130-3. [http://dx.doi.org/10.1126/science.278.5346.2130] [PMID: 9405350]

[9] Keefer CL, Baldassarre H, Keyston R, *et al.* Generation of dwarf goat (*Capra hircus*) clones following nuclear transfer with transfected and nontransfected fetal fibroblasts and *in vitro*-matured oocytes. Biol Reprod 2001; 64(3): 849-56.

[http://dx.doi.org/10.1095/biolreprod64.3.849] [PMID: 11207200]

[10] Park KW, Cheong HT, Lai L, *et al.* Production of nuclear transfer-derived swine that express the enhanced green fluorescent protein. Anim Biotechnol 2001; 12(2): 173-81.
[http://dx.doi.org/10.1081/ABIO-100108344] [PMID: 11808633]

[11] Lai L, Park KW, Cheong HT, *et al.* Transgenic pig expressing the enhanced green fluorescent protein produced by nuclear transfer using colchicine-treated fibroblasts as donor cells. Mol Reprod Dev 2002; 62(3): 300-6.
[http://dx.doi.org/10.1002/mrd.10146] [PMID: 12112592]

[12] Lai L, Prather RS. Creating genetically modified pigs by using nuclear transfer. Reprod Biol Endocrinol 2003; 1: 82.
[http://dx.doi.org/10.1186/1477-7827-1-82] [PMID: 14613542]

[13] Cibelli JB, Stice SL, Golueke PJ, *et al.* Cloned transgenic calves produced from nonquiescent fetal fibroblasts. Science 1998; 280(5367): 1256-8.
[http://dx.doi.org/10.1126/science.280.5367.1256] [PMID: 9596577]

[14] Brink MF, Bishop MD, Pieper FR. Developing efficient strategies for the generation of transgenic cattle which produce biopharmaceuticals in milk. Theriogenology 2000; 53(1): 139-48.
[http://dx.doi.org/10.1016/S0093-691X(99)00247-2] [PMID: 10735069]

[15] Brophy B, Smolenski G, Wheeler T, Wells D, LHuillier P, Laible G. Cloned transgenic cattle produce milk with higher levels of beta-casein and kappa-casein. Nat Biotechnol 2003; 21(2): 157-62.
[http://dx.doi.org/10.1038/nbt783] [PMID: 12548290]

[16] Takahashi K, Yamanaka S. Induction of pluripotent stem cells from mouse embryonic and adult fibroblast cultures by defined factors. Cell 2006; 126(4): 663-76.
[http://dx.doi.org/10.1016/j.cell.2006.07.024] [PMID: 16904174]

[17] Okita K, Ichisaka T, Yamanaka S. Generation of germline-competent induced pluripotent stem cells. Nature 2007; 448(7151): 313-7.
[http://dx.doi.org/10.1038/nature05934] [PMID: 17554338]

[18] Kang L, Wang J, Zhang Y, Kou Z, Gao S. iPS cells can support full-term development of tetraploid blastocyst-complemented embryos. Cell Stem Cell 2009; 5(2): 135-8.
[http://dx.doi.org/10.1016/j.stem.2009.07.001] [PMID: 19631602]

[19] Zhao XY, Li W, Lv Z, *et al.* iPS cells produce viable mice through tetraploid complementation. Nature 2009; 461(7260): 86-90.
[http://dx.doi.org/10.1038/nature08267] [PMID: 19672241]

[20] Bousquet D, Blondin P. Potential uses of cloning in breeding schemes: dairy cattle. Cloning Stem Cells 2004; 6(2): 190-7.
[http://dx.doi.org/10.1089/1536230041372373] [PMID: 15268795]

[21] Agca Y, Critser JK. Assisted Reproductive Technologies and Genetic modifications in Rats. In: Weisbroth SH, Franklin CL, Eds. The Laboratory Rat Suckow, M A. MA, USA: Elsevier Academic Press Burlington 2003; pp. 165-90.

[22] Wilmut I, Beaujean N, de Sousa PA, *et al.* Somatic cell nuclear transfer. Nature 2002; 419(6907): 583-6.

[http://dx.doi.org/10.1038/nature01079] [PMID: 12374931]

[23] Wolf DP, Mitalipov S, Norgren RB Jr. Nuclear transfer technology in mammalian cloning. Arch Med Res 2001; 32(6): 609-13.
[http://dx.doi.org/10.1016/S0188-4409(01)00324-1] [PMID: 11750737]

[24] Totey SM, Singh G, Taneja M, Pawshe CH, Talwar GP. *In vitro* maturation, fertilization and development of follicular oocytes from buffalo (*Bubalus bubalis*). J Reprod Fertil 1992; 95(2): 597-607.
[http://dx.doi.org/10.1530/jrf.0.0950597] [PMID: 1518014]

[25] Madan ML, Chauhan MS, Singla SK, Manik RS. Pregnancies established from water buffalo (*Bubalus bubalis*) blastocysts derived from *in vitro* matured, *in vitro* fertilized oocytes and co-cultured with cumulus and oviductal cells. Theriogenology 1994; 42(4): 591-600.
[http://dx.doi.org/10.1016/0093-691X(94)90376-T] [PMID: 16727565]

[26] Das GK, Jain GC, Solanki VS, Tripathi VN. Efficacy of various collection methods for oocyte retrieval in buffalo. Theriogenology 1996; 46: 1403-11.
[http://dx.doi.org/10.1016/S0093-691X(96)00319-6]

[27] Samad HA, Khan IQ, Rehman NU, Ahmad N. The recovery, *in vitro* maturation and fertilization of nili-ravi buffalo follicular oocytes. Asian-Aust J Anim Sci 1998; 11: 491-7.

[28] Gasparrini B, Neglia G, Palo RD, Campanile G, Zicarelli L. Effect of cysteamine during *in vitro* maturation on buffalo embryo development. Theriogenology 2000; 54(9): 1537-42.
[http://dx.doi.org/10.1016/S0093-691X(00)00473-8] [PMID: 11191875]

[29] Kumar A, Solanki VS, Jindal SK, Tripathi VN, Jain GC. Oocyte retrieval and histological studies of follicular population in buffalo ovaries. Anim Reprod Sci 1997; 47(3): 189-95.
[http://dx.doi.org/10.1016/S0378-4320(96)01588-6] [PMID: 9329860]

[30] Boni R, Rovelli S, Gasparrini B, Langella M, Zicarelli L. *In vitro* production of buffalo embryos in chemically defined medium. Buffalo J 1999; 15: 115-20.

[31] Galli C, Duci R, Crotti G, Lazarri G. Embryo production by ovum pick up in water buffalo. Theriogenology 1998; 49: 400.
[http://dx.doi.org/10.1016/S0093-691X(98)90753-1]

[32] Vittoria A. Anatomy of the female genital tract in the buffalo. Proceedings of the 3rd course on biotechnology of reproduction in buffaloes. 15-20.

[33] Singh R, Majundar AC. Chronological changes of buffalo follicular oocytes maturation *in vitro*. Indian J Anim Sci 1992; 62: 205-9.

[34] Chauhan MS, Singla SK, Palta P, Manik RS, Madan ML. *In vitro* maturation and fertilization, and subsequent development of buffalo (*Bubalus bubalis*) embryos: effects of oocyte quality and type of serum. Reprod Fertil Dev 1998; 10(2): 173-7.
[http://dx.doi.org/10.1071/R97080] [PMID: 9801269]

[35] Westhusin ME, Burghardt RC, Ruglia JN, *et al.* Potential for cloning dogs. J Reprod Fertil Suppl 2001; 57: 287-93.
[PMID: 11787163]

[36] Amano T, Kato Y, Tsunoda Y. Full-term development of enucleated mouse oocytes fused with embryonic stem cells from different cell lines. Reproduction 2001; 121(5): 729-33. [http://dx.doi.org/10.1530/rep.0.1210729] [PMID: 11427160]

[37] Kühholzer B, Hawley RJ, Lai L, Kolber-Simonds D, Prather RS. Clonal lines of transgenic fibroblast cells derived from the same fetus result in different development when used for nuclear transfer in pigs. Biol Reprod 2001; 64(6): 1695-8. [http://dx.doi.org/10.1095/biolreprod64.6.1695] [PMID: 11369597]

[38] Dinnyés A, De Sousa P, King T, Wilmut I. Somatic cell nuclear transfer: recent progress and challenges. Cloning Stem Cells 2002; 4(1): 81-90. [http://dx.doi.org/10.1089/153623002753632075] [PMID: 12006159]

[39] Willadsen SM. Nuclear transplantation in sheep embryos. Nature 1986; 320(6057): 63-5. [http://dx.doi.org/10.1038/320063a0] [PMID: 3951549]

[40] Bansal ML, Gupta N, Yadav AS, Ahlawat SP, Gupta SC. Karyological profile of nuclear donor skin fibroblast cell lines at different passages. Indian J Anim Sci 2010; 80: 570-1.

[41] Parnpai R, Tasripoo K, Kamonpatana M. Development of cloned swamp buffalo embryos derived from fetal fibroblasts: comparison *in vitro* cultured with or without buffalo and cattle epithelial cells. Buffalo Journal 1999; 15: 371-84.

[42] Heyman Y, Chavatte-Palmer P, LeBourhis D, Camous S, Vignon X, Renard JP. Frequency and occurrence of late-gestation losses from cattle cloned embryos. Biol Reprod 2002; 66(1): 6-13. [http://dx.doi.org/10.1095/biolreprod66.1.6] [PMID: 11751257]

[43] Yanagimachi R. Cloning: experience from the mouse and other animals. Mol Cell Endocrinol 2002; 187(1-2): 241-8. [http://dx.doi.org/10.1016/S0303-7207(01)00697-9] [PMID: 11988333]

[44] Bonk AJ, Cheong HT, Li R, *et al.* Correlation of developmental differences of nuclear transfer embryos cells to the methylation profiles of nuclear transfer donor cells in Swine. Epigenetics 2007; 2(3): 179-86. [http://dx.doi.org/10.4161/epi.2.3.4844] [PMID: 17965590]

[45] Campbell KH, Fisher P, Chen WC, *et al.* Somatic cell nuclear transfer: Past, present and future perspectives. Theriogenology 2007; 68 (Suppl. 1): S214-31. [http://dx.doi.org/10.1016/j.theriogenology.2007.05.059] [PMID: 17610946]

[46] Gasparrini B, De Rosa A, Attanasio L, *et al.* Influence of the duration of *in vitro* maturation and gamete co-incubation on the efficiency of *in vitro* embryo development in Italian Mediterranean buffalo (Bubalus bubalis). Anim Reprod Sci 2008; 105(3-4): 354-64. [http://dx.doi.org/10.1016/j.anireprosci.2007.03.022] [PMID: 17481834]

[47] Laowtammathron C, Lorthongpanich C, Ketudat-Cairns M, Hochi S, Parnpai R. Factors affecting cryosurvival of nuclear-transferred bovine and swamp buffalo blastocysts: effects of hatching stage, linoleic acid-albumin in IVC medium and Ficoll supplementation to vitrification solution. Theriogenology 2005; 64(5): 1185-96. [http://dx.doi.org/10.1016/j.theriogenology.2005.02.001] [PMID: 16125561]

[48] Smith LC. Membrane and intracellular effects of ultraviolet irradiation with Hoechst 33342 on bovine

secondary oocytes matured *in vitro*. J Reprod Fertil 1993; 99(1): 39-44. [http://dx.doi.org/10.1530/jrf.0.0990039] [PMID: 8283450]

[49] Lagutina I, Lazzari G, Duchi R, *et al.* Somatic cell nuclear transfer in horses: effect of oocyte morphology, embryo reconstruction method and donor cell type. Reproduction 2005; 130(4): 559-67. [http://dx.doi.org/10.1530/rep.1.00772] [PMID: 16183874]

[50] Polejaeva IA, Campbell KH. New advances in somatic cell nuclear transfer: application in transgenesis. Theriogenology 2000; 53(1): 117-26. [http://dx.doi.org/10.1016/S0093-691X(99)00245-9] [PMID: 10735067]

[51] Schurmann A, Wells DN, Oback B. Early zygotes are suitable recipients for bovine somatic nuclear transfer and result in cloned offspring. Reproduction 2006; 132(6): 839-48. [http://dx.doi.org/10.1530/REP-06-0054] [PMID: 17127744]

[52] Simon L, Veerapandian C, Balasubramanian S, Subramanian A. Somatic cell nuclear transfer in buffalos: effect of the fusion and activation protocols and embryo culture system on preimplantation embryo development. Reprod Fertil Dev 2006; 18(4): 439-45. [http://dx.doi.org/10.1071/RD05079] [PMID: 16737637]

[53] Vajta G. Handmade cloning: the future way of nuclear transfer? Trends Biotechnol 2007; 25(6): 250-3. [http://dx.doi.org/10.1016/j.tibtech.2007.04.004] [PMID: 17434218]

[54] Tatham BG, Dowsing AT, Trounson AO. Enucleation by centrifugation of *in vitro*-matured bovine oocytes for use in nuclear transfer. Biol Reprod 1995; 53(5): 1088-94. [http://dx.doi.org/10.1095/biolreprod53.5.1088] [PMID: 8527512]

[55] Peura TT, Lewis IM, Trounson AO. The effect of recipient oocyte volume on nuclear transfer in cattle. Mol Reprod Dev 1998; 50(2): 185-91. [http://dx.doi.org/10.1002/(SICI)1098-2795(199806)50:2<185::AID-MRD9>3.0.CO;2-G] [PMID: 9590535]

[56] Oback B, Wiersema AT, Gaynor P, *et al.* Cloned cattle derived from a novel zona-free embryo reconstruction system. Cloning Stem Cells 2003; 5(1): 3-12. [http://dx.doi.org/10.1089/153623003321512111] [PMID: 12713696]

[57] Tecirlioglu RT, French AJ, Lewis IM, *et al.* Birth of a cloned calf derived from a vitrified hand-made cloned embryo. Reprod Fertil Dev 2003; 15(7-8): 361-6. [http://dx.doi.org/10.1071/RD03052] [PMID: 14984692]

[58] Du Y, Kragh PM, Zhang Y, *et al.* Piglets born from handmade cloning, an innovative cloning method without micromanipulation. Theriogenology 2007; 68(8): 1104-10. [http://dx.doi.org/10.1016/j.theriogenology.2007.07.021] [PMID: 17889304]

[59] Ritchie WA, Taylor JE, Gardner JO, *et al.* Live lambs born from zona-pellucida denuded embryos. Cloning Stem Cells 2005; 7(3): 178-82. [http://dx.doi.org/10.1089/clo.2005.7.178] [PMID: 16176127]

[60] Akshey YS, Malakar D, De AK, *et al.* Hand-made cloned goat (*Capra hircus*) embryos—a comparison of different donor cells and culture systems. Cell Reprogram 2010; 12(5): 581-8. [http://dx.doi.org/10.1089/cell.2009.0120] [PMID: 20818994]

[61] Shah RA, George A, Singh MK, *et al.* Pregnancies established from handmade cloned blastocysts

reconstructed using skin fibroblasts in buffalo (*Bubalus bubalis*). Theriogenology 2009; 71(8): 1215-9. [http://dx.doi.org/10.1016/j.theriogenology.2008.10.004] [PMID: 19168209]

[62] Takahashi K, Tanabe K, Ohnuki M, *et al.* Induction of pluripotent stem cells from adult human fibroblasts by defined factors. Cell 2007; 131(5): 861-72. [http://dx.doi.org/10.1016/j.cell.2007.11.019] [PMID: 18035408]

[63] Yu J, Vodyanik MA, Smuga-Otto K, *et al.* Induced pluripotent stem cell lines derived from human somatic cells. Science 2007; 318(5858): 1917-20. [http://dx.doi.org/10.1126/science.1151526] [PMID: 18029452]

[64] Stadtfeld M, Nagaya M, Utikal J, Weir G, Hochedlinger K. Induced pluripotent stem cells generated without viral integration. Science 2008; 322(5903): 945-9. [http://dx.doi.org/10.1126/science.1162494] [PMID: 18818365]

[65] Okita K, Nakagawa M, Hyenjong H, Ichisaka T, Yamanaka S. Generation of mouse induced pluripotent stem cells without viral vectors. Science 2008; 322(5903): 949-53. [http://dx.doi.org/10.1126/science.1164270] [PMID: 18845712]

[66] Page RL, Ambady S, Holmes WF, *et al.* Induction of stem cell gene expression in adult human fibroblasts without transgenes. Cloning Stem Cells 2009; 11(3): 417-26. [http://dx.doi.org/10.1089/clo.2009.0015] [PMID: 19622035]

[67] Jacenko O. Strategis in generating transgenic mammalis. In: R Tuan (ed) Methods in Molecular Biology vol 60 Recombinant Gene expression protocols Humana Press, Totowa, NJ. 1997; 11: pp. 399-424.

[68] Gordon JW, Ruddle FH. Integration and stable germ line transmission of genes injected into mouse pronuclei. Science 1981; 214(4526): 1244-6. [http://dx.doi.org/10.1126/science.6272397] [PMID: 6272397]

[69] Jaenisch R. Germ line integration and Mendelian transmission of the exogenous Moloney leukemia virus. Proc Natl Acad Sci USA 1976; 73(4): 1260-4. [http://dx.doi.org/10.1073/pnas.73.4.1260] [PMID: 1063407]

[70] Gossler A, Doetschman T, Korn R, Serfling E, Kemler R. Transgenesis by means of blastocyst-derived embryonic stem cell lines. Proc Natl Acad Sci USA 1986; 83(23): 9065-9. [http://dx.doi.org/10.1073/pnas.83.23.9065] [PMID: 3024164]

[71] Wang B, Zhou J. Specific genetic modifications of domestic animals by gene targeting and animal cloning. Reprod Biol Endocrinol 2003; 1: 103. [http://dx.doi.org/10.1186/1477-7827-1-103] [PMID: 14614774]

[72] Bordignon V, Keyston R, Lazaris A, *et al.* Transgene expression of green fluorescent protein and germ line transmission in cloned calves derived from *in vitro*-transfected somatic cells. Biol Reprod 2003; 68(6): 2013-23. [http://dx.doi.org/10.1095/biolreprod.102.010066] [PMID: 12606490]

[73] Polejaeva IA, Chen SH, Vaught TD, *et al.* Cloned pigs produced by nuclear transfer from adult somatic cells. Nature 2000; 407(6800): 86-90. [http://dx.doi.org/10.1038/35024082] [PMID: 10993078]

[74] Rideout WM III, Wakayama T, Wutz A, *et al.* Generation of mice from wild-type and targeted ES

cells by nuclear cloning. Nat Genet 2000; 24(2): 109-10.
[http://dx.doi.org/10.1038/72753] [PMID: 10655052]

[75] Jang G, Bhuiyan MM, Jeon HY, *et al.* An approach for producing transgenic cloned cows by nuclear transfer of cells transfected with human alpha 1-antitrypsin gene. Theriogenology 2006; 65(9): 1800-12.
[http://dx.doi.org/10.1016/j.theriogenology.2005.10.014] [PMID: 16303172]

[76] Palmer TD, Hock RA, Osborne WR, Miller AD. Efficient retrovirus-mediated transfer and expression of a human adenosine deaminase gene in diploid skin fibroblasts from an adenosine deaminase-deficient human. Proc Natl Acad Sci USA 1987; 84(4): 1055-9.
[http://dx.doi.org/10.1073/pnas.84.4.1055] [PMID: 3493485]

[77] Bosch P, Hodges CA, Stice SL. Generation of transgenic livestock by somatic cell nuclear transfer. Biotecnol Apl 2004; 21: 128-36.

[78] Van Reenen CG, Meuwissen TH, Hopster H, Oldenbroek K, Kruip TH, Blokhuis HJ. Transgenesis may affect farm animal welfare: a case for systematic risk assessment. J Anim Sci 2001; 79(7): 1763-79.
[http://dx.doi.org/10.2527/2001.7971763x] [PMID: 11465364]

[79] Margawati ET. Transgenic animals: Their benefits to human welfare. http://wwwactionbioscienceorg/biotech/margawatihtml 2003.

[80] Vajta G, Gjerris M. Science and technology of farm animal cloning: state of the art. Anim Reprod Sci 2006; 92(3-4): 211-30.
[http://dx.doi.org/10.1016/j.anireprosci.2005.12.001] [PMID: 16406426]

[81] Wall RJ, Powell AM, Paape MJ, *et al.* Genetically enhanced cows resist intramammary *Staphylococcus aureus* infection. Nat Biotechnol 2005; 23(4): 445-51.
[http://dx.doi.org/10.1038/nbt1078] [PMID: 15806099]

[82] Clark J, Whitelaw B. A future for transgenic livestock. Nat Rev Genet 2003; 4(10): 825-33.
[http://dx.doi.org/10.1038/nrg1183] [PMID: 14526378]

[83] Wadhwa N, Kunj N, Tiwari S, Saraiya M, Majumdar SS. Optimization of embryo culture conditions for increasing efficiency of cloning in buffalo (*Bubalus bubalis*) and generation of transgenic embryos *via* cloning. Cloning Stem Cells 2009; 11(3): 387-95.
[http://dx.doi.org/10.1089/clo.2009.0003] [PMID: 19594388]

[84] Resnick JL, Bixler LS, Cheng L, Donovan PJ. Long-term proliferation of mouse primordial germ cells in culture. Nature 1992; 359(6395): 550-1.
[http://dx.doi.org/10.1038/359550a0] [PMID: 1383830]

[85] Verma V, Gautam SK, Singh B, *et al.* Isolation and characterization of embryonic stem cell-like cells from *in vitro*-produced buffalo (*Bubalus bubalis*) embryos. Mol Reprod Dev 2007; 74(4): 520-9.
[http://dx.doi.org/10.1002/mrd.20645] [PMID: 17034054]

[86] Anand T, Kumar D, Singh MK, *et al.* Buffalo (*Bubalus bubalis*) embryonic stem cell-like cells and preimplantation embryos exhibit comparable expression of pluripotency-related antigens. Reprod Domest Anim 2011; 46(1): 50-8.
[http://dx.doi.org/10.1111/j.1439-0531.2009.01564.x] [PMID: 20042025]

[87] Huang B, Li T, Wang XL, *et al.* Generation and characterization of embryonic stem-like cell lines derived from *in vitro* fertilization Buffalo (*Bubalus bubalis*) embryos. Reprod Domest Anim 2010; 45(1): 122-8.
[http://dx.doi.org/10.1111/j.1439-0531.2008.01268.x] [PMID: 19144015]

[88] Sritanaudomchai H, Pavasuthipaisit K, Kitiyanant Y, Kupradinun P, Mitalipov S, Kusamran T. Characterization and multilineage differentiation of embryonic stem cells derived from a buffalo parthenogenetic embryo. Mol Reprod Dev 2007; 74(10): 1295-302.
[http://dx.doi.org/10.1002/mrd.20592] [PMID: 17290421]

[89] Mueller S, Prelle K, Rieger N, *et al.* Chimeric pigs following blastocyst injection of transgenic porcine primordial germ cells. Mol Reprod Dev 1999; 54(3): 244-54.
[http://dx.doi.org/10.1002/(SICI)1098-2795(199911)54:3<244::AID-MRD5>3.0.CO;2-5] [PMID: 10497346]

[90] Ginis I, Luo Y, Miura T, *et al.* Differences between human and mouse embryonic stem cells. Dev Biol 2004; 269(2): 360-80.
[http://dx.doi.org/10.1016/j.ydbio.2003.12.034] [PMID: 15110706]

[91] Rui R, Shim H, Moyer AL, *et al.* Attempts to enhance production of porcine chimeras from embryonic germ cells and preimplantation embryos. Theriogenology 2004; 61(7-8): 1225-35.
[http://dx.doi.org/10.1016/j.theriogenology.2003.06.007] [PMID: 15036957]

[92] Sasaki E, Hanazawa K, Kurita R, *et al.* Establishment of novel embryonic stem cell lines derived from the common marmoset (*Callithrix jacchus*). Stem Cells 2005; 23(9): 1304-13.
[http://dx.doi.org/10.1634/stemcells.2004-0366] [PMID: 16109758]

[93] Srirattana K, Lorthongpanich C, Laowtammathron C, *et al.* Effect of donor cell types on developmental potential of cattle (*Bos taurus*) and swamp buffalo (*Bubalus bubalis*) cloned embryos. J Reprod Dev 2010; 56: 49-54.

[94] Pandey A, Gupta SC, Singh N, Rana JS, Gupta N. Efficiency of scnt buffalo (*Bubalus bubalis*) embryos in different culture medium and analysis of mrna expression of insulin-like growth factors during embryogenesis. Reprod Domest Anim 2009; 45: 786-95.

[95] Suteevun T, Parnpai R, Smith SL, Chang CC, Muenthaisong S, Tian XC. Epigenetic characteristics of cloned and *in vitro*-fertilized swamp buffalo (*Bubalus bubalis*) embryos. J Anim Sci 2006; 84: 2065-71.

[96] Kitiyanant Y, Saikhun J, Chaisalee B, White KL, Pavasuthipaisit K. Somatic cell cloning in Buffalo (*Bubalus bubalis*): effects of interspecies cytoplasmic recipients and activation procedures. Cloning Stem Cells 2001; 3: 97-104.

[97] Muenthaisong S, Laowtammathron C, Ketudat-Cairns M, Parnpai R, Hochi S. Quality analysis of buffalo blastocysts derived from oocytes vitrified before or after enucleation and reconstructed with somatic cell nuclei. Theriogenology 2007; 67: 893-900.

[98] Yang CY, Li RC, Pang CY, *et al.* Study on the inter-subspecies nuclear transfer of river buffalo somatic cell nuclei into swamp buffalo oocyte cytoplasm. Anim Reprod Sci 2010; 121: 78-83.

[99] Shah RA, George A, Singh MK, *et al.* Hand-made cloned buffalo (*Bubalus bubalis*) embryos: comparison of different media and culture systems. Cloning Stem Cells 2008; 10: 435-42.

SUBJECT INDEX

C

D

E

H

I

K

L

M

R

S

T

U

V

W

Y

Z

Made in the USA
Las Vegas, NV
03 November 2026

57424104R00297